In loving memory of my husband Frank V. Hill,
who died suddenly October 24, 2011.

With gratitude to our three children, Michael, Keith, and Valerie,
who grew up to be honorable, productive, caring people. Not
to be forgotten is Frank's trusty friend, Shaman.

Signe S. Hill

To my Aunt and Godmother, Catherine L. Zunzer,
for her love, support, and ever-present thoughtfulness.

Helen S. Howlett

Success in Practical/ Vocational Nursing

From Student to Leader

Signe S. Hill, RN, BSN, MA
Formerly Instructor, Practical Nurse Program
Northeast Wisconsin Technical College
Green Bay, Wisconsin

Helen Stephens Howlett, RN, BSN, MS
Formerly Instructor, Practical Nurse Program
Northeast Wisconsin Technical College
Green Bay, Wisconsin

7th Edition

ELSEVIER

http://evolve.elsevier.com

ELSEVIER
SAUNDERS

3251 Riverport Lane
St. Louis, Missouri 63043

SUCCESS IN PRACTICAL/VOCATIONAL NURSING:
FROM STUDENT TO LEADER

ISBN: 978-1-457-70335-7

Notices

Knowledge and best practice in this field are constantly changing. As new research and experience
broaden our understanding, changes in research methods, professional practices, or medical
treatment may become necessary.

Practitioners and researchers must always rely on their own experience and knowledge in
evaluating and using any information, methods, compounds, or experiments described herein. In
using such information or methods they should be mindful of their own safety and the safety of
others, including parties for whom they have a professional responsibility.

With respect to any drug or pharmaceutical products identified, readers are advised to check the
most current information provided (i) on procedures featured or (ii) by the manufacturer of each
product to be administered, to verify the recommended dose or formula, the method and duration
of administration, and contraindications. It is the responsibility of practitioners, relying on their
own experience and knowledge of their patients, to make diagnoses, to determine dosages and the
best treatment for each individual patient, and to take all appropriate safety precautions.

To the fullest extent of the law, neither the Publisher nor the authors, contributors, or editors,
assume any liability for any injury and/or damage to persons or property as a matter of products
liability, negligence or otherwise, or from any use or operation of any methods, products,
instructions, or ideas contained in the material herein.

Library of Congress Cataloging-in-Publication Data
Hill, Signe S.
  Success in practical/vocational nursing : from student to leader / Signe S. Hill, Helen Stephens
Howlett. – 7th ed.
      p. ; cm.
  Includes bibliographical references and index.
  ISBN 978-1-4557-0335-7 (pbk. : alk. paper)
  I. Howlett, Helen A.   II. Title.
  [DNLM: 1.   Nursing, Practical. 2.   Nurse's Role. 3.   Nursing Theory. 4.   Vocational Guidance.
WY 195].
  610.73'0693–dc23   2012007385

Executive Content Strategist: Teri Hines Burnham
Associate Content Development Specialist: Heather Rippetoe
Publishing Services Manager: Deborah L. Vogel
Project Manager: John W. Gabbert
Designer: Ashley Eberts

Printed in China

Last digit is the print number: 9   8   7   6   5   4   3   2   1

Acknowledgments

- Terri Hines Burnham, Executive Content Strategist, Nursing, provided guidance and support in planning and developing the 7th edition of *Success in Practical/Vocational Nursing: from Student to Leader.*
- Heather Rippetoe, Associate Content Development Specialist, was quick to respond to our questions and requests. She was encouraging and provided straightforward feedback and queries on our chapters as she prepared the book for publication.
- Jennifer Shropshire, Associate Content Development Specialist, who got us started while she was working on the most important project of her life.
- John Gabbert, Project Manager, whose patience and prompt and courteous assistance helped us get across the finish line.
- Reviewers provided useful feedback for us to consider prior to beginning the writing process and for each chapter as it was completed. We thank them for their thoroughness and consider them partners in updating the information and suggesting additions and deletions for this edition.
- Peggy Callantine, RN, former CNO, Sheridan Memorial Hospital, Sheridan WY. Board member and Operations Chair of Alternative Elder Living, Inc., a.k.a. Green House Living for Sheridan, wrote the section on Green House in chapter 18.
- Susan deWit, always willing to encourage, laugh, and share. She has continued to share her expertise and new information with us.
- Fr. John W. Girotti, Rector and Pastor of Saint Francis Xavier Cathedral, Green Bay, WI, for his timely review and suggestions for "Catholicism" in Chapter 17.
- Elizabeth Timmons, Library Director, and staff, Muehl Public Library, Seymour, WI, for their gracious and timely retrieval of relevant articles.
- Diane Hall, Technology and Consulting with Eide Bailly, was there to provide answers to computer problems: some large, some small. Diane did so willingly, and promptly responded to requests for HELP!
- Jason Gile, Senior Consulting Engineer, Heartland Business Systems, Little Chute, WI, who again outdid himself in timely response to the few problems the Mac presented and introduced the benefits of the iPad, a very helpful tool.
- Michael S. Hill MS, CRC, ABDA, author of Chapter 22, *Finding a Job: What Works, What Doesn't.* Mr. Hill's vocational experience has included compliance with federal and state laws, stakeholder training, market research, development and successful college training plans, job development/placement, labor market and wage surveys, job seeking skills training, litigation review and court testimony experience, short and long term disability plan administration, Family Medical Leave Act (FMLA) administration, and American with Disabilities Act (ADA) consultation.
- A special thank you to our husbands: Frank Hill and George Howlett. The 7th edition of *Success in Practical/Vocational Nursing: From Student to Leader* was completed through your support. You provided special memories, endless encouragement, humor in just the right measure, and made yourselves scarce when necessary. You will forever be in our hearts.

Contributor and Reviewers

CONTRIBUTOR

Michael S. Hill, MS, CRC, ABDA
Rehabilitation Policy Specialist
State of Minnesota - Department of Labor and Industry
Safety & Workers Compensation Unit
St. Paul, Minnesota

REVIEWERS

Korbi Kidd Berryhill, RN, MSN, CRRN
Vocational Nursing Program Director
South Plains College
Lubbock, Texas

Kathy Lynn Burlingame, MSN
Academic Dean - Director of Nursing
Minnesota State Community and Technical College
Detroit Lakes, Minnesota

Evadne A. Harrison-Madu, PhD, MSN, RRT, RN
Practical Nursing Program Coordinator
Essex County College
Newark, New Jersey

Monica Iaquinta, RN, MSN, MS, BSN
Coordinator of Practical Nursing
United Technical Center
Bridgeport, West Virginia

Lauralee S. Krabill, MBA, RN, C, CNOR
Director
Sandusky Career Center School of Practical Nursing
Sandusky City Schools
Sandusky, Ohio

Beth Moss, MSN, RN, BA
Program Chair, Practical Nursing
Des Moines Area Community College
Newton, Iowa

Cate Rongish, RN, MSN
Assistant Professor
Clarkson College
Omaha, Nebraska

Peggy Valentine, RN, BSN, MSNC, DON
Director of Nursing
Skyline College
Roanoke, Virginia

Sandy Westhoff, BSN, RN
Instructor
Washington School of Practical Nursing
Washington, Missouri

James Floyd Williamson, RN
LPN Coordinator/Instructor
School of Practical Nursing
Mingo Career & Technical Center
Delbarton, West Virginia

LPN Threads

Standard LPN Threads series features incorporated into *Success in Practical/Vocational Nursing: From Student to Leader*, 7th edition make it easy for students to move from one book to the next in the fast-paced and demanding LPN/LVN curriculum. The following features are included in the LPN Threads:

- A **reading level evaluation** is performed on all LPN texts to increase the consistency among chapters and ensure the text is easy to understand.
- **Full-color design, cover, photos,** and **illustrations** that are visually appealing and pedagogically useful.
- **Objectives** (numbered) begin each chapter, provide a framework for content and are important in providing the structure for the TEACH Lesson Plans for the textbook.
- **Key Terms** with phonetic pronunciations and page number references are listed at the beginning of each chapter. Key terms appear in color in the chapter and are defined briefly, with full definitions in the **Glossary.** The goal is to help the student reader with limited proficiency in English to develop a greater command of the pronunciation of scientific and non-scientific English terminology.

- A wide variety of **special features** relate to critical thinking, leadership and management, and more. Refer to the To the Student and Instructor section of this introduction on page ix for descriptions and examples of features from the pages of this textbook.
- **NCLEX Review Questions** and **Critical Thinking Scenarios** presented at the end of chapters give students opportunities to practice critical thinking and clinical decision-making skills with realistic student/patient scenarios.
- **Key Points** at the end of each chapter correlate to the objectives and serve as a useful chapter review.
- A full suite of **Instructor Resources** including TEACH Lesson Plans, Lecture Outlines, and PowerPoint Slides, Test Bank, Image Collection, and Open-Book Quizzes.
- In addition to consistent content, design, and support resources, these textbooks benefit from the advice and input of the **Elsevier LPN/LVN Advisory Board**.

LPN Advisory Board

To the Student and Instructor

We are pleased to introduce you to the 7th edition of *Success in Practical/Vocational Nursing: From Student to Leader*. The changes and additions to this edition are based on instructor evaluation of the 6th edition. Their suggestions, student letters to us, current trends in nursing, and new information related to nursing have all been carefully evaluated. As always, we attempt to present you with the most up-to-date information at the time of writing.

From Whiteboards to Smart Boards, paper course outlines to Course Management Systems, Instructor comments indicate that use of electronic and mobile devices by practical/vocational nursing students and programs is as diverse as the students and programs themselves. As co-authors who have adopted smartphones and iPads, we, too, have diverse styles. Signe will cautiously and carefully get her ducks in a row before diving into the electronic pond while Helen gleefully cannonballs in, then wonders where the ducks went. Students and instructors experienced in the use of the electronic and mobile world need patience and the desire to share knowledge and skill with those just coming aboard.

Because of our awareness of student time constraints and changes in learning techniques, we have made the information more readily available by using bulleted information where appropriate and adding interactive learning exercises and critical thinking exercises. Our chapter summaries are more complete, and additional critical thinking scenarios and test questions that challenge you to practice utilizing the information you are learning are included. Professional Pointers have been added to almost every chapter as cues to professional behavior. Some materials have been placed in *Evolve*.

Chapter 1, *The Adult Learner: Hints to Succeed.* For personal and economic reasons, students and instructors encounter all age groups in the classroom and clinical areas. Chapter 1 introduces the topic of "The Four Generations" to increase awareness of characteristics and learning preferences of each age group. Critical thinking scenarios track a Generation X student throughout Unit 1.

Chapter 4, *Studying and Testing* emphasizes the need to comprehend (understand) information from readings and class situations in order to be able to apply this information to the clinical area.

Chapter 5, *Using Available Resources* stresses individual responsibility, despite prior library experience, for discovering nursing resources in the Learning Resource Center. The professional use of mobile devices, social media, and social networking is discussed. The need for current, relevant, and accurate nursing information is stressed.

Chapter 7, *How Practical Nursing Evolved: From 1836 to Present.* At the request of instructor reviewers, we have added information about nurses through the current wars. You will discover nurse heroes that have done their work well, won meritorious awards, and yet, are seldom covered in the news.

Chapter 10, *Nursing Theory, Research, and Evidence-Based Research* is a chapter new to the 7th edition as requested by reviewers to be an introduction to topics to which practical/vocational nursing students are exposed in practice. Nursing theories of Nightengale, Orem, Leininger, Peplau, Roy, and Watson, as well as Maslow and Rosenstock are discussed in an easy-to-understand format. The importance of nursing research is stressed and a description of quantitative and qualitative research given. The chapter describes the "background of" and "nursing's role in" Evidence-Based Practice (EBP) and how best evidence for practice guidelines is determined. Also included is *Spirit of inquiry*, the National League for Nursing (NLN) competency for practical/vocational nursing that addresses nursing research and evidence-based practice.

Chapter 11, *Ethics Applied to Nursing: Personal vs. Professional Ethics* looks at what you *ought* to do. It helps you differentiate between personal ethics and nursing ethics. In nursing, personal ethics are put aside in order to care for persons whose values may conflict with yours.

Chapter 12, *Nursing and the Law: What Are The Rules?* assists you in becoming aware of what you must do *legally* in nursing, with an emphasis on knowing your *State Nurse Practice Act*.

Chapter 15, *The Health Care Team: Where the Practical/Vocational Nurse Fits In* includes descriptions of the educational preparation of all nurses on the nursing team from the Certified Nursing Assistant to the Chief Nursing Officer in addition to other health care workers. The chapter also presents patient-centered care as a philosophy of care.

Chapter 16, *Cultural Uniqueness, Sensitivity, and Competence* discusses the appropriate use of texts with information about different cultural groups.

Chapter 17, *Spiritual Needs, Spiritual Caring, and Religious Differences* discusses how religion affects patient care. Ten additional scenarios addressing cultural differences can be found on *Evolve*.

Chapter 19, *Health Care System: Financing, Issues, and Trends* has been revised to include explanation of aspects of The Affordable Care Act. Two reports of the Institute of Medicine—*To Err is Human* and *Crossing the Quality Chasm*—focus on the quality, safety, and cost of health care. The chapter also explores how practical/vocational nurses play a role in improving these areas.

Chapter 20, *Leadership Skills: Empowering Self and Others* emphasizes the need to be aware of your state's Nurse Practice Act when considering nursing in your expanded role. Along with Chapter 22, these chapters can be used to help you legally and safely evolve to an expanded role.

Chapter 21, *LPN/LVN Charge Nurse Skills: Management Including Assignment and Delegation.* Long-term care continues to be a much-utilized site of employment for practical/vocational nurses with additional preparation and experience. Chapter 21 differentiates between assignment and delegation and assists graduates to carry out these functions legally and safely.

Chapter 22, *Finding a Job: What Works, What Doesn't* was again contributed by Michael Hill, MS. He has included sensible internet usages, electronic and traditional resumes, functional letters, interview questions with to-the-point answers, an intensive job application to complete, and considerations when faced with drug testing and background checks. The examples Mr. Hill provided are straightforward, easy to apply, and have successfully produced jobs. We are pleased to include information by a professional whose work within non-profits, private-for-profit, union, and state government has helped individuals obtain competitive jobs.

Chapter 23, *NCLEX-PN® Examination: Meeting Minimum Requirements* has been updated for the 2011 Examination. Website addresses are included in the chapter to make it easy for you to obtain the most current information on the examination including a Candidate Bulletin that explains: costs, how and when to apply to take the examination, sites, what you may and may not bring along to the examination site, and how you will be notified about your examination result.

Chapter 24, *Future Career Decisions: Choosing What is Right for You* realistically explains that the LPN/LVN may need or choose to take courses for certifications or go on to become an RN. Reasons are discussed such as personal choice, lack of jobs in the area you wish to live in, a desire for additional challenges, or a financial need. The *Transition to Practice* proposed program of the National Council of State Boards of Nursing, piloted in 2012, is introduced.

TEACHING AND LEARNING PACKAGE

We provide a rich, abundant collection of supplemental resources for both instructors and students

FOR THE INSTRUCTOR

The new, comprehensive Evolve Resources provide a wealth of material to meet your teaching needs. Instructors will have access to all of the student resources as well as the following:

- An ExamView Test Bank contains NCLEX-PN® Examination-style questions that include multiple-choice and alternate format item questions.
- TEACH PowerPoint Presentations (including Audience Response Questions) include approximately 1,100 slides with annotations.
- TEACH Lesson Plans in the new updated TEACH format which are based on textbook chapter objectives. These lesson plans provide a roadmap to link and integrate all parts of the educational package and can be modified or combined to meet your scheduling and teaching needs.
- An Open-Book Quiz is provided for each chapter in the textbook.

FOR THE STUDENT

- Evolve Student Learning Resources include NCLEX-PN® Examination-style interactive review questions that test your knowledge and help you prepare for licensure.
- Helpful Phrases for Communicating in English and Spanish are also provided.
- Additional ancillary material to supplement the content of the chapters.

We welcome your comments and suggestions. You can contact us in care of the customer service department at Elsevier (support.elsevier.com). We wish you well in your school year.

Signe S. Hill
Helen Stephens Howlett

Reading and Review Tools

Objectives introduce the chapter topics.

Key Terms are listed with page number references, and difficult medical, nursing, or scientific terms are accompanied by simple phonetic pronunciations. Key terms are considered essential to understanding chapter content and are defined within the chapter. Key terms are in color the first time they appear in the narrative and are briefly defined in the text, with complete definitions in the Glossary.

Each chapter ends with a *Get Ready for the NCLEX-PN® Examination!* **section** that includes (1) **Key Points** that reiterate the chapter objectives and serve as a useful review of concepts, (2) a list of **Additional Resources**, (3) a set of **Review Questions for the NCLEX-PN® Examination** with answers located in the back of the book, and (4) **Scenarios** with answers located on the Evolve site.

References and Suggested Readings in the back of the book provide resources for enhancing knowledge.

CHAPTER FEATURES

 Keep in Mind Boxes – introduce the reader to the underlying theme of the chapter.

 Critical Thinking Boxes – encourage problem-solving for both academic and personal situations.

 Coordinated Care Boxes – are presented in four ways to introduce the reader to leadership and management in nursing:
- Management Tools – provide practical instructions and resources and have the reader apply learned concepts to specific situations.
- Management Hints – provide tips for handling management situations.
- Leadership Activities – provide students with exercises to practice their leadership skills. Instructions and needed resources are provided.
- Leadership Hints – give helpful hints to follow and remember when in a leadership situation.

 NEW! Professional Pointers – give readers advice on nursing best practices in the professional arena.

 Try This Boxes – challenge students to imagine, visualize and think outside the box.

Contents

chapter

1

The Adult Learner: Hints to Succeed

evolve

http://evolve.elsevier.com/Hill/success

Objectives

On completing this chapter, you will be able to do the following:

1. Using your birth date, identify your generation and its characteristics.
2. Identify yourself as a traditional adult learner, returning adult learner, or recycled adult learner.
3. Identify personal areas of strength that will help you ensure success in the practical/vocational nursing program.
4. Identify personal areas that could interfere with your success in the practical/vocational nursing program.
5. Explain in your own words three rights of learners.
6. Discuss personal responsibility for learning and active participation in the learning process as learner responsibilities.
7. Identify the purpose of evaluation in the practical/vocational nursing program.
8. Discuss 10 learner responsibilities.

Key Terms

active learning (ĂK-tĭv LĔRN-eng, p. 7)
constructive evaluation (kŏn-STRŬ K-tĭvē ē-VĂL-ū-ā-shŭn, p. 8)
facilitator (fă-SĬL-ĭ-TĀ-tŏr, p. 6)
First Amendment (ă-MĔND-mĕnt, p. 6)
formal education (FŎR-măl, p. 3)
generalization (GĔN-ĕ r-ă-lĭ-ZĀ- shŭn, p. 3)
generational personality (GĔN-ĕr-Ā- shŭn -ăl, p. 1)
informal education (ĭn-FŎR-măl, p. 3)
learner (LĔR-nĕr p. 1)

paradigm (PĂR-ă-DĪM, p. 6)
performance evaluation (pĕr-FŎR-măntz ĭ-văl-ū-Ā-shŭn, p. 7)
positive mental attitude (PŎS-ĭ-tĭv MĔN-tăl ĂT-ĭ-tood, p. 4)
recycled adult learner (rē-SĪ-kăld, p. 2)
referral (rĭ-FŬR-ăl, p. 9)
returning adult learner (rē-TŬRN-ĭng ă-DŬLT LĔRN-ĕr, p. 2)
self-directed learner (SĔLF-dĭ-RĔCT-ĕd LĔRN-ĕr, p. 3)
self-evaluation (SĔLF-ē-VĂL-yoo-ā-shŭn, p. 8)
teaching (TĒCH-ĭng, p. 6)
traditional adult learner (p. 2)

DIVERSITY OF THE ADULT LEARNER

The adult learner (one who acquires knowledge and skills) comes in all ages, and it is possible to have learners from four generations in your nursing class. Depending on birth year, generational groups can be characterized. Time frames and names for the four generations vary among authors, but each generation is separated by approximately 20 years (Box 1-1).

Try This

The Four Generations

Using Box 1-1, identify your generation.

People born around the same time generally develop a generational personality of how they think and what they value. This personality is shaped by a common history of cultural events, images, and experiences. Income, religion, education, and geography also enter the picture in forming your generational personality. When you understand the views of different generations, you will be better able to communicate and collaborate with the students in your class. In addition to your classmates, the people with whom you will be working as a licensed practical/vocational nurse quite possibly will also be of several generations.

Your goal is be aware of each generation's shared experiences. Avoid stereotyping individuals of a specific generation as their experiences may be viewed differently. A stereotype is a false assumption. It is an expectation that all individuals within a specific group will act exactly the same because they are members of that group. Stereotypes ignore the individual differences that occur within a specific group—for example, a generational group. See Box 1-2 for characteristics of each generation.

Box 1-1   The Four Generations

- Matures (The Silent Generation) born before 1946
- Baby Boomers (Boomers) born between 1946 and 1964
- Generation X (Gen X) born between 1965 and 1982
- Generation Y (Millennials/Net Generation) born after 1982

Data from Halfer D, Saver C: Bridging the generation gaps. *Nursing Spectrum/ Nurse Week*, 2008.

Box 1-2   Characteristics of the Four Generations

MATURES (THE SILENT GENERATION)
- Depending on birth year, generational personalities may be shaped by the Great Depression, World War II, and/or the Korean War.
- Are more conservative, prefer formal titles, are more formal with intrapersonal interactions, seek conformity.
- Do not like ambiguity or change, prefer to learn in formal, structured ways, oriented to past but are adaptable.
- Digital immigrants. May be reluctant to use advanced technology; need more time and hands-on to learn modern technology devices and protocols.

BABY BOOMERS
- Depending on birth year, generational personalities may be shaped by Watergate, the Vietnam War, the space race, civil rights, women's liberation, and the assassinations of John and Robert Kennedy and Martin Luther King.
- Dedicated, highly motivated and hard-working, idealistic.
- Prefer learning in a relaxed, organized, and respectful atmosphere; like group discussions.
- Digital immigrants and have varying technology skills.

GENERATION X (GEN X)
- Depending on birth year, generational personality may be shaped by the *Challenger* explosion, the end of the Cold War, MTV, and AIDS.
- Accept diversity, less judgmental, pragmatic (practical), flexible, self-reliant (had Boomer parents), multitask well, used to change, informal.
- Intolerant of busywork, like small chunks of information, prefer self-study.
- Digital immigrants and are technically literate.

GENERATION Y (MILLENNIALS)
- Depending on birth year, generational personality may be shaped by Columbine, 9/11, and the Afghanistan and Iraq wars.
- Dynamic, confident, straightforward, opinionated, optimistic, sociable, embrace change, multitask, like group discussion.
- More tolerant of people different from them—for example, race and sexual orientation.
- Digital natives (Net Generation); grew up using cell phones and computers.

Data from Halfer D, Saver C: Bridging the generation gaps. *Nursing Spectrum/ Nurse Week*, 2008; Hartner K. Generational diversity. *ADVANCE Newsmagazines for LPNs*, February 20, 2007. Retrieved September 20, 2007, from http://lpn. advanceweb.com/Common/Editorial/PrintFriendly.aspx; Olson M: The millennials: first year in practice. *Nursing Outlook* 57:10-17, 2009; Billings D, Halstead J: Teaching in nursing: a guide for faculty, St. Louis, 2009, Elsevier/Saunders; Mehallow C: Generational conflict in nursing: how to relate to colleagues across generations. Retrieved July 14, 2011, from http://career-advice.monster.com/ in-the-office/workplace-issues/generational-conflict-in-nursing/article.aspx.

 Try This

Your Generational Personality

Using Box 1-2, Characteristics of the Four Generations, identify the characteristics of your generation that do/do not apply to you.

The **traditional adult learner** comes to an educational program directly from high school or from another program of study. They are in transition from late adolescence to young adulthood. In addition to their own developmental tasks, these students are being propelled into situations of responsibility for others. Traditional adult learners grew up in a digital, wireless world and are known as the Net Generation/ Millennials.

The **returning adult learner** has been out of school for several years. Many of these learners have not taken any courses since high school. Returning adult learners include Generation Xers, Baby Boomers, and Matures. Returning adult students are experiencing many different life transitions. Perhaps an employer shut down a business, or a layoff occurred, resulting in a need for job training. Because of retirement, extra income and health insurance benefits may be needed. Although retired from one's job, "retirement" may provide time to pursue "I always wanted to be a nurse." Because of valued life and work experiences, returning adult learners have built a strong foundation for the personal commitment and transitions needed in nursing school and practical/vocational nursing.

Adult learners with prior education beyond high school are also an important part of practical/vocational nursing. This learner shares some of the characteristics of both traditional and returning adult learners. However, this adult learner might have technical school or college experience or an undergraduate or graduate degree in a discipline other than nursing. Because these adults are starting a new cycle in their lives, we call them **recycled adult learners**. Reasons for choosing to enroll in the practical/vocational nursing program include the following:

- Desire to change careers
- Attraction to nursing
- Desire to acquire new job skills
- Possible lack of jobs in area for which person has a degree
- Outlook for a full-time job with benefits is more promising in practical/vocational nursing

Regardless of the reason for enrolling in the 9-month to 1-year practical/vocational nursing program, recycled learners find that this program meets their needs in both time and cost. In addition to the characteristics of returning adult learners, the recycled learner brings experience in tackling a challenging educational program, including use of the learning resource center (library). Just as recycling is good for the environment, recycled learners are good for practical/vocational nursing programs. Nursing in general, and practical/vocational nursing in particular, are benefiting from the maturity, focus, and experience of returning and recycled adult learners.

? Critical Thinking

Which Type of Adult Learner Am I?

Which type of adult learner are you? Survey your classmates. Determine which ones consider themselves to be traditional, returning, or recycled adult learners.

FORMAL AND INFORMAL EDUCATIONAL EXPERIENCES

Generalizations can be made about each type of learner. Keep in mind that generalizations are broad, sweeping statements. The characteristics of each type of adult learner are not found in every individual.

- Traditional adult learners are accustomed to formal education. The practical/vocational nursing program in a vocational-technical school, junior college, or private school is an example of a program of formal education.
- Returning adult learners might not have been in a classroom for some time, but they have been learning. They have had informal education experiences every day of their lives. Examples of their informal educational experiences include using a new cell phone, filling out a new income tax form, and handling a new family problem. These experiences can be helpful when learning new material.
- Recycled learners may have recently graduated from college. Some may have entered the practical/vocational nursing program after a career in another field of work. Recycled learners have many formal and informal educational experiences that help them in a practical/vocational nursing program.

◎ Try This

Informal Educational Experiences

List at least five informal educational experiences you have had since high school.
1.
2.
3.
4.
5.

GEARED FOR SUCCESS

All adult learners have things going for them that allow them to succeed in the practical/vocational nursing program.

Traditional adult learners:
- Are at their prime physically, are filled with energy and stamina, and often have fewer out-of-school responsibilities to distract them from their studies.
- Are experts at educational routine and have been given the opportunity to develop reading, writing, studying, and test-taking skills.
- Are digital natives who have always had cell phones and computers in their lives. They know how to register for classes and take tests online. When they need information, they "Google," and when they want to contact a friend, they send a text message.

Returning adult learners:
- May feel they have used up their energy in finding a parking space, and once they do, they may be puzzled about how to find their way to their assigned classroom.
- Have had responsibilities and life experiences that help them relate well to new learning, make sense out of it, and get the point quickly. These serious learners are ready to work.
- Are digital immigrants who have had to learn to live in a digital world. Some find it easy to adapt, but others may find it more difficult to do so. When these learners need information, they go to the library or reach for the telephone directory. To stay connected with friends and family, they use their landline, cell phone, or email.
- Are mature, motivated, and self-directed learners who have set goals for themselves. Many have made economic, personal, and family sacrifices to go back to school.

Recycled learners:
- Are also experts in educational routine, and they too have had the opportunity to develop reading, writing, studying, and test-taking skills.
- Are digital immigrants, and because of prior formal learning experiences, they are skilled in searching the Internet for academic information.
- Are serious, motivated, and self-directed learners.

? Critical Thinking

Reasons I Can Succeed

Identify and list three attributes you possess that will help you succeed in the practical/vocational nursing program.
1.
2.
3.

LIABILITIES AND HIDDEN DANGERS

All adult learners are geared for success, and each group has its own strong points. However, each group also has some liabilities—things that could stand in the way of success.

HIDDEN DANGER SHARED BY ALL ADULT LEARNERS

One of the greatest liabilities shared by all adult learners is the fear of failure. Fear of anything is a very strong motivator, but in a negative sense. Fear of failure in school is a feeling that usually develops as a result of past negative experiences with learning situations. Perhaps you did not do well in some high school or college classes. Maybe you did not study, studied the wrong way, or allowed yourself to be put down by teachers or professors in the past. Maybe you allowed yourself to underachieve because of peer pressure. Regardless of the cause, you may look at school in a negative, threatening way.

Your past is history. You have a clean slate ahead of you! Many adult learners with the same history and fears as you have succeeded in their educational programs. You are an adult in an adult educational experience. Begin to picture in your mind the rewards of succeeding in the practical/vocational nursing program. Forget the failures and setbacks you may have suffered in high school and other educational experiences. Replace your fear of failure with the desire for success. Keep your thoughts positive, and practice these positive thoughts continuously. Watch the content and tone of your thoughts and words. Negative thoughts and words can play like a tape. As surely as you learned this negative script, you can learn a positive script. However, it does take time. Replace your "I cannot" and "I never could" with "I want to," "I can," "I will," and "I am going to." Avoid dwelling on the past and look to the future. Go all the way with PMA—positive mental attitude. If you consistently expect to succeed, and combine this expectation with hard work in your studies, you *will* succeed. Did you know that your brain believes anything you tell it? If it learned to believe you could fail, it also learn to believe you can succeed. Start today to engage in positive self-talk.

Sometimes students who have not succeeded in other nursing programs enroll during midterm in the practical/vocational nursing program. Reasons for not making it in prior nursing programs are varied, personal, and confidential. These students may feel the need to be on their guard. They may behave in a defensive manner, especially if there were teacher-student conflicts in the prior nursing program. It is good for these students to remember that the past is history. All that counts is their performance in the present. For them, it is possible to start over with a clean slate.

DANGERS FOR THE TRADITIONAL ADULT LEARNER

The following examples of dangers for traditional adult learners are examples of generalizations. They may or may not apply to the traditional adult learners you know.

Grade Inflation

A grade of C on a test or for a nursing course surprises some traditional adult students because, despite the effort put into studying in high school, they always received As. The same studying routine will not lead to success in your nursing program.

Traditional adult learners often have fewer outside responsibilities to distract them from their studies. Some traditional adult students lack time-management skills or motivation when it comes to studying. Some may still be in the same habits they became comfortable with in high school. Study time required to master content in a practical/vocational nursing program is personal to each student. However, if you are accustomed to receiving an A in high school for minimal effort, you will not experience this reward in the practical/vocational nursing program.

Social Activities

Some traditional adult learners may allow social activities and recreation to compete with school and study time. In a 24/7/365 wired/wireless world, they are accessible at all times to friends, family, and the Internet. Set limits by sharing your class and clinical schedules with family and friends, and restrict being contacted to emergencies only during those times. Develop awareness of the chance to get distracted when online and for valuable time to slip away.

Employment

The amount of time occupied by employment outside of school hours may be another interference for some traditional adult learners. Ask yourself, "How much of the time that I am employed outside of school is necessary for food, shelter, and other realistic expenses?" Many explanations can be given for the liabilities listed here for traditional adult learners. Some traditional adult learners may still be working at developing an awareness of who they are and what life is all about for them. Some may lack a sense of direction and have no clear goal or idea of what they really want to do in life. Some may lack inner motivation to be a practical/vocational nurse. These learners can succeed by taking responsibility for making decisions about priorities and personal use of time that will help them meet the goals they have established for themselves.

DANGERS FOR THE RETURNING ADULT LEARNER

Physical

Returning adult learners may experience difficulties with academic behavior. Their reading, writing, test-taking, and study skills may be rusty. Computer and other skills for an electronic information society may be lacking. Physical changes occur as adults age and can affect learning. The senses of vision and hearing are at their peak in the adolescent years and decline very gradually through the adult years.

As the decades go by, these adults may notice the need for more illumination when they read. They also may experience problems with reading small print. Some returning adults note that they are not as energetic as they once were.

Social and Family Responsibilities

Returning adult learners have many roles to play outside of school. They may be husbands, wives, significant others, mothers, fathers, daughters, sons, grandparents, employees, and/or volunteers. Generally they are very busy people. Returning to school may result in feelings of guilt because they know it will affect their relationships and routines outside of school.

Because of their many roles, returning adult learners have more demands placed on them. Some families may not support their parent's choice to continue their formal education. Spouses/significant others may object to the extra demands placed on them. In many cases the returning adult learner must struggle with learning how to juggle the worlds of learner and head of the family.

Despite these demands, returning adult learners, like traditional and recycled adult learners, need to learn how to manage their time. They need to learn how to concentrate when time for concentration is made available. Sometimes, returning adult learners set unrealistic goals for themselves and have to readjust their game plan. Although past experience can be an asset, returning adult learners may have to rethink and possibly unlearn some things they have learned in the past. They might have allowed some of these things to become habits.

When faced with obstacles, some adults may decide to throw in the towel and write off school as a bad idea. This book can help you avoid this negative way of thinking and go on to succeed.

DANGERS FOR THE RECYCLED ADULT LEARNER

The recycled adult learner shares the same liabilities as do traditional and returning adult learners. Depending on their age and personal responsibilities, recycled adult learners may feel an energy crisis as they pursue their academic life.

Attitude

Some recycled adult learners may have a mindset that because they earned a degree or have some college experience, the practical/vocational nursing program will be a breeze to get through. Be aware of the difference between obtaining a college degree and obtaining a technical college education. In college a student might have no practical experience with his or her major subject until junior or senior year or after graduation, if fortunate enough to be hired for the first job applied for in the chosen field. In the practical/vocational nursing program in a technical college, the application of current learning is stressed continuously. Students

need to apply theory continuously to the clinical area. What you learn on Monday will be used in the clinical area on Tuesday. And you will be expected to consistently apply learning from past nursing classes. Perhaps poor time management resulted in cramming for examinations. Cramming is an ineffective strategy for long-term learning. This measure will be useless in the practical/vocational nursing program because of the consistent expectation of application of theory to the clinical area.

 Critical Thinking

Personal Needs for Improvement

Identify and list three things that could stand in your way of success in the practical/vocational nursing program.

1.
2.
3.

SPECIAL CHALLENGES FOR PRACTICAL/ VOCATIONAL NURSING STUDENTS

No matter what type of adult learner you are, some learners have special challenges to success in practical/vocational nursing. Learners with a spouse/significant other at home may be extremely busy with school and family affairs. Learners with aging parents may be involved with their needs for assistance. Single parents may feel overwhelmed when the learner role is assumed in addition to all their other roles. It may be good for learners with spouses/significant others to imagine what it would be like to be a learner without these individuals to offer support.

Practical/vocational nursing students who speak English as their first language sometimes indicate the difficulty of course work and the amount of time it takes to complete assignments. It may be insightful for these learners to imagine being responsible for the same amount of course work when English is their second language. Learners who speak English as a second or additional language need to strive continually to understand content presented in a language that is different from their native tongue. Reading assignments need to be translated by these students to their native language to be understood. Taking a test requires extra effort, as these students may need to translate test directions and items to their native language for understanding before answering an item. This is comparable to presenting English-speaking learners with textbooks and tests written in Spanish or Russian with the need to translate both to English.

We have met many learners facing the preceding challenges and commend them for the good job they have done, against great odds, in the practical/vocational nursing program. They are a testimonial that success is within your reach, even if you are faced with these special challenges.

LEARNERS HAVE RIGHTS

As an American citizen, you need to start thinking about some fundamental rights that you have been granted through the U.S. Constitution that will affect you as a learner. The First Amendment gives you freedom of expression as long as what you want to express does not disrupt class or infringe on the rights of your peers. So when your instructor asks you to join in a discussion, do not be afraid to do so. Instructors want your input in a class session. They have no intention of holding your comments against you. The Fourteenth Amendment assures you due process. Due process means that if you are charged with a violation of policies or rules, you will be presented with evidence of your misconduct and will be entitled to state your position. So relax. The institution in which you are enrolled cannot terminate you at whim, nor does it want to. It exists to help you succeed. A more detailed account of these two rights can probably be found in your school's student handbook. If you do not have a copy of the student handbook, download an online copy or obtain one from the student services department. An important learner's right is the right to have an organized curriculum and a responsible instructor who is prepared to teach it. You have the right to know the requirements of each course and how you will be graded for each course. Although your tuition and fees do not pay for all the services you receive through your school, you are the most important person in the educational system. You are the reason the instructor was hired. You do not interfere with the instructor's work—you are the focus of it.

RESPONSIBILITIES OF LEARNERS

The first responsibility of learners is to learn. The authors of this book want you to test your knowledge about the process of learning before you read any further. Read the following four statements and decide if they are true or false. As the chapter continues, these statements will be discussed. You will be expected to check the accuracy of your responses. Remember, your answers are for your eyes only.

 Critical Thinking

Responsibilities of Learners

Read the following four statements, and indicate whether each is "true" or "false."
1. The instructor has the responsibility for my learning.
2. If I fail, it is the responsibility of the instructor.
3. If I succeed, the credit for my success should go to the instructor.
4. My instructor has the responsibility to pass on to me all the information I will need to know in my career as a practical/vocational nurse.

TEACHING VERSUS LEARNING

Years ago, a wonderful thing happened in the area of adult education. Teachers were exposed to the difference between teaching and learning. Great emphasis was placed on the role of the learner. Changing emphasis from teaching to learning is called a paradigm (a way of thinking) shift. Learners need to be aware of the exciting world of learning and the roles of teaching and learning in that process. In doing so you will know what is expected of you as an adult learner.

Passive Learners

Many of us (and this includes the authors and some of your instructors) have had educational experiences in the past that encouraged dependency and passivity on the part of the learner. Think back to the educational experiences you have had. Did they involve sitting in classes in which the teacher did most of the talking and you just took notes? Did you view the teacher as someone who possessed knowledge and somehow was going to pass it on to you? And, if you did not pass, did you say, "The teacher flunked me"? When you think about it, these situations are characterized by the adjectives *dependent* and *passive*.

The last time you were dependent from necessity was when you were an infant. Even then you were far from passive. When you became a toddler, you became very independent and began to learn about the world in earnest. You very actively pursued your learning—that is, the acquiring of new knowledge and skills. And you did it with gusto! Now you are an adult learner. How unfair of an instructor to expect you to become dependent and passive in your learning. This is especially true because studies have proved that people learn best when they are actively involved in their own learning and have an interdependent relationship with the instructor.

Instructors—Facilitators of Learning

You have already learned that it is the instructor's responsibility to set up a curriculum. Your state's board of nursing dictates the content of the curriculum in a school of nursing. It is then up to the faculty of your school to decide how that content will be included in the nursing program. Some practical/vocational programs might use the general structure of the NCLEX-PN® examination in developing a curriculum. Instructors are facilitators because they are responsible for creating a learning environment in which learning can take place. They do this by arranging for a variety of activities and experiences. Part of that learning environment involves being available to you when you encounter questions and problems you cannot solve. Instructors also have the responsibility to evaluate learning. They do so by testing and observing learners.

As a student, you have not only the right but the responsibility to talk to an instructor when you have a concern about your relationship with him or her. Under rules of assertiveness, always go to the source. The same rule applies if you have a problem with a classmate. Approach the classmate, not another student.

Active Learning

To "learn" is to acquire knowledge and skills. The verb *acquire* means to obtain or gain by your own effort. As a learner in a practical/vocational nursing program, you need to be your own agent of knowledge and skill acquisition. You have the personal responsibility to acquire the knowledge and skills needed to be a practical/vocational nurse. Active learning is not a passive activity. As a learner, you must open yourself up, reach out, and stretch to gain knowledge and skills. To be successful, you must be personally involved in your learning. It is impossible for instructors to pour knowledge and skills into your head. You need to become self-directed and curious in your learning. You need to use critical-thinking skills to help you comprehend what you read in texts and journals, what you see on PowerPoint presentations and DVDs, and what you hear in class discussions. Instructors will not hover over you and guide your every step. Instructors are there to help you along when you need it.

Do not expect the instructor to assume your skill for you, be your medical dictionary, or reteach Chapter 2 in *Anatomy and Physiology* because you did not have time to study. Instead, expect your instructor to observe you while you are trying to work through a difficult skill. The instructor will make suggestions and demonstrate a point here and there to help you along. If you are having trouble, expect your instructor to help you put a definition of a medical term in your own words. Expect the instructor to answer specific questions you may have about Chapter 2 in *Anatomy and Physiology*. These are the roles of teacher and learner and examples of their interdependency. If you are to learn and succeed in practical/vocational nursing, you need to become actively involved in your own learning. You say you are too old to learn? You say you cannot teach an old dog new tricks? Much study has been done in this area. To date, studies of adult learning clearly indicate that the basic ability to learn remains essentially unimpaired throughout the life span. Now review the answers to your true/false questions from the Critical Thinking exercise on p. 6. Are there any answers you want to change before looking at the key?

1. *False.* You have the responsibility for your own learning. You must become actively involved in the learning process.
2. *False.* If you fail, it is your own fault. Adult educational programs are geared for success. You are geared for success. Although you could list many reasons why you might not succeed, the teacher flunking you is not one of them. Learners sometimes allow themselves to flunk.
3. *False.* When you succeed (and you are perfectly capable of doing so), only you can take credit for the success. You were the person who assumed responsibility for your own learning. You became actively involved in the learning process.
4. *False.* Instructors have had much experience in nursing. They do not know all the experiences you will have in your career as a practical/vocational nurse. Even if they did, there would be no time or way to transfer this knowledge to you. Instructors help learners learn how to learn. This is important in an ever-changing field such as nursing. Your instructors will encourage you to develop critical-thinking and problem-solving skills, which will enable you to handle new situations as they arise in your nursing career.

If you had no wrong answers, you should be an expert on learning. Now put your expertise to work for you. If you had one or more wrong answers, the authors suggest you reread the "Teaching versus Learning" section in this chapter. Chapters 3, 4, and 8 will help you to become an active learner and a critical thinker and be successful in the practical/vocational nursing program, on NCLEX-PN®, and as a candidate for an LPN/LVN nursing position.

ROLE OF EVALUATION

The second responsibility of learners is to receive and participate in evaluation. Evaluation plays an important role in your education in the practical/vocational nursing program and throughout your career. You have set a goal to become a practical/vocational nurse. As the year goes on, your instructors will evaluate you in several different ways to determine whether you are progressing in the achievement of that goal. When you graduate, you will be evaluated periodically while on the job, sometimes as a means of determining whether you are to receive a salary increase. At other times you will be evaluated to see if you are functioning well enough to keep your job. Evaluation in the practical/vocational nursing program generally occurs in two areas: written tests that measure your knowledge of theory and performance evaluations that measure your ability to apply your knowledge in the clinical area. Evaluation in these areas is a learning experience in itself.

Theory Tests

Learners and instructors look at test results very differently. Learners focus on the number of items they answered correctly. They need to identify what they did right on a test so they can apply the process of getting the right answer to future tests and apply this information in the clinical area. Instructors focus on the specific items the learner got wrong. Wrong items indicate critical knowledge the learner does not have. Do not just ask for your grades. Try to arrange time with your instructors to review your tests. It is inaccurate to say that grades do not count. You must earn the minimum grade established by your nursing program. But consider this: If you got 80% on a test, it means you did not answer 20% of the questions correctly. Now place yourself in the patient's slippers. What about the 20% of the test questions your nurse got wrong? Was it something the nurse should have known to care for you safely? For this reason, try to look at tests as learning experiences. Be as interested in your wrong answers as you are in your correct answers. Take time to look at your tests with the goal of understanding why the correct answers are correct and why the wrong answers you gave are wrong.

Clinical Performance Evaluations

The most meaningful evaluations you will receive during the year will be the performance evaluations given while you are in the clinical area. Because these evaluations give you an opportunity for career and personal growth, it is important to understand this form of evaluation and the responsibilities you have with regard to it. Clinical performance evaluations also provide an example of how to evaluate others in your expanded role.

In the clinical area, instructors will be observing you as you care for patients. They are observing you to discover the positive things you are doing to reach your goal of becoming a practical/vocational nurse. These behaviors are to be encouraged. They indicate that learning has taken place, you are applying your knowledge, and you are growing and progressing toward your goal. Instructors are also observing you to discover behaviors that stand in the way of reaching your goal. These behaviors are to be discouraged. Your instructor will update you daily on your progress in a verbal or written manner. At the end of a clinical rotation, you will receive a written performance evaluation during a conference with your clinical instructor.

From the start you need to look at performance evaluations as a two-sided coin. The instructor is on one side, and you are on the other. As part of their job, instructors have the responsibility of evaluating your performance. As a learner, you have the responsibility of being aware of your clinical behaviors. You are responsible for **self-evaluation**. Practical/vocational nursing students, at the time of graduation, should be able to look at their nursing actions and be aware of their strong behaviors and behaviors that need improvement. Developing the ability to be aware of one's behaviors begins with day one in the practical/vocational nursing program, including the skills laboratory. A learner does not automatically have this skill. Learners must consistently work at viewing themselves objectively. Instructors will help in this area. For example, when learning how to make a bed, ask yourself, "Is the finished product as good as I had intended it to be when I started?" Do not wait for the instructor to identify areas of success or areas that need improvement.

Professional Pointer

Objective awareness of one's own behaviors is an important skill to have as an employee.

Think back to when you received comments from your teachers and parents about your behavior in grade school and high school. How did you feel when you received these comments? Many people grow up with bad feelings about these episodes of criticism and even about the word itself. Criticism means evaluation. Some people attach a negative meaning to criticism and view it as a put-down.

The phrase "constructive criticism" may evoke negative feelings. The phrase "constructive evaluation" is frequently used instead. This choice of words may help you look at evaluation of your behaviors in a positive way. It is important to distinguish what is being evaluated. You must separate your behaviors or actions from yourself, the person.

Constructive evaluation directed toward your behaviors has no bearing on your value as a person. Look at your behaviors either as being positive and helping you to reach your goal or as needing improvement. Behaviors that need improvement need to be modified so that you can reach your goal of being a practical/vocational nurse.

As you progress in the nursing program, you will learn about a systematic way of conducting patient care called the "nursing process" (see Chapter 8). An important part of the nursing process is evaluation of patient goals while giving patient care. If your actions are not helping patients reach their goals, they need to be modified. Knowledge of the nursing process will help you develop your ability to look at your actions and evaluate them. Comments from instructors will help your self-awareness.

A good way to start learning self-evaluation is to look at yourself in everyday life. Ask yourself how you look through the eyes of others:
• How would you like to be your own spouse?
• How would you like to have yourself as a learner?
• How would you like to be your own mother or father?
• How would you like to be your own nurse?

If you would not like to be any of these people, identify the reasons why.

Another good exercise is to make two lists: a list of your assets or strong points and a list of your liabilities or areas that need improvement. When asked to evaluate themselves, learners traditionally rate themselves more negatively. They tend to neglect their strong points. Identifying strong points is not proud or vain behavior. It is dealing with yourself honestly and openly. After you have identified assets and liabilities, review your assets periodically. Make an effort to continue these strong points while modifying your liabilities. Work on one liability at a time. If you do so, your assets list will grow and your liabilities list will shrink.

A good place to start self-evaluation in nursing is in the skills lab of your basic nursing course. Observe the results of your actions. Are you using a drape during procedures to avoid chilling and invading the patient's privacy? Are you aware of the effect of the tone of your voice on your instructors and peers?

Evaluation is an ever-present reality in any career. Getting into the practice of self-evaluation early in your program of study will help you to develop a skill you will use daily in your career and personal life.

? Critical Thinking

Self-Evaluation

List one of your strong areas that you have identified as a new practical/vocational nursing learner. (Review your answers to Critical Thinking: Reasons I Can Succeed on p. 3.)

List one area needing improvement that you have identified as a practical/vocational nursing student. (Review your answers to Critical Thinking: Personal Liabilities on p. 5.)

? Critical Thinking

Plan to Eliminate My Areas That Need Improvement

Write a plan that will help you eliminate one of your areas that need improvement. How can you convert this area to a strong area?

DEALING WITH REFERRALS

If you are evaluated by your instructor as having areas that need improvement, the instructor might refer you to a counselor at school. Examples of areas that require a referral are a grade below passing in a major test and frequent absences from class. Counselors at technical colleges and junior colleges are academic counselors who have expertise in helping students identify reasons for academic problem areas. A referral to a counselor is an attempt to help you succeed. These counselors can help students set up a plan of action to remedy the problem. We have seen some students resist going to the counselor because they think it is a waste of time.

? Critical Thinking

Referral to Counselor

What could be one reason for thinking that an appointment with the counselor is a waste of time? How could keeping an appointment with the counselor be helpful to a student?

OTHER RESPONSIBILITIES OF LEARNERS

In addition to assuming responsibility for your own learning, becoming actively involved in the learning process, and receiving and participating in evaluation, it is necessary to be aware of some other responsibilities you have as a learner:

1. Be aware of the rules and policies of your school and the practical/vocational nursing program. Abide by them.
2. When problems do develop, follow the recognized channels of communication both at school and in the clinical area. The rule is: Go to the source. Avoid "saving up" gripes. Instead, pursue them as they come up. Deal with them in an assertive manner (see Chapter 14).
3. Be prepared in advance for classes and clinical experiences. You expect teachers to be prepared, and they expect the same of you. When you are unprepared for classes, you waste the time of the instructor, your peers, and yourself. When you are unprepared for clinical experiences, you are violating an important safety factor in patient care. When you are scheduled for the clinical area, your state board of nursing expects you to function as a licensed practical/vocational nurse would function under your state's Nurse Practice Act.
4. Prepare your own assignments. In postconference use your peers and the experiences and knowledge they have and learn from one another.
5. Seek out learning experiences at school and in the clinical area. Set your goals higher than the minimum.
6. Seek out resources beyond the required readings. Examples of these resources can be the learning resource center, information from past classes, and the Internet.
7. Assume responsibility for your own thoughts, communication, and behavior. Avoid giving in to pressure from your peers. BYOB—be your own boss.
8. Be present and on time for classes and clinical experiences. Follow school and program policies for reporting absences. Getting into this habit will prepare you to be a favored employee.
9. Enter into discussion when asked to do so in class.
10. Treat those with whom you come into daily contact with respect. Be mindful of their rights as individuals.

11. Seek out your instructor when you are having difficulties in class or the clinical area. Often instructors can tell when students are having problems. More important are the times when they cannot tell, and only the student knows a problem exists. Do not be afraid to approach your instructors. They are there to help you.

12. Keep a record of your grades as a course proceeds. At the beginning of a course the instructor and/or your course syllabus will explain the method of calculating your final grade. You are responsible for knowing how you stand grade-wise in a course at any point in time.

Get Ready for the NCLEX-PN® Examination!

Key Points

- Adult learners have diversity in age resulting in differing ways of thinking and valuing.
- The adults in your class could be Matures (The Silent Generation), Baby Boomers, Generation Xers, and Generation Ys (Millennials).
- Adult learners can be classified as traditional adult learners, returning adult learners, or recycled adult learners.
- Each category of adult learner possesses characteristics that can help the learner succeed in the practical/vocational nursing program.
- Each group of adult learners also possesses characteristics that can prevent success.
- Liabilities occur in areas in which learners have control over their solutions. They do not stand in the way of success.
- Although learners have rights, they also have responsibilities. The most important of their responsibilities are the personal responsibilities for learning, taking an active part in the learning process, and participating in the evaluation of their learning and growth.

Additional Learning Resources

evolve Go to your Evolve website (http://evolve.elsevier.com/Hill/Success) for the following FREE learning resources:
- Answers to Critical Thinking Scenarios
- Additional learning activities
- Additional Review Questions for the NCLEX-PN® exam
- Helpful phrases for communicating in Spanish and more!

Review Questions for the NCLEX-PN® Examination

1. Select the appropriate behavior for the student practical/vocational nurse.
   1. To accept responsibility for personal success, including grades, in the nursing program.
   2. To be as passive a learner as you can possibly be both in classes and in the clinical area.
   3. To learn everything from the nursing instructors that is needed to function as a PN/VN.
   4. To blame the nursing instructor for any failures that occur in class or the clinical area.

2. A practical/vocational nursing learner has been referred to the counselor because of a failing grade on the last test in Nursing Fundamentals. Which of the following learner responses indicates the student understands the purpose of the referral?
   1. "The instructor does not like me and wants me to quit the program."
   2. "This is a warning that I will be asked to withdraw from the program."
   3. "The purpose of a referral is to help me identify problems to avoid failure."
   4. "A psychologist will evaluate me for psychological problems that may be interfering with success."

3. A practical/vocational nursing student has just received the end-of-course clinical evaluation. Which of the following attitudes is most appropriate regarding the role of evaluation of students in the clinical area?
   1. Instructors and SPN/SVN students have the responsibility to identify positive behaviors and those that need improvement.
   2. It is the job of the instructor only to identify positive clinical behaviors and behaviors that need improvement.
   3. When SPN/SVN students identify positive behaviors, it indicates that they are proud and vain individuals.
   4. When behaviors that need improvement are identified, clinical evaluation may destroy self-esteem in the SPN/SVN student.

4. Four practical/vocational nursing students were absent the day tests were returned and reviewed in a pediatric course. Which of the following students has a plan that will benefit the student in future testing and clinical situations?
   1. The student who on the next class day will ask the instructor for the grade on the test for personal records.
   2. The student who on the next clinical day asks the instructor to schedule time to go over test items that were correct.
   3. The student who thinks that because the test is history, it is unnecessary to review test items, since the grade is final.
   4. The student who asks when there is time to go over all the test items so the reasons for wrong answers can be identified.

Alternate Format Item

1. Which of the following students is *not* demonstrating behavior for success in the practical/vocational nursing program? *(Select all that apply.)*

   1. A recent high school graduate who expects the instructor to teach her everything she needs to know.
   2. A student who is a mother of four and spends time in the library each afternoon reviewing class notes.
   3. A student who has not been in school for 20 years and seeks out the instructor when content is not understood.
   4. A student with college experience who works part-time and joins a group that crams before each examination.
   5. A student who speaks English as a second language and studies every night in preparation for class and clinical.

2. Olivia, 37, just started the practical nursing program at the local technical college. Her class is composed of students in their late teens, twenties, thirties, fifties, and one retired man. From the following list of generalized characteristics, select those that describe Olivia's generational age. *(Select all that apply.)*

   1. Accepts diversity in the members of her class.
   2. Is more formal when approaching classmates.
   3. Works long hours to get the job done.
   4. Does not readily use the computer lab.
   5. Is self-reliant when learning nursing skills.

Critical Thinking Scenario

Amy, 36, has been accepted for the next practical nursing program at her local technical college. Having gotten over her initial excitement at being accepted to prepare to be a practical nurse, Amy begins to have concerns: "Can I really do this? I have three kids, am a single parent, and haven't had any classes since high school! And high school was a bad dream for me. I never got along with my teachers. And how am I going to be able to afford school both in time and money? I work full-time now and have a hard time making ends meet in time and money. And I heard you have evaluations of what you do when taking care of patients. I don't like people being critical of me." What can you suggest to Amy to help her with her concerns?

Objectives

On completing this chapter, you will be able to do the following:

1. Discuss three benefits of time management for an adult learner.
2. Using the four phases of the nursing process as a guide, develop a personal time management plan to be used as a student practical/vocational nurse.
   a. List the activities of the various roles you fill in daily life.
   b. Arrange the list of various roles according to whether they are high priority or low priority.
   c. Keep at least a 1-day activity log to determine the present use of your time, including social networking.
   d. Devise a semester schedule and a weekly schedule to reflect present commitments.
   e. Make a daily "to-do" list.
   f. Carry out weekly and daily schedules for 2 weeks.
   g. Evaluate the effectiveness of your personal time management plan and modify it, if necessary.
3. Identify right-brain techniques to use in time management.

Key Terms

data collection (DĀ-tă, p. 14)
delegate (DĚL-ĭ-GĀTE, p. 19)
effectiveness (ĕ-FĔK-tĭv-nĕss, p. 13)
efficiency (ĕ-FĬSH-ĕn-sē, p. 13)
evaluation (ĭ-văl-ū-Ā-shŭn, p. 20)
habit (hă-bĭt, p. 14)
implementation (ĬM-plĕ-mĕn-TĀ-shŭn, p. 18)
long-term goal (p. 14)

minitask (mĭn-ĭ-tăsk, p. 19)
planning (plăn- ĭng, p. 14)
priorities (prī-ŌR-ĭ-tēz, p. 13)
procrastination (prō-KRĀS-tĭ-NĀ-shŭn, p. 19)
short-term goal (p. 20)
social networks (SŌ-shŭl, p. 18)
support system (sŭ-PORT SĬS-tĕm, p. 15)

 Keep in Mind

Invest your limited time carefully in the fast-paced PN/VN program. Not only will you be preparing for a successful NCLEX-PN® experience, but you will also have some time to enjoy yourself during your student year.

Have you noticed at school and in your personal life that some people seem to get more done than others? Worse yet, some of the busiest people are the ones getting the most done. To add insult to injury, all of us are given the same amount of time—168 hours a week—in which to get the job done. How can some individuals get the job done and some not? The answer does not lie in the fact that some people have fewer responsibilities and less to do in a week's time. The answer lies in their ability to manage their time.

WHY CAN'T I GET ORGANIZED?

There are several explanations for being disorganized and managing time poorly:

- Trauma in one's personal life: Organizing may be the last thing on your mind if you have experienced a divorce or a death in the family.
- Disorganized upbringing: Disorganization may be the style one grew up with, and this style may be a source of comfort.
- Lack of commitment to be a practical/vocational nurse: Disorganization could be a symptom of discontent with your choice of career.

Regardless of the reason for disorganization, millions of dollars are spent annually to hire time management experts to help people get organized. Millions more are spent on gadgets and devices that promise the same organization. This chapter contains free information and tips that can help you get organized and manage your time more efficiently and effectively. If you follow the suggestions, they will help make what could be a challenging year more tolerable for you.

SELF-TEST OF TIME MANAGEMENT

Time management is a major skill that contributes to learner success. It is also a necessary skill for practical/vocational nurses to better manage their time in the clinical area to meet patient outcomes. To start this chapter, take a self-test of time management so you will know how you stand with regard to this important skill. If you are going to be responsible for managing clinical time, you need to be able to manage personal time.

The answers to the self-test are the ones suggested by time management experts. Although different time management techniques work for different people, these suggested answers reflect basic techniques that could help you succeed in the practical/vocational nursing program.

 Try This

Self-Test of Time Management

Answer "yes" or "no" as you read each of the statements, and apply them to your personal use of time.

1. I keep a semester or course calendar to reflect requirements and due dates of work for all my classes.
2. I keep a weekly plan of everything that must be done at school and in my personal life.
3. I keep a daily list of things I must do at school and in my personal life.
4. Daily I list and rank in importance my priorities for using school and personal time.
5. After listing and ranking my daily priorities for school and personal life, I stick to the list.
6. I use my best working time during the day for doing high-priority schoolwork.
7. I plan to do lower-priority schoolwork before higher-priority schoolwork.
8. I start school tasks before thinking them through.
9. I stop a school task before I have completed it.
10. I spend the few minutes before class talking to my classmates about anything other than the class.
11. I have trouble starting a major task for school.
12. I become bored with the subject I am studying.
13. I have a hard time getting started when I sit down to study.
14. Sometimes I avoid important school tasks.
15. I find myself easily distracted when I study.
16. I always try to get everything done in my personal life that must be done.
17. I frequently engage in social networking instead of doing schoolwork.
18. I manage to turn a short coffee break into a long coffee break.
19. I study nightly for my classes.
20. I frequently have to cram for examinations.

The following are the suggested answers to the self-test:

1. Yes	8. No	15. No
2. Yes	9. No	16. No
3. Yes	10. No	17. No
4. Yes	11. No	18. No
5. Yes	12. No	19. Yes
6. Yes	13. No	20. No
7. No	14. No	

Count the number of statements you disagree with and plug yourself into one of the following categories:

1–5 Disagree with	You deserve the *Alan Lakein** award.
6–10 Disagree with	Hang in there! With a little guidance, you will get on the right track.
11–20 Disagree with	We know you must be exhausted, but keep on reading—quickly!

*Alan Lakein is a famous time management expert. In 1973 he first published a very readable book entitled *How to Get Control of Your Time and Your Life*. Except for technology, the key to using time wisely has not changed since the first edition was published.

BENEFITS OF TIME MANAGEMENT

Time management is a technique designed to help you not only do the things you have to get done but also the things you want to finish in a definite time period. Time management can put you in control of your life rather than making you a slave to it. You will have to give up some of the things you were accustomed to doing before you became a practical/vocational nursing student. Time management techniques can help you gain some personal time for your family and yourself so you will not feel that there is time only for school. Time management can help you work smarter, not harder. It will not give you more hours in the week but will help you use what hours you do have more efficiently and effectively. **Efficiency** will help you get things done as quickly as possible. Time management does not deal solely with efficiency like the efficiency experts of the 1950s. The efficiency of the 1950s can bring images of robot-like individuals working to get every task done in the shortest time possible in a machine-like manner. Efficiency needs to be balanced with **effectiveness**. Effectiveness involves setting **priorities** among the tasks that need to be done and doing them the best way possible and choosing the most important task to do and doing it the right way. Efficiency involves doing things as quickly as possible.

REVIEW OF PERSONAL GOALS

How did you score on the time management self-test? If you are a typical adult, you are probably reading quickly right now to find out how to improve your time management. Take heart: Very few of us get the Alan Lakein award. Most of us could stand to learn how to use our time more efficiently and effectively. Ineffective use of personal time is learned behavior, better known as a **habit**. Any behavior that is learned can be unlearned if you work at it, and new habits can be acquired.

If you have set a goal to be a practical/vocational nurse, you are already on the right track in time management, no matter what you scored. This is your **long-term goal** and the bull's-eye to which you will direct your efforts for the next year. It would be beneficial to write that goal on an index card and place it where you will see it often, such as your car visor, the bathroom mirror, or the refrigerator door. Be specific when you write your goal.

GETTING ORGANIZED WITH THE NURSING PROCESS

DATA COLLECTION

Data collection in time management involves two areas:

- Discovering what roles you fill in your daily life
- Collecting data on how you actually spend your time

Enrollment in a vocational-technical program, whether you are single, divorced, widowed, or married, requires some degree of change in the activities in which you were involved before entering the program. Regardless of your state in life, all the roles you fill can be classified into any of five general categories: school, job, family, community, and recreation.

The activities involved in a practical/vocational nursing program are structured:

- Face-to-face classes and clinical experience are at a specific time.
- Online classes need to be structured by the student.

When you are enrolled in a vocational-technical program such as practical/vocational nursing, your school day is chock-full. Seldom do you have the choice of when you will take a specific course.

Your Roles and Activities

The same structure as your class day is not evident in four additional roles you have. In these other roles you might be involved in some activities that you either did not plan to do, do not enjoy doing, do not have time to do, or feel do not need to be done. Complete the Try This exercise: My Personal Roles and Activities on Evolve. A blank form is included to collect data about your personal roles and activities for the data collection portion of time management.

Your Personal Time Use

You are now ready to document how you actually use your personal time. Ideally, a time log should be kept for approximately 1 week to document how you use your personal time. Because time is marching on, a 1-day time log for a class day can give you a general idea of how you use your time at present. Complete the Try This exercise: Use of Personal Time on Evolve.

Supply one more piece of information, and your data collection will be complete. List below one activity you wish you had time for. The activity could have been listed under your roles, but maybe it was not listed at all. Remember, the sky's the limit as long as your wish is something that is really important to you.

 Critical Thinking

My Special Wish

My special wish is . . .

_____
_____
_____

BEFORE YOU CONTINUE

How students use their time is partly a result of which side of the brain is dominant. Chapter 3 discusses the difference between right- and left-brain dominance. You may note personal brain dominance in your behavior. Chapter 3 gives you the opportunity to assess your specific dominance on p. 23. Time management systems generally reflect the left-brain thinking style. This style is linear (prefers a step-by-step, methodical approach), compared with right-brain thinkers who are nonlinear (see and do in an unstructured manner). Traditional tools of time management are directed to left-brain thinkers because they process information in sequence. Right-brain thinkers look at the picture as a whole. Right-brain thinkers prefer their own tools/ideas for time management and are good at devising them. Neither system of thinking is good or bad. Both sides of the brain work together and complement each other.

The challenge of time management for practical/vocational nursing students is to find the side of your brain in which the dominance lies. Use the strengths of this side, but strive to use the resources of both sides of your brain. We will provide some right-brain strategies in the planning stage. Right-brain thinkers will be able to develop tools with which they are more comfortable.

PLANNING

When you have completed data collection, you will be ready to proceed to the **planning** stage.

- A plan helps to keep you honest. It reflects the face-to-face classes you must attend and the studying you need to do to reach your long-term goal. It is your blueprint for action.
- With a plan you will avoid the roller-coaster phenomenon all too familiar to students: falling behind in school and then trying to catch up.
- Planning helps you include time for friends and family. It helps you avoid overlooking an important part of your well-being: recreation.
- Planning helps you avoid the danger of allowing extracurricular activities to come before schoolwork, which is the major reason for failure in postsecondary educational programs.

- The planning phase of time management will result in a blueprint for action. In this phase you will learn how to plan the use of your precious 168 hours a week.
- Planning involves thinking about setting priorities (most important tasks), but these thoughts need to be recorded in some manner to be successful.
- You need to devise a plan for yourself so that you can program your time on a monthly, weekly, and daily basis. The plan should include the activities that are part of all the roles you fill and not just your role as a student. Your plan needs to reflect the total of your activities.

Arguments Against Planning

At this point some individuals will say they do not have time to plan and will pass off the suggestion about planning their time. Individuals who are too busy to plan are the very persons who need to be planning. If you do not plan, you will overlook priorities and possibly miss some available free time. For the small amount of time planning takes, the benefits are great. Some persons who say they do not have time to plan really do not want to find time to get priority work done. They may use lack of time as an excuse. Some individuals look at planning as leading to inflexibility and loss of freedom. They want to "hang loose" and go in different directions as the opportunities arise. Flexibility of this sort can result in disorganization and the accomplishment of few, if any, important tasks. As imposed deadlines near, guilt, frustration, and anxiety appear. These individuals wind up being a slave to time instead of being its master. A plan developed in accordance with the principles of time management will help you to be a master of time. The plan will be developed with flexibility in mind, and you will be able to trade time with yourself when unexpected events come up.

Old Habits Die Hard

Unlearning old habits and learning new habits are not easy tasks. Although it takes work in the form of self-discipline and determination to drop old, comfortable ways, it is possible. Studies have revealed that it takes at least 21 days of consistently repeating a new habit to break an old habit. Be sure to practice the new habit whenever the opportunity presents itself. In doing this, the new habit will eventually become a part of you. Oh, no! You say you slipped up and reverted to the old habits? Do not give up! Reinstate your plan and try again.

Scheduling Time

The only special equipment you need for planning is some form of calendar. You need a device, paper or electronic, that has blank spaces for each date so you can list activities. Examples of methods used for planning include the following:

1. A calendar on your personal computer—for example, iCal, Google Calendar, or your cell phone.
2. A personal digital assistant (PDA). A hand-held device with lots of memory can hold your daily plan, to-do lists, calendar, and anything else to keep you organized.
3. Calendars. Some school bookstores provide a semester calendar for students. You can also make your own monthly calendar by copying a current calendar.
4. When using a print calendar, index cards, or sticky notes for each activity, use one color card or note for roles and another color for activities. Pile the cards or stick the notes on a wall. This method also helps put activities in appropriate categories or roles.
5. Use a timeline for planning instead of a calendar.

Setting Priorities

To plan your time, you need to be able to set priorities and assign activities.

- The Try This exercise: Setting Personal Priorities on Evolve helps you decide which of your activities are most important and which activities need to come first.
- When setting priorities, remember that there is a difference between importance and urgency. Not everything that is urgent is important. A good example is a cell phone call during mealtimes.
- Suggestions to help you differentiate between what is urgent and important regarding priorities can be found at http://www.couns.uiuc.edu/brochures/time.html/ under Self-Help Brochures/Time Management.
- To have a successful year in the practical/vocational nursing program, teamwork is important. Identify the people in your life who make up your team. This is your support system. Inform them of the goals and priorities you have set for yourself for this school year.

? Critical Thinking

My Personal Support System

List the people in your personal support system on the following lines, a piece of paper, index cards, or sticky notes.

_____

_____

_____

Assigning Activities

Some of your activities can be assigned to specific individuals on your team. Box 2-1 lists examples of tasks that can be assigned in this manner. Taking growth and development into consideration, the tasks listed for children are excellent ways for them to learn responsibility.

Box 2-1   Tasks That May Be Delegated

SPOUSE/SIGNIFICANT OTHER
- Pay bills
- Help clean
- Take charge of car maintenance
- Mow the lawn
- Paint
- Do small repairs
- Prepare meals
- Start laundry
- Transfer laundry to dryer
- Shovel snow

PRESCHOOL AND EARLY SCHOOL-AGE CHILDREN (4 TO 8 YEARS)
- Put dirty clothes in designated area
- Fold laundry
- Make clean laundry piles
- Deliver laundry to correct room
- Clear dishes from table (not the good dishes)
- Make own bed (avoid criticizing outcome of efforts)

SCHOOL-AGE CHILDREN (9 TO 12 YEARS)
- Cook simple meals
- Wash dishes
- Dry dishes
- Put dishes away
- Start laundry
- Shop for a few food items as indicated on list
- Dust
- Run vacuum
- Pack own lunches
- Water plants
- Weed
- Shovel snow
- Make own bed
- Sweep

ADOLESCENTS (13 TO 18 YEARS)
- Run errands with family car if they have a license
- Wash car
- Plan menus

- Prepare grocery list within budget
- Put away groceries
- Mow the lawn
- Paint
- Make own bed
- Clean
- Wash clothes
- Iron if necessary or desired
- Sew on missing buttons

FRIENDS
- Substitute for you at bowling the night before a big examination
- Feed you occasionally

RELATIVES
- Substitute for Mom or Dad at Scout meetings, PTA meetings, or school activities
- Spend time with children
- Holiday baking or shopping

RATIONALE FOR ACTIVITIES CHOSEN FOR:
Preschool and early school-age children. Children in these age groups are experiencing muscle development and noticing their psychomotor development; they want to try new things. Make-believe rides high with these kids, and they love to play house. Capitalize on this.

School-age children. These children are adults-in-training. Muscles continue to develop, and psychomotor skills are increasing. They need tasks of the real world to engage in and should be encouraged to carry them through to completion.

Adolescents. Sometime during adolescence the ability to think as an adult will develop, allowing this age group to budget and apply principles of basic nutrition to everyday life. One of the tasks of adolescence is to become independent. Encourage its development by assigning meaningful activity to this age group.

School-age children and adolescents can also do activities in the column preceding their column but would probably prefer the specific activities listed for their age group.

Assigning to Children. As in the study of growth and development, these suggested activities apply to the typical child in each age group. The suggestions may or may not apply to your children, but do not underestimate them. You will be able to come up with some ideas that do fit your children and can be added to the list. At first it may take some time to instruct your children, but in the long run it will be worthwhile. Have you ever heard the saying "You have to spend money to make money"? Well, in time management sometimes it takes time initially to teach the people near you what is expected of them. In the long run it will pay off handsomely in time saved. In addition, your child benefits by learning responsibility, skills, and independence.

The same principle will be used in patient care. It may take time to teach patients how to master a skill for themselves. Once they learn the skill, it will save

you time, and as a bonus, the patients gain independence. These suggestions are a wonderful way to help a child become independent and develop lifelong skills.

Dealing with a Spouse/Significant Other. Are you having trouble getting your spouse/significant other to cooperate? Here are some thoughts:
- Avoid interpreting stubbornness as laziness or lack of love. Did your spouse/significant other grow up in an environment in which household chores were divided by sexual orientation? The spouse/significant other may feel that assuming new tasks jeopardizes his masculinity or her femininity.
- Decide on the areas in which you think your spouse/significant other could be most helpful during this hectic time of your life. Talk with your spouse/significant other (only you know the best

time and situation for this). Hopefully, you both agree that you should be going to school and have identified the positive features of this endeavor for both of you. Review these positive features. Collaborate on solutions to ease your lack of time.

- Establish some precious "spouse/significant other only" time to be honored during your hectic year at school. You do not want to create the feeling of being left out during this whole experience.

You can find the Try This exercise: Assigning Activities on Evolve. This exercise will help you decide the personal roles and activities that can be assigned, which you can indicate on your paper, index cards, or sticky notes.

Try This

Semester, Weekly, and Daily Planning

SEMESTER PLANNING

Time Involved: Approximately 10 minutes

On your planning calendar/system, list the things that must be done during this time frame. The following are examples of activities to include:

- Your class/clinical schedule
- Dates of major examinations
- Dates papers are due
- Dates of doctor/dental appointments
- Dates for haircuts, shopping, and so on

Include activities that are assigned. Indicate them by circling/highlighting the activity on your calendar/planning system. If using paper, write the name of the person who is responsible for it. Post these sheets, one month at a time, on your refrigerator for you, your family, or your roommate or significant other to see. The semester schedule needs to be done only once, in pencil. Additions or corrections are made as needed. This is also a way of communicating your new life to those with whom you live. Keep in mind that if you do live with other people, your new schedule is something to which they must get accustomed. And if you record your schedule on an electronic device that requires a password, make sure those who need access to the schedule have the password.

WEEKLY PLANNING

Time Involved: Approximately 10 minutes

- A blank form, Time Management: Weekly Schedule, can be found on Evolve.
- A blank weekly calendar can also be downloaded at www.bucks.edu/%7especpop/weekly-sch.htm.

Fill in all your classes and other fixed activities for the week, or paste/tape your cards or sticky notes here. Photocopy as many sheets as there are weeks in the semester or time period of your current classes. Use some time each weekend to plan your week. Be sure to include in your planning the time you spend before and after classes. As assignments are made, add them to your weekly plan. Your weekly plan not only will reflect study time, but it will also specify what needs to be studied and when. The following are some suggestions to keep in mind when planning your week:

1. Plan studying for your prime time. Prime time is the time at which you are most effective in doing a task. High-priority courses need to be studied during personal prime time.
2. Plan blocks of time for studying by identifying your personal attention span for various school activities. For example, when reading, note the time you start reading and when you begin to lose your concentration. Note the amount of time that has passed. Do this for several sessions of studying. You will begin

to see patterns in your attention span. Take a 3- to 5-minute break at this point in your studying. Vary your activity.
3. Some people may find they have a 20-minute attention span, whereas others may have an attention span of 1 hour. The important thing is to not let your break extend beyond a few minutes. Condition yourself to get right back to work, without the need for start-up time.
4. It is impossible to tell you exactly how much time you will need for studying for each of your classes. This will vary from student to student and from class to class. Does the face-to-face class meet daily? If so, you will have a daily assignment. The old suggestion of 2 hours of study for each hour of class will be just right for some classes, too much for others, and not enough for the rest.
5. Identify small blocks of time and make them work for you. They are important sources of time. These minutes can add up quickly to large time losses. These small blocks of time usually occur between face-to-face classes. Try doing the following during these small blocks of time:
   - Get up.
   - Stretch.
   - Take deep breaths if staying in the same classroom.
   - Walk briskly while taking deep breaths to get to your next class.
   - Review in your mind the class you just attended.

   These activities will force more oxygen into your bloodstream and help it circulate to your brain. This results in better thinking and a fresher state of mind. One of the worst things to do is to grab a soda or a cigarette. The soda, if nondiet, will quickly elevate your blood sugar level and encourage insulin to be deposited in the blood. The insulin will quickly lower the sugar content of your blood, leaving you with a tired, dragged-out feeling. Smoking constricts your blood vessels and decreases the amount of oxygen carried to your brain. Your brain needs oxygen to help you think and to keep you alert.
6. While waiting for your next face-to-face class, select one of the following activities:
   - Review your notes from the class you just finished. This will allow you to fill in any gaps you may have in your notes. You will aid your retention and understanding of the material by reviewing it in this way.
   - Mentally prepare for your next class. Review your assignment. If it is an autotutorial class, review your plan of activities for the class.
   - Discuss an assignment with a peer. School is a social activity, but do not waste time by fooling around during all of your small blocks of free time. The more you get done at school, the less you will have to do at home.
7. Include only what is essential on your plan. Details take too much time to record and are a real turnoff.
8. Plan for three meals a day with appropriate snacks, based on what you have learned in your nutrition course. Eating properly and keeping up your fluid intake will help avoid fatigue and irritability. With a busy schedule, you need to avoid being tired and irritable at all costs.
9. Plan for adequate sleep. Individuals have personal sleep patterns. Try to get in tune with yours. Do you ever wake up before your alarm? The next time you do, calculate how many hours of sleep you have had. Odds are your hours of sleep are some multiple of 1.5 hours. Brain research has shown that you will function better if you get up after 6 or 7.5 hours of sleep rather than after 7 or 8 hours. Apparently, we repeat a sleep cycle every 1.5 hours. If you get up a half hour into your next cycle, you could be very sluggish. Think of this when you set your alarm. When the alarm goes off, resist the temptation to hit the snooze button.

Continued

Try This

Semester, Weekly, and Daily Planning—cont'd

10. Remember, although some sacrifices must be made, your life is more than just school. Review "My Special Wish" on p. 14 of this chapter and include it on your weekly schedule.

DAILY PLANNING

Time Involved: Approximately 5 minutes

This schedule could prove to be the most important one as far as getting things done. Alan Lakein (1973) calls the daily plan a "to-do" list. He states that both successful and unsuccessful people know about to-do lists. Successful people use such a list every day to make better use of their time. Unsuccessful people do not. This is the simplest schedule to make.

1. Make a to-do list on your cell phone or a 3 × 5-inch card. List the items you plan to accomplish. Be sure to include the high-priority activities for school and your personal life that you identified on Evolve. Refer to your weekly calendar/planning system to refresh your memory about your assignments and their due dates. Rank (prioritize) your activities so that you can handle first things first. Use numbers, highlighting, or colored sticky notes to indicate priority.
2. Map a to-do list.

Professional Pointer

Make a to-do list every day to make better use of your time.

Decide for yourself the best time of day for preparing your to-do list. Some people like to prepare this list while eating breakfast as a way to get into the activities of the day. Some people like to prepare the list right before they go to bed. These people may be getting an extra benefit that they are not aware of. Their subconscious will be able to go over the list while they peacefully sleep and renew themselves. Carry your list with you. Stick to the activities and priorities you have listed. Delete/cross off/tear off the activities when you have completed them. Ah, what a feeling!

Planning takes so little time. It can be fun and not a chore. Just think of all the benefits that come out of taking 10 minutes to plan each month, 10 minutes to plan each week, and 5 minutes to plan each day. What great returns for so little effort! And by composing your plans and lists, you have freed your brain from one more source of clutter and saved it for all the learning you need to do.

IMPLEMENTATION

Implementation is the part of your time management program in which your plans become action. The only value of a plan lies in its being used. Thanks to the planning you have done, you now have an incentive to get started because you already know exactly where you have to be and what you have to do. Here are some hints on how to follow that plan.

- As you begin to follow your personal plan, you may notice that some of your peers at school are not planning their time. They may even give you static for attempting to plan yours.

- Even if it means leaving some peers in the shuffle, have the intestinal fortitude to follow your schedule. You paid your tuition and have your own personal time problems to contend with to get full mileage out of that tuition.
- If you paid your tuition with money from a scholarship or grant, look at that money as the paycheck received for working a 40-hour week. School is your job.
- There may be some students who put their efforts into social networking instead of scholastic pursuits. They might think they will look better if others do not succeed. You will recognize these students when they tell you straight out that your efforts will make them look bad.
- Make sure you never miss a face-to-face class, regardless of peer pressure or any reason other than an emergency.
- If an emergency does make it necessary to miss a face-to-face class, you spend more time trying to obtain the missed information than if you had attended the class. You may never capture all of it.
- In actually carrying out your schedule, be aware of a danger that can occur when you assign a specific time to a task. Sometimes the time it takes to do a task, whether for home or school, can stretch out to fill whatever time you have assigned to it.
- Practice setting realistic time limits in which to complete tasks so you do not fall into this trap.

Critical Thinking

Return on Your Investment

Write a few sentences about what *your* tuition is buying for *you*.

_____

_____

Procrastination

You know what you have to do and when it must be done, but do you ever find yourself putting off high-priority tasks to sometime in the future?

Critical Thinking

High-Priority Task That I Have Put Off

List one high-priority task that you have put off this week.

_____

How did you feel about postponing this task? Such action usually leads to tension. Fear of failure may cause students to put off things to the last minute. Putting off provides the student with an excuse for not doing well. What is causing your reluctance?

- Reevaluate the task you have been avoiding. Is it really a high-priority task? Remember, your planning needs to be flexible.

- The priority status of tasks can realistically change. Be careful if you find yourself using this explanation too often.
- Besides fear of failure, other causes for putting off what is important are ill health (you do not have the energy), laziness (you do not have the motivation), and past successful episodes of procrastination (if you did not do it, someone else did or nobody cared).
- Regardless of the cause, we all procrastinate to some degree. Some people make more of a habit of it than others do.

Minitasking

If you look truthfully at the tasks you keep postponing, odds are they are unpleasant, difficult, or time consuming. It seems we never postpone things that are fun or simple to do. In fact, sometimes we avoid high-priority tasks and do a bunch of low-priority ones. This action gives us an immediate yet false feeling of accomplishment.

Whatever the cause of your procrastination, if you are behind in your work, you are behind in success. Most times it takes more time and energy to escape the task than to do it in the first place.

A sure way to finish those unpleasant, difficult, and time-consuming tasks is to reduce the entire task to a series of minitasks.

- Minitasks will get you involved in starting the task in a less painful way. Just starting a task, even in a minimal way, is a positive force. Getting started takes more effort than keeping momentum.
- A minitask needs to be simple to do and take no more than 5 minutes of your time.
- Minitasks need to be readily at hand for quick reference to be effective.
- Many students fear upcoming major tests and put off studying for them. Some examples of minitasks for this situation could include:
  - Before and after each face-to-face class, review your current class notes and related material covered previously.
  - Write the more difficult information you must know for the test on index cards. For example, write a term on one side of the card and its definition on the other. List causes of, consequences of, prevention of, and differences between items of class content, and have these cards handy for quick reference whenever you have a spare minute.
  - Follow the same procedure for items you got wrong on quizzes.
  - Talk to a peer about course content.

Refer to Chapter 3 for information on identifying your personal learning style preference. Now write some minitasks for the high-priority task you identified in the Critical Thinking exercise, High-Priority Task That I Have Put Off on p. 18.

Refer to Chapter 3 for information on identifying your personal learning style preference. Now write some minitasks for the high-priority task you identified in the Critical Thinking exercise, High-Priority Task That I Have Put Off on p. 18.

? Critical Thinking

Minitasks for a High-Priority Task

1. _____
2. _____
3. _____

Hints for Handling the Home or Apartment

No matter how much you delegate, if you are a spouse and parent, a single parent, or a single adult, you must realize that your house or apartment is not going to be as spic and span as usual while you are a student. A few hints may help ease the transition. Some of these hints are also helpful for those who are helping out while a spouse or significant other goes to school and for single adults who might be living on their own for the first time.

- Your grandmother always told you to tidy up to make it look like you really cleaned. Pick up papers and magazines as you pass through a room.
- If you do not have time to wash dishes, rinse and stack them to be done later, rather than just collecting them on the kitchen counter. If you have a dishwasher, scrape dishes and stack.
- Make your bed each morning when you first get up. It only takes a few seconds and improves the appearance of the bedroom dramatically. Smooth out the top covers before you get out of bed and then slither out.
- Place dirty clothes in a laundry basket in your bedroom or bathroom instead of just heaping them on the floor. Hang up other clothing instead of just draping it over furniture.
- Clean the tub or shower after use by soaping up your washcloth and washing the sides of the tub or shower walls while they are still warm, then rinsing. (Be sure to put your washcloth in the laundry and get out a clean one.) Or while it is still wet, spray the shower with a product that eliminates the need for later scrubbing.
- Put away any hair dryer, cool curling iron, or similar devices after use, or collect them in a basket to reduce clutter.
- If you live in a two-story home, put a box at the top of the stairs and another one at the bottom for objects that need to go upstairs or be brought downstairs. There is always something coming or going, and this will save extra trips.
- Having trouble with the family remembering their assigned chores?
  - Record your schedule on a family calendar on your computer.
  - Or draw the shape of a house on cardboard, draw 31 windows on the house, and number them in sequence. Cut three of the four sides of each window so that it opens up. Place the cardboard over a piece

of shelf paper. On the paper write names and chores for each day. Paste this chore sheet in place and tape up the windows. The first month takes the most time, but the chore list is a snap after that. Be sure to include a surprise or treat occasionally.

- A fun and fast way for an adult or child to dust is to wear a washed sock. Briefly spray the sock with furniture polish and go to it.

The sky's the limit as far as creative ideas for saving time at school and in your personal life. You will come up with some ideas out of sheer necessity as the year goes by. When you do, be sure to share them with your peers and authors (send them in care of the customer service department at Elsevier: support.elsevier.com).

EVALUATION

Evaluation of your time management program will take place continuously from the minute you start implementing your plan.

- Evaluation involves determining how well your plan is working and how you are progressing toward meeting your short-term goals and long-term goal. It is a crucial part of time management. Why continue with a plan if it is not helping you reach your goals?
- If the plan is not working, modify it. Ask yourself, "What changes should I make in my plan so that it will help me reach my goals?"
- The best gauge you have for evaluating your plan is your test grades. Grades will tell you if you are devoting as much time as needed to make the grade in a course.
- How is your daily participation in class?
- Do you have assignments completed when they are due? Are you even aware that you had an assignment?
- Did you forget the test was on Thursday because you didn't mark it on your weekly calendar/planning system?
- Are you lapsing into the habit of procrastination?
- Not only will evaluation help you see how well you are progressing toward your goal, but it will also help you develop the evaluation and modification skills you will need as a practical/vocational nurse.

Get Ready for the NCLEX-PN® Examination

Key Points

- Time management is the efficient and effective use of personal time to meet goals.
- Techniques of time management can help you gain control over your life rather than being a slave to it, and they can help you work smarter, not harder.
- Most systems of time management are geared to the left-brain style of thinking. Students with a right-brain thinking style need to adapt time management systems to styles that reflect their interests and strengths.
- By using elements of the nursing process, you can set up time management techniques to fit your personal life and style.
- Data collection includes the activities in the various roles you fill and collecting data about present personal time use, including social networking.
- Planning involves composing semester, weekly, and daily plans to include high-priority activities.
- Implementation involves carrying out your plan.
- Evaluation involves deciding whether your plan is helping you meet your short-term goals and long-term goal of completing the practical/vocational nursing program and modifying your plan accordingly.

Additional Learning Resources

evolve Go to your Evolve website (http://evolve.elsevier.com/Hill/Success) for the following FREE learning resources:
- Answers to Critical Thinking Scenarios
- Additional learning activities
- Additional Review Questions for the NCLEX-PN® exam
- Helpful phrases for communicating in Spanish and more!

Review Questions for the NCLEX-PN® Examination

1. Developing an action blueprint of time use is an example of which stage of time management?
   1. Planning
   2. Evaluation
   3. Implementation
   4. Data collection

2. Which of the following statements most appropriately describes the benefits of time management for the practical/vocational nursing student?
   1. Time management reduces the need to give up any activities in a student's personal life while in school.
   2. Time management helps students manage classroom responsibilities and manage time with patients in clinical area.

3. Time management requires students to get responsibilities at school and at home completed as quickly as possible.

4. Time management eliminates the need to develop short-term and long-term goals for class and clinical rotation.

3. A practical/vocational nurse failed the first two major tests in the nursing program. The student claims there is no time for study and admits that personal responsibilities are overwhelming. To set up a time management program, select the intervention this student needs to adopt initially.

1. Write a plan to show how time will be spent in the next month at school.

2. Follow the personal plan for use of time while in school and in clinical area.

3. Review personal daily responsibilities and document present use of time.

4. Determine how much progress is being made to reach the goal of graduation.

4. Which of the following behaviors is a priority of effectiveness in time management?

1. Finish low-priority tasks on a personal to-do list as quickly as possible, and then study.

2. Complete your reading assignment for tomorrow's practical/vocational class.

3. Start a low-priority task you love to do before beginning to work on a class paper.

4. Before studying for a test on Friday, complete a two-page paper that is due next month.

Alternate Format Item

1. Which of the following practical/vocational nursing students used principles of the planning stage of time management during their student year? *(Select all that apply.)*

1. Matt arranged for his mother-in-law to take his three children for their physicals so they can participate in sports.

2. Sophia had the family reunion at her home as a means of taking her mind off the fact that she is flunking everything.

3. Elizabeth took time to teach 3-year-old Alexander how to fold his laundry when it comes out of the dryer.

4. Dominic contacted all the people in his support system and told them about his priorities for this year.

5. Because of the system he developed using sticky notes, Danti did not miss a class assignment all year.

2. List the steps of the nursing process in the correct order of priority.

1. Planning

2. Implementation

3. Evaluation

4. Data collection

Critical Thinking Scenarios

Amy, continued . . .

Amy is now in her third week of the practical nursing program. She has been late for class two times and has been absent one time because her son had a dental appointment. What suggestions would you give Amy to help her improve attendance?

Learning Methods and Skills: How Do You Learn?

Objectives

On completing this chapter, you will be able to do the following:

1. Discuss brain dominance and its effect on learning.
2. Discuss characteristics of left-brain-dominant and right-brain-dominant learners.
3. Explain the relationship of two learning styles to brain dominance.
4. Describe three major perceptual learning styles.
5. Explain how your major learning style relates to your thinking style.
6. List and describe seven identified intelligences that affect learning.
7. Speculate on how your personality pattern influences your learning.
8. Explain what is meant by the following terms that are alternatives to linear note taking: *mapping, clustering, idea sketches, diagramming, engaging in mental imagery.*
9. Explain how a student with an undependable learning system such as untreated adult ADHD can learn successfully.
10. Discuss ways of dealing with additional barriers to learning.

Key Terms

adult attention deficit hyperactivity disorder (ADHD) (p. 29)
auditory learner (ĂW-dǐ-TŎ-rē, p. 24)
bodily/kinesthetic learning (kǐn-ǐs-THĔ-tǐk, p. 26)
clustering (p. 27)
global thinkers (p. 23)
hardwiring (p. 22)
idea sketches (p. 27)
interpersonal learner (ĬN-tĕr-PĔR-sŏn-ăl, p. 26)
intrapersonal learner (ĬN-tră-PĔR-sŏn-ăl, p. 26)
kinesthetic/tactual learner (TĂK-chū-ăl, p. 24)
left-brain-dominant (lĕft brănd DŎM-ĭ-nĕnt, p. 23)

linear thinker (p. 23)
linguistic learner (lĭng-GWĬS-tĭk, p. 26)
logical learner (LŎG-ĭ-kăl, p. 26)
mapping (p. 27)
mental imagery (MĔN-tăl ĬM-ăj-rē, p. 29)
musical learner (MŪ-sĭ-kăl, p. 26)
perceptual learning style (pĕr-SĔP-choo-ăl, p. 23)
right-brain-dominant (rīt brănd DŎM-ĭ-nĕnt, p. 23)
spatial learner (SPĀ-shăl, p. 26)
visual learner (VĬS-ū-ăl, p. 24)
visual linguistic (VĬS-ū-ăl, p. 24)
visual spatial (VĬS-ū-ăl SPĀ-shăl, p. 24)

 Keep in Mind

Identify your learning style(s): Make them work for you in learning, comprehending, retaining, and applying information in the care of patients.

Everyone learns differently. Some practical/vocational nursing students take voluminous notes. Some just listen. Others learn best by hands-on activities and group instruction. Listen to student conversations about studying to get clues on different styles of learning. For example, "I like absolute silence"; "I like my music blaring"; "I study best in the wee hours of the morning"; "I like to munch when I study"; "I make up rhymes to help me remember"; "I read on a treadmill";

and so on. All students can be equally successful. There are many theories about what affects learning style.

 Try This

Take a few minutes to list your "favorites" when studying.

Brain dominance impacts the way you think. Your thinking style impacts the way you learn. Your learning style is the way you receive information most efficiently and effectively.

BRAIN DOMINANCE

The battle of biology (hardwiring) versus socialization (how you are raised) in brain development is finally backed by scientific evidence. Originally, biology alone was credited for male/female differences in areas such as learning and behavior. For a number of years, until the late 1980s, the importance of socialization became the focus. It was thought that men and women became what they are based on their specific socialization. Looking back, it has not worked out this way, and boys and girls have paid dearly for this singular emphasis.

RIGHT AND LEFT SIDES OF THE CEREBRUM

The two sides of the brain are designed to form a partnership. It is accepted that the left hemisphere of the brain is verbal and processes in sequence. The right hemisphere recognizes negative emotions faster, whereas the left hemisphere is more active when experiencing positive emotions. The left side of the brain is verbal and fluent, and without the help of the right side to add tone and inflection, it would make our speech robot-like. In school, the left side of the brain helps break down information so we can master it. The right side gives a total picture of our learning (Table 3-1).

RIGHT-BRAIN-DOMINANT INDIVIDUALS

Primarily right-brain-dominant individuals tend to be intuitive, imaginative, and impulsive. They prefer to start out with a broad idea and then pursue supporting information. They learn best by:

- Seeing and doing in an informal, busy, somewhat unstructured environment.
- Simulations, group discussions, panels, and activity-based learning.

LEFT-BRAIN-DOMINANT INDIVIDUALS

Left-brain-dominant learners tend to be analytical, rational, and objective. They learn best by:

- Putting together many facts to arrive at an understanding.
- Having traditional lectures, demonstrations, and assigned readings.

THINKING STYLE

Usually one side of the brain is dominant and affects the way you process information. The two most common styles are linear and global. Linear thinkers (also known as left-brain-dominant):

- Prefer a very structured approach to learning. They are most comfortable doing things in order. For example, when going to their first day of the nursing program, linear thinkers will have checked ahead of time the route they will take, which door to go in, where the room is located, the time they are expected to arrive, and what supplies they are expected to bring.
- They will review the information carefully *before* leaving home.

Global thinkers (also known as right-brain-dominant):

- Are more comfortable going to the nursing program their first day by accessing information and relating it to their overall goals. They will just get into their vehicle and drive, without any preplanning, on that first day.

LEARNING STYLES

Learning takes place in different ways. It is important not to pigeonhole anyone, including yourself. Everyone is capable of learning with any learning style and will use another style to reinforce learning.

PERCEPTUAL LEARNING STYLES

Perceptual learning style refers to our three main sensory receivers:

- Visual (learn primarily with their eyes)
- Auditory (learn primarily by listening)
- Kinesthetic/tactual (learn primarily by hands-on tasks)

The majority of individuals in Western countries prefer the visual learning style. The next most natural is auditory, and the smallest percentage learn through movement (kinesthetic) and tactile (touch) styles.

Table 3-1 Left and Right Hemispheres of the Cerebrum	
LEFT HEMISPHERE	**RIGHT HEMISPHERE**
Processes in sequence	Processes spatially
Trained musicians	Beginning music student
Verbal/fluent side	Among left-handed people, nearly half use right hemisphere for language
Robot-like speech	Adds tone and inflection to our voice
	Higher-level mathematicians
More active during positive emotion	Chess players, problem solvers have more activation during tasks
Puzzles over missing part, such as a shaven beard	Recognizes negative emotions faster
Breaks down new information into bits and pieces so it can be mastered	Recognizes face in the crowd even if beard is shaved off
	Gives a total picture of our learning

Try This

Self-Evaluation of Sensory Learning Style Directions

Underline the symbol that is most accurate for each statement.

	Yes	Sometimes	No
Prefers to talk rather than read.	•	Δ	□
Likes to touch, hug, and shake hands.	Δ	□	•
Likes to brainstorm in groups.	•	Δ	□
Uses finger spelling as a way to learn words.	Δ	□	•
Prefers written directions.	□	•	Δ
Sings or talks to self.	•	Δ	□
Likes to take notes for studying.	□	•	Δ
Remembers best by doing.	Δ	□	•
Likes or makes charts and graphs.	□	•	Δ
Learns from listening to lectures and tapes.	•	Δ	□
Likes to work with hands.	Δ	□	•
Might say, "I don't see what you mean."	□	•	Δ
Good at jigsaw puzzles and mazes.	□	•	Δ
Has a good listening skill.	•	Δ	□
Presses pencil down hard when writing.	Δ	□	•
Learns words by repeating out loud.	□	•	Δ
When traveling, prefers to have oral directions.	•	Δ	□
Plays with objects during the learning period.	Δ	□	•

Count all of the symbols. The highest number indicates the sensory reading preference.

KEY

□ = visual • = auditory Δ = kinesthetic/tactile

Adapted from the Barsch Learning Style Inventory, Penn State Learning Style Inventory, and the University of Georgia Education Technology Center Learning Style Inventory.

 Critical Thinking

Summarizing Your Learning Styles

After you have completed the Self-Evaluation of Sensory Learning Styles(s) exercise, make two columns on a piece of paper. Label the columns "A" and "B." Write the statements you answered as "Yes" or "No" in column "A," and write the statements you answered as "Sometimes" in column "B." You have identified your sensory learning style. The "Perceptual Learning Style Preference" section tells you how the information can be helpful to studying.

PERCEPTUAL LEARNING STYLE PREFERENCE

People think differently. They think in the system corresponding to the sense of vision, hearing, or kinesthetic/tactile.

- **Observers:** Visual learners have two subchannels: visual-linguistic and visual-spatial. Visual-linguistic learners learn best through reading and writing. They tend to remember what they read. They like to write down directions and pay better attention to traditional lectures if they watch them on video or a PowerPoint presentation. Visual-spatial learners do less well with reading generally, and they learn best through charts, demonstrations, videos, and other visual materials. They can easily visualize faces and places and seldom get lost in new surroundings. Observers tend to say, "I see what you mean" or "I think you mean. ..."

- **Listeners:** Auditory learners think in terms of hearing, talk to themselves, or hear sounds. They may move their lips and read out loud. They learn best by hearing and tend to have difficulty with reading and writing assignments. Listeners tend to say, "I hear what you are saying."

- **Doers:** Kinesthetic/tactual learners have two subchannels: movement and touch. They tend to lose interest during class if there is no movement or external stimulation. Kinesthetic learners experience feelings in regard to what is being thought about. They learn best by moving, doing, touching, experiencing, or experimenting. Sometimes learners with this style are categorized as slow learners because the information is not presented in their learning style.

Being identified as a specific type of learner does not mean that a learner thinks exclusively in any one of these overall systems. What it means is that most people think more in one system than another. There are ways to enhance learning by supporting the overall system. No learning preference is better than another. It is usually easier to feel connected to someone who shares a similar learning preference: "We think in the same language."

 Critical Thinking

Think about instructors you have had from the lower grades to the present. Which instructor was your favorite? What was their teaching style? Did it match your favorite style of learning?

Professional Pointer

A learning preference is just that. There are ways to make it work for you.

Visual Learner

If you are a visual learner, you learn best by watching a demonstration first. Make this preference work for you by using the following techniques:

- Sit in the front seat of a face-to-face class.
- Stay focused on the teacher's facial expression and body language.
- Take notes in class, and highlight, color code, and use mind maps to process and learn content.
- Rewrite notes in your own words as a form of studying (e.g., write notes or draw pictures in the margin of your book or as a note on the screen).
- Use index cards for review or memorization.
- Review films or videos, DVDs, podcasts, and so on.
- Look for reference books that contain pictures, graphs, or charts, or draw your own.
- Request demonstrations and observational experiences before practicing a new skill.
- Try to "picture" a procedure rather than just memorizing steps.

Auditory Learner

If you are an auditory learner, you learn best by hearing. Make this preference work for you by using the following techniques:

- Listen carefully if the instructor summarizes what you will be learning, points out what is important to remember, and summarizes what has been covered during class.
- Read aloud or mouth the words. Concentrate on hearing the words, especially when reading test questions.
- When attending a lecture, listen to the words instead of taking notes during class. Tape the presentation and discussion if the instructor and students grant permission. Play the tapes back several times.
- Find a "study buddy" or group with whom to discuss class content. Compare notes and verbalize the information to aid in learning the material.
- Request permission to make audiotapes or oral reports (instead of written reports) for credit.
- Make up silly rhymes or songs (mnemonic clues) to remember key points.
- Request a verbal explanation of illustrations, graphs and diagrams.

Kinesthetic/Tactual Learner

If you are a kinesthetic learner, you learn best by touching, moving, or hands-on tasks. Traditional lectures, in which one is required to sit, read, or listen for long periods of time, may be difficult for you. It is a problem to process both visual and auditory input.

Using your muscles by gesturing can help improve memory of information by matching a gesture to information that needs to be remembered. When the gestures and word are associated in your mind, performing this gesture can retrieve the word. Physical motion can jog memory and promote recall. You should see the motions students go through during an examination. Make this preference work for you by using the following techniques:

- Handle the equipment before you practice a nursing procedure.
- Move while reading or reciting facts (e.g., rocking, pacing, or using a Stairmaster or stationary bike).
- Change study positions often. During traditional lectures, you may want to sit in back in order to stand up and take notes without being too obvious.
- Use background music of your choice when studying away from school.
- Take short breaks and do something active during that time.
- Offer to do a project as a way of enhancing a required classroom presentation. For example, if you have been asked to explain how oxygen gets out of a capillary and carbon dioxide gets in, develop a project to use as the basis for your explanation.
- Use arrows to show relationships when taking notes. Use flash cards, games, mnemonic clues, and other game-like activities to reinforce content of long reading assignments.
- Highlight key concepts; make diagrams and doodles.

 Try This

Enhance Your Learning

List suggestions that you think will help enhance your learning.

_____

_____

_____

CATEGORIES OF MULTIPLE INTELLIGENCES

Gardner (1999) described what he termed "multiple intelligences" as being more accurate than the single measure of the intelligence quotient (IQ) that most people are familiar with. The seven identified intelligences include the following:

1. Linguistic
2. Logical/mathematical
3. Spatial
4. Musical
5. Bodily/kinesthetic
6. Interpersonal
7. Intrapersonal

This knowledge provides additional information that will further enhance your learning.

IDENTIFYING AND USING THE INTELLIGENCES

LINGUISTIC LEARNER (THE WORD PLAYER)

If you are a linguistic learner, you learn best by saying, hearing, and seeing words. You like to read, write, and tell stories. You are good at memorizing names, places, dates, and trivia. Make this preference work for you by using the following techniques:

- Take notes when you read this text and reduce the number of words you have included in the notes. Your love of words and vocabulary may cause you to become distracted from the key points. Use these notes as your study source.
- Review all written work before handing in the assignment. Delete extra words and phrases that are not directly related to the topic.

LOGICAL/MATHEMATICAL LEARNER (THE QUESTIONER)

If you are a logical learner as well, you learn best by using an organized method that involves categorizing, classifying, and working with abstract patterns and relationships. You are good at reasoning, math, and problem solving. Make this preference work for you by using the following techniques:

- Take the time to organize a method of study that fits you personally.
- Redo your notes to fit your study method, categorizing the material under titles.

SPATIAL LEARNER (THE VISUALIZER)

If you are a spatial learner, you learn best by visualizing, dreaming, working with colors and pictures, and studying diagrams, boxes, and special lists in the textbook/e-text. You are good at imagining things, sensing changes, puzzles, and charts. Make this learning preference work for you by using the following techniques:

- Make your own diagrams, boxes, or lists when they are not available in the text/e-text.
- Redo your notes using key concepts only.
- Box key information in the text. Highlight in your e-text.

MUSICAL LEARNER (THE MUSIC LOVER)

If you are a musical learner, you learn best by humming, singing, or playing an instrument. You are good at remembering melodies, rhythms, and keeping time. Make this preference work for you by using the following techniques:

- Play your favorite music, or hum while studying. Remind yourself which music relates to the content you are studying.
- Play an instrument while reviewing information in your head.

BODILY/KINESTHETIC LEARNER (THE MOVER)

If you are a bodily/kinesthetic learner, you learn best by touching, moving, and processing knowledge through bodily sensations. You are good at physical activities and crafts. Make this preference work for you by using the following techniques:

- Move around when studying. If you work out on a treadmill, stationary bike, or Stairmaster, it becomes a good time to read or review notes.
- Dance or act out concepts you are studying to experience the sensations involved.

INTERPERSONAL LEARNER (THE SOCIALIZER)

If you are an interpersonal learner, you learn best by sharing, comparing, cooperating, and interviewing. You are good at understanding people, leading others, organizing, communicating, and mediating. Make this preference work for you by using the following techniques:

- Organize and/or participate in a study group.
- Compare your understanding of material with that of other students.

INTRAPERSONAL LEARNER (THE INDIVIDUAL)

If you are an intrapersonal learner, you learn best by working alone, self-paced instruction, and having your own space. You are good at pursuing interests and goals, following instincts, understanding yourself, and being original. Make this learning preference work for you by using the following techniques:

- Work on individualized projects.
- Trust your instincts in regard to study needs.

(Gardner & Hatch, 1990; Miller & Babcock, 1996.)

Be aware of the type of learner you are, but do not limit yourself to those styles. Try out suggestions listed under other preferences. Some of them will further enhance your learning

 Critical Thinking

Implementing Suggestions

Make a realistic plan involving learning styles that you think will work for you. Include observable, desired outcomes; a plan of action; and dates by which you will accomplish this plan. Remember that the dates are just educated guesses based on intimate knowledge of how you function. Be sure you note how you will determine progress toward a behavioral change. Use a format that works for you: columns, clustering, doodling, pictures, and so on.

 Professional Pointer

Identify your patient's learning style and use it as a basis to support teaching started by the RN or physician.

HOW WE LEARN

Scientists are not exactly sure how the brain can rewire itself with each new stimulation, experience, or behavior and cause learning. One idea is that a stimulus occurs and is processed in the brain at several different areas. Neural pathways (traces) become more and more efficient when a learning exercise, such as reviewing notes, is repeated. This is done through myelination (coating) of the neurons. Stimulation occurs when you learn something new. The mental or motor stimulation lights up the brain in several areas, producing even greater beneficial energy—for example, you receive a new assignment or have a new clinical experience.

The brain gets its energy for learning primarily from blood—about 8 gallons per hour. Remember to keep up your water intake. According to Jensen (1998), "Dehydration is a common problem in school classrooms, leading to lethargy and impaired learning." Other factors that impede long-term memory include lack of sleep, multitasking, distraction, and lack of focus during class.

MAPPING (CONCEPT MAP)

Brain researchers have suggested an alternative to the linear method of note making (see Chapter 4 for a discussion of the difference between note taking and note making). It encourages using the *right side* of the brain, with its emphasis on images. Color and drawings are processed by the right side of the brain and are important components of mapping. Information presented in a linear manner, as in traditional note taking, is not as easily understood as information presented by key concepts. The use of key concepts is the primary way in which the brain processes information. The brain takes these key concepts and integrates them in relationships. So if the brain does not work in lines or lists, the method of note making called mapping can enhance your ability to understand, review, and recall this information. Mapping is a method in which information is organized graphically so it is seen in a visual pattern of relationships. Mapping is most meaningful to the person who draws the map. Box 3-1 gives hints for note making, using the mapping method. Figure 3-1 is an example of a summary using clustering, a basic form of mapping that helps simplify topics. Clustering is especially helpful for *visual* learners.

Some nursing programs have found mapping helpful in developing critical-thinking skills by having learners use this format to develop nursing care plans as concept maps, instead of the traditional column format.

VISUAL STRATEGIES TO ENHANCE UNDERSTANDING

Your scholastic world is bombarded with words, sentences, and paragraphs. One of the most beneficial techniques to comprehend (understand) and remember all new information is to balance this verbal mixture with visual strategies. Each of the following visual strategies will help you understand and ultimately remember information better. They deal with the right side of the brain. You will be tapping a resource that possibly you have not used often. If you have right-brain dominance, your understanding will be improved by adopting left-brain strategies of organizing information. If you have left-brain dominance, your understanding will be improved by adopting right-brain strategies of organizing information. These strategies include improving the general organization of material and writing and restating new information in your own words.

Draw Idea Sketches

These drawings will probably be comprehensible only to you. The emphasis of idea sketches is not on the quality of the drawing but on the process you must go through to take a verbal concept and represent it graphically, without words. To go through this process, you must understand the verbal concept. You can even set it up as a cartoon. Use stick figures and describe the concept verbally. Figure 3-2 is an idea sketch illustrating the function of the drug Lanoxin (digoxin), which is used to slow and strengthen the heartbeat.

Use Color in Whatever Form of Note Making You Use

Use different color print, highlighters, crayons, or colored pencils. Avoid merely underlining or highlighting the sentences. Use the different colors to help capture and direct your attention to information that fits in different categories. Different colors will help your brain organize and retrieve information.

Make Your Own Diagram as You Read

If you commit to memory by using words only, you are using only half of your brain's resources—those of the left side. If you also produce a sketch of that

---

Box 3-1   Hints for Note Making: Mapping Method

Start with your note paper in a horizontal position.
- Start with a small circle in the middle of the paper.
- Put the main topic of activity in the circle.
- Add branches off the circle for important ideas and subtopics. Arrange these branches like the spokes of a wheel. Use a different-colored pen for each of the branches. Draw more branches off branches as needed for each topic. Draw a picture to go with each key topic or idea. Artistic ability does not count here. What is important is that the picture gives meaning to you!

FIGURE 3-1 Clustering.

FIGURE 3-2 Idea sketch: Lanoxin (digoxin).

idea, you will have brought the right side of your brain into use. Using both sides of the brain encourages the storage and retrieval of information. Those who rely solely on pictures of ideas benefit by also using words.

Engage in Mental Imagery

Engaging in mental imagery will help you remember material because it demands that you understand the information. When you use mental imagery, you become the idea that you are having difficulty understanding. The right side of your brain generates pictures of the idea, and the left side supplies the script to explain what is going on in the pictures (and always in your own words). Box 3-2 provides a mental image developed by a practical nursing student to give herself a simple understanding of the function of insulin, a hypoglycemic agent that increases glucose transport across muscles and fat cell membranes. Notice how she uses the senses of hearing and feeling and also body movement to help achieve understanding. She also uses a metaphor to tie it into something she is trying to learn. The student recites the image to herself while she closes her eyes and visualizes it. First she had her roommate read the story while she visualized the scenario.

Perhaps a physiologist would wince at this description. However, it is nothing to be ashamed of if it helps you understand a concept. Plus, mental imagery can be fun.

Critical Thinking

Increasing Understanding of Concepts

Choose a concept you are having trouble understanding in one of your nursing classes or text/e-book readings, and try to increase understanding by using the following:
1. Draw an idea sketch.
2. Use mental imagery.
   Which strategy was most useful for the concept you chose?

UNDEPENDABLE MEMORY AND LEARNING SYSTEM

Some average and above-average individuals with potential talent embrace failure messages, low self-esteem, and loss of hope. Some of these people are part of a population that continues to live with untreated adult attention deficit disorder (ADHD). Among the characteristics are an undependable memory and learning system and problems with self-regulation and self-motivation. The individual may have problems with procrastination, distractibility, organization, prioritization, and impulsive decision making. Because of previous poor performance at school or work, they may have been labeled as "lazy," "stupid," or "crazy."

POSSIBLE BEHAVIORS

- Procrastination
- Indecision, difficulty recalling and organizing details required for a task
- Poor time management, losing track of time
- Avoiding tasks or jobs that required sustained effort
- Difficulty initiating tasks
- Difficulty completing and following through on tasks
- Difficulty multitasking
- Easily bored
- Impatient
- Easily irritated
- Impulsive

Adults with ADHD have experienced a lot of pain due to repeated failure resulting in embarrassment, self-blame, and a loss of hope. Intelligence is not affected in ADHD. Excellent information is available in books like *You Mean I'm Not Lazy, Stupid, or Crazy?!*, by Kelly and Ramundo (1993). Hallowell and Ratey (2010) provide tips on managing ADHD in their article "Adult ADHD: 50 Tips on Management" at http://www.addresources.org/article.

SOME SUGGESTIONS FOR THE STUDENT WITH ADHD

- Educate yourself about ADHD. Understanding the disorder is a useful tool in learning to manage symptoms.
- Get a coach—a person near you (not a spouse) who will keep you on task but always with humor.

| Box 3-2 | Mental Images Depicting the Function of Insulin: I Am Insulin—a Job Description |

I am Insulin, and I am shaped like a canoe. In fact, I am a green canoe. My job is to make sugar or glucose in the blood available to most of the cells of the body for energy. I like my job. I like things that are sweet, but not too sweet, so normal blood sugar is just my thing. Sometimes after the person who owns the pancreas where I am stored in my canoe rack eats a meal, a whistle blows, and I know this is a signal to launch myself into the bloodstream. As I ride the currents of blood, I rock gently back and forth, and the sugar in my bloodstream jumps right in to be a passenger in the canoe. Blood sugar likes me. I think it is because I am green, but I might be wrong. When I am pretty full, but not full enough to swamp, I pass through the blood vessels, paddle through the sea of tissue fluid (boy, it smells salty) around the cells, and pass through the cell membrane. Then I deposit the sugar by making these molecules jump out of the green canoe and into the fluid inside the cell. I feel pretty important in my job. Without me, the blood sugar molecules would be unable to pass through the cell membranes. Because of this, I am given the official job title of hypoglycemic agent. I lower the level of sugar in the blood.

Excuse me! There goes the whistle.

A coach assists you in staying organized, encourages you, and reminds you to get back to work.

- Making a list of tasks to be accomplished is a helpful way to focus on what you need to do. Break down tasks into manageable ones. Attach deadlines to the smaller tasks. Prioritize your lists so the most important assignments are accomplished first.
- Procrastination is a major issue. Be alert to the possibility, and discipline yourself to avoid procrastination.
- Color coding: The adult with ADHD is often visually oriented. Color helps to focus attention and also makes what you are looking at memorable. Use color in your text/e-book as you read to bring out important points. Highlight as you read. Do the same with your files and schedules. Sometimes laying a color transparency over the page you are reading or placing a brightly colored poster board on your desk will hold your attention.
- Pay attention to the different learning styles you read about in this chapter and try out the styles that appeal to you. The student with ADHD may need to multitask in order to study successfully (for example, listening to a study tape while jogging). Since physical activity is generally a part of ADHD, you may discover that reading or reviewing notes works best for you when you are on a Stairmaster, stationary bike, or other apparatus that moves. Having music may help drown out distracting noises when studying.
- Be alert to what time of day works best for you for studying. Decorate your personal study environment to inspire you. Invent your own way of studying. Do what works for you even if other students study differently.
- Note what is important and jot down ideas that invariably show up. Daydreaming is an important part of ADHD, and noting ideas may be a way of staying on task while studying.
- When studying, give yourself a mini-time-out before you switch to a different subject. Transition is often difficult for the student with ADHD, and a little break will help in the transition.
- Find ways to recharge your batteries without guilt.

Try This

All students need to "blow off steam" periodically. List three positive ways you accomplish this task.

1.
2.
3.

MORE BARRIERS TO LEARNING

Barriers may or may not be of your own making. Regardless of the reason for their existence, they belong to you now. It is up to you to identify if the barriers exist and if they affect your learning. It is also up to you to seek help in dealing with the barriers, if needed. Two such barriers are racial bias in textbooks and a type of illiteracy that involves the inability to comprehend the content of what you have read. Recognizing and reading words with fluency (speed and accuracy) are not the issues.

RACIAL BIAS IN TEXTBOOKS

Textbook content is based on the authors' interpretation of resources used as the basis of their research for writing. Multicultural resources may or may not have been part of the preparation, even if desirable for a particular topic. A lack of multicultural information in areas such as cultural differences and spiritual practices may give the reader a one-sided viewpoint, especially when the information is being presented as being factual—for example, "This race (culture, religion) always . . ."

According to Byrne (2001), six categories of bias in textbooks include the following:

1. *Invisibility:* The majority culture is used as the only example in the narrative and in all illustrations. This may result in the student of a nondominant culture feeling less than significant culturally.
2. *Stereotyping:* The writing preference oversimplifies the behavior and traits, such as physical appearance, intelligence, personality characteristics, social roles, and ambition. A sense of being misunderstood and undervalued is common.
3. *Imbalance and selectivity:* The majority culture's viewpoint is presented as the only "truth."
4. *Unreality:* Unpleasant realities and topics are avoided, which can promote racial tension by not providing the opportunity to openly discuss cultural practices and behaviors that differ.
5. *Fragmentation and isolation:* Information on nondominant cultures is separated from mainstream content, supporting feelings of insignificance.
6. *Linguist bias:* Cultural and ethnic groups are presented as being exotic or primitive.

Try This

Text/e-Book Authority

Briefly summarize a time you questioned text/e-book authority.

Critical Thinking

Text/e-book Authority

Identify which of the six categories triggered the concerns that led to the prior question. What did you do with your concern? Did the outcome of the experience influence the way you looked at yourself as a member of a cultural group? If so, how and why? What would you do differently if given the opportunity to repeat the experience?

The authors of this book encourage you to question textbook authority whenever you are sincerely concerned. One way to do this is to check out the authors' list of references and suggested readings. The references provide a list of the materials that were used to prepare each chapter.

INABILITY TO UNDERSTAND (COMPREHEND) CONTENT

Almost everyone in the United States can read and recognize words, but not everyone understands the meaning of the words they read. Years ago, a reading researcher identified the stages we must go through in order to comprehend what we read. They are still valid. They are as follows:

- Before a child starts grade school, the foundation for reading and learning has been laid. By being read to, a child learns what books are for and how they are used.
- In grades 1 and 2, a child learns to translate written letters and symbols into sounds and words.
- In grades 3 and 4, the school-age child develops speed and accuracy in reading (fluency). The child has not yet learned to comprehend what is being read.
- In grades 4-8, the school-age child masters vocabulary and learns how to pick out the main parts when reading. This is the beginning of reading for content.
- In high school, students learn to weigh evidence in messages they are reading and evaluate and make judgments about what they read. These behaviors demonstrate the ability to read for content and understand what is being read.
- By the end of high school, adolescents have reached a stage in which they are able to manage their own learning process, choosing what to read and knowing how to use what they have learned in areas of interest.

Many people in the United States have not reached the level of comprehending what they read. Memorization is not the same as comprehension (Clinton, 2000).

[?] Critical Thinking

Review the six bulleted statements in the "Inability to Understand (Comprehend) Content" section and identify how the levels apply to your ability to comprehend and apply information. If you identify gaps in comprehension, whom will you approach for assistance? Make a plan as though you are making it for a classmate.

PUTTING IT ALL TOGETHER

Quality education encourages you to explore and apply alternative thinking, multiple answers, and creative thoughts. You can become a self-directed learner using the following techniques:

- Practice thinking critically (see Chapter 8).
- Identify your major and specific learning styles. Studying becomes easier.
- Understand basic right- and left-brain functions and how they work together. It helps you appreciate your capacity for learning.
- Do your part to prevent dehydration when studying and participating in classes. Water is a major ingredient of blood, which motivates the brain.
- Maintain a positive attitude as you continue to learn and apply what you are learning.
- Set realistic goals and evaluate the results to see whether these goals were met.

It is an obstacle to learning to believe learning can take place without effort.

- Remember that established preferences of learning may not be working for you. Learning styles can be changed or modified as needed. It is also worth it to try suggestions from other styles to see if the suggestions enhance your learning.
- Tie in new learning to previous lessons and experiences. This gives the material meaning and makes it easier to remember.
- Seek help when it is needed. Sometimes being alone is best; sometimes it is best to study with others.
- Identify your reading level and make sure you reach your potential.
- Learn beyond the point necessary for doing or performing a skill. Keep reviewing and practicing the skills you learned. Practice, practice, practice.
- Fit new information into what you already know.
- Question what you do not understand and question the source of information when you have reason to believe it is incorrect.
- Remember that whatever your learning style is, the best memory is to write it down.

According to a Chinese proverb, "the weakest link lasts longer than the strongest memory."

Get Ready for the NCLEX-PN® Examination

Key Points

- Brain dominance impacts thinking style, which in turn impacts the way you learn.
- Each side of the brain processes things differently. It is accepted that the left hemisphere is more verbal and processes in parts and sequences. The right hemisphere is nonverbal and sees a total picture. A connection between the right brain and music has been established.
- The two most common thinking styles are linear (left-brain-dominant) and global (right-brain-dominant).
- Some people think in pictures (visual learners). Some hear sounds (auditory learners). Some experience a feeling in regard to what they are thinking about and learn best by doing (kinesthetic/tactile learners). Each learning style can be enhanced, and it is possible to use more than one learning style to reinforce learning.
- Multiple intelligences translate into learning styles. Identifying whether you are a linguistic learner (likes words and new vocabulary), a logical learner (organized and consistent), a spatial learner (prefers boxes and diagrams to words), a musical learner (likes to hum, sing, or play a musical instrument), a bodily/kinesthetic learner (likes touching and moving), an interpersonal learner (likes sharing, comparing, and cooperating), or an intrapersonal learner (likes working alone, self-paced instruction) further enhances your learning ability.
- Your personal attitude toward learning also influences the learning process. Attitude is closely related to whether you are a reactive learner who expects to be taught or an active learner who takes charge of his or her own education.
- Clustering, a form of mapping, is a method of note making.
- Visual strategies such as drawing idea sketches, using color in whatever form of note-making works for you, diagramming information so it makes sense to you, and using mental imagery are all additional ways of study to assist in developing long-term memory of what you are studying.
- Almost everyone in the United States can recognize words and read with fluency and accuracy. Because of being able to read with fluency and accuracy, there is an assumption that the person understands what they are reading. Studies show that many people in the United States have not progressed past the fourth-grade level in reading.
- ADHD does not affect intelligence. There are numerous effective techniques to help the person succeed.

Additional Learning Resources

Review Questions for the NCLEX-PN® Examination

1. What does the term *kinesthetic* mean?
   1. Experiences feelings about what is being taught.
   2. Good at reasoning, mathematics, and problem solving.
   3. Good at imagining things, sensing changes, puzzles, and charts.
   4. Learns best by first watching a hands-on demonstration.

2. How do you determine if you process information primarily on the left side of your brain?
   1. When learning a new procedure, you pay more attention to what the total information is rather than focusing on the steps.
   2. You break down information into smaller units and work to understand each step before proceeding to the next step.
   3. You have a tendency to give up on reading because it feels like too much of an overload.
   4. You would rather talk the procedure through to yourself rather than having someone else show you how the procedure is done.

3. Your instructor is involving all of the students in the teaching/learning process. You will work in groups of four. Your group decides to divide the responsibility based on each student's major learning preference. Which student will be responsible for preparing the demonstration materials?
   1. Darius is a visual learner.
   2. Carlos is an auditory learner.
   3. Tom is a tactual learner.
   4. Jill is a logical/mathematical learner.

4. You find yourself discussing the new definition of *illiteracy* that you have just learned. Your friend does not believe you are correct and challenges you to give him an example. Which of the following examples would be most appropriate in this situation?
   1. Your inability to understand me is a perfect example of illiteracy.
   2. The new definition of illiteracy relates primarily to the kind of teaching that is taking place in less privileged schools.
   3. The new definition is not really that important in practical/vocational nursing because we are not responsible for decision making.
   4. The new definition of illiteracy recognizes the focus on learning to read and develop fluency in reading during the first 4 years of school. The next step is comprehension.

Alternate Format Item

1. Which of the following statements is *not* true regarding racial bias in textbooks? *(Select all that apply.)*

   1. It toughens up the student for the real world.
   2. It creates a sense of feeling culturally insignificant.
   3. It presents minority cultures as being significant.
   4. It avoids unpleasant topics that could be discussed.

2. List three visual strategies that assist the brain in developing long-term memory for a topic you are attempting to understand.

   1.
   2.
   3.

Critical Thinking Scenarios

Scenario 1

Amy has just completed her second week of the practical nursing program. All she can see are words and more words. It all seems overwhelming. Her major problem seems to be how to take notes that make sense to her. Amy has been recopying her class notes nightly. She has discovered that recopying notes word for word is time consuming, and it is not helping her to understand and recall the information.

Provide some advice to assist Amy. Describe some alternative methods of note making compared to the note taking that Amy is doing during classes.

Scenario 2

A new student who has been diagnosed with ADHD insisted on being in the back of the classroom and would walk around during class. A couple of the other students would periodically make a sarcastic comment directed at him. The instructor decided to change the order of chapters to be discussed in class, and today's discussion was about different learning styles and how to identify your personal style(s). When the instructor started talking about undependable learning styles, Joe began to listen. There were parts of what she said that sounded like him. The instructor also talked about impulsive behaviors, and Joe recalled his dad telling him many times that he keeps jumping into things without first thinking it through. Now it was this nursing program, and Joe already doubts his decision. Maybe there was finally information he could use. Feeling there was no hope for him is getting old. How would you suggest he get started and where he can get some support?

Using Your Methods and Skills: Studying and Testing

Objectives

On completing this chapter, you will be able to do the following:

1. Use techniques in learning situations that will:
   a. Increase your degree of concentration.
   b. Improve your listening skills.
   c. Enhance your comprehension (understanding) of information needed for critical thinking as a practical/vocational nurse.

d. Develop your ability to store information in long-term memory.
   1) Form neural traces to store information for recall.
2. Use hints for successful test taking when taking tests in the practical/vocational nursing program.

Key Terms

active listener (ĂK-tĭv LĬS-ĕn-ĕr, p. 36)
comprehension (KĂM-prĭ-HĔN-shŭn, p. 37)
distracters (dĭ-STRĂK-tĕrz, p. 41)
external distractions (ĕks-TŬRN-ăl dĭ-STRĂK-shŭns, p. 34)
internal distractions (ĭn-TŬRN-ăl dĭ-STRĂK-shŭns, p. 34)
key (p. 41)

key concepts (kē kŏn-sĕpts, p. 36)
mnemonic devices (nĭ-MŎN-ĭc, p. 39)
options (ŎP-shŭns, p. 41)
passive listener (PĂ-sĭv LĬS-ĕn-ĕr, p. 36)
stem (stĕm, p. 41)
understanding (ŬN-dĕr-stăn-dĭng, p. 37)

 Keep in Mind

Spruce up your study skills and sail through test days at school stress free. This includes NCLEX-PN®. After this biggest of tests, you will say, "That wasn't so bad after all!"

Many educational institutions offer courses in how to study before learners enter a program and have departments that offer study skills services after a learner has enrolled. There are millions of Internet sites that provide information about study skills. Google "Pageburst," take a guided tour, check out the text and study skills, and see what can help you the most. Despite these resources, lack of study skills, including test-taking skills, is a major factor for failure or dropping out of a nursing program. Learners who need these services are not always aware that they need them. Learners cannot assume they have the study skills necessary to succeed in the practical/vocational nursing program because they have attended high school or college. It takes time and effort to comprehend, store, and recall the knowledge and skills needed for critical thinking in your chosen career.

GENERAL HINTS FOR LEARNERS

CONCENTRATION

Concentration is the ability to keep your mind completely on the task at hand. The major enemy of concentration is distraction. Many distractions in a learner's life compete with the need to buckle down to school assignments. These distractions can be summarized as two types: external distractions, which are those that come from outside yourself, and internal distractions, which are those that come from inside yourself. Strive for a study environment that meets your learning style preference (see Chapter 3).

External Distractions

External distractions occur in your physical and social environments. An obvious distraction is hunger. Be sure you have met your hunger needs before settling in to study. Nutritious snacks can provide a reason for needed breaks.

Personal Study Area. Your physical environment can be a potential enemy of concentration. Here are some tips to avoid distractions:

- Identify the type of environment that allows you to get the most out of your study time. Your grades will be the criteria by which you can judge whether your environment is helping or hurting.

- Locate realistic indoor and outdoor areas for studying that are associated with learning.
- Alternating areas where one studies can improve retention of information. The learning resource center can be used between classes and after school. At some schools, study rooms can be reserved.
- Have on hand the tools you use with a print or e-book.
- You will save yourself a lot of time and aggravation if you do not have to look for your study tools each time you sit down to study.

Lighting. Eyestrain can occur if lighting allows glare, shadows, or flicker to exist in your study area.

- eReaders may require additional external lighting.
- Reading lamps are available that advertise natural white light and a light grid to reduce eye-tiring glare.
- If a ceiling light is available, turn this on in addition to your table lamp to reduce shadows.
- A table lamp with a properly seated bulb needs to be shaded to reduce flicker.
- Your writing surface needs to be a light color to reflect light and reduce glare.
- If you experience symptoms of eyestrain, such as headaches, dizziness, tiredness, or blurred vision, while reading after you have tried to eliminate glare, shadows, and flicker, it may be time to have an eye examination to rule out the need for corrective lenses.
- Some learners discover they need glasses only after they enroll in an educational program that demands much reading, such as the practical/vocational nursing program.

Background Noise

- Television, iPods, and so forth can be distracting background noise to some learners, but others find that they study best with these devices.
- If these habits are interfering with your concentration and test grades, establish new habits.

Internet and Social Networking. Being online offers a vast amount of resources for all your classes.

- It is easy to get distracted by the information available on the Internet and social media sites.
- If you use search engines, Facebook, and Twitter for personal and recreational purposes, you now need to learn how to use the Internet and social media professionally (see Chapter 5).
- Watch your time when you are online for educational, personal, or professional reasons because hours can slip by before you know it.

Your Peers. Peers could be a possible external distraction. The energy devoted to any of the following behaviors can seriously deplete the energy needed to achieve success in the practical/vocational nursing program and can create unneeded stress and frustration. Answer "Yes" or "No" to the following questions about your peers in the practical/vocational nursing program.

1. Are the people you associate with at school encouraging your progress in the practical/vocational nursing program?
2. Do you and your peers support and encourage one another?
3. Do you pick a special person to sit with in class so you can privately chat while others are talking?
4. Do you seek out other students who have negative attitudes? If so, what are the conversations you engage in during a supposedly relaxing coffee break?
5. Do the people you associate with love to belittle, complain, and tear down the instructor, the course, and various students in your group?
6. Does your anxiety level increase when you carpool with certain students on test days?

 Try This

Personal Distractions

List any external physical distractions that are affecting your concentration.

_____

_____

What can you do to eliminate these distractions?

_____

_____

Internal Distractions

You can have the study space, lighting, noise level, equipment, and peers for studying but still not be able to keep your mind on the task at hand. The culprit may be distractions arising from inside you. Common examples of internal distractions and suggestions for overcoming them follow.

Complaints of Mental Fatigue. Some learners confuse boredom with fatigue.

- Avoid studying one subject so long that you get bored with it.
- Keep up your physical self with proper food, sleep, and exercise.
- At the first sign of getting tired, take a short break and come back to new material so that you can get your mental second wind.

Daydreaming. Daydreaming can be a creative adventure or wasted time.

- Every time you find your mind wandering from the topic at hand, try putting a check mark on a piece of paper that you keep at your side. This may remind you that you are drifting off and need to get back to work.
- Students who use this technique find that the number of check marks decreases dramatically with time.

◎ Try This

Daydreaming

List four topics that you daydream about when studying.

_____
_____
_____
_____

LISTENING/VIEWING

The Active and Passive Listener/Viewer

Whether you are involved in a minilecture or a discussion, viewing DVDs or watching a PowerPoint presentation as part of course assignments, you are going to miss a lot if your mind wanders. Listening/viewing is much more than the mechanical process of hearing or seeing. There are two kinds of listeners/viewers. Which type are you?

- The passive listener/viewer receives sounds or sees words with little recognition or personal involvement.
- Passive listeners/viewers may be doodling, staring out the window, staring at the instructor, aimlessly trying to copy everything—all the while thinking about where to eat after class.
- The active listener/viewer is always thinking, not just hearing or seeing words.
- Active listeners/viewers listen and look with full attention, are open-minded and curious, and are always asking themselves questions about content.
- The active listener/viewer, who really listens to hear and thoughtfully looks to see, is searching for relevant information, strives to understand it, and is always trying to figure out how content fits into the big picture, as you will also do on the clinical area.
- Active listeners/viewers realize that listening and seeing are important means of gathering information, and they work at developing these skills. The skills are also used on the clinical area.
- The active listener/viewer searches for ways in which the words can be put to practical use regardless of the student's level of interest in, or degree of, fondness for the instructor or the instructor's dress or mannerisms. Box 4-1 gives you hints on how to become an active listener/viewer.

◎ Try This

Active Versus Passive Listener/Viewer

Identify and list behaviors that indicate you are an active or passive listener/viewer.

My active listening/viewing behaviors:

_____
_____

My passive listening/viewing behaviors:

_____
_____

Box 4-1 Hints for Active Listening/Viewing in Classes

- Be well rested for class or activity.
- Complete assignments, extra readings, and exercises before class or activity.
- Focus on what is happening with the lesson. Listen and/or look for key information, central ideas, examples, and study hints.
- Capture key points of the PowerPoint presentations.
- Ask questions before, during, and after class.
- Make eye contact with the speaker.
- Listen when other students are speaking.
- Seek help when a difficult concept is not understood.

Note _Making_ Versus Note Taking

An important part of listening/viewing is remembering what you have heard or seen. Some students say that taking notes interferes with their listening/viewing skills. They are correct if they are in the business of taking notes. Research has shown that a student remembers only 50% of a 10-minute lecture when tested immediately afterward and only 25% of that lecture when tested 2 days later. You can improve those percentages to as much as 80% to 90%. Whether using your tablet or paper and pen, the secret is to engage in note _making_ whenever you are listening/viewing. Because instructors derive test questions from minilectures, discussions, activities, DVDs, PowerPoint presentations, and texts, that 80% to 90% of a specific learning activity could translate into a comparable test score. Note _making_ will help you to pay attention, concentrate, and organize your ideas.

Note Making Hints

- Never try to capture every spoken or written word . This is note _taking_, and it is impossible.
- Actively listen/look for the main ideas. Capture them in a way that reflects your personal learning style or styles. You are recording ideas or key concepts that you will later add to, correct, and study. Your goal is to understand the information, _not_ memorize it.
- Engage in note _making_, formulating condensations of what is said or seen in a text-like manner.
- Develop your own personal symbols, abbreviations, and/or shorthand of sorts to help you capture the main ideas, yet retain readability without having to completely transcribe the notes.
- With practice, notes will improve. Your goal is a set of notes you can use as part of test preparation.
- Outlining is a structured form of note making that starts with major points and indents supporting points. Numbers or letters can be used to outline but are not necessary. Indentations will do. Box 4-2 contains hints for note making.

Some students think that making notes alone will help them to retain the material. Active and frequent review of your notes is an important step in retention of material so that you can recall it at a later time.

Box 4-2	Hints for Note Making

- When using a tablet or pen and paper, include the date and general topic of class/activity at the top of the page and any assignments that are given.
- Place specific topics of the class to the left of the page.
- Indent points as they are presented to explain/discuss the topic.
- Leave spaces between topics to add information to clarify the topic as needed.
- After class, in the left margin of a paper page, record any questions to clarify your understanding of the content.
- At the bottom of the page, summarize the content of the notes on that page, *in your own words*. This summary forces you to think about the ideas in your notes. You are critically thinking about the information, not passively copying it to be memorized later.

HOW TO UNDERSTAND (COMPREHEND) INFORMATION

READING ASSIGNMENTS

"I read the material four times and got a D. My friend read the material once and got an A. It isn't fair." The learner who is speaking is correct. It takes a lot of time to read material four times for a test. The missing ingredient is the lack of understanding (comprehension) of information that is read.

- To think critically in nursing, you must have information.
- To acquire information, you must be able to read with understanding.
- Reading with understanding makes possible retention of the information.
- Retention ensures recall.

Earning only a D by merely reading words is a poor return on your time investment. Did you ever drive somewhere without remembering how you got there? That is the same as reading the text four times or getting to the end of a page and not knowing what you read. These readers have zoned out and have mindless reading. As they read, their minds will be somewhere else. They may be hungry, thirsty, tired, need to go to the restroom, or thinking about other things. Their comprehension of the information is low to absent, and test scores will suffer.

Because you are responsible for large amounts of reading in the practical/vocational nursing program, the ability to read with understanding is a necessary skill. Most of us are able to read printed words on a page. However, the reading demanded of a learner and future employee requires understanding of the meaning of the words read. Reading to learn and understand involves a rate of speed and degree of understanding that are effective.

You probably had to take a reading test as part of your preentrance tests for the practical/vocational nursing program. Generally these tests are brief. If you scored low, you were referred for help with this skill. Perhaps you were one of those who achieved an acceptable score on these short-reading tests but could use some hints on how to increase your reading efficiency. Evaluate your reading habits by answering "Yes" or "No" to the questions in the following Try This exercise.

Try This

Reading Habit Evaluation

Circle the reading habits that apply to you.
1. Do you ever reread a sentence before you come to the end?
2. Do you ever have trouble figuring out the main point of an author?
3. Do you stop reading every time you come across a word you cannot define and look up the word immediately?
4. Do you read novels, popular magazines, newspapers, and textbooks at the same speed?
5. Do you ever have trouble remembering what you read?
6. Do you have trouble understanding what you read?
7. Do you ever think of other things while you read?
8. Do you read every word of a sentence individually?
9. Do you focus on details when you read?
10. Do you tire quickly when reading?
11. Do you skip uncommon words when you read?

If you answered yes to any of the previous questions, you could benefit from help with your reading. A trip to your school's study skill center or consulting with your instructor for assistance with reading can help improve your skill in reading more efficiently and effectively.

Reading Effectively
- Read in phrases, a few words at a time, rather than word by word. Although the brain can view only one word at a time, it understands only when words are in phrases. For better understanding, you should read as you speak (i.e., in phrases).
- Put expression into your reading. You do not speak in a monotone, so why read that way? Musical learners can benefit by singing what they read.
- Be aware of your reading assignments that are technical or scientific in nature and vary your reading speed accordingly. The more recreational your reading material (e.g., novel or magazine), the faster you can read. For more technical or scientific material you must slow down. Regardless of your learning style, when the going gets tough in a paragraph of assigned reading, reading the difficult material aloud may help clear up more challenging information.
- Highlight unfamiliar words as you read. When you are finished reading, copy the words on an index card and look them up in the appropriate dictionary. Most of the unfamiliar words you come across will be medical terms, which can be found in a medical

dictionary. At first you will think these words are Greek, and you are right. Quite a few of them are derived from the Greek language. The rest are derived from Latin.

- Write the definition on the other side of the card. Break down the word with vertical slashes into its prefix (the word beginning), root (core word), and suffix (word ending) so you can begin making associations with other words that have the same prefix, root, or suffix. If your medical dictionary does not include this information with each word, the information can be found in medical terminology texts or as part of a computer program of medical terminology.

- Nursing involves learning a new language. Regardless of learning style, include your own drawing to represent the definitions of these words with the verbal definition. This may help you recall the meaning of the word. Using index cards allows your language development to progress because you can take the cards wherever you go. Learning can occur whenever you have a few minutes to spare.

- Highlight key phrases or write notes in the margin. Make a note if using your computer. Highlighting will keep you active and result in the identification of key concepts for study and review.

- See Evolve for the modified *PQRST Method of Textbook Study* if you want to be sure you will pass tests.

Remember, an important part of any textbook is the index at the back of the book. This index will help you locate information quickly. The glossary (alphabetical listing of boldfaced terms in this text) at the back of the book will provide the definition of these words.

? Critical Thinking

Improving Reading Habits

Write your plan to increase your reading comprehension. Note how you will determine progress.

REMEMBERING AND FORGETTING

We all can recall things from the past, indicating that our brains have the ability to store information. But how many times have you said, "I forgot" or "I cannot remember"? Possible causes of forgetting include a negative attitude toward the subject, which interferes with the motivation to remember. Valid as this cause of forgetting may be, perhaps the most common reason why students cannot remember is that they never understood and stored the information in the first place. They really did not internalize the information and comprehend it to begin with. Perhaps they did not listen/view actively, or they just read words and created a mental blur.

FROM TEMPORARY TO PERMANENT MEMORY BY WAY OF A NEURAL TRACE

Once you understand information, you need to store that information so that you can recall it when needed on the clinical area (and on tests!). To store information in your long-term memory, a neural trace or record of the information must be laid down. It takes 4 to 5 seconds for information to move from the temporary, or short-term, memory to the permanent, or long-term, memory. To form a long-term memory of information, you must strive to understand that information. In doing so, you will give your brain the chance to lay down a neural trace. Presto! You have created a memory of that information. Short but frequent study periods with concentration will help you understand information and store it in your long-term memory. Then it is ready for recall.

Remember that a positive mental attitude is a factor in learning, allowing you to understand and remember. Remind yourself that all the basic courses in your nursing program are essential. They are the building blocks for all the remaining courses you will take in the practical/vocational nursing program. The following techniques help increase understanding of your studies by allowing neural traces to be recorded in your brain.

- As you listen or read, seek out key concepts, basic principles, and key ideas. Be selective and learn to sift out and reject unnecessary details. The activity of being selective helps you lay down neural traces. Emphasize accuracy, not speed. You want correct information to make a clear neural trace. It is difficult to unlearn wrong information and replace it with correct information. You cannot memorize everything. If you could, you would not have an understanding of anything. The student who memorizes has difficulty in applying course information and solving problems in the clinical area.

- Short study periods followed by short rest periods are better than long study marathons. This type of study will reenergize you and allow neural learning to continue during rest periods. It seems that cramming for examinations is treated like a rite of passage among some students. Brain research has shown that short but frequent study periods help you store information in long-term memory. This will make the information available for testing and for application in the clinical area.

- Regardless of your learning style, use as many body senses and as much body movement as possible when trying to learn new information. Recite the information aloud as you read, using your own words. If you can explain it, you must understand it and will know it. Hearing you say the information aloud is an additional channel that allows neural traces to be recorded.

- Write down the information in your own words. This muscle action will help you clarify ideas and improve thinking. *Do not copy word by word from a book.*

The techniques of using body senses and body movement are all elements of tactual learning (see Chapter 3) and help lay down a neural trace. Try them, and see if they work for you. Adopt the suggestions that help you understand the material in your classes. They will increase your long-term memory of that information.

MEMORY AIDS

Mnemonic devices are examples of memory aids. Some examples include the following:

- *Rhymes*
  Thirty days hath September . . .
  I before *e* except after *c* . . .
  In fourteen hundred and ninety-two . . .
- *Acronyms*
  Every good boy does fine (to remember the line notes of the treble clef in music)

There are also devices in nursing that can help you remember information. For example:

- *CMTSP* (for assessment of the nerve and blood supply to an extremity)
  C = color
  M = motion
  T = temperature
  S = sensation
  P = pulse
- *PERRLA* (for assessment of the pupils)
  P = pupils
  E = equal in size
  R = round
  R = regular in shape
  L = react to light
  A = accommodation (pupils constrict)

Memorizing these acronyms can help the practical/vocational nurse remember groups of information. They do not take the place of or help you to understand the information.

SUCCESSFUL TEST TAKING

The majority of items on the NCLEX-PN® examination are written at the application or higher levels of cognitive ability (NCLEX-PN® Examination, 2011). You can anticipate application-level or higher types of questions as part of theory tests in the practical/vocational nursing program.

Test-taking skills are divided into three general areas: preparing for the test, actually taking the test, and reviewing the test. The following sections address these areas.

PREPARING FOR THE TEST

- Preparation for test taking begins the first day of class with striving to understand information to both do well on the test and for clinical performance.
- Clarify content to be covered on the test and the form of the test. The instructor will be measuring your understanding of all the objectives that the test covers.
- Clarify the types of questions that will be asked on the tests. For example, will the test be multiple choice and/or short answer? Specific hints for taking multiple-choice, fill-in-the-blank, multiple-response, and prioritizing questions are included in this chapter.
- To store information in your long-term memory, review class information periodically.
- In study groups, write practice questions and share them to formulate complete accurate answers.
- Cramming—last-minute studying of material for a test—sometimes results in short-term memory of material that might help you pass a test. However, because you did not engage in repetitions spaced over days, storage in long-term memory will not occur and application of the material to the clinical area will be difficult.
- Cramming for an examination is like packing your suitcase for a vacation at the last minute. You wind up with a suitcase filled with things you do not need and a whole list of things you forgot to bring.
- Do not reread the textbook. You have already completed your reading with understanding. Because you have studied the material periodically since the last test and used study skill techniques, all you need to do at this point is focus on your highlights, margin writings/onscreen notes, and index cards to check your understanding and retention of the information.
- The night before the test, go to bed at your usual time.

TAKING THE TEST

- If it is a group scheduled test, arrive at the classroom with plenty of time to get your favorite seat.
- Beware of peers who try to make you nervous by saying things like "You didn't study *that*, did you?" or "You mean you *didn't* study that?"
- If an online test, follow the rules for testing.
- You organized your time and systematically reviewed for the test. Keep a positive mental attitude. Take slow, deep breaths to reduce tension.
- Avoid spending large amounts of time on difficult questions and avoid getting upset about them. Both of these activities waste time and do not earn points. Go on to the next question and return to the skipped item later. However, be aware that on the NCLEX-PN® examination, you will not be able to skip items and then go back to them. For the NCLEX-PN® examination, you need to answer each item as it comes up on the test.
- Take the full time for the test. If you finish early, try to answer the questions you skipped.

- Make sure you have not missed an item or group of items.
- If it is a paper multiple-choice examination with an answer sheet, make sure your answers match up with the proper slot on the answer sheet. The instructor cannot possibly know you put the answer to number 37 in the slot for number 36. If you are using a separate answer sheet that will be machine corrected, be sure you erase your first answer completely if you change answers.
- Should you change an answer? Although research has shown that test scores are generally improved by changing answers, we have seen some learners decrease their test scores by the same action. If you have given the item further thought and feel it should be changed, change it. Test by test, keep tabs on your test scores to see whether changing answers is helping your final score and modify your behavior accordingly.

REVIEWING YOUR TESTS

Remember, tests are a learning tool. When the examination is corrected and returned to you, do the following:

- Read the items you missed. Why are they wrong? Did you make a careless mistake? Did you know the material? Can you correct the item without looking in your textbook or notes? If not, look up the answer.
- Read the items you answered correctly. What did you do right to get credit for these items?
- Decide which of your study skills and test-taking techniques are and are not working to your benefit. Modify your test-taking strategies accordingly.
- After reviewing their tests, some students realize that they need to study more, study differently, and/or read the test questions more analytically in order to succeed.

Some students who have organized their notes and their time, systematically reviewed and understood the material have nevertheless done poorly on tests. A reason for this could be that they did not follow the directions on the test. How well do you follow directions? Take out a blank sheet of paper and do the exercise in the Try This box on this page.

How did you do? If you did not follow the directions, do you feel tricked? You were not. The directions were clear, and you simply did not follow them. Listen meticulously to oral directions and read the written directions completely before each test. To those of you who did follow the directions for this exercise, keep up the good work! If directions are ever unclear, ask the instructor before proceeding. Clarify the time limit of the examination. Now you are ready to begin. The hints in the following sections will come in handy for test taking.

 Try This

How Well Do You Follow Directions?

Directions: Read the following directions carefully. You will have 1 minute to do the exercise after reading the directions. Be sure to write legibly. When you have finished, check your answers against the directions before handing in the paper. Be sure to read the entire exercise before beginning.

1. On a sheet of paper, print your name in the upper left-hand corner, last name first.
2. Under your name, write the last four digits of your Social Security number.
3. In the upper right-hand corner, write the name and number of the course for which you are taking this exercise.
4. In the lower left-hand corner of the paper, write today's date.
5. In the lower right-hand corner, write your instructor's name, last name first.
6. Fold your paper in half lengthwise.
7. Number the left half of your paper 1 to 6, skipping three lines between each number.
8. Number the right half of your paper 7 to 12, skipping three lines between each number.
9. Now that you have read all the steps in this exercise, do only number 1 of the exercise and hand your paper to the instructor.

REDUCING ANXIETY BEFORE TESTING

Research shows that if a person does not do well on tests, odds are that he or she is less intelligent than the average student, has poor study habits, or has weak test-taking skills. Less intelligence does not apply or you would not have been admitted into the nursing program. Poor study habits do not apply if you established good study habits, organized your study time as suggested in this chapter, and made use of your personal learning style to comprehend course content as suggested in Chapter 3. If poor study habits are an issue, you would notice it by poor test grades and seek help.

Normal anxiety is your friend. This type of anxiety actually makes you sharper and more alert during a test. Only when anxiety overwhelms you does it become your enemy. Accept the energy resulting from normal anxiety as your partner. Total personal comfort is not the key. Normal anxiety leaves you somewhere between too much relaxation and too much tension—perfect for testing.

Make the days before testing work for you through your positive thinking. Think about what you think about. Are you in the habit of seeing yourself failing or just squeaking by? Because everyone daydreams and sets the stage for their reality, daydreaming is a natural way to practice being confident and successful. Visualization may be helpful. For additional ways to relieve anxiety, see the suggestions in Chapter 6.

Spend the evening before the test doing what works best for you prior to a test. For some it is reviewing select notes. For others it is relaxing. Little will be accomplished by worrying or by last-minute cramming. Read something light and entertaining, watch television, or do what you already know works for you.

Get a good night's sleep by going to bed at your usual time (whatever meets your sleep requirements). It is believed that sleep restores memories that were lost during a hectic day. Going to bed extra early and not falling asleep may just result in a new worry. Follow through with your usual morning habits. Avoid forcing your system to adjust to a demand that is not a usual part of your routine.

 Try This

Relax!

Make a *tentative* plan for what you will do the evening before any test examination.

HINTS FOR SPECIFIC QUESTIONS

The types of tests you will be taking in the practical/vocational nursing program, including the NCLEX-PN® examination, are achievement tests. They measure how much you have learned. Following are four types of questions found on the NCLEX-PN®. The same types will be used during testing in the practical/vocational nursing program.

Multiple-Choice Questions

- Multiple-choice questions are called items. Each multiple-choice question includes a stem, three distracters, and a key.
- The stem is the first line of a multiple-choice question.
- It defines the situation for which the learner must pick out the correct answer. The stem is presented as a statement or a question.
- Four statements, called options, follow the stem. Three of the options are incorrect answers and are called distracters. One of the options is the correct answer and is called the key.
- Distracters are presented to test whether you really have learned the material and can apply it.
- The format of the NCLEX-PN® examination is multiple-choice questions, most of which measure application or higher levels of nursing knowledge. Box 4-3 gives general hints for taking multiple-choice tests.

Box 4-3   Multiple-Choice Test Hints

- Read over all the options given before making any decision.
- Eliminate the options you know are definitely wrong.
- Remember the course subject matter for which you are being tested.
- Eliminate options that are not related to the subject.

 Try This

Multiple-Choice Questions

Choose the appropriate option (the key) for the following multiple-choice statements. There is only one answer to each multiple-choice statement.

1. Multiple-choice questions are examples of:
    1. Sentences for which one-word answers are required.
    2. Questions or sentences with four options for answers.
    3. Two vertical columns that must be matched item by item.
    4. Statements that require a sentence on the answer sheet.
2. When answering multiple-choice questions, it is *not* necessary to:
    1. Read all of the directions.
    2. Eliminate wrong options.
    3. Read each of the options.
    4. Ignore any negative words.

ANSWER TO MULTIPLE-CHOICE QUESTIONS

1. Key = 2. A question or sentence is given with four options. Only one option, the key, is correct. The rest of the options are distracters—that is, options that are there to test whether you really have learned the material and can apply it. Option 1 describes fill-in-the-blank items, option 3 describes matching tests, and option 4 describes short-answer items.
2. Key = 4. This multiple-choice item contains a negative word in the stem that can complicate things. Read the stem without the negative word to get some meaning out of it, and then read the options. One option should not fit in with the others. Now reread the original stem with the negative word and see whether the option you have already isolated fits in. Items with negative words in the stem are sometimes accused of being more of a reading test than a test of understanding of content. Although the test begins with directions, there may be additional directions before individual multiple-choice questions. These directions may ask you to select one best answer or select what is most important of four correct answers. *Do not stop reading when you think you have the correct answer.* There may be a better option yet to come. Options 1, 2, and 3 are true.

Multiple-choice questions are not "multiple-guess" questions. Think through each response thoroughly before choosing your answer. Should you ever guess? To be able to make a decision about guessing, you must know whether you will be penalized for wrong answers. Even if you are penalized, figure out the odds. If you can eliminate one distracter for certain, you have a better chance of answering correctly. Can you eliminate two out of four distracters? Your chances are now even better. You make the decision. Remember, on the NCLEX-PN® examination you will have to answer every item as it comes.

Alternate Item Formats
Fill-in-the-Blank. These questions require you to calculate an item—for example, a medication dosage or intake and output. You may be asked to round the answer to the nearest whole number or the nearest tenth.

Try This

Fill-in-the-Blank Questions

The LVN needs to chart intake for a patient. The patient drinks 8 ounces of coffee, a slice of toast, and 8 ounces of water. Record the intake in ccs. (Fill-in-the-blank questions will be used in your courses with a clinical component.)

Answer: Intake is 480 ccs. Thirty ccs equals one ounce.

Multiple-Response. A question is presented and you need to select all the options that relate to the information in the question. No partial credit is given. If there are five correct options and you select only four, you do not receive credit.

 Try This

Multiple-Response Questions

1. Indicate the strategies to improve reading comprehension. *(Select all that apply.)*
   1. Read text word by word.
   2. Highlight key information.
   3. Read quickly to complete the assignment.
   4. Avoid writing in book margins.
   5. Draw pictures to explain concepts.

Answer: 2, 5

Prioritizing. A nursing situation is presented and you need to prioritize (choose what you would do first, second, third, etc.) from a list of given steps or interventions. You would order the answer options from the first to the last step or priority. This is also called an ordered-response question.

 Try This

Prioritizing Question

Michael has decided he wants to be a practical nurse and work in long-term care. Prioritize the actions Michael must take to reach his goal.
1. Pass all nursing courses.
2. Obtain a job as a practical nurse.
3. Pass the NCLEX-PN®.
4. Investigate practical nursing.
5. Be admitted to the nursing program.
6. Graduate from the nursing program.

Answer: 4, 5, 1, 6, 3, 2

Get Ready for the NCLEX-PN® Examination

Key Points

- Learning how to learn is important because study skills enable the SPN/SVN to understand (comprehend) and store in long-term memory the theory and skills required to be a practical/vocational nurse.
- When theory and skills are stored in long-term memory, they can be retrieved or recalled as the basis for critical thinking.
- Perhaps your most important skill for success in the practical/vocational nursing program is your reading skill.
- There is no easy way to learn information.
- Techniques that have been proved effective in increasing your level of concentration are creating personal study areas, evaluating the influence of peers, and decreasing daydreaming.
- Improving your listening/viewing skills requires you to be an active, rather than a passive, listener/viewer.
- Effective note *making* may enhance your ability to understand information.
- Using the suggestions in this chapter, including hints for test taking, can help you succeed in the practical/vocational nursing program.

Additional Learning Resources

evolve Go to your Evolve website (http://evolve.elsevier.com/Hill/Success) for the following FREE learning resources:
- Answers to Critical Thinking Scenarios
- Additional learning activities
- Additional Review Questions for the NCLEX-PN® exam
- Helpful phrases for communicating in Spanish and more!

Review Questions for the NCLEX-PN® Examination

1. Select the type of question that presents the student with a stem and several options from which to choose the correct answer.
   1. Matching
   2. Essay exam
   3. Short answer
   4. Multiple-choice

2. Which of the following statements describes the "S" step of the PQRST method of textbook study?
   1. Repeat, in your own words, the main points.
   2. Survey all of the material in the assignment.
   3. Periodically check to see what you remember.
   4. Carefully read charts, tables, figures, and boxes.

3. A student in the practical/vocational nursing program frequently daydreams during classes that use group discussion as a learning strategy. What is the most important behavior for this student to improve listening skills?

   1. Tweet to focus on what is being said.
   2. Stare at the student who is speaking.
   3. Listen with attention to the speaker.
   4. Focus on instructor mannerisms to stay alert.

4. Which of the following strategies is most effective to increase reading comprehension?

   1. Put concepts in the form of a drawing.
   2. Avoid writing notes in shorthand form.
   3. Make a timeline of important concepts.
   4. Use textbook terms to explain concepts.

Alternate Format Item

1. Understanding information that is read in the practical/vocational nursing program is necessary to save that information in long-term memory so it can be retrieved when needed for critical thinking. Which of the following students are using strategies that help in accomplishing this task? (Select all that apply.)

   1. Cole, while previewing a reading assignment, formulates questions from chapter titles that he can answer while reading the assignment.
   2. Juan takes a concept that he is having difficulty understanding and creates a story in his own words while visualizing the story.
   3. Cheyenne repeats what she reads in her own words after completing the assignment and again several times after the initial reading.
   4. Levi takes a verbal concept that he is having difficulty understanding and, without using words, draws a picture to explain the concept.

2. Which of the following are behaviors of active listeners during a class discussion in a medical/surgical class? (Select all that apply.)

   1. Daisy listens with full attention to whoever is speaking.
   2. Pao questions the content of the discussion.
   3. Sage thinks about the speaker's hairstyle.
   4. Isabella tries to relate this discussion to her last clinical assignment.
   5. Clay wonders how to ask the speaker for a date.

Critical Thinking Scenario

Amy visited the counselor at school and discussed some time management strategies. Her situation at home has improved. While on a class break, Amy tells you she has improved how she manages her time but Amy earned a C in the first Fundamentals quiz and flunked the second quiz. She says she can't make sense of her notes and the night before the test is too late to clarify with peers what went on in class a week ago. What advice can you give Amy regarding study habits and reading assignments?

Learning During School: Using Available Resources

Objectives

On completing this chapter, you will be able to do the following:

1. Identify your knowledge of your school's learning resource center (LRC), including:
   a. Available print and digital resources
   b. Available technology
   c. Procedures to locate print and digital resources
   d. How to use technology to access digital resources
2. Discuss the value of reading assignments in periodicals.
3. Use a periodical index; locate an article related to nursing.
4. Discuss six hints used to gain full value from minilectures and PowerPoint presentations.
5. Compare learner responsibilities for each of the following means of delivering practical/vocational nursing classes/courses.
   a. Face-to-face class
   b. Distance learning
6. Discuss your responsibilities for each of the following learning strategies:
   a. Minilecture, discussion
   b. Discussion buddy
   c. Cooperative learning
   d. Technology use during learning activities
7. Discuss the use of the following resources in your personal learning:
   a. Syllabus, course outline, Course Management System (CMS)

b. Nursing skills lab
c. Study skills lab
d. Study groups
e. Tutoring
f. Audiovisual materials
g. Internet
h. Electronic device (laptop, smartphone, iPad [or other tablet], iPod Touch, etc.)
i. Computer-assisted instruction (CAI)
j. Simulation
   1) Case scenarios
      a) Paper
      b) Computer
   2) Static mannequins
   3) Electronic mannequins
   4) Virtual clinical excursion
8. Describe how the following resources help you stay current in practical/vocational nursing:
   a. Periodical indexes
   b. Nursing organizations
   c. Community resources
   d. Guest speakers
   e. Mobile devices
9. Discuss professional use of social media/social networking.

Key Terms

app (p. 52)
audiovisual (AV) materials (ĂW-dē-ō-VĬZH-ū-ăl, p. 46)
blended course (BLĔN-dĕd, p. 49)
bucket theory (BŬK-ĭt, p. 47)
call number (kăl, p. 46)
case scenario (kas sĕn-ÂR-ē-ō, p. 52)
community resources (kă-MŪ-nĭ-tē RĒ-sŏr-sĕs, p. 54)
computer-aided instruction (p. 52)
computer simulation (SĬM-ū-LĀ-shŭn, p. 52)
cooperative learning (kō-WŎP-ĕr-ă-TĬV, p. 48)
copyright laws (KŎP-ē-rīt, p. 47)
Content Management System (CMS) (p. 49)
course outlines (kŏrs ŎWT-līn, p. 50)
digital databases (DĀT-ă-bās, p. 54)
discussion buddy (dĭs-KŬ-shŭn, p. 48)
distance learning (DĬS-tăns, p. 49)
electronic devices (Ē-lĕk-trŏn-ĭc, p. 51)

electronic simulation (p. 52)
guest speakers (gĕst, p. 54)
interlibrary loan services (p. 47)
Internet (p. 47)
learning resource center (LRC) (p. 45)
lecture-discussion strategy (p. 48)
librarian (p. 46)
mobile devices (p. 51)
nursing organizations (NŬR-sĭng ŏr-gă-nĭ-ZĀ-shŭns, p. 54)
nursing skills lab (NŬR-sĭng skĭlz, p. 50)
online catalog (p. 46)
peer-reviewed (p. 51)
periodical index (PĬR-ē-ŏd-ĭ-kăl ĭn-DĔKS, p. 53)
periodicals (PĬR-ē-ŏd-ĭ-kălz, p. 53)
podcast (PŎD-căst, p. 51)
reference materials (RĔF-rĕnts mă-TER-rē-ăls, p. 47)
simulation (SĬM-ū-LĀ-shŭn, p. 52)

social media (SŌ-shŭl ME-dē-ăh, p. 54)
social networking (SŌ-shŭl NĔT-wŏrk-ēng, p. 54)
stacks (p. 47)
static simulation (p. 52)
study group (STŬ-dē groop, p. 50)

study skills lab (STŬ-dē skĭlz, p. 50)
syllabus (p. 49)
tutoring (TOO-tŏr-ēng, p. 50)
virtual clinical excursions (VĔR-choo-ăl, p. 53)

 Keep in Mind

Knowing where and how to access nursing information makes keeping up-to-date for patient care and passing the NCLEX-PN® less stressful. It will protect your nursing license, too.

The focus of this chapter is to provide information about additional resources for information used in practical/vocational nursing. Because you are never done learning, suggestions are given to help you stay up-to-date in nursing for clinical, for the NCLEX-PN®, and as a graduate. Even if you have past experience in an educational program of study, you will find information in this chapter that will help you adjust to and succeed in the practical/vocational nursing program with less stress and frustration.

YOUR SCHOOL'S LEARNING RESOURCE CENTER

If you are a returning adult student, you know the learning resource center (LRC) as the library. Today, some students walk to the library to access what they need, and others just point their mouse and click. LRC reflects the increased scope of the library in the twenty-first century. The center consists of a lot more than books. How do you feel when you find out you must use the learning resource center? If you have some negative feelings, perhaps it is because you are unfamiliar with the sources of information contained in this resource and how to access and use them.

DIFFERENT STUDENT SKILL LEVELS AND DIFFERENT RESOURCES OF THE LEARNING RESOURCE CENTER

All LRCs have *similar* print and digital resources or access to these resources. However, not all LRCs are *equal* in technology. The LRC is a large item in any school budget. States face huge budget deficits. These deficits may affect which technology and resources your LRC contains. Some of you are skilled at using the LRC and its resources (Box 5-1). We recognize your ability. If you are skilled in this area, be aware that some of your peers may not be as skilled in using the LRC and its general resources and technology. They will find the hints in this chapter helpful. Because of the differences in your LRC, compared to the LRC of other programs and student differences in skill level, this chapter focuses on what tasks you need to be able to do as a

practical/vocational nursing (SPN/SVN) student in your LRC to obtain nursing information for class and clinical (Box 5-2).

- Box 5-1 includes a checklist of tasks you need to carry out to fully use the **general** print and digital resources and technology of your LRC for your student year and as a graduate.
- Box 5-2 includes a checklist of tasks you need to carry out to fully use the **nursing** resources and technology of your LRC for your student year and as a graduate.

 Box 5-1 | Checklist of Tasks Needed to Fully Use Learning Resource Center General Resources and Technology

Identify which of the following tasks you are able to carry out in your LRC by writing "Yes" next to them. Write "No" next to the tasks you are unable to carry out.

- Does the LRC staff provide tours and/or orientation to services in person or online?
- Are library staff available to provide support by phone, email, and/or real-time online?
- How does my LRC classify all of its print and digital holdings (books, videotapes, periodicals, CD-ROMs, DVDs, etc.)?
- How can I find the call number of a specific item?
- Once I have the call number, how can I locate a specific item?
- Where do I check out a specific item for home use?
- Can I access resources in my LRC from my home computer?
- How do I check out AV equipment for home use?
- How can I access needed resources that are not in my LRC?
- How can I access reference materials? (These would include an English dictionary, medical and nursing dictionaries, encyclopedias, almanacs, yearbooks, atlases, handbooks, and other similar categories of books.)
- Can I access learning resources in other schools' LRCs?
- Where is the circulation desk?
- Where are the copying machines?
- Are there computers for personal use? Do they have Internet access?
- Where can I study in the LRC?
- How can I reserve a room for group study?
- Where are pamphlets located?
- Is there a Wi-Fi hot spot for a personal laptop, smartphone, iPod Touch, or iPad (or other tablet)?

Box 5-2	Checklist of Tasks Needed to Fully Use LRC Nursing Resources and Technology

Identify which of the following tasks you are able to carry out in your LRC and write "Yes" next to them. Write "No" next to the tasks you are unable to carry out.

- How do I access print and digital nursing periodical listings?
- How do I access periodical indexes for nursing topics?
- How do I access current print and digital nursing journals and periodicals?
- How do I access back issues of print and digital nursing journals and periodicals?
- How can I obtain a copy of articles in back issues of nursing journals and periodicals?
- How can I obtain a print or digital copy of an article in a nursing journal or periodical if my LRC does not subscribe to the publication?
- Does my LRC have online databases for nursing and general information?
- Where are the nursing texts located in the stacks?
- What is the procedure for accessing nursing materials that have been put on reserve for nursing classes?
- Are mobile devices available for use in the clinical area? If so, what nursing information is available for use with these devices?
- Are handheld computers available for class/clinical use?
- Are earphones supplied?

Despite prior LRC experience, you need to identify and correct any deficiencies in regard to using nursing resources and technology in your school's LRC. Knowing how to carry through the tasks will save you energy, time, and frustration.

 Try This

Checklist—General and Nursing Resources and Technology

On index cards or notepads, list the general and nursing LRC tasks from Boxes 5-1 and 5-2 with which you are *not* familiar.

WHERE TO START

Investigate your learning resource center. You need to know the physical layout of the LRC and general hours of operation. Is a tour available in person or online? Touring the LRC can save you many wasted hours and much frustration later in the school year. Is an informational brochure available? You will find that your LRC contains a wealth of services that will help make your time in the practical/vocational nursing program easier and less stressful. Ask the librarian the best way for you to find the answers to items on your checklists with which you are unfamiliar. LRC staff are available to answer questions. Because the LRC is a learning area, you need to help to keep it a quiet environment. **A simple "please" and "thank you" for staff efforts will be appreciated.**

 Critical Thinking

Filling in the Gaps in My Learning Resource Center Knowledge

On the index cards or notepads you used for the previous learning exercise (Boxes 5-1 and 5-2), list the solutions to the tasks you could not carry out but found by investigating the LRC. To save time when using the LRC, refer to these notes as needed.

General Information About Resources of the Library

Librarian. This is perhaps the best resource in the whole school. The librarian is a college-educated specialist who knows what the library has to offer in the area of information and where that information can be found. Look at the librarian as a professional educator about information for learning and as a person who is always ready to assist you. Is the librarian available by email or real-time online to answer questions? When you ask for assistance in person, be sure to watch the process the librarian uses to obtain the information you need. The next time, you will be able to help yourself!

Circulation Desk. The circulation desk is the area where library materials that can be checked out are processed. If materials that can be checked out are reserved by your instructor, they will probably be found here. They can be checked out for short periods, along with audiovisual equipment to use with the material, if needed. Materials are returned to this desk.

Online Catalog. You can obtain a lot of information about your LRC by yourself once you understand the cataloging system. Most LRC's card catalogs are online (computerized) catalogs. All print and digital materials found in your LRC are indexed in this computerized system. In addition to books, cataloged materials also include audiovisual materials (audiorecordings, videos, CD-ROMs, DVDs, etc.). You can search for desired materials by subject, title, or author. The LRC may also have access to free or purchased access to digital databases. If the LRC does not have the material you are searching for, but another LRC on the online system does, this information might also be included.

In some systems students are able to access the online catalog and digital resources from home via computer, user name, and password. This system of cataloging saves students valuable time and energy.

LOCATING IN-HOUSE RESOURCES

Libraries may choose to use either of two systems to classify in-house materials so they are easy to locate: the Dewey Decimal system and the Library of Congress classification system. Regardless of the system your library uses, the call number shown on the author, title, or subject screens is the same number as that on the material itself. Copy, in order, all the letters and numbers in the call number.

The Stacks

Armed with the call number, you can proceed to the stacks—the place where the majority of materials that can be checked out are located. The books are placed in call number order according to academic disciplines. When you do find the material you are looking for, note that materials covering the same subject are shelved in the same area. You might find additional useful material on the same shelf.

Reference Materials

Reference materials include dictionaries and other similar categories of books, including medical and nursing dictionaries, almanacs, yearbooks, atlases, encyclopedias, and handbooks. Some of these resources can be found online. You will find up-to-date information on any subject in this area. Print reference books generally do not circulate. Information from print reference materials may be copied on a copy machine if the book cannot be checked out. Online information can be printed.

Interlibrary Loan Services

Interlibrary loan services allow your LRC to borrow materials you need that are not in your library's holdings. Print books and audiovisual materials are available through this service. A link for a digital full-text version of an article may be provided. If your LRC does not have the periodical in which an article you need is located or an electronic subscription to the source, a photocopy of the article or a link, free of charge, might be obtained from a library that does have some form of the periodical.

Vertical Files (Pamphlet Files)

Vertical files contain pamphlets of various subjects arranged in alphabetical order by topic.

Professional Journals

Practical/vocational nurses need to be aware of sources that will provide up-to-date, relevant, and accurate information on nursing topics. Professional journal articles give you the opportunity to stay on top of the latest research in nursing and its application. In addition to articles that are assigned reading, practical/vocational nurses need to be self-directed in finding and using articles that pertain to selected nursing topics and nursing problems occurring in the clinical area. Professional journals of interest to practical/vocational nurses include, but are not limited to, *The Journal of Practical Nursing*; *Nursing Made Incredibly Easy*; *Nursing2012* (*the year in the title changes as the year changes*); and *The American Journal of Nursing*.

Try This

Nursing Periodicals

Identify the location of the aforementioned nursing journals in your LRC. Determine which of them will help you keep up-to-date in nursing. Identify the location of other nursing periodicals.

Articles

All learners are looking for the perfect textbook, the one that is complete and self-contained. It does not exist! Specific journal articles may be assigned to give you up-to-date information to supplement the readings in your textbooks. Use the same hints for reading textbooks when reading these articles.

Copyright laws prohibit the instructor from copying an article for each of you. For this reason the required reading articles may be available on a reserve basis in the LRC by photocopy or digitally by a link within a Course Management System (CMS). Because copyright laws allow you to have one copy of an article, photocopy or print the reserve article for your own use. Underline, highlight, write in the margins, or type a note on your copy. Remember, the instructor knows you are busy. Articles are not busywork but a necessary part of any career education to keep current in your discipline.

Magazines and Newspapers

Include newspapers and popular magazines as sources of information on health-related topics. Magazine articles never replace professional journal reading, but they do provide information that your patients read. As one practical nursing student said, "I had better be up-to-date and understand what my patients are reading." Be aware of the author's expertise. This will help you evaluate the accuracy of the information on the topic and suitability for health care.

RESPONSIBLE USE OF LEARNING STRATEGIES

Face-to-Face Class

Lectures/minilectures. Some of your teachers may have been taught using the "bucket theory" of education. The bucket theory suggests that merely by lecturing, a teacher can transfer knowledge from the teacher's mind to the mind of the student. This teaching method evolved from Aristotle's day. The teacher was considered the source and the vehicle of transmission of information—similar to a sage on the stage. Of course, the printing press, computers, and the Internet had yet to be invented!

Research has shown that students learn best from methods other than traditional lecture. Although traditional lecturing is an outmoded form of instruction, *brief lectures* (minilectures) can be valuable as a means of enhancing your assigned readings and clarifying information. A minilecture situation is a brief episode, taking only a portion of class time. Minilectures are intended to enhance your reading assignment, not replace it. A minilecture reflects the fact that the teacher spent time searching, reading, selecting, and organizing information for your benefit. The instructor has done all the work and has become smarter in the process. However, minilectures are passive learning experiences that do not actively involve you in the learning process. During minilectures you have the responsibility to apply all of the active learning suggestions found in Chapter 4. You need to remain especially alert and actively involved. The instructor may introduce various techniques—for example, Clickers—to keep you actively involved during minilectures as well as class in general.

Lecture-discussion. In the lecture-discussion strategy, the instructor shares several ideas with the class and then stops to let the class discuss the ideas. Sometimes the instructor may say that the next class will be nothing but discussion of the assignment. The instructor then acts as a discussion leader. An example of a learning strategy to help keep the discussion focused on course objectives includes the following:

- Box 5-3: an example of a learning strategy used in minilectures called discussion buddy.
- Box 5-4: hints for participating in discussions and related activities.

Box 5-3   Learning Strategy: Discussion Buddy

1. You may be assigned to a discussion buddy before class.
2. The two of you will be given a discussion task.
3. Focus carefully on the minilecture so you will be able to formulate an answer to the discussion task.
4. After the minilecture, discussion buddies share their answers with one another. A new answer is formulated from both your responses.
5. The instructor will choose students at random to share their newly composed answers with the class.

Box 5-4   Hints for a Discussion Class

- Be prepared to participate in the discussion by completing your assignment before class. This will allow you to be an active participant.
- Be sure you have made a list of questions about the assignment. Discussions are the perfect time to clear up questions.
- While other learners are speaking, listen to what they have to say. Some learners make the mistake of using other learners' speaking time to formulate their own comments.
- You may disagree with others during a discussion. Do so assertively and firmly. Avoid yelling matches. It enriches your world to listen to another's point of view before responding.

Cooperative Learning. Cooperative learning is a technique that emphasizes individual accountability for learning a specific academic task while working in small groups. Cooperative learning encourages you to:

- be actively involved in your learning.
- develop critical-thinking skills.
- develop positive relationships with your peers.
- develop the ability to work in a team situation—a skill an employer is looking for in an employee.
- use the suggestions listed under the previous lecture-discussion section to help you get full mileage out of this strategy.

What goes on in the classroom is just as important as what goes on in a reading assignment. There is, however, one great difference between the two: *You can repeat a reading assignment, but you can never repeat a missed face-to-face class.* Here are some hints to help you learn from any face-to-face class situation:

- Before taping a class activity, clarify if taping is allowed.
- Never skip a face-to-face class unless an emergency arises. Some students skip class to get another hour's sleep, use the time to prepare for another class or an examination, or get in their legal number of cuts (if legal cuts are in your school's policies). When an emergency does make it necessary for you to miss class, photocopying notes is not the answer to catch up on what you missed. Ask a peer to go over his or her notes and tell you about the class. Recall what you learned in Chapter 3 about personal learning styles.
- Come to class prepared. By having the assignment completed before class, key terms and concepts will be familiar to you. You will be ready to participate in learning activities. You will save yourself embarrassment by avoiding questions that are answered easily by the readings. Unless your learning style requires it, heading for the last row is heading for distractions and lower grades.
- Listen for verbal cues that will inform you of key points during minilectures (see Box 5-5). Keep vigilant for nonverbal cues given by the instructor that will also inform you of key ideas. Examples are raising the hands; a long, dramatic pause; raising or lowering the voice; and leaning toward the class. Be sure to copy everything that is written on the whiteboard/smartboard.

Box 5-5   Verbal Cues for Key Ideas in Minilectures, Discussions, and Online Activities

"The most important difference is . . ."
"The major principle in this situation is . . ."
"To sum up . . ."
"The main point is . . ."
"Finally, . . ."
"In conclusion, . . ."
"Moreover, . . ."
"To repeat . . ."

- The instructor speaks at a much slower rate than you are capable of thinking. The fact that you can think faster than the instructor can speak allows you to relate this new information to information you have learned in the past and to formulate questions that need clarification or for content you do not understand. Ask these questions in class, or seek out the instructor after class. It is *your* responsibility to question what you do not understand.
- Look over your notes as soon after class as possible. Use the hints given in Chapter 4. Follow these techniques to comprehend the information you learned in class and place it into your long-term memory.
- Be present while in class. Avoid using class time to work on other projects. Be an active listener.

Distance Learning. Some of the courses in your practical/vocational nursing program or parts of courses may be available through distance learning. In this learning strategy, the student and teacher are separated by physical distance. The course could take part in "real time," in which all of the students in the course and the instructor participate simultaneously by means of interactive TV. A blended course (hybrid course) combines face-to-face instruction with online learning. A popular alternative is instruction in which students can choose when and where they will attend class. Online resources carry out this type of distance learning.

- Have the equipment needed, *or access to* equipment needed, to complete course assignments. Depending on the distance learning course, the equipment list *could* include any of the following:
  - Computer with adequate hard disk space or a device that uses the cloud via Wi-Fi (wireless connection to the Internet)
  - Word processor
  - Modem
  - Fax machine
  - Internet service provider—broadband, if available
  - Cable TV connection
  - CD/DVD player if this is not available with your computer
- You are in charge of your schedule. As with any class, self-discipline and motivation are important tools for success. The time management information in Chapter 2 will help you establish a weekly class and study schedule. The nature of the course requires you to have access to email, Facebook, and/or Twitter. Check these sites daily for messages from instructors and fellow students. You also may be required to post items and/or participate in chat rooms as class assignments.
- Study skills are a must. Chapter 4 emphasizes the need for the proper study skills, including a study environment required by your learning style. Distance learning courses require much reading. The ability

| Box 5-6 | Technology Courtesy for Learning Activities |

- Check school policy for the use of cell phones, smartphones, iPod Touch, iPad, laptops, and so on.
- If cell phones are allowed, turn off the ringer and put it on vibrate.
- If it is necessary to return a call, leave the immediate area, quietly make your call, and quickly complete it.
- Avoid emailing, texting, tweeting, instant messaging, and playing games during class activities.
- Avoid surfing the Internet during class activities.
- Avoid listening to music on your iPod during class activities.

to understand information by means of the written word is important. Chapter 3 helped you determine your personal learning style and can help you decide if distance learning is right for you.

- Because distance learning requires you to communicate by methods such as posting, email, and/or fax, Chapter 13 will help you organize your thoughts so that you can present them in a concise manner and communicate your intended message. These hints will be especially useful if you are taking an Internet course sponsored by a school that participates in real-time discussion and/or postings by students and teachers on electronic bulletin boards and in chat rooms.

Distance learning has proved to be at least as effective as traditional methods of instruction. Positive features include the fact that students become more active in personal learning and have more involvement in and control over the learning process.

TECHNOLOGY USE DURING LEARNING ACTIVITIES

Class time requires active listening and participation in learning activities. Avoid using class time for snoozing, talking to friends, or any of the activities listed in Box 5-6. Your time in the practical/vocational nursing program gives you the opportunity to sharpen (bring to an excellent level) professional behavior that is appropriate for your job as a practical/vocational nurse.

OTHER LEARNING RESOURCES

SYLLABUS AND COURSE OUTLINES

A syllabus is an up-to-date course document available by handout or online as part of a Content Management System (CMS) at the beginning of a course. At a minimum, the syllabus includes a course description, course objectives, course requirements for a passing grade, required textbooks, grading scale, instructor information (office location, how to contact the instructor, office hours, response times for emails, etc.), course policies, and testing policies.

Your school may have course outlines for each course. These outlines are a great help to an adult learner. They contain unit-by-unit course objectives and content areas, which indicate what the learner must know to pass the course. Each objective begins with a verb. Watch the verb carefully because it tells you the level of understanding you must achieve to meet the objective. If an objective states you must *list* something, that task is quite different from having to *compare* and *contrast* the same information. Instructors develop their test questions from the course objectives and course content. The course outline will include a list of resources indicating where the information to answer the objectives is found. Supplementary material in the form of worksheets, charts, activities, and additional reading may be included to round out your learning. A CMS contains complete online course content and includes, for example, a syllabus, library links, learning modules, a calendar for quizzes, tests, and assignments, chat rooms, and other features.

STUDY GROUPS

Do you have a desire to achieve better grades? Do you need to study more effectively? Do you need a little support? Joining a study group could be the strategy for you. Students usually form their own study groups out of need. Studies have shown that despite each person's preferred learning style, *actively* participating in a study group can improve academic performance. Notice we said *actively* participating. Sometimes students join a study group thinking that the group will help them pass, and they avoid active participation; these students are similar to freeloaders. Study groups work when students use them to become actively involved in their own learning. The group provides an outlet for oral rehearsal of material, which promotes retention. Active study group members usually develop questioning and reasoning skills on a higher level.

TUTORING

Tutoring is a very select study group. For best results, the student arranges tutoring through a special department by means of instructor referral or self-referral. The purpose of tutoring is to help a student understand the material better and pass the course. We guarantee one thing in tutoring: The tutor will probably get an A. Students who need tutoring *sometimes* have learning disabilities. In these situations, because of an excellent attitude on the part of these students and their active participation in the tutoring process, tutoring can be beneficial. Students without learning disabilities who actively participate in the tutoring process also are successful in passing courses.

We are concerned about students at risk for failure who expect the tutor to "learn for them." These students do not actively participate in the tutoring process. We have also seen some privately arranged tutoring situations fail because the tutor felt that the student at risk needed to be "saved." Please note: Students cannot be saved. Nothing can replace active participation on the part of the learner. If you want to pass a course, you must become actively involved in your own learning.

NURSING SKILLS LAB

The nursing skills lab is a resource that will allow you to practice and develop your physical nursing skills. It is to be used throughout your nursing program. This lab contains the physical items needed to make the practice area as similar to the workplace as possible. *Skills must be practiced.* Reading about skills, watching a film, and watching other students practice are only the first steps in developing a physical skill. **Practice until you are proficient in each skill so you will feel comfortable performing these tasks in the clinical area or with simulation.** Remember that you recall 10% of what you hear, 20% of what you see, 50% of what you read, and 90% of what you do, so do all that you can. The Teton Lakota Indians have a proverb that summarizes how practical/vocational student nurses need to approach the skills component of their nursing program: "Tell me and I'll listen. Show me and I'll understand. Involve me and I'll learn."

You will be required to make appointments to give a return demonstration of skills. This routine will give you an opportunity to organize your time. This is what is expected of the practical/vocational nurse as part of patient care. When you make an appointment with the skills lab, you are entering into an agreement with the lab personnel. Your responsibility is to practice the skill until you can perform it in the time frame of your appointment. If you are unable to keep your appointment, inform the lab personnel. This will allow them to schedule other students into lab time for skills testing.

STUDY SKILLS LAB

If your school has a study skills lab, it is available to help you with academic problem areas. Examples of areas in which help is available are study skills, time management, reading (including vocabulary and comprehension), listening skills, math skills, test-taking skills (especially situation tests), note making, writing, and any other academic problem you may have. You can go to the skills lab on your own or by referral from your instructor or counselor.

 Critical Thinking

No Time for Tutoring or the Skills Center

Some students who need tutoring or the study skills center state they do not have time to go for help. Comment about this response.

AUDIOVISUAL MATERIALS

In addition to minilectures, discussions/activities, textbooks, and articles, the instructor may have included videos, CDs, DVDs, PowerPoint presentations, and podcasts as part of your assignment. Audiovisual (AV) materials are not considered extra or additional assignments. They are a significant part of all areas of learning. These learning resources give faith to the saying "A picture is worth a thousand words." AV materials provide an additional sensory channel for learning, compared with reading. In some nursing courses, especially autotutorial skills courses, the AV medium is the course. The student progresses independently, attending periodic lecture-discussion classes and seeking out the instructor when questions arise. Approach the AV material as you do a class. Realize that you have the option of repeating all or part of the material when you do not understand it.

INTERNET

The Internet offers unlimited resources on many subjects. The Internet is the physical infrastructure that allows the electronic circulation of billions of sites of information to Internet-ready computer users. An Internet provider charges a monthly fee and is a computer user's link to the Internet. Provider services can be dial-up modems, dedicated service lines (DSL), or broadband (high-speed Internet), meaning that you have instant access when your computer is turned on. An example of a broadband provider service is instant access RoadRunner. The iPad is a tablet that is available in two models with Wi-Fi only or Wi-Fi and choice of two phone companies that offer data plan subscriptions that provide connection to the Internet. When people are linked to the Internet, they are said to be "online."

The World Wide Web (www) is the most effective means of providing access to the vast amount of information available on the Internet. Everything on the Internet has an address (called a URL) that helps in locating a specific site. Most addresses begin with http://www, followed by a dot. The next letters in the address are specific to the site you wish to access; for example, www.nclex indicates the site that provides information about the LPN/LVN licensing exam. This is followed by three letters, called a domain name, which denote the site's source. For example, the complete address for the site for information about your licensing exam is www.nclex.org. The following are common domain names and their meanings:

- com: for-profit sites
- gov: the U.S. federal government
- edu: colleges and universities that grant 4-year degrees
- org: usually reserved for nonprofit organizations
- net: network organizations
- mil: military

Search engines are programs that can help students zero in on the exact information for which they are searching. Search engines periodically scan the web and index it. Therefore, search engines are like the telephone book. A popular search engine is Google.com. On Evolve are suggestions of Internet sites that can be used by practical/vocational nursing students as learning resources and for patient teaching resources.

It is necessary for the practical/vocational nurse to develop information literacy in finding health information for your patients and yourself. Although the Internet provides the means of obtaining that information, it is up to you to evaluate if that information is recent, accurate, and relevant. Wikipedia, known as a free online encyclopedia, is an example of a source that nursing students should *not* use to obtain information for class or clinical. Wikipedia is written by volunteers, and the articles can be edited by anyone with site access. The quality, accuracy, and appropriateness of Wikipedia articles are not checked by scholars in the articles field (peer-reviewed).

Box 5-7 contains guidelines for gathering Internet information for your use or to share with patients. Let the user beware: Students can spend a lot of time on the Internet. To save time, take a few minutes to read the section that gives hints for using a specific site. Stay focused on your purpose. Avoid getting sidetracked.

 Try This

Peer Assistance with Computer/Internet

If you do not have computer/Internet experience, ask students in your class who are familiar with using computers for hints on using this technology and information resource.

MOBILE DEVICES

Because of Wi-Fi, your educational institution and/or clinical site may provide wireless access to the Internet. Mobile devices with Internet capabilities are useful for obtaining information for class and the clinical area. Before utilizing the following information, clarify the policy of your school and clinical area for using computers and mobile devices while on the clinical area.

- **You must separate your private and professional uses of mobile devices.** If your device is capable of taking photos or videos, do not use these functions with patients. HIPAA requirements (see Chapter 12) prohibit the use of electronic devices for these purposes. If you are a student, you could be dropped from the program. If you are licensed, you could receive a sanction regarding your license if you take photos or videos of patients on the clinical area.

Box 5-7 **Guidelines for Gathering Internet Information**

- The Internet is not regulated in any way. Anyone can publish anything they want on the Internet. When searching the Internet, you can find the most recent and accurate information, as well as the most inaccurate and out-of-date information.
- Let the user beware: People can spend a lot of time on the Internet. To save time, take a few minutes to read the section that gives hints for using a specific site. Stay focused on your purpose. Avoid getting sidetracked.
- Check the professional credentials and qualifications of the author of the information.
- Determine the organization, group, agency, company, and so on that created the site. This will help you evaluate the credibility of the information. The domain name is helpful in evaluating credibility. For example, a site that has a ".gov" domain name may be more credible than a ".com" site that may be promoting a product.
- Check the date the information was created and last modified. This will ensure up-to-date material.
- What are the objectives of the author of the material? Does the author express opinions? Does the author have a personal bias?
- When conducting searches, supply key words to help the search tool narrow the document results to just the ones you want to see.
- When using key words for a search engine, use phrases or single words that are pertinent to your topic and describe it objectively.
- Use nouns only, and put the most important words that describe your topic first.
- When searching with a phrase (e.g., "study skills"), surround the phrase with quotation marks. This forces the database to search for words that are next to each other.
- Plus signs (+) or the word "AND" identify words that must appear in the search (e.g., nursing+practical).
- Minus signs (–) or the word "NOT" exclude words from the search (e.g., NCLEX-PN®, NOT NCLEX®-RN).

- Nursing-based software that contains drug information, laboratory values, disease processes, and a medical dictionary is available as a subscription to be downloaded on your mobile device.
- Reference e-books for downloading on your mobile device can be purchased.
- Apps can provide instant clinical reference materials at the point of care for drugs, lab studies, and medical/surgical conditions. Some apps are free, but others charge a fee. Check the app store of your device.
- Check the appropriateness of selected software/apps with your instructor.
- Sites that provide information for mobile devices can be found on Evolve.

COMPUTER-AIDED INSTRUCTION

Computer-aided instruction (CAI) has the following benefits:

- Allows learners to be actively involved in their learning.
- Encourages problem solving, a skill that employers expect of practical/vocational nurses.
- Provides immediate feedback by quickly evaluating answers and decision-making strategies.
- Provides an opportunity to develop the ability to follow directions.

Learning by CAI is enhanced for students with right-brain dominance. CAI can also be used effectively by any student to master new material. It simplifies concepts and reinforces skills that have been presented previously. If you do not have computer skills and CAI is used in your practical/vocational nursing program, you will be taught the skills necessary to use this type of teaching strategy. The process is simple even if you do not have any computer experience. Many of you will use the computer in the clinical area to store and retrieve patient information. And in less than 1 year, all of you will be taking the NCLEX-PN® examination by computer.

SIMULATION

Simulation is a learning activity that uses imaginary patient situations that mimic the reality of the clinical environment. The learner has the opportunity to think like a nurse and gather data, set priorities, plan, implement, and evaluate care in a virtual (reproduced/replicated by a computer) patient situation without risk to the patient. Simulation encourages decision making and critical thinking.

Simulation can take many forms:

- Case scenarios can be delivered in a printed format or by computer. In each type, an imaginary patient story will bring reality to theory in the form of a clinical situation. Both forms may be used when the patient census is inadequate for patient assignments, when a desired patient situation is unavailable, or when enhanced learning of specific concepts is desirable.
- Computer simulation can be a learning situation on CD inserted into a computer. The computer-patient simulation changes, as it would in the clinical area. This requires the student to evaluate the situation and plan new assessments (data collection) and interventions.
- Static simulation uses mannequins that are full-size body models or models of specific parts of the body made to be realistic. These mannequins are used for practicing skills before reaching the clinical area and returning demonstrations of procedures—for example, urinary catheterization, insertion of intravenous lines, and application of colostomy bags.
- Electronic simulation uses mannequins that are high-tech, more costly simulation models that can be programmed to set up different patient situations and allow practice of nursing procedures and data collection (assessment).

- **Virtual clinical excursions** are computer programs that electronically (controlled by a computer) provide a virtual hospital floor and patients. This experience provides a patient record, Kardex, medication administration record, drug guide, medical dictionary, and textbooks learners can access to collect data, set priorities for care, administer medications, manage patient care problems, and document care. These excursions encourage students to critically think and problem solve in a safe and secure environment (deWit, 2009).

STAYING CURRENT IN PRACTICAL/VOCATIONAL NURSING

PERIODICALS

Because nursing magazines are published weekly, monthly, and quarterly (i.e., periodically), they are called periodicals. They are also referred to as journals—publications that contain news or material of current interest to a particular discipline. Professional journals contain articles that include the most recent information available for a specific subject and subjects that are too new to be included in texts. This is the reason periodicals are important resources for a learner in a field that is changing as quickly as nursing and health care. The titles and authors of various articles cannot possibly be included in the online catalog of the LRC. These can be found instead in two forms: bound books called print periodical indexes and digital databases.

Print Periodical Indexes

Entries in periodical indexes are listed by author, title, and subject. Read/view the help sections to ease your use of these resources. The following are two periodical indexes/databases that are of special value to practical/vocational nursing students:

1. *Readers' Guide to Periodical Literature*. This comprehensive index includes over 200 popular American nontechnical magazines. This guide is useful for recreational reading of specific topics, such as setting up a workshop, growing herbs, and learning about the Internet. The *Readers' Guide* is useful for practical/vocational nursing students because technical data on health topics are presented in understandable language for the general public.

2. *Cumulative Index to Nursing and Allied Health Literature* (CINAHL®—the red book). This comprehensive and authoritative periodical index contains current listings for nursing and allied health fields and for others interested in health care issues, including biomedicine, consumer health, and alternative medicine. Nursing, allied health, and related journals are reviewed and indexed for over 11,000 topics. A videotape and CD-ROM are available to provide instruction on how to use the print index.

Figure 5-1 illustrates the information found in a typical entry in the CINAHL® print edition. Some schools have purchased access to online CINAHL® databases. CINAHL® will be your primary source for current, accurate, and relevant articles used for patient care.

Your LRC will have a periodical listing that includes the professional journals and magazines and the dates of the issues that are found in your library. If the article you need is in a journal or magazine that is not held in your library in some form, see the librarian. The librarian can locate the article online in another library and arrange for you to receive a link or photocopy by interlibrary loan. If your library has the date and issue you need, go to the section of the library that contains the periodicals. If the issue you need is not there, refer to the LRC notes that you completed at the beginning of this chapter to find out how to access the issue.

Understanding how to use a periodical index is a necessary skill. How well do you understand the information found in a print periodical index entry? Each CINAHL® book/database contains directions for using the source. Use the following CINAHL® print entry to test your understanding of CINAHL® citing. Answer the questions found underneath the entry. Refer to Figure 5-1 if you need help in reading the CINAHL® citation.

 Try This

Using the CINAHL® Print Edition

Using the following citation, supply the information requested.

Put a Cap on Community-Acquired Pneumonia (Kent, V.) (ceu exam questions) Nursing Made Incredibly Easy 2011 March/April 9:2 34-45 (13 ref.).

Author:
Title of article:
Volume and number of periodical:
Name of periodical:
Date of article:
Pages:
Additional information found in article:
Are there references in the article? If so, how many?

1– Patient Safety 2– What Frontline Nurses Need to Know
3– McKeon, L. and Cardell, B. 4– (tables/charts)
5– Nursing Made Incredibly Easy 6– Jan./ Feb. 2011
7– 9(1) 8– 44-53 9– (11 ref)

Key: 1. Subject. 2. Title of the article. 3. Authors of the article. 4. Additional information found in article. 5. Periodical in which the article appears. If the periodical is abbreviated, the periodical index in the front of the book will have a list of periodical abbreviations and the full name of the journal for which those abbreviations stand. 6. Date of publication. 7. Volume and number of periodical. 8. Page numbers of article. 9. Number of references used.

FIGURE 5-1 Explanation of an entry from the printed *Cumulative Index to Nursing and Allied Health Literature.*

Digital Periodical Databases. The process of keeping "up-to-date" has been simplified as far as finding information is concerned. Digital databases are expensive sources of information. If your LRC has this technology available for student use, be sure to use it. The systems are user friendly. Combined with a helpful LRC staff, you cannot lose! Because *digital* databases are costly, some schools of practical/vocational nursing may share a computer system with a health care institution. Inquire if student access is available.

NURSING ORGANIZATIONS

Nursing organizations organize speakers, seminars, and workshops on up-to-the-minute nursing topics and related health care topics. These programs are frequently made available to students. Specific practical/vocational nursing organizations are discussed in Chapter 24.

COMMUNITY RESOURCES

The city library and museums sometimes sponsor programs and exhibits on topics of interest and of use to practical/vocational nursing students. Additional community resources are health care facilities, such as hospitals and clinics, that offer lecture series.

GUEST SPEAKERS

Nurses and other health professionals are sometimes invited to visit nursing classes as guest speakers or to make presentations via video. These speakers donate their time to present current information on their areas of expertise and updates on specific nursing topics. Often their employers have released them to visit nursing classes. Regardless of the method of presentation, students need to treat these speakers with attention and respect.

SOCIAL MEDIA (ELECTRONIC MEDIA) AND SOCIAL NETWORKING

Nurses are now using Facebook and Twitter, the most commonly used social media networks for communicating with family and friends, to communicate and collaborate with nursing organizations and keep up-to-date with colleagues. Professional organizations also use these networks to allow nonattendees to follow conventions, seminars, and so on. The interactivity of these sites allows one to consume as well as contribute information. However, a practical/vocational nurse needs to develop awareness of the professional versus personal use of these sites. The 2011 National Council of State Board Examiners (NCSBN) white paper "A Nurse's Guide to the Use

of Social Media" states that 46 Boards of Nursing (BON) were surveyed by the National Council, and 33 boards reported receiving complaints about nurses who violated patient confidentiality/privacy by posting patient information on social networking sites. Sanctions ranged from a letter of concern, mandatory continuing education, to suspension of license.

- Violation of patient privacy is a violation of HIPAA and can result in a fine for your employer and sanctions for you from your State Board of Nursing.
- Violation of patient confidentiality is also a violation of your professional code of ethics. (See Chapter 11.)
- Whether or not you engage in social media is a personal choice. If you choose to participate, carefully check the privacy policy of the site. Thoughtfully develop a profile and carefully set your privacy settings.
- Avoid putting on the Internet *anything* you would not put on television or the front page of a newspaper. Prospective employers may Google you.
- LinkedIn is the biggest professional site, and interactions are more formal. This is a site for posting resumes, education, work history, accomplishments, and professional memberships. The goal is to connect with or remain connected with colleagues (Duffy, 2011). **If you list your employer, remember that you are then a representative of that agency.**
- The NCSBN (2011) White Paper: A Nurse's Guide to the Use of Social Media and video are references to guide you. It is available at NCSBN.org.
- The Nurse's Social Media Advantage (Fraser, 2011) provides information about professional use of social media for novices as well as those who are social media savvy.
- The American Nurses Association (ANA) has compiled a resource guide that nursing students can use to learn about professional use of social networking. See Social Networking Principles Toolkit for tips and a fact sheet @ana.org.

 Professional Pointer

Presentation of self on social media requires professional behavior.

 Try This

Social Media Policies

Investigate social media policies developed by your school, clinical areas, State Board of Nursing, and the National Council of State Boards of Nursing.

Get Ready for the NCLEX-PN® Examination

Key Points

- The hints for using learning strategies and resources found in this chapter will help you obtain the information you need to get better grades on tests and achieve your goal of becoming a practical/vocational nurse.
- The LRC is your most valuable resource for learning as a student and for keeping up-to-date as a graduate.
- In addition to textbooks, minilectures, lecture-discussions, and cooperative learning are specific course learning strategies that are used by the practical/vocational nursing student.
- Methods of delivering instruction, such as distance learning, make learning more student-oriented.
- Additional learning resources include articles from periodicals, the syllabus, course outlines, Content Management Systems (CMS), study groups, tutoring, audiovisual materials, the Internet, computer-aided instruction, web-based classes, and simulation.
- Staying current in practical/vocational nursing is made possible by using print or digital periodical indexes, CD-ROM databases, the Internet, skills labs, nursing organizations, community resources, and guest speakers.
- It is necessary for practical/vocational nurses to distinguish between personal and professional use of social media.
- After learning the information you need to be a practical/vocational nurse, you must demonstrate that learning has taken place by your performance in the clinical area and on tests.

Additional Learning Resources

evolve   Go to your Evolve website (http://evolve.elsevier.com/Hill/Success) for the following FREE learning resources:
- Answers to Critical Thinking Scenarios
- Additional learning activities
- Additional Review Questions for the NCLEX-PN® exam
- Helpful phrases for communicating in Spanish and more!

Review Questions for the NCLEX-PN® Examination

1. Select the activity that is the *least* suggested learning strategy in an SPN/SVN program.
   1. Distance learning
   2. Lecture-discussion
   3. Instant messaging
   4. Nursing skills lab

2. A nursing instructor suggests that a practical/vocational nursing student receive help with study skills at the school's Skills Center. Which student response most accurately indicates that the student understands the purpose of the Skills Center?
   1. "I cannot afford the fee to attend study programs in the Skills Center at my school."
   2. "In high school, only students with learning disabilities attended the Skills Center."
   3. "It will take too much time out of my limited study time to go for help with studying."
   4. "Even a few visits to the Skills Center can help me get more out of my study sessions."

3. Classes in a practical/vocational nursing program may be conducted in a lecture-discussion format. Select the student behavior that is *least* effective for this learning strategy.
   1. When time is needed to study for a test in a different class, arrange for a peer to take notes for you in your absence.
   2. Complete all assignments before going to class and prepare questions you have about parts of readings that are unclear.
   3. If you disagree with a student during a discussion, assertively present your point of view after the student finishes speaking.
   4. Listen while instructors and students are speaking; avoid using this time to prepare your comments to add to the discussion.

4. Four practical/vocational nursing students are commenting at break time about the personal/vocational assignment to arrange a tour of the LRC. Select the statement that indicates understanding of the purpose for this assignment.
   1. "Knowing the location of nursing journals in the LRC will save me time and frustration when they are assigned."
   2. "I know a library's resources and how they are organized because I took business courses in college last year."
   3. "Because taxpayer money funds the learning resource center and its holdings, nursing faculty need to encourage its use."
   4. "I have a part-time job and a family, and I do not have time in my schedule to tour the learning resource center."

Alternate Format Item

1. A variety of learning resources and strategies are used in a practical/vocational nursing program. Which of the following students are using these resources and strategies to their advantage? *(Select all that apply.)*
   1. Alberto joined a study group that meets every day after school to review and discuss class notes.
   2. Marta frequently skips lectures to study for a test in another class and to play video games for relaxation.
   3. Instead of watching assigned AV materials, Julia borrows notes of the materials from friends who viewed them.
   4. Because of a long commute, Thai signed up for a distance learning class to save more study time.

2. Choose which of the following practical/vocational nursing students is using their electronic devices appropriately during class. *(Select all that apply.)*

   1. Cora follows school policy for using her BlackBerry in class.
   2. Chett catches up with his emails and tweets during class discussion.
   3. Allie listens to music on her iPod during PowerPoint lectures.
   4. Jarian turns off his Android and puts it on vibrate during class.
   5. Heather quickly takes a call from her son's day care center.

Critical Thinking Scenario

Amy is present daily for class. Her grades have shown a steady improvement. While changing classes, Amy tells you she doesn't go to the LRC because she can't find anything she is looking for. Give Amy some suggestions for using the LRC.

Personal Health Promotion: A Role Model for Patients

Objectives

On completing this chapter, you will be able to do the following:

1. Develop a reasonable healthy eating and physical activity plan for yourself using the Dietary Guidelines for Americans 2010 (http://www.health.gov/dietaryguidelines/dga2010DietaryGuidelines2010.pdf).
2. Explain why the June 2011 MyPlate.gov (http://www.choosemyplate.gov/) is easier to comprehend and use as a mealtime food guide than MyPyramid.
3. List six how-to messages to guide healthy eating as a part of healthy food guidelines.
4. Explain why proper body mechanics help but do not prevent all back, shoulder, and other injuries nurses may develop.
5. Locate items on the clinical unit available to assist you with moving and lifting patients.
6. Differentiate between stress and burnout.

7. Develop a realistic plan to assist you in dealing with overwhelming stress or feelings of hopelessness during the school year.
8. Identify possible clues that may indicate a nurse is chemically impaired by alcohol and/or other drugs while on duty.
9. Explain the difference between codependency and conscientious nursing.
10. Discuss the difference between recreation and relaxation.
11. Describe which source of relaxation is most effective for you to use during class or on clinical.
12. Explain methods you will use to prevent the spread of infection among patients and from the clinical setting to your home and into the community.

Key Terms

burnout (p. 62)
chemical dependency (dĭ-PĒN-dĕn-sē, p. 65)
codependency (KŌ-ddĭ-PĒN-dĕn-sē, p. 65)
CRKP (p. 62)
C. difficile (p. 61)
Dietary Guidelines for Americans 2010 (p. 58)
empathy (ĔM-pă-thē, p. 63)

health care–associated infections (HAIs) (p. 61)
MRSA (p. 62)
MyPlate icon (p. 58)
nutrient-dense foods (p. 58)
subungual zone (sūb-ŪNG-gwăl, p. 62)
sympathy (SĬM-pă-thē, p. 63)

 Keep in Mind

Make time for yourself. Build some pleasure into every day.

NEW LOOK AT NUTRITION AND HEALTH

As food, shelter, clothing, and their availability have improved, longevity has increased for past generations. Predictions are that longevity will not increase for the children of the current generation. The reasons given relate to lack of exercise and poor eating habits. Obesity and related health issues have become a serious issue not just for adults but for children as well.

The U.S. Department of Health and Human Services (HHS) has expressed concern about the high rate of obesity in all age groups. The U.S. Centers for Disease Control and Prevention (CDC) underwrote an analysis that showed obesity to be a major factor in America's rising health care costs. The CDC recommended that obesity be targeted as aggressively as smoking. Because government and ultimately the taxpayer are financing half the economic burden of obesity, it is no longer seen as just a personal or societal issue.

Low-fat snacks got the public's attention after the release of the 1992 USDA Food Guide Pyramid. The assumption was that if the label says "low-fat," it is healthy to eat the snack without further investigation. Although many people want to be healthy, the influx of contradictory information, powerful advertising, and availability of tempting low-fat, high–refined carbohydrate foods has made choices confusing and overwhelming. Some people hook onto the low-fat label and often do not feel satisfied after they eat. They compensate by eating larger quantities. Restaurants and fast-food establishments have increased serving sizes. Studies show that the more food there is on our plate or on the table, the more we eat at the time.

2010 DIETARY GUIDELINES FOR AMERICANS

The 2010 Dietary Guidelines for Americans are based on the most recent scientific evidence review. The guidelines provide "information and advice for choosing a healthy eating pattern—namely, one that focuses on nutrient-dense foods and beverages and that contributes to achieving and maintaining a healthy weight." The guidelines link poor nutrition and lack of physical activity to major causes of illness and death. Also included is information on food safety principles. The guidelines are reviewed by the Department of Agriculture (USDA) and the U.S. Department of Health and Human Services (HHS) every five years and updated as new scientific information emerges. As the epidemic of obesity and related illnesses continues, it is important that Americans have information to make better choices in their eating habits and lifestyles.

INTRODUCTION TO THE MYPLATE ICON

Because of the rise in childhood obesity and related illnesses, the 2010 White House Child Obesity Task Force requested that reasonable advice be developed to help facilitate easier healthy food choices. The 2010 guidelines are helpful, but both adults and children have had difficulty understanding and using the MyPyramid icon. As a result, the MyPlate icon was designed to replace MyPyramid (Figure 6-1). In June 2011, First Lady Michelle Obama and Secretary of Agriculture Tom Vilsack introduced the new icon. The White House is playing a leading role by coordinating the USDA guidelines with Michelle Obama's "Let's Move" initiative.

FIGURE 6-1 MyPlate. The 2010 MyPlate recommends the following: Avoid oversize portions; make half your plate vegetables and fruits; make at least half your grains whole grain; protein is the smallest part of the plate; switch to fat-free or low-fat (1%) milk; look for lower-sodium soup, bread, and frozen meals; and drink water instead of sugary drinks.

How-To Messages to Guide Healthy Eating
- Enjoy your food, but eat less.
- Avoid oversize portions.
- Make half of your plate fruits and vegetables.
- Make half of your plate grains and proteins.
- Make at least half of your grains whole grain.
- Protein is the smallest part of the plate.
- Switch to fat-free or low-fat (1%) milk.
- Look for lower-sodium soup, bread, and frozen meals; choose foods with lower numbers.
- Drink water instead of sugary drinks (http://www.chosemyplate.gov).

Expect to see the new icon in many places: supermarkets, restaurants, schools, television, businesses, and so on. A broad-based partnership is involved in reducing childhood and adult obesity and related illness.

 Try This

Making Good Food Choices

Make a list of favorite foods (and portions) that you are currently eating. Modify your current eating pattern based on the MyPlate icon.

 Professional Pointer

Patients form an opinion of your competency as a nurse based on your *physical appearance* the first time they see you. You never get a second chance to make a good first impression.

MAKING TIME FOR PHYSICAL ACTIVITY

It takes more than information on the importance of a healthy diet and daily exercise, and the increase in chronic disease and death, to improve health. We know from studies what works, but what will provide the personal motivation to make it happen in your life as a lifelong activity? The motivating factor for individuals is something personal: "What is in it for me?"

 Try This

Making Room for Exercise

Make a list of the activities that you are involved with that count as exercise. Rate the activities on a scale of 1 to 5 as light, moderate, or heavy, with 1 being the lightest and 5 being the heaviest.
1. How often do you do each activity?
2. Does the activity increase flexibility?
3. Does the activity increase muscle strength?
4. Does the activity reduce stress?
5. Does the activity make you feel better about yourself?

MODERATE PHYSICAL ACTIVITY

A pleasant surprise is that any amount of exercise is helpful. As little as 30 minutes a day of moderate activity on most or all days of the week will make a noticeable difference in your health.

- The 30 minutes of activity can even be divided into 10-minute increments. Ten-minute bursts of activity have been shown to be as effective as continuous exercise. The important thing is to choose an activity that you like and that fits in with your busy lifestyle.
- Brisk walking (meaning 3.5 miles per hour) is probably the easiest for most people to incorporate into a busy day. If possible, walk to work, or park your car farther away from your destination.
- Use stairs rather than the elevator.
- Walk with a coworker during your lunchtime, or volunteer to be the one to go to another part of the building to pick up something.
- If you are fitting in a walk with a friend at lunchtime, a few minutes of slower walking at the beginning can be a useful preparation for more brisk walking. Slow your pace for a cool-down toward the end of the walk (Table 6-1).

START THE DAY WITH A STRETCH AND FLEX

Stretching and flexing cannot be overemphasized for the nurse.

- Before getting out of bed, start your day with *stretching*. Think of how a cat or dog stretches before they get busy with their activities. Follow their lead and prepare your sleepy muscles for the day by stretching while still in bed.
- If the back muscles are feeling uncomfortable, *lying on your back and drawing the knees to your chest* may be helpful. Stay that way until you sense some relief.
- The lower back may benefit from a *low-back stretch*. You are already lying flat with the previous exercise. Bend your knees slightly and keep your feet on the bed. Roll your knees to the side and back to the center. Reverse to the other side, keeping your back flat.
- *When ready to get up,* roll to the side with your knees bent. Use your elbow and arms to push yourself up gently. This is much easier on the back than bolting upright or jumping out of bed.

Table 6-1	Examples of Moderate Activity	
ACTIVITY	**TIME**
Bicycling	5 miles in 30 minutes
Walking	2 miles in 30 minutes
Social dancing (fast)	30 minutes
Swimming laps	20 minutes
Walking stairs	15 minutes
Gardening	30-45 minutes
Playing volleyball	45 minutes
Pushing stroller	1.5 miles in 30 minutes
Shooting baskets	30 minutes
Running	1.5 miles in 15 minutes
Raking leaves	30 minutes

MAKING MINIMAL EFFORT PAY OFF AT WORK

Items you bring to work can enable you to strengthen certain groups of muscles. Here are some examples:

- If you work at a desk for much of the day, a small, latex-free hand exerciser in the shape of a ball can be squeezed when one hand is free. It is useful for strengthening the muscles in the lower arm and hand.
- Even easier is to pick up something from the desk, such as a stapler, and flex your lower arm.
- Resistive, nonlatex exercise tubing is color-coded according to the resistance desired. The tubing (or band) can be rolled up and takes limited space to transport. You can do any stretching exercise without it. The tubing just provides more resistance.

Once you are at work, stretching is essential for different reasons. Take a few minutes to stretch (warm up) the muscle groups before beginning patient care. Relax and breathe deeply while you stretch. It is worth finding stretching exercises that you can work in periodically throughout the day. They should become increasingly pleasant and soothing. Here are some examples:

- **Improve circulation and prevent muscle cramps** by doing a gentle, seated spinal twist. Sit up straight with your upper thighs at the edge of the seat. Cross your right leg over your left leg. Place your left hand on the inside of your left knee. Twist to the right as you exhale. Bring your right elbow or shoulder around toward the back of the chair. Hold the stretch for four to five breaths, twisting deeper when you exhale. Do this gently. Return to the starting position. Repeat in the opposite direction, crossing your left leg over your right leg, and so on.
- **Correct poor posture.** Nurses often assume poor posture to do the work that they do. In fact, few of the tasks involved in direct patient care permit you to maintain good posture. Poor posture is hard on the spine, interferes with breathing, and increases the risk of shoulder and back pain. Stand up straight. Clasp your hands behind you at your buttocks. Press your shoulder blades toward each other. Have your elbows bent slightly. Breathe deeply, and then exhale. Press your knuckles toward the floor, straightening your arms. Do not arch forward; keep the back straight. Breathe in. Lift your chest, lengthening your spine. Straighten your arms a little as you exhale. Hold the stretch for five breaths. Release. After some practice, this stretching exercise will be easy to do and feel great on the back.
- **Deep breathing** periodically throughout the shift helps to relieve tension in the lower back, neck, and shoulders. Place a hand on the abdomen and the other on the rib cage. Inhale deeply and feel the abdomen rise. As you exhale, feel the air move to the ribs and on up. Do this three to four times.

- A **head roll** helps to relieve tension in the neck, upper shoulders, and back. *Do not roll the head all the way around.* Instead, drop your head down, roll the neck to the right over the shoulder, and then back to the left shoulder. Repeat, reversing the direction.
- **Back stretches while sitting** stretch the back, neck, and arm muscles. Sit fully in a chair. Bring your torso over your knees and touch the floor with your hands. Sit up gently, raise your arms, and reach as high as you can with your fingers. Do this two to three times.
- **Relieve back pain** by sitting on the edge of a chair. Bend forward slightly. Lift a weight you are comfortable with, first with one arm and then with the other. Repeat several times.
- **Side stretches** may relieve tensed arm, hip, and lower back muscles. Stand with your feet apart. Hold a towel or tubing overhead and stretch your arms up and to the right side. Keep the hips still and facing front during the stretch. Switch sides and repeat.

Use exercises that you use to stretch muscles before working out. Obviously you will have to limit your exercises to those you can do while standing or sitting. Nursing is a form of working out and deserves the same thoughtful preparation you would use for an exercise activity.

[?] Critical Thinking

Making Exercise a Daily Activity

1. What is in it for you to incorporate exercise, including stretching, into your daily routine? Think in terms of both home and work.
2. What are your reasons for exercising?
3. Make a plan that fits your need and works with your lifestyle.
4. Involve children as well if they are a part of your current life.

BACK INJURIES IN NURSING: WHAT WE DID *NOT* KNOW

Nurses have been taught body mechanics in the belief that if done properly during patient care, injury to the nurse can be avoided. If this is entirely true, why is the rate of back injuries in nurses double that among construction workers? According to Nelson and colleagues (2003), "Manual lifting and other patient-handling tasks are high-risk activities for both nurses and patients. The prevalence of work-related back injuries in nursing is among the highest of any profession internationally; annual prevalence rates of nursing-related back pain range from 35.9% in New Zealand to 47% in the United States to 66.8% in the Netherlands." There are many related factors involved, including the rising rate of obesity in nurses and other staff who handle patients. As reported by the Associated Press (2007), "Duke University researchers found that the fattest

| Box 6-1 | The 16 Most Physically Stressful Tasks for Nurses |

1. Transferring a patient from toilet to chair
2. Transferring a patient from chair to toilet
3. Transferring a patient from chair to bed
4. Transferring a patient from bed to chair
5. Transferring a patient from bathtub to chair
6. Transferring a patient from chair lift to chair
7. Weighing a patient
8. Lifting a patient in bed
9. Repositioning a patient from side to side in bed
10. Repositioning a patient in a chair
11. Changing an absorbent pad
12. Making a bed with a patient in it
13. Undressing a patient
14. Tying supports
15. Feeding a bedridden patient
16. Making a bed without a patient in it

Used with permission. From Nelson A, Fragala G, Menzel N. (2003). Myths and facts about back injuries in nursing. *AJN* 103:22-41.

workers had 13 times more lost work days due to work-related injuries, and their medical claims for those injuries were seven times higher than their fit co-workers." This study was based on data from 11,728 people employed by Duke and its health system.

Body mechanics do help reduce the rate of nurse injury, but it is not enough by itself. Interestingly, body mechanics were based on studies with men. Yet, nursing remains primarily a female occupation. Women often have less upper-body strength than their male counterparts. Some of the early rationale was based on lifting boxes with handles, bending the knees, and keeping the back straight. In our experience, we have never had patients who came complete with handles for lifting! Other roadblocks are bedside clutter and small, confined spaces. Many nursing tasks involve unnatural positions, such as bending forward with the torso twisted. In their article, Nelson and colleagues offered the 16 most stressful handling tasks in order of rank (Box 6-1).

PREVENTING INJURIES

The ANA launched a "Handle with Care" campaign in 2003. The purpose is to reeducate nurses in principles of safe handling and movement of patients in a way that prevents injury to both the patient and the nurse. In the fall of 2005, a safe patient handling and movement (SPHM) pilot curriculum was funded in 26 nursing programs. Multiple pieces of ergonomically correct lifting devices were provided for the projects. The cost of such equipment has been a factor in initiating similar programs across the country. In 2005, Texas, Ohio, and New York approved laws. In 2006, the state of Washington enacted legislation mandating the development of policies and the acquisition of lifting devices, and allowing tax credits for the cost of equipment (Crocker, 2006).

Back (gait) belts were initially thought to be a partial answer, but intensive study by the National Institute of Occupational Safety (NOSHA) has not been able to prove the claims. Lifting devices have proved to be of help when used properly, but not all lifting devices are created equal. An ergonomically correct device must be chosen for a particular lift, and the nurse must know how to operate it properly. Sometimes nurses avoid using a lift, even if that would be the best choice, because it is stored away from the area or improperly maintained. Sometimes nurses have forgotten how to use the device because of a time lapse. If properly used, mechanical devices can minimize injury. Ceiling lifts have become popular and are installed in the ceiling of a patient's room.

An interesting factor is that many nurses experience injury as a result of accumulative trauma—slowly over a period of time with repeated stress. Administration is paying more attention to long-term cost savings. Having an ergonomic evaluation of their agency, buying the correct mechanical lift devices for their service, and training nurses to use the devices correctly have proved cost effective by decreasing the number of back and shoulder injuries. Compared with lost nursing days, insurance, medical costs, workers' compensation costs, and so forth, the benefits far outweigh the cost of the mechanical devices.

? Critical Thinking

Preventing Injury in the Clinical Area

Investigate what devices are available for you to use in the clinical area to minimize potential back, shoulder, and other injuries. Where are they located? Do you know how to properly use all of the assists available? Who will train you to use the devices? Under what circumstances is each appropriate to use?

Do you currently have a back or other injury that will benefit from strengthening exercises? Who is available to teach you exercises and how to do them so the exercises do not cause additional injury?

HEALTH CARE–ASSOCIATED INFECTIONS (HAIs): AN ISSUE OF SAFETY FOR THE PATIENT, YOUR FAMILY AND YOU

According to the Centers for Disease Control (CDC) estimates, roughly 1.7 million health care–associated infections (HAIs) from all types of bacteria combined kill about 99,000 Americans each year. HAIs are infections patients develop in the hospital or other health facility, usually within 48 hours after admission or within 30 days after discharge. Usual methods of transmission include airborne or personal contact. The most common types involve the urinary tract, lungs (pneumonia), skin, and surgical wounds. Health care workers commonly spread the infections. Physicians, nurses, and other health care workers move from patient to patient

and become a means of transmitting infections. These are not infections patients would have developed anyway. Hand hygiene carried out properly between care of patients is a major deterrent to the spread of infection. Hand washing or using hand sanitizer is a simple procedure. When done improperly it sets the stage to pass on the organism to the next patient. Hands must be washed with soap and water or cleaned with hand sanitizer. Hand sanitizer, however, is not enough when hands are contaminated with any of the following:
- Blood
- Body fluids
- Secretions
- Excretions

Equipment, articles, tables, and so on that are contaminated by blood, body fluids, secretions, or excretions must also be cleaned using the solution specific to the contamination.

Gloves play an important part in preventing the spread of organisms. Hands must be washed before applying gloves and after gloves are removed. Gloves must be removed and new gloves applied between patients.

** Try This**

During clinical, count the number of staff you notice going from one patient to another without changing gloves.

Use of gowns and disposable aprons prevents doctors and nurses from spreading germs on clothing. Also needed is meticulous cleaning of equipment used for patient care, including the blood pressure cuff, stethoscope, ventilators, and so on. Sanitizing surfaces with the proper cleanser for the organism is also needed. The recent widespread deployment of waterless, alcohol-based hand antiseptics has made this task even easier for harried caregivers. The CDC has recommended that health care workers use ethyl alcohol–based hand rubs for "routine" hand cleansing (referring to situations in which the hands are not visibly soiled or contaminated with blood or other body fluids).

Yet, compliance with hand hygiene remains poor in most institutions—often in the range of 40% to 50%. Patients are encouraged to request that family members and friends not visit if they are ill to prevent transfer of germs from outside sources. Patients and visitors are also asked to be alert to breaks in technique, such as a nurse not washing the hands before coming into contact with the patient, and they should not be afraid to request that caregivers wash their hands before touching the patient.

Clothes and uniforms worn while bending over a patient can pick up germs. *Clostridium difficile* (*C. difficile*) is often caused by fecal material from one patient entering another patient's mouth (for example, the combination of emptying bedpans and delivering food trays). Using an alcohol-based hand antiseptic does not destroy this organism when it is in the spore form. Frequently, stethoscopes, blood pressure monitors, and other equipment are contaminated with live bacteria. If not cleaned between patient uses, the germs are passed on to the next patient and, in the case of sharing equipment, to the caregiver.

The British Medical Association has encouraged physicians to not wear neckties, which can be a bug haven, and other functionless clothing to work. Ties are rarely washed, and lab coats are often hung up at the end of the day and put on the next day. Also of concern is what nurses wear to work. Nurses are encouraged to change into work shoes when they arrive at work. Wearing the shoes the caregiver wears at home, to the store, and back to clinical, transports organisms from all the places they go and then back into their home environment. Uniforms worn to places of business also provide a means of transporting community organisms to the hospital and hospital organisms home and into the community. Long hair that hangs down provides another transport method, and it is thought that germs from the hair may enter areas like a wound when doing a sterile procedure such as a dressing change or inserting a catheter.

Yamamoto and Marten (2007) call methicillin-resistant *Staphylococcus aureus* (MRSA) "the original superbug: dangerous, deadly, and highly transmissible. It can survive on hands, clothing, environmental surfaces, and equipment, so it is easily transmissible in health care settings." When "resistant" is used in the name, it designates that the organism name that follows can no longer be destroyed by that medication (once the drug of choice for treatment). MRSA was first reported in the 1960s, and it is now estimated that 46 of 1000 patients have MRSA. Patients already weakened by disease or illness are most susceptible. There is also a community version of MRSA know as community-associated MRSA. This variety tends to cause skin and soft tissue infections such as boils, abscesses, and blisters, accompanied by fever, pain, and purulent drainage. What looks like a spider bite may actually be an early sign of MRSA. Once again, fastidious infection control such as hand hygiene, environmental cleaning, and use of best practices with central lines and ventilators are nursing methods of prevention.

Carbapeneme-resistant *Klebsiella pneumoniae* (CRKP) is another drug-resistant bacteria that is known to cause pneumonia, bloodstream infections, and meningitis and is resistant to almost all antibiotics. CRKP is related to a high morbidity and mortality rate of 30% to 57%. Most patients are elderly, critically ill, and have been hospitalized for a longer time. Invasive devices such as ventilators and central venous lines and unrecognized carriers are a factor. Long-term acute hospitals and nursing homes generally have the highest rates.

CRKP was first described in North Carolina in 1999 but has now been identified in 30 states (CDC, 2009). Routine infection control (hand hygiene) and contact precautions are important preventative factors for nurses.

Research has shown that another major culprit in the spread of health care–associated infection is artificial nails and exceptionally long natural nails (Barber, 2003). As early as 2002, the CDC recommended that health care workers not wear artificial nails or extenders when having contact with high-risk patients. Specific cases causing severe infection or deaths have been traced to nurses with artificial nails and long natural nails. Most handborne pathogens collect in the crook between the fingertip and the nail (i.e., subungual zone). Artificial nails, long natural nails, and nails with chipped nail polish are difficult to clean properly. Long natural nails can become a source of infection directly or through a glove that is punctured by a long nail. Even after careful hand washing or use of surgical scrubs or hand rubs, these personnel often harbor substantial numbers of pathogens in subungual spaces. Although the studies focus primarily on the serious hazard to the patient, artificial nails, long natural nails, and nails with chipped polish are also a way to take home pathogens to your friends and family. Some health facilities have banned long natural fingernails and artificial nails. There is additional concern about pierced fingernails.

DIFFERENTIATING BETWEEN BURNOUT AND STRESS

Burnout is different from stress. Although burnout can be the result of unrelenting stress, it is not the same as stress. In fact, your world can seem perfect—beautiful home, great job, lots of friends—and one day you realize that you feel empty and hopeless. Stress is related to too many physical and mental demands. The person cares too much and thinks if he or she can just do it right and do more, everything will be okay. The person who is stressed is aware of the stress, whereas the person with burnout may not be aware of being burned out.

Some reasons for burnout include having unrealistic expectations imposed on you by yourself or someone else, being required to perform tasks that are against your personal values, working under severe rules, being bored by work that does not challenge you, or feeling trapped for economic reasons in a job or other life situation. Someone else may be pointing out that your attitude and behavior have changed. What is being identified is the cynicism, sense of hopelessness, detachment from others, and negative attitude toward patients and patient care. The major damage to the person with burnout is emotional. Table 6-2 provides a comparison of stress and burnout.

Table 6-2	Stress Versus Burnout
STRESS	**BURNOUT**
Characterized by overengagement	Characterized by disengagement
Emotions are overactive	Emotions are blunted
Produces urgency and hyperactivity	Produces helplessness and hopelessness
Exhausts physical energy	Exhausts motivation, drives, ideals, hope
Leads to anxiety disorders	Leads to paranoia, detachment, depression
Causes disintegration	Causes demoralization
Primary damage is physical	Primary damage is emotional
Stress may kill you prematurely; you won't have enough time to finish what you started	Burnout will never kill you, but life may not seem worth living

From http://www.helpguide.org/mental/burnout_signs_symptoms.htm.

 Try This

Your Life Choices and Burnout

When people asked you why you wanted to study nursing, what was your response? Is this statement related to burnout?

PREVENTING BURNOUT

Empathy Versus Sympathy

Differentiating between feelings of empathy and sympathy in regard to your patient is a major consideration in preventing burnout. Empathy is a respectful, detached concern. As a nurse you understand what your patient is experiencing, but you do not experience the emotion. Patients entering a medical facility are out of their own element. You can pick up the stress they experience as a sympathetic response, having lost perspective of the nurse-patient relationship.

The patient may be demanding a magical, dramatic change in his or her condition. Regression (retreat to an earlier, less stressful style of development) is almost always present in the patient. Needs are often expressed indirectly, perhaps through irritable comments or requests. The patient's emotional responses may elicit negative emotional responses in a sympathetic nurse.

Some patients do not respond to treatment no matter how hard they, and you, try. They may continue to go downhill to the point of death. Meanwhile other patients may not cooperate, and your sympathetic response of anger and frustration will get in the way of a therapeutic relationship with them. Some patients are negative in their responses to staff or constantly ask questions in a challenging way. Maybe you are beginning to think in terms of who does and does not deserve care. Nonassertive and aggressive verbal and nonverbal communication styles can have other devastating effects.

Sympathy is a reaction that leaves you vulnerable to identifying with and experiencing the emotion along with the patient. This means that you are no longer in control of the situation, and your therapeutic value as a nurse is limited. A long-term sympathetic response is very stressful. What starts out as a caring relationship can become detrimental to you and your patient because of being overinvolved.

Detached Way of Evaluating Self

Another significant step in preventing burnout is to develop a detached way of evaluating your daily performance. Waiting for a patient, doctor, or nurse manager to notice your performance is rarely helpful or rewarding. Perhaps they notice only what is missing. However, a detached, daily evaluation of your performance leaves you free to credit yourself for what you have done well. Furthermore, it alerts you to areas in which you need more study, assistance, or practice. Be your own most effective CEO!

Time Management

Time management is another important factor in dealing with both personal and professional areas of your life. Because of its significance, Chapter 2 is devoted to this topic.

Humor

Do not forget humor! No matter how seriously you take yourself, you are never going to get out of this life alive. So lighten up.

1. Humor shows you care.
2. Nurses are accepted better when they have a sense of humor.
3. Humor shows you your patient's personality with their defenses down.
4. Humor reduces tension and helps you get on with your work.
5. Humor makes us equals because we laugh at the same things (Balzer-Riley, 2000).

Remember that using humor with a patient is funny only if the patient thinks so, too. Many things happen in a nursing situation that can be lightened up through humor. Case in point: The nursing instructor walked into the room to see how the student nurse was doing with the patient. As the instructor approached the patient, she extended her hand and greeted the patient by name. As the patient opened his mouth to speak, he simultaneously expelled flatus—a thunderous clap! The patient's eyes opened wide, there was momentary silence, the student looked shocked, and then the instructor chuckled! "It happens," she said with a shrug. Soon all three were laughing; the embarrassment was gone. The real issue of the patient's condition and nursing care was again the priority.

Maintaining Nursing Skills

Maintaining nursing skills throughout your career is essential. Even if you are in a situation that requires less hands-on care, make time to perform nursing procedures. Learn how to perform new procedures as they are introduced to your facility. This helps feed your self-worth and makes you a more valuable employee. Both issues are closely related to burnout. Chances are that if you do not maintain nursing skills, you will develop a secret fear of being put on the spot and perhaps find a way out of requests to demonstrate or assist with a procedure.

Here are a few more tips for reducing stress and preventing burnout:
1. Be clear about the reasons you want to be a nurse.
2. Set clear goals with realistic expectations.
3. Know your limits. Learn when to say "no."
4. Work within your team structure.
5. Keep in mind that you cannot be all things to all people.
6. Maintain a clear understanding of what constitutes a professional, caring relationship. The patient needs a nurse, not a buddy.
7. To experience less guilt and anger, do not personalize the patient's response to you. Keep the patient in the patient role. See that the patient responds out of the patient's own needs.
8. Maintain a positive attitude (i.e., warm, caring, and hopeful), even if the patient is dying. The patient and the family will feel less hopeless.
9. Understand your own needs, both personally and professionally. Maintain a balance and a clear distinction between your work and your personal role. It is necessary to tell the patient who wants to be involved in your personal life by calling and visiting that "I will do my best as a nurse while I am at work, but my personal life is separate. You may *not* call my home or visit me in my home." Furthermore, developing personal relationships with patients is unprofessional and violates the Nurse Practice Act in many states.
10. Be alert to signs of burnout. Lack of caring for your patient is a real danger signal.
11. Maintain perspective about your role as a nurse. Sometimes the whole world looks ill and grim! Remind yourself that you have a choice: *Nursing can be a limited part of your life or the dominant feature in your life.* You get to choose.

 Critical Thinking

Where Am I Headed?

1. Inventory your feelings and physical health. Are friends making comments regarding your attitude and behavior?
2. Do you find yourself frequently focusing on home issues at work and work issues at home?
3. Are you often talking about work when you are with friends and family?
4. If your answers indicate that there are issues, do something about it now before you are overwhelmed physically and/or mentally.

SECONDARY TRAUMATIC STRESS

We want to briefly touch on this important issue of secondary traumatic stress. Nurses in burn units, emergency departments, neonatal intensive care units, or other high-stress environments are constantly exposed to traumatic horrors that may cause this type of stress. After a while, some nurses will respond with hypertension, gastritis, peptic ulcers, and fatigue. There may be more sick days, problems with decision making, isolation, withdrawal, or behavioral outbursts. The result will be a decrease in staff morale and errors in judgment, which will affect not only the patients but the employer as well.

RECOGNIZING SIGNS OF SECONDARY TRAUMATIC STRESS

It is important to recognize signs of oncoming secondary traumatic stress and not attempt to hide it. Too often nurses think that they are not entitled to their feelings and that they must be kept to oneself. It is important that nurses are alert to their feelings, thoughts, and physical changes and how they are functioning with patients and other staff.

Sometimes journaling is a way to get the feelings out and identify the seriousness of what is happening for the nurse. When journaling, remember to include things you did that were right. Nurses tend to focus on the negative outcomes of traumatic situations. Remember that sometimes, no matter how many things we do that are correct, the patient still dies or ends up with a lifelong disability. That is just the way it is.

PREVENTION

It helps to get sufficient rest, which is not easy if you become focused on the negative outcomes. Proper diet and personal relaxation techniques such as meditation or imagery may be helpful. It is important to have positive relations with peers and to have people with whom you can share your feelings and concerns honestly.

If all these efforts do not work, then ask for a change in assignment to another nursing area. There is nothing wrong with requesting a change; it is not a sign of failure. Keep your options open for getting professional help. Sometimes what has happened now has ties to the past, which will need professional assistance to unravel, heal, and make necessary changes. Participating in employer-sponsored or privately arranged support groups or counseling is helpful to many nurses.

CHEMICALLY DEPENDENT NURSES

Chemical dependency refers to abuse of alcohol and/or other drugs. Alcohol is listed separately to emphasize that it is the most commonly abused drug. Between 2% and 18% of nurses become chemically dependent on alcohol and/or other drugs (Weiss, 2005). These nurses tend to be perfectionists and often have a family history of chemical dependency. Nurses work taking care of others and frequently ignore their own needs. The health care system uses medication to deal with symptoms and illness. Nurses diagnose themselves and begin to "treat" their symptoms. It often starts as an alcoholic drink or other drug to unwind at the end of a work shift. Gradually more of the alcohol or other drug is needed to attain the same effect. Finally the drug controls the user.

Eventually, the nurse may divert drugs from patients or ask physician friends for "hallway prescriptions." If the user is a nurse, the nurse is considered impaired when use of the drug(s) extends to the quality of work. When the impairment is discovered, there is so much humiliation for a nurse: The nurse is expected to know better. There is also the possibility of losing their nursing license and, as a result, their livelihood. According to the National Council of the State Boards of Nursing (NCSBN), most state nursing board sanctions are drug related. If the nurse has been caught stealing drugs, he or she may face criminal proceedings.

Because of the prevalence of alcohol use, we will speak specifically about alcohol. The list of telltale signs that we list later applies to all chemical dependency. Alcohol is a drug that acts like a depressant. Unlike food, alcohol does not have to be digested. It is absorbed directly into the bloodstream from the stomach and small intestine, reaching the brain within 5 minutes. At first alcohol stimulates you. If you continue to drink, it depresses you and may put you to sleep. However, the sleep may be short. Alcohol interferes with the necessary sleep cycle needed for a restful sleep. When combined with other drugs (e.g., sedatives, antianxiety medication, and some over-the-counter [OTC] medications), alcohol will have a multiplying effect. **This means that the combined effect is more than 1 + 1.** Accidental overdoses can occur this way.

A telling sign of any chemical dependency in nurses is a gradual decline in performance, which usually

Box 6-2	**Telltale Signs of Chemical Dependency in Nurses**

Behaviors that need to be checked out include the following:
- Complaints by staff, students, and patients
- Accidents, errors in documentation, a greater number of injuries caused while moving patients or equipment, errors in practice, and poor judgment
- Increased visits to the employee health department or emergency room; increased volunteering to take calls for others (especially true for evening and night shifts if there is less staff; makes stealing patient drugs easier)
- Arriving early or staying late to assist in the narcotic count
- Frequent absenteeism after days off and for personal emergencies, especially on a Monday
- Irritability and mood swings
- Performing only the minimum amount of work required
- Inability to perform psychomotor skills owing to intoxication or tremors

becomes noticeable within 3 to 6 months (Box 6-2). Most important, you have a duty to the patient and, in many states, a legal duty to report the use of alcohol or other drugs.

 Critical Thinking

How Am I Doing?

1. Do I turn to alcohol or other drugs for relief from pain or job stress on a regular basis?
2. If the answer to question number 1 is yes, to whom will you go to seek intervention?
3. If you realize that a coworker or someone else on the health care team is drinking or is impaired by other drugs while on duty, consider the following questions:
   What is your responsibility to the coworker?
   What is your responsibility to the patient?
   What is your responsibility to your school or employer?
   What is your responsibility to your State Board of Nursing (Nursing Commission)?

CODEPENDENCY: A PATHOLOGIC NEED

 Try This

Codependency: A Pathologic Need

Before you read any further, answer the following questions:
1. What is your reason for making nursing your career choice?
2. Who supplies the most important critique of your day's work?
3. How do you feel if the patient or instructor does not tell you that you did a good job?

Codependency is when a person has a pathologic need to be needed by others. The behavior of others affects them in a way that causes them to be obsessed about "fixing" the behavior (i.e., the need to control the behavior of others). Some writers have speculated that a large number of nurses may be codependent. Helping others is a way of meeting their own codependency needs. Codependent nurses become overinvolved in their patient's life and go to extremes to serve both their patients and coworkers. They react too quickly to feelings with a sense of intensity and urgency. Patients (and others) in their life are viewed disrespectfully (i.e., they are thought to be incapable of participating in their own care). This viewpoint takes away a sense of personal control.

The codependent nurse may think that no one else can give the patient care that is required. The codependent nurse readily accepts a patient's statement that "no one has ever given (me) such wonderful care (or understood me)." The nurse is equally devastated by any perceived criticism by the patient (e.g., "How can they say that after all I did?"). Codependent nurses give the message that the patient, family, or staff member is more ill (or helpless) than initially perceived. For some codependent individuals, a painful childhood that included sexual abuse, violence, or chemical abuse may have paved the way to codependency (Table 6-3).

Beattie (1992), a notable author on the subject of co-dependency, has compared codependent behavior to the sides of Karpman's drama triangle (victim, rescuer, persecutor). Because codependent persons are caretakers or rescuers, they rescue, persecute, and ultimately end up feeling victimized. Beattie's self-help book *Codependent No More* presents specific information on codependent characteristics and how to change the behaviors.

DEALING WITH NEGATIVE STRESS: SOME IDEAS

Try This

Avoid Negative Stress

List some things that cause excessive negative stress in your life.

It is interesting to note that it is *our reaction to a situation, rather than the situation itself* that causes stress. Everything that happens to you—either pleasant or unpleasant—creates stress. Interpretation of stress as distress or negative stress is dependent on personal problem-solving skills and the intensity and duration of the situations involved. Ironically, a time of boredom and understimulation is accompanied by high adrenaline levels in the body, as is a time of high stress during overstimulation. In other words, individuals seem to do best with a moderate amount of stress in their lives. What is defined as moderate stress varies from person to person.

As a nurse you probably have better coping skills than most. You accept that acute stress is part of the vocation you are preparing for. During your clinical rotations, instructors assign you to increasingly more

? **Critical Thinking**

Codependency: A Bothersome Behavior

Codependent behavior can be modified. As with any behavior that is bothersome, the sooner it is recognized, the easier it is to modify. Ask yourself:
1. Do any of the behaviors described in Table 6-3 apply?
2. Circle the behaviors that apply.
3. Choose one behavior that you think will cause the most difficulty as a nurse.
4. Make a plan for change that is attainable, measurable, and time-referenced.

Table 6-3 Some Codependent Characteristics and Behaviors	
CHARACTERISTICS	**BEHAVIORS**
Says "yes"—really means "no"	Agrees to help another staff member and then complains to someone else about being taken advantage of
Feels the fate of nursing care rests on their shoulders	Takes on nonnursing duties that belong to other departments
Feels responsible for solving other people's problems	Sympathetic rather than empathetic response to patients and other staff
Competes for attention rather than supporting coworkers	Engages in one-upmanship and intershift rivalries over patient care
Often feels angry, unappreciated, and used	Comes in early and works late; works extra shifts to "help" coworkers
Does not support patient's need for autonomy and return to self-confidence	Does for the patient what the patient needs to do to regain optimal health and self-sufficiency
Makes excuses and conceals negative practices rather than working for change	Feels powerless; takes on extra duties because of chronic understaffing
Shows feelings of anger indirectly	Pouts, procrastinates, forgets, gets sick, or is late
Perfectionist: gossips and judges	Unrealistic expectations of others
Avoids conflict	Too nice, loving, and forgiving
	Smiles when having negative feelings

difficult tasks. They remain on the unit to assist you in dealing with the expected and unexpected situations as they occur. The clinical experience gives you an opportunity to experience the real world of nursing—an incredible plus in building your coping skills. However, you continue to be vulnerable to stress, and many factors can add to the vulnerability: a nursing shortage; patient acuity and rapid discharge; complexity of new medications, treatments, and equipment; personal issues not separated from work; and so on. The belief that good nurses are self-sacrificing has many nurses focusing on care for others (work and family) and ignoring their own needs.

 Try This

Find a Good Role Model

Who will be a positive role model for you? Find someone who does a good job as a nurse and also finds time to focus on personal needs (good nutrition, exercise, recreation, relaxation, etc.).

RELAXATION

Relaxation training is one way to manage stress. During a relaxed state, the pulse and respiratory rates decrease, the metabolic rate and blood pressure are lowered, and muscular tension is decreased. Along with the positive physical changes experienced by all except 3% of the population, you also experience a sense of well-being. If you are part of the 3% that become more stressed during a relaxation exercise, there is nothing wrong with you. It just is, so think about what does bring about the physical changes for you, as previously described. For example, a student shared that relaxation exercises and soothing music made her "ready to climb the walls," whereas hard rock had a calming effect on her. Knowing this, she insisted on listening to hard rock during labor.

Many relaxation methods are available and need to be tailored to your lifestyle. Decide on a regular practice time. Some of you will want to start your day with a relaxation exercise. Some of you will want to end your day this way. Overall relaxation is accomplished most readily before meals or at least 2 hours after a meal because of the stimulant effect of food on the body. Caffeine-containing drinks, such as regular coffee and some soft drinks, are best avoided before a training session.

MEDITATION

For meditation, you need a quiet environment, a mental device, a passive attitude, and a comfortable position.

- A **quiet environment** helps eliminate distractions and permits you to concentrate on a mental device of your choosing.

- A **mental device** is any sound, word, or phrase that evokes a sense of calm in you as you repeat it.
- **Repeat the device silently or aloud** with your eyes closed. If you prefer to keep your eyes open, you can fix your gaze on an object. Either way, your mind is focusing on one thing. If you are feeling uncomfortable with your eyes closed, open them, look around, and close them again when satisfied, and return to the mental device.
- **Concentrate on your normal breathing pattern.** It enhances your repetition of the mental device. Breathe through your nose when you breathe out.
- A **passive attitude** is considered most significant for eliciting a successful relaxation response. Distracting thoughts may occur; simply let them pass and return to repetition of the mental device. Trying too hard usually creates tension.
- A **comfortable position** prevents added muscular tension. Sit with good posture, wear loose-fitting clothes, take off your shoes, and keep your feet on the floor. Lying down is not encouraged because you tend to fall asleep (unless that is your intent).
- To begin, breathe in and out (mental device), then repeat.
- To stop, sit for a while, note how you are feeling, open your eyes, look around, get up slowly, and continue your day.

IMAGERY

Imagery is an excellent way of learning to relax and, once learned, can be done in less structured settings, such as during break time. It is also a way of protecting yourself against situations you may face in the future, by visualizing the situation and how you will move through it successfully. It is also creative and fun. You already do it; you did so before embarking on your present career by imagining the steps to becoming a nurse and seeing yourself as a licensed practical/vocational nurse.

This kind of imagery is not the guided imagery that is used in psychotherapy, requiring a trained psychotherapist to deal with the symbolic material that may emerge. Some of you are better at imagining than others. Some may only see shadowy figures, whereas others see vivid, Technicolor images. Images need not be particularly vivid to be effective.

- Begin with a brief relaxation exercise if you are very tense.
- Once relaxed, follow the imagery.
- Two or three deep breaths are helpful before the imagery. In practicing the imagery, it is important to take sufficient time to include enough detail so you can get into the imagery.
- When ready to conclude the imagery, count from 1 to 10, sit for a while with your eyes closed, open your eyes, and then stretch.

Box 6-3 Imagery: Relieving Anxiety

- Design your own favorite place—whatever is your idea of complete peace, harmony, and joy.
- See yourself appropriately dressed in the setting you have created.
- Take time to look around and visualize your surroundings with great detail.
- Use all of your senses to experience the sight, sound, smell, touch, and taste available in your special hideaway.
- See yourself staying there and feeling peaceful and calm. Remember that it is a safe place and that you can return there to rest daily.
- When you are ready to leave, take one look back, knowing that you can return anytime.
- You will continue to feel relaxed and happy as you return to your daily activities.

It is worthwhile to remember that if you experience anxiety anytime during the imagery, you need only to open your eyes and continue with the imagery. Some of you will be comfortable with your eyes open during the entire process and do not seem to have any problems visualizing. Imagery, like other relaxation techniques, takes self-discipline; therefore, daily practice sessions are suggested. Modify the instructions to meet personal needs. Instructions for using imagery to relieve anxiety are found in Box 6-3.

BRIEF RELAXATION

Brief relaxation techniques are useful as a method for relieving anxiety or preparing your body for relaxation techniques like imagery. For example, say you have been contacted to go see your instructor with no further explanation or you are getting ready for a test. The first two techniques in Box 6-4 can be done without anyone being aware that you are quieting your anxiety.

Personal Stress Management

Design a personal stress management plan for yourself. Include the date you will start and where you will seek instruction, if necessary.

SLEEP

All the methods of dealing with personal stress can be sabotaged unless you develop a regular pattern of sleep. Be aware that you can create your own insomnia by taking your worries to bed. Tell yourself firmly that you have done your best for the day and will not think about the issues until you awaken. Some put their left-over worries into the hands of a Supreme Being at the end of the day or put them on a bookshelf. To make the best use of this information, do the following:

Box 6-4 Brief Relaxation

- **Brief Relaxation.** This exercise prevents the rush of thought. It can be used to induce on-the-spot relaxation in a public place or to promote sleep. Directions: Part your lips slightly. Place the tip of the tongue behind the lower teeth. Keep it there without pressure for a while. Continue with normal breathing. Place: Walking down the hall, in the bathroom, in class, in a meeting (not in front of the boss or instructor), during break, while studying.
- **Yawning.** This is a 1-minute tension release exercise. The lungs expand; the back, jaw, mouth, and tongue relax. More oxygen comes into the system. Directions: Drop your jaw gently until it feels large enough to take in a whole fruit. As you begin to yawn, it feels as though it will never end. As you yawn, you are taking in a deep breath. When the yawn ends, you feel relaxed clear down to your stomach. Your lungs have expanded and your back begins to release its tension. Place: Nice to do near an open window.
- **Do Nothing.** Take 5 to 10 minutes to sit quietly and do nothing. Pay attention to the sounds around you, your emotions, and any tension in your body (Jaret, 2003).
- **Breathe Easy.** Take 5 minutes to slow down your breathing to approximately six deep abdominal breaths a minute; inhale for 5 seconds, then exhale for 5 seconds (Jaret, 2003).

- Go to bed at the same time; listen to what your body is telling you. Going to bed extra-early or later than your usual bedtime is not doing your body a favor.
- Most important, when you naturally awaken, get out of bed. Better yet, do the stretching exercises and then get out of bed.
- Be alert to the number of hours you slept and if you feel rested. You will recognize a pattern if you track your sleep hours for several days.
- No doubt you have at some point decided to treat yourself to a few extra minutes of sleep and ended up feeling tired much of the day. Research seems to indicate that the body is set on a 25-hour clock, and when you get up at a different time, the body tries to "reset" the clock throughout the day. (No wonder the treat you offered yourself did not work!)
- Nurses still work different shifts in some agencies. If there are many changes within a week, the body is struggling to reset its clock throughout the time that the change is taking place. A "next best thing" if you are missing regularly scheduled sleep is to lie down for a 20-minute nap when you get home or take a quick catnap on days when the 20-minute nap is not possible.

Get Enough Sleep

Evaluate your sleep habits. Do you feel rested most of the time?

Get Ready for the NCLEX-PN® Examination

Key Points

- The Dietary Guidelines for Americans 2010 provide updated information on eating, physical activity, and food safety.
- The MyPlate icon released in June 2011 replaces the MyPyramid.
- MyPlate divides a plate in fourths with one-half fruits and vegetables, at least half of your grains whole grain; protein is the smallest part of the plate.
- As little as 30 minutes of moderate exercise, such as brisk walking, on most days of the week will affect personal health in a positive way. The 30 minutes of exercise can be broken down into three 10-minute periods, if necessary.
- Nurses are among the highest of any profession internationally to have work-related back injuries.
- Practicing good body mechanics alone cannot prevent all back injuries. Ergonomic evaluation of needs, taking time to use the right lifting device for the task, and keeping your body healthy, trim, strong, and flexible are all helpful in preventing back injuries.
- Hand washing is the single most important prevention technique for containing spread of infection.
- Artificial and long fingernails are linked to patient infection and deaths.
- Burnout and stress are not the same. With stress, the nurse cares too much and is trying to work harder to solve the situation. Burnout leaves the nurse feeling hopeless, helpless, and cynical. Burnout is experienced emotionally, and the sense of caring for patents is blunted.
- Nurses who work in settings such as burn units, emergency departments, or neonatal units are constantly exposed to traumatic horror. These nurses are especially susceptible to developing secondary traumatic stress.
- About 2% to 18% of nurses become dependent on alcohol or other drugs. The effort to self-medicate gets out of hand when additional amounts of the alcohol or drug are needed to attain the same effect.
- Codependent persons have a pathologic need to be needed by others. They become overinvolved in the patient's life and go to extremes to serve the patient.
- Our reaction to a situation, rather than the situation itself, causes stress in our lives.
- Limit work as one part of your life; enjoy a full personal life that includes friends, family, recreation, relaxation, other activities, and so on.
- Relaxation works to relieve both psychological and physical stress. Choose relaxation that fits into your lifestyle and meets your needs.
- Regular sleep habits help to avoid the fatigue caused by the body's attempt to reset the body clock when sleep patterns are disrupted.

Additional Learning Resources

evolve Go to your Evolve website (http://evolve.elsevier.com/Hill/Success) for the following FREE learning resources:
- Answers to Critical Thinking Scenarios
- Additional learning activities
- Additional Review Questions for the NCLEX-PN® exam
- Helpful phrases for communicating in Spanish and more!

Review Questions for the NCLEX-PN® Examination

1. What symptom has become the most important factor in developing a chronic disease?
   1. Accidents
   2. Hypertension
   3. Obesity
   4. Alcohol

2. What is the most important way to protect patients from health care–associated infection?
   1. Use of masks during patient care
   2. Consistent hand hygiene during patient care
   3. Reporting infractions in infection control
   4. Dispensing antibiotics 20 minutes before beginning care

3. What explanation will you offer when a nonnurse friend asks you why so many nurses have back problems?
   1. Nurses are unable to consistently use good body mechanics because many nursing tasks cause unnatural positions.
   2. Lifting devices are stored too far from the central area of work and nurses do not have the time to dig them out.
   3. Nurses are expected to be strong and flexible, and many nurses perceive it as a sign of weakness to ask for help.
   4. Nursing shortage creates an atmosphere of urgency on the unit, so nurses have little time to care for themselves.

4. Select the priority strategy that would help the LPN/LVN stay alive and well in nursing.
   1. Ask for daily feedback from your immediate boss.
   2. Make patients and staff the focus of your daily life.
   3. Keep in mind that nurses have better coping skills than most.
   4. Monitor yourself as you learn and make changes.

Alternate Format Item

1. You are the charge nurse on a unit in the nursing home. A staff nurse mentions that patients are not worth the time spent on them: "They just complain and finally die no matter what we do." Which of the following apply to this situation? *(Select all that apply.)*

   1. We are all in the same situation.
   2. Working here is your own choice.
   3. Get over it. What did you expect?
   4. When did this feeling start?
   5. You are a poorly prepared nurse.

2. It has been brought to your attention that your best friend in the program (also on the same clinical rotation as you) is not following proper procedure with hand sanitation. The word is that he is rinsing the tips of his fingers only when he washes his hands. *(Select all that apply.)*

   1. You talk to the instructor and have her confront him.
   2. You ask him to meet you for coffee after work.
   3. You tell him directly what the conversation will be about.
   4. If unwilling to listen, ask the instructor to fail him in this course.
   5. Ask him to explain why he is only rinsing the fingertips.
   6. Demonstrate proper cleansing if he is willing to watch.

Critical Thinking Scenarios

Scenario 1: Patients and Family Members Can Help

Bill was admitted to the hospital for gastric surgery. The surgeon reassured Bill that the surgery had gone well and recovery should be smooth. When his sister Amy arrived at the hospital, she noted several things that bothered her. The man washing the foyer floor was mopping the floor in slow motion with what appeared to be dirty water. As she walked through the hallway to locate her brother's room, she noted several rooms that had ISOLATION signs posted on the door. Amy saw nurses and NAs with patient gowns covering their uniforms go from room to room to give medications, adjust IVs, check oxygen, and so forth. Although there was a sink, soap dispenser, and towels in the hallway, she did not observe anyone wash their hands.

Her brother was alert and relieved with the positive report he received from the surgeon. After greeting her brother, Amy asked about the patient in the other bed. Bill said he had not met his roommate because the curtain had been drawn since he arrived. Later in the day, Amy watched a nurse adjust her brother's IV and then go to the roommate's bed. Later that day she watched as a nurse left the other patient's area, carrying soiled dressings in her hands.

What are the breaks in technique that you noted? What would you advise Amy to do in order to protect her brother? To whom should Amy speak about her observations? Write an ending to this story (it is based on a factual experience).

Scenario 2: Relieving Test Anxiety

The same old problem: Another test is coming up this Friday. I have a history of not doing well on tests. I spend most of the night studying and get up early to study some more. Class projects are due Wednesday, and I have decided to face this problem head-on.

- Provide an outline for the result I expect.
- Summarize what I learned during my research.
- Explain what I will do differently Thursday night.

How Practical/Vocational Nursing Evolved: 1836 to the Present

Objectives

On completing this chapter, you will be able to do the following:

1. Identify the year and place the first school of practical nursing was founded.
2. Name the school's most famous pupil.
3. Discuss the contributions of this most famous nurse.
4. Name the year in which licensing for practical nursing first began.
5. Present the rationale for your personal stand on entry into nursing practice.
6. Name one contribution of war nurses to overall nursing:
   - Crimean War
   - World War I
   - World War II
   - Korean Conflict
   - Vietnam War
   - Afghanistan war
   - Iraq war

Key Terms

Clara Barton (p. 77)
Cadet Nurse Corps (p. 80)
Mildred I. Clark (p. 82)
Jane Delano (p. 78)
Dorothea Lynde Dix (p. 76)
Glenna Goodacres (p. 83)
Anna Goodrich (p. 78)
Lystra Gretter (p. 76)

Anna Mae Hays (p. 82)
Lenah S. Higbee (p. 79)
Lillian Kinkela-Keil (p. 81)
Florence Nightingale (p. 73)
Notes on Nursing (p. 75)
M. Adelaide Nutting (p. 78)
Mary Seacole (p. 74)
Lillian Wald (p. 77)

 Keep in Mind

The first nurses were practical nurses, and you are part of that proud heritage.

The length of the course for the modern practical (or vocational) nurse is approximately 9 months to 1 year in most states. There is some variation in the actual number of weeks. Historically speaking, all nurses had less educational preparation for their work than do current licensed practical/vocational nurses (LPN/LVN).

MODERN PRACTICAL NURSES

Nursing has experienced many changes throughout its history (Table 7-1), and the changes continue. Two major changes that have occurred in practical nursing are a gradual increase in the required formal knowledge base and a requirement for licensing to practice practical nursing. Unlike the historically untrained or poorly trained practical nurse, who had unlimited and unsupervised freedom to practice, the present practical nurse is now often a hybrid. Today's practical/vocational nursing student (SPN/SVN) is being taught basic skills during the nursing program. After licensing, the LPN/LVN is permitted to perform complex nursing skills as assigned by the registered nurse (RN) and allowed by their state's nurse practice act. Assigning is allowed as long as the LPN/LVN feels confident performing the skill or the following requirements are met:

- An RN is willing to teach the skill.
- An RN observes the return demonstration.

See Chapter 21 for information on assigning and delegation.

Table 7-1 Practical Nursing Milestones

PERIOD IN HISTORY	EVENT
1836	First real school of nursing, in Kaiserswerth, Germany. Florence Nightingale attended for 3 months. Eighteen years later, after start of Crimean War, Nightingale nursed wounded with 38 self-identified (untrained) nurses.
1860	Nightingale established a school of nursing in England. She wrote several books. The most famous was *Notes on Nursing.*
Civil War (1861-1865)	In the South: Most nursing done by infantrymen assigned to the task. Southern women volunteered services. In the North: Dorothea Lynde Dix, a teacher, was appointed Superintendent of Nurses and organized a corps of female nurses (untrained).
1864	Clara Barton, a teacher, collected supplies for soldiers. This led to her appointment as Superintendent of the Department of Nurses for the Army.
1881	Clara Barton established the first chapter of the American Red Cross in Danville, New York.
1892	First class for formal training of practical nursing: YWCA, Brooklyn, New York.
1893	Nightingale Pledge written by Canadian-born Lystra Gretter, principal of Farrand Training School in Detroit. Henry Street Settlement founded by Lillian Wald, a social worker who graduated from a nursing program. Practical nurses pioneered in this new public health movement. They went into homes and taught the basics of cleanliness and control of communicable diseases to families in New York slums.
1893	Ballard School for Practical Nursing opened in New York.
1907	Thompson School for Practical Nursing opened in Brattleboro, Vermont.
1914	Mississippi is the first state to pass a law to license practical nurses.
1917	Standardization of nursing requirements for practical nursing by National League of Nursing Education (now the National League for Nursing [NLN]).
World War I (1914-1918)	Shortage of practical nurses. Army School of Nursing established. Highlighted the need for more and better-prepared nurses. Smith Hughes Act of 1917 provided money for developing additional schools of practical nursing.
1920s	Acute shortage of practical nurses. Many did not return to nursing after the war.
1920-1940	Most practical nursing limited to public health agencies and visiting nurse associations.
1938	New York only state to have mandatory licensure.
World War II (1939-1945)	Shortage of RNs created need for LPNs. At home, practical nurses worked in clinics, health departments, industries, and hospitals. In the war, they ventured into hardship tours in Europe, North Africa, and the Pacific.
1940	The number of practical nurses peaked in 1940 at 159,009.
1941	NAPNES (National Association of Practical Nurse Education and Service), a nation's professional organization dedicated exclusively to practical nursing, was founded.
1943	Cadet Nurse Corps was founded; two-and-a-half-year courses to become nurses.
1944	Comprehensive study of practical nursing by U.S. Department of Vocational Education. This was the first time that tasks of practical nursing were agreed upon.
End of World War II	Nursing shortage saw movement of practical nurses into hospitals and gradually increasing responsibilities.
1949	NFLPN (National Federation of Licensed Practical Nurses) was founded to provide structure nationwide through which LPNs could promote better patient care and act on behalf of LPNs. The NFLPN-organized Joint Committee on Practical Nurses and Auxiliary Workers in Nursing Services recommended use of the title "licensed practical nurse" and differentiated between tasks of registered nurses and LPNs.
Korean Conflict (1950-1953)	Nurses finally became part of the military.
1951	*Journal of Practical Nursing* published by NAPNES (now *Practical Nursing Today*).
1952	Approximately 60% of the nurse workforce was made up of practical nurses.
1955	All states had licensure laws for practical/vocational nurses.
1957	NLN established a Council of Practical Nursing Programs.
1960	By 1960, every state had a nurse licensure law.
1961	NLN began offering accrediting services for practical nursing programs.

Table 7-1	Practical Nursing Milestones—cont'd
PERIOD IN HISTORY	**EVENT**
Vietnam War (1961-1973)	Military nurses were assigned to Vietnamese hospitals, MASH units, as flight nurses, and hospital ships.
1965	ANA (American Nurses Association) first moves toward two distinct levels in nursing: professional and technical.
1975	1315 state-approved PN programs. More than 45,000 PN graduates. After 1975, number of PN programs and graduates declined.
1979	NLN published first list of competencies for practical/vocational nursing programs.
1980s	Resurgence of ANA moves toward two distinct levels of nursing. This resulted in some states adopting two levels of nursing and then rescinding their decision because of the nursing shortage.
1984	Creation of ALPNA (American Licensed Practical Nurses Association).
1989	The American Medical Association (AMA) initiated and subsequently dropped the registered care technician (RCT) proposal.
1990s	Unlicensed personnel are used for patient care. The number of hospital nursing jobs has decreased. The primary employment site has moved into the community.
1994	First computerized adaptive test (NCLEX-PN®) available to practical/vocational nursing graduates.
1995	Full-time nursing positions in hospitals decreased. Patient/nurse ratios increased. Primary employment in community continues.
1996	Long-term care certification examinations for LPNs/LVNs by National Council of State Boards of Nursing with the National Association for Licensed Practical Nurse Education and Service.
2000	Increased demand for LPNs/LVNs in nursing homes and extended care; demand down in hospitals.
2001— Afghanistan war	Military nurses help set up surgical teams, MASH units, air evacuation, combat support units in Afghan and Iraqi hospitals.
2003—Iraq war	
2007	Nursing programs are turning students away because of the shortage of instructors.

FIRST SCHOOL OF NURSING (1836)

The first real school of nursing was founded by the Lutheran Order of Deaconesses under the supervision of a German pastor, Theodor Fleidner, in Kaiserswerth, Germany. The year was 1836. The purpose of the program was to teach principles of nursing care to the Lutheran Order of Deaconesses. Many of the graduates of Kaiserswerth Deaconess Institute settled in other parts of the world and established similar programs. The school's most famous pupil was the English-woman Florence Nightingale, the founder of modern nursing. She attended the school for 3 months and studied under Caroline Fliedner.

FLORENCE NIGHTINGALE (1820–1910)

Florence Nightingale was born in Florence, Italy. Her parents named her after the city and called her "Flo." Nightingale's parents were wealthy, influential, and accepted in society. Florence was presented at court and was expected to follow the social pattern of other women of her day. Women were considered intellectually inferior to men. Education for middle- and upper-class women often consisted of lessons in etiquette, dancing, music, manners, embroidery, painting, and modern languages. Instead of being tutored by

governesses or in a private school, Nightingale's father tutored her in modern and ancient languages, history, composition, philosophy, and mathematics, including statistics. He was a strict disciplinarian, but she was an eager student (LeVasseur, 1998).

Nightingale turned down a proposal of marriage from a man her sister later married. Early on, Nightingale knew she had a purpose in life to fulfill. She begged her parents to permit her to go into the nurses' training program in Kaiserswerth, Germany. Her parents were not pleased, since nursing was seen as a job suitable only for lower-class women. As we know, Nightingale got her way. Upon graduation, she became superintendent for the Institution for the Care of Sick Gentlewomen in Distressed Circumstances, now the Harley Street Nursing Home in London (Romanoff, 2006). She began to take steps to make the work of nurses who served the gentlewomen easier. Dumbwaiters were installed so the nurses did not have to carry heavy trays up and down stairs. Nightingale also developed a system of call bells that could be seen in hallways to identify which person was summoning. Because the institution discriminated against Catholics and Jews, she dropped religion as a requirement for admission. Some of the governing board members were not happy with her changes.

The following year, as Nightingale was planning to become superintendent of King's College Hospital in London, the Crimean War broke out. She sent a letter to the Secretary of War offering her services. She did not know that he had also sent a letter to her requesting her assistance.

CRIMEAN WAR 1853–1865

Shortly after the start of the 1853 Crimean War (in which Britain, France, Turkey, and Sardinia fought Russia for control of access to the Mediterranean from the Black Sea), information about the neglect and poor care of casualties began to reach England. A correspondent for the *London Times* newspaper wrote vivid accounts of the deplorable conditions and lack of medical and nursing care for the British troops. The Sisters of Mercy tended Russian troops, the Sisters of Charity tended the French, and the wounded of England were almost completely neglected. The correspondent's charges were so persistent that a commission was sent to investigate. As a result, the Secretary of War decided that England, too, should have a group of women nurses to tend the war casualties.

The Secretary of War contacted Florence Nightingale and explained the situation to her. Because she had both nursing and administrative experience, the secretary perceived her as the one nurse in England capable of organizing and supervising care in a foreign land.

Being appointed to the task organizing and supervising nurses during the Crimean War gave Nightingale an unexpected opportunity for achievement. She left for Crimea, taking with her 38 self-proclaimed nurses of limited experience, 24 of whom were nuns. On arrival, they found overcrowded, filthy hospitals with no beds, no furniture, no eating utensils, no medical supplies, no blankets, no soap, no linens, and no lamps. Wounded soldiers lay on the filthy floor in their battle uniforms (Figure 7-1). Soldiers were more likely to die from infected wounds than the wound itself. Nightingale took charge. Using the supplies she brought, and raising funds, she purchased supplies that doctors could not obtain for the army. Nightingale hired people to clean up the "hospitals" and established laundries to wash linens and uniforms and prepare nutritious meals. She expected a great deal of herself and those who worked with her. It was not an easy task. A major prejudice that had to be overcome was that of medical officers, who considered the nurses intruders. The hours were long and difficult for Nightingale and her nurses. An additional concern was that sometimes nurses became more involved in converting patients to their particular faith than in giving general care. Nightingale hired tutors to teach convalescing soldiers how to read and write. Many soldiers had family following them, and recreation rooms were set up for their use. She believed that the best nurses were those who had good character,

FIGURE 7-1 Florence Nightingale ministering to soldiers at Scutari (lithograph).

who experienced a sense of calling, and who were well trained to meet the physical needs of patients. The barracks, a 4-mile labyrinth of cots meant for 1700 patients, packed in 3000 to 4000 patients. She did not want her nurses on the wards after dark and could often be seen after hours making additional rounds with her lamp to check on patients. The soldiers fondly referred to her as "Birdie." These extra efforts earned her the title "the Lady with the Lamp" as immortalized in Longfellow's poem "Santa Filomena" (Box 7-1).

MARY SEACOLE; HONORED FOR HER WORK

Nightingale had help during many of those nights. Mary Seacole, a nurse from Jamaica, also played an important role in the history of nursing. She used her own money to build a lodging house in Crimea and turned the second floor of it into a hospital, where she nursed the soldiers. Seacole was especially knowledgeable about tropical medicine and used herbs and natural plant medicines to treat patients with cholera, yellow fever, malaria, and diarrhea. At the end of her day, she would go to the barracks hospital and offer her help to Nightingale. They worked side by side caring for the soldiers. Both Seacole's government and the British Commonwealth honored her for the lives she saved (Cherry and Jacob, 2011).

DEATH RATE DROPS; NIGHTINGALE DECORATED

After 6 months, it was obvious that the efforts of Nightingale and her nurses were paying off. The death rate among the wounded dropped from 420 deaths per 1000 casualties to 22 per 1000. She stayed through the war and was the last to leave. Many of her nurses had become ill during the war and were sent home to recover. Nightingale became ill with Crimean fever, probably typhus, and almost died. When she returned home, Queen Victoria decorated her for her efforts in the war.

Box 7-1	Santa Filomena

Whene'er a noble deed is wrought,
Whene'er is spoken a noble thought,
Our hearts, in glad surprise,
To higher levels rise.
The tidal wave of deeper souls
Into our inmost being rolls,
And lifts us unawares
Out of all meaner cares.
Honor to those whose words or deeds
Thus help us in our daily needs,
And by their overflow
Raise us from what is low!
Thus thought I, as by night I read
Of the great army of the dead.
The trenches cold and damp,
The starved and frozen camp—
The wounded from the frozen plain,
In dreary hospitals of pain—
The cheerless corridors,
The cold and stony floors,
Lo! in the house of misery,
A lady with a lamp I see
Pass through the glimmering gloom,

And flit from room to room.
And slow, as in a dream of bliss,
The speechless sufferer turns to kiss
Her shadow, as it falls
Upon the darkening walls.
As if a door in heaven should be,
Opened, and then closed suddenly,
The vision came and went—
The light shone and was spent.
On England's annals, through the long
Hereafter of her speech and song.
That light its rays shall cast
From portals of the past.
A lady with a lamp shall stand
In the great history of the land,
A noble type of good,
Heroic womanhood.
Not even shall be wanting here
The palm, the lily, and the spear.
The symbols that of yore
Saint Filomena bore.

—*Henry Wadsworth Longfellow*

NIGHTINGALE ESTABLISHES FIRST SCHOOL OF NURSING IN ENGLAND

One of Nightingale's major goals was to establish a school of nursing in England. An overwhelming number of physicians opposed such a school. Their opposition was that "because nurses occupied much the same positions as housemaids, they needed little instruction beyond poultice making, the enforcement of cleanliness, and attention to their patients' personal needs" (Kalish and Kalish, 1995). In 1860, Nightingale established the Nightingale Training School at St. Thomas Hospital in England. It was a 1-year program. She chose this site because of the hospital's reputation for progressive medical care. The school was independent from the hospital and financially independent as well. She believed nurses should work only in hospitals, not in private duty. Nightingale had strict admission standards that emphasized high moral character and intelligence. She was strict with her nursing students. They were locked up at night as a way to assure the middle-class parents that their daughters were safe from harassment. Upon graduation, she gave the nurses gifts of books and invited them to tea. When her graduates went to work in far-off places, she sent flowers to welcome them to their new home (Romanoff, 2006).

Nightingale's personal and nursing decisions reflected the influence of works by Plato and Hippocrates. Examples include her decision to remain single, her sense of mission, her concern with patient environment, her focus on the whole patient, and her belief in the need for keen observation and assisting nature to heal the patient (LeVasseur, 1998). Nightingale wrote over 200 publications, the most famous of which is *Notes on Nursing*. Although she was reclusive, she was influential in matters of military and public health policy because she kept such precise notes, which included statistics. She even advised the American secretary of war how to set up hospitals for the wounded during the Civil War.

NIGHTINGALE'S CORE BELIEF ABOUT NURSING

The core of Nightingale's spirituality was a belief in perfection. To her, nursing was a sacred calling, a commitment to work for mankind, not a business. Other Victorian women like her shared the sense of the sacredness of time and belief that wasting time was a sin. Nursing became a way for Florence Nightingale to work toward the perfection of mankind and her personal salvation. She was against licensure. To her it was too much like nurses being in a union. She eliminated prejudice against a better class of women entering nursing and created a push toward the development of nursing as a respectable vocation.

Nightingale was intelligent, well educated, and skeptical. This combination made her the foremost critic of the meaning of nursing and the nursing role. She continued to be involved in health policy well into her eighties. She was the first woman to receive the Order of Merit from the King of England. In 1910, she died in her sleep of heart failure at age 90. The government offered to bury her at Westminster Abbey, but according to her wishes, she was buried in the family plot at East Wellow, Hampshire. The marker reads, "F.N. Born 12 May 1820. Died 13 August 1910."

In 1893, Lystra Gretter, the principal of Farrand Training School in Detroit, and a committee modified the Hippocratic Oath. They named it the "Nightingale Pledge" as a token of esteem for the founder of modern nursing. It continues to be recited in many schools during graduation, primarily because of the mistaken belief that Nightingale wrote it. It reads as follows:

> I solemnly pledge myself before God and in the presence of this assembly, to pass my life in purity and to practice my profession faithfully. I will abstain from whatever is deleterious and mischievous, and will do all in my power to maintain and elevate the standard of my profession, and will hold in confidence all personal matters committed to my keeping and all family affairs coming to my knowledge in the practice of my calling. With loyalty will I endeavor to aid the physician in his work, and devote myself to the welfare of those committed to my care.

? Critical Thinking

Nightingale Pledge and Nursing

Review the Nightingale Pledge. Does it apply to the practical/vocational nurse in the twenty-first century? If you were to make changes, what would they be?

NIGHTINGALE MUSEUM ON THE SITE OF HER SCHOOL OF NURSING

In the spring of 1989, the Florence Nightingale Museum opened in London on the grounds of St. Thomas Hospital, the site of the Nightingale School of Nursing. The museum is a tribute to this nursing leader, despite the fact that she wrote in her journal, "I do not wish to be remembered when I am gone." Despite her great and courageous contributions to nursing, Florence Nightingale saw only her own faults and her failures.

? Critical Thinking

Nursing—Vocation or Profession?

What would Florence Nightingale say to nurse applicants today who say they are entering nursing to "help" people, to get a job, or to make money? Have we matured as a vocation or as a profession? What do you think?

EARLY TRAINING SCHOOLS IN AMERICA

Nurses in America were scarce and poorly trained. In 1849, Pastor Fliedner of Germany, who helped establish the first hospital and nursing school in Europe, came to America with four of his highly trained deaconesses. While Pastor Fliedner was involved with establishing the first Protestant hospital in America, the deaconesses started the first formal training program for nurses in the United States. The hospital, known as the Pittsburgh Infirmary, still exists in Pennsylvania as the Passavant Hospital. The training program was separate from the hospital with the intent being to educate nurses.

As the nursing shortage continued, hospital-based schools of nursing emerged as a cost-effective (i.e., free) labor force for the hospitals. The living conditions and the long hours required a great deal of physical and emotional endurance of the students.

CIVIL WAR (1861—1865)

In the 1800s, women who worked in hospitals, particularly in the South, were victims of deep prejudice from men in general and especially from the medical profession. As one southern woman put it, "It seems strange that what the aristocratic women of Great Britain have done with honor is a disgrace for their sisters on this side of the Atlantic to do" (Kalish and Kalish, 1995).

Casualties were high on both sides during the Civil War. Many soldiers died right on the field, and others died because of a poorly trained medical corps. Southern women offered their services as volunteers, but most of the nursing was done by infantrymen assigned to do a task they did not want to do. It was many months before the Confederate government recognized southern women for their contributions (Figure 7-2).

In the North during the Civil War, women offered their services as nurses to the government. One hundred women were selected to take a short training course from doctors in New York. Dorothea Lynde Dix, a teacher by profession, was appointed Superintendent of Nurses. Her task was to organize a corps of female nurses. She would recruit only women who were younger than age 30 and plain looking; they wore simple brown or black dresses and were forbidden

FIGURE 7-2 Nursing in the Civil War (wood engraving).

to wear hoop skirts or jewelry. Women who did not meet these criteria nursed anyway but without official recognition or pay from the government.

When they examined the nursing during the Civil War, doctors decided that the nursing system was defective. They did not approve of the women involved. However, it was a success in the eyes of the wounded soldiers. A longtime advocate for better conditions for those who suffered from mental illness, Dix went on to establish the first hospital for the mentally ill.

CLARA BARTON

Clara Barton, a teacher by profession, was one of the first civilians in the Civil War to round up army supplies. She rented a warehouse, filled market baskets, and encouraged friends to send food, blankets, and other supplies for the soldiers. Her efforts resulted in her being appointed Superintendent of the Department of Nurses for the Army in 1864. Clara Barton's efforts frequently found her on the front lines, and she nearly lost her life on two occasions. After the war, President Andrew Johnson commissioned her to do what she wanted to do: find missing prisoners of war. Later, while visiting in Europe for health reasons, she met J. Henri Dunant, founder of the International Red Cross. He asked for her help in introducing the Red Cross to America. Through Barton's efforts, the first chapter of the American Red Cross was established in Danville, New York, in 1881.

Critical Thinking

What is the relationship between the American Red Cross and nursing?

FORMAL TRAINING: PRACTICAL NURSING

In 1893, the Ballard School under the auspices of the YWCA opened the first formal practical nurse program in Brooklyn, New York. The course lasted 3 months and focused on home health care for the chronically ill, invalids, children, and the elderly. It included cooking, nutrition, basic sciences, and basic nursing procedures. The graduates were referred to as attendant nurses. Other similar schools include the Thompson School for Practical Nursing, which opened in Brattleboro, Vermont, in 1907 and still operates and is accredited by the NLN, and the Household Nursing Association School of Attendant Nursing, which opened in Boston in 1918. The Household School later changed its name to the Shepard-Gill School of Practical Nursing. The focus continued to be home nursing and light housekeeping duties. Hospital experience was not a part of the early programs. Before 1940, there were few controls, little education, practically no planning, and minimal supervision.

Critical Thinking

The name for practical and vocational nursing has changed through the years. If you could change it one more time, what would you name it?

NURSING IN THE HOME

Before World War I, most nursing done by practical nurses was home nursing, primarily because most people were cared for in the home. Even operations were performed in the home. There is some truth to how old Western movies portrayed surgery on the kitchen table. The nurse's 24-hour schedule included such procedures as cupping and applying leeches; preparing stupes for relief of abdominal distention, mustard plasters for relief of congestion, and poultices for drawing out pus from infections; and administering enemas. These were often nutritive enemas that contained eggnog with brandy or chicken broth. Intravenous infusions did not exist. Some practical nurses also assumed the then-accepted role of midwife. They taught new mothers the basics of cleanliness, diet, and child care (Figure 7-3). Approximately 1700 midwives attended 30% of all births in New York in 1919.

FROM HOME TO PUBLIC HEALTH NURSING

By the end of the nineteenth century, there was renewed interest in charitable work and concern for the sick. Practical nursing began to expand from home nursing to public health nursing, care of patients in the slums, school nursing, industrial nursing, and well-baby care. Once again, practical nurses pioneered in this new public health movement.

One of the best-known centers in 1893 was the Henry Street Settlement in New York. Lillian Wald, a social worker, graduated from nursing school and

FIGURE 7-3 Public health nursing follow-up visits.

intended to become a doctor. Wald taught home nursing to immigrants and was so impressed by their need for medical care that she left medical school to begin a nursing service, the Henry Street Settlement. Practical nurses who were members of the Henry Street Settlement taught families in New York slums the basics of cleanliness and control of communicable diseases. There was a decrease in school absenteeism because the spread of childhood illness was reduced. School nurses visited schools and new mothers and their babies. They taught mothers the basics of preventing the summertime killer of infants: cholera infantum. It was estimated that their efforts resulted in the survival of 1200 more babies than usual during the hot summer months. Another original contribution of the nurses was the development of "Little Mother Leagues" in the slums, in which all girls older than age 8 were taught how to take care of their younger siblings, including the infants.

TWENTIETH CENTURY

Practical nursing evolved to meet the nursing shortage and to make better use of nursing personnel. By 1903, states began to take steps that ultimately led to monitoring of practical nursing. During this period, nursing organizations were developed. The National League of Nursing Education (now the National League for Nursing, or NLN) took the most influential step. In 1917, the league developed a nationwide system of standardization of nursing requirements for practical nursing.

MISSISSIPPI: FIRST TO LICENSE PRACTICAL NURSES

In 1914, Mississippi was the first state to pass a law licensing practical nurses. This was an important event because the public had no way of knowing who was providing nursing care. For centuries self-proclaimed nurses were responsible for the majority of the nursing that was done. Licensing, however, was not mandatory, and by 1938, New York was the only state to have mandatory licensure.

> ### ? Critical Thinking
>
> **State License**
>
> Does your state have mandatory licensure? What year did it begin?

WORLD WAR I NURSES 1914-1918

The history of nursing is also the history of war and hard-fought women's rights. Women were considered fragile and delicate and kept at home to raise their babies and keep house. World War I made it necessary for women to work outside the home so men could go to war. Poster campaigns depicted the glamour of war in order to get young women to sign up as doctors and nurses to help with the war effort. Women were encouraged to be tough, but they still struggled with those who did not want women working outside of the home. Nurses had been part of wars in the past but never as part of the military. World War I was the first war where nurses had professional training in order to serve. America declared war on Germany in 1917, and it was evident that there were not enough nurses to serve. Jane Delano of the American Red Cross began to recruit nurses and train and equip them for overseas duty. About 20,000 nurses were assigned to go overseas, and many of them stayed overseas after the war to help with the postwar relief programs (Figure 7-4).

The U.S. government insisted that only trained nurses could be sent to France with the Army. The reality was there were not enough nurses to meet both war and domestic needs. National nursing leaders M. Adelaide Nutting, Anna Goodrich, and Lillian Wald met and formed the National Emergency Committee on Nursing. As a result, the Vassar Training Camp was created to train college graduates in an intensive 3-month program to enter schools of nursing. Soon other universities began to offer similar nursing programs. In 1918, the Army School of Nursing was established at Walter Reed hospital in Washington, D.C. It extended similar programs to other military hospitals throughout the United States.

World War I nurses were not allowed to serve at the advanced dressing stations on the front lines, although some nurses showed up there. They served primarily in hospitals organized for treating the wounded: field hospitals, which were sometimes just behind the front; clearing hospitals (known as evacuation hospitals) that were 10 miles back from the front; and base hospitals, where all the wounded were eventually sent. They dealt primarily with communicable diseases, wounds, infections, shock, hemorrhage, and poison

FIGURE 7-4 The Sacred Twenty: the first 20 Navy nurses appointed in 1908.

gas inhalation, and they even performed minor surgeries. The work was long and exhausting, with deplorable conditions and few supplies. Young nurses were exposed to horrors the like of which they had never experienced—not the glamour that had been advertised on the posters.

At the peak of the war, 23,000 (some sources say 30,000) nurses were in service, and none held a military rank. Although governed by military discipline, they were neither officers nor enlisted personnel. Because of this, they had no authority to direct corpsmen or orderlies or to take on administrative duties. After the war, through an amendment to the National Defense Act, the Army Nurse Corps was given officer status. This did not increase their pay or allowance to that of their male counterparts.

There is no record of a nurse dying because of combat, but about 260 nurses died because of the influenza epidemic of 1918. Many women were recognized for their service with awards. Three nurses received the Distinguished Service Award, and four Navy nurses were awarded the Navy Cross. In her book *Nursing, the Finest Art*, Donahue (1985) states, "One of the four, Lenah S. Higbee, the second Superintendent of the Corps, from 1911 to 1923, had a destroyer named in her honor on January 1945. This was the first time a fighting ship was named after a woman in the military service."

World War I emphasized what nurses of that time were capable of accomplishing. It also highlighted the need for more and better-prepared nurses. Moving nursing into colleges and universities was a major step for nursing education. Admission standards for nursing schools were raised, and the expectations of graduates were increased.

It was the service of women in the military that gave the big push for women's rights: the Nineteenth Amendment, which was ratified in 1920. President Woodrow Wilson made a passionate plea to the Senate to pass the amendment. He pointed out how women were expected to work hard and make sacrifices without the privileges and rights men enjoyed.

An interesting accidental benefit of World War I was the invention of Kotex. A German-American chemist developed the item to use as dressings and bandages for European field hospitals. Red Cross nurses began to use the product as sanitary napkins and the idea caught on with a Neenah, Wisconsin company. They began manufacturing the product as a sanitary napkin in 1921 and sold it as uKotex.

Canadian Nurses in World War I

Unlike American nurses in the military, the Canadian nurses were given the designation of lieutenants in the army and were stationed at nursing care wards. Canadian nurses worked around the clock to treat the wounded, who were brought in on stretchers or just dragged in because no stretchers were available. They had thousands of wounded to care for and try to prevent the onset of infections. Many lives were saved because of the nurses' diligence.

The shortage of beds in the military hospitals often made it necessary to put the wounded on the floor. These men were the victims of the many hungry rats that overran the hospital and were hungry and fearless and not afraid to bite the wounded soldiers. A Hall of Honor was built in Ottawa, Canada, to remember and honor the Canadian nurses who stood so strong in times of such difficulty.

SMITH HUGHES ACT OF 1917

The home front was facing a battle of its own in 1917 and 1918, with a major epidemic of pneumonia in 1917 and a worldwide epidemic of Spanish influenza in 1918. The mortality rate was high, especially in 1918. The Smith Hughes Act of 1917 provided money for developing additional schools of practical nursing. The first high school vocational/practical nursing program opened at the Minneapolis Girls Vocational High School in 1919. However, the new schools could not supply nurses quickly enough to meet the severe shortage in the United States.

NURSES RETURN HOME: ACUTE NURSING SHORTAGE FOLLOWS WORLD WAR I

After the war, many nurses did not continue nursing. Some stayed overseas to help with relief efforts. This led to an acute shortage of nurses in the 1920s. Many more hospitals opened schools of nursing. Their real purpose was to provide staffing. Hospitals without schools were staffed heavily with untrained help.

From 1920 to 1940, six states made laws licensing practical nurses, but only a small number of practical nursing schools existed in the United States. Much of the nurse's work continued to be in public health agencies and visiting nurse associations.

DEPRESSION OF THE 1930s

During the Great Depression in the 1930s, many nurses lost their jobs or worked in hospitals for room and board rather than a salary. When it became fairly obvious that America was becoming involved in World War II, nursing leaders began to prepare for the need for nurses at all levels. They did not want to face the nursing shortage experienced during World War I. This was a monumental task because nursing had decreased in popularity as a vocation.

WORLD WAR II 1939–1945

Although World War II began in 1939, the United States was unofficially involved by offering Lend Lease, which gave war materials to Allied countries in exchange for being allowed to use Allied bases. Initially noncombatants, American aircraft and warships escorted merchant ships and protected them against U-boat attacks. When Pearl Harbor was attacked, the United States declared war the following day. World War II involved about 50 countries and resulted in major changes throughout the world.

When Pearl Harbor was bombed on December 7, 1941, there were fewer than 12,000 nurses on duty in the Army Nurse Corps. Few of them had military experience and knowledge of Army protocol. Fifteen 4-week training programs were developed for new nurses. The programs stressed Army protocol; military customs and courtesies; field sanitation; defenses against air, chemical, and mechanized attacks; personnel administration; requisitions and correspondence; and property responsibility. More than 27,330 newly inducted nurses graduated from the 15 programs.

It became quickly obvious that there were not enough trained personnel to administer anesthesia. More than 200 nurses enrolled in the 6-month course on how to administer inhalant anesthesia, blood and blood derivatives, and oxygen therapy and how to recognize and treat shock. Nurses specializing in psychiatric care were in great need. One of 12 patients in Army hospitals was admitted for psychiatric care. A 12-week course was developed by the surgeon general to teach nurses how to care for and medicate combatants with psychiatric disorders.

Approximately 59,000 American nurses served in the war. Army and Navy nurses served in both the European and Pacific theaters. They were closer to the front than in past wars. Nurses were assigned to field hospitals, evacuation hospitals, hospital ships, and as flight nurses on medical transport planes. Because of the care combatants received in field hospitals or during evacuation, fewer than 4% died from wounds or disease. The demand for nurses in the Army and Navy Nurse Corps helped create a nursing shortage at home. In 1943, Congress passed the Bolton Act, which became the basis for the Cadet Nurse Corps. The government subsidized schools that were willing to teach primary nursing skills in 2½ years. More than 150,000 nurses graduated from these programs. The Cadet Nurse programs were discontinued in 1948, but the public considered these programs a great success.

When the war ended, the Army was still segregated and still had a quota system for black nurses. Only 479 nurses of the 50,000 serving in the Army Nurse Corps were black nurses, and they were limited to taking care of black troops in black hospitals. The Army dropped its quota system in 1944 because of the negative public reaction. By the end of the war, black nurses had served in Africa, England, Burma, and the Southwest Pacific. Federal funding for the Cadet Nurse Corps made it possible for 2000 black students to enroll in the Cadet Nurse program.

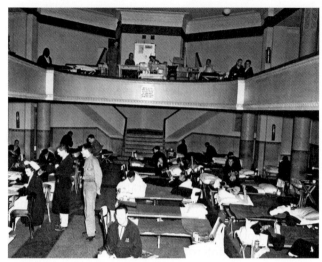

FIGURE 7-5 Eighth Evacuation Hospital situated in the auditorium of a former Italian school, Casablanca, French Morocco.

Practical nurses played a significant role both at home and in World War II. At home, practical nurses worked in clinics, health departments, industries, and hospitals. At the battlefields, practical nurses and registered nurses could be found in both the European and Pacific theaters (Figure 7-5). Some officers were initially reluctant to have nurses assigned at combat zones. The dedication, organization, and professionalism proved their worth and won the respect of doctors, corpsmen, patients, and military command. Nurses adjusted to long hours with little rest, loss of electricity, bombings, kamikaze attacks, frequent moves and setting up of field hospitals, internment in concentration camps, deaths of patients and other nurses, wounds and diseases, and dealing with members of numerous cultures. It was noted that nurses adjusted to difficult and dangerous situations with a minimum of complaints.

Nurses received 1619 medals, citations, and commendations during the war, 16 of them posthumously to nurses who died as a result of enemy fire. After the war, nurses were eligible for the G.I. Bill of Rights that entitled them to continue their education paid for by the government.

PRACTICAL NURSING RESPONSIBILITIES INCREASE AFTER WORLD WAR II

The end of World War II saw a continuing shortage of nurses. This shortage helped practical nurses play an important part in hospital nursing. Most hospitals gradually increased the responsibilities designated for the practical nurse. By the 1940s, there were nearly 50 approved practical nursing programs in the United States. The number of practical nurses in America peaked at 159,009 in 1940. By 1944, practical nursing was already experiencing a decline.

PRACTICAL NURSING DUTIES OUTLINED

In 1944, the U.S. Department of Vocational Education made a comprehensive study of practical nursing. This marked the first time that tasks of practical nursing were agreed on. Extensive specific duties were outlined, with an emphasis on maintaining aseptic technique. The phrases "to judge," "to appraise," "to recognize," and "to determine" were often used to describe the scope of the practical nurse's job.

RN AND LPN TASKS DIFFERENTIATED

Other important changes followed. In 1949, the Joint Committee on Practical Nurses and Auxiliary Workers in Nursing Services recommended use of the title "licensed practical nurse." Furthermore, the committee differentiated between the tasks of the RN and the LPN. They saw the LPN as being under the supervision of the RN. The committee also suggested that practical nurses organize to make decisions on their salary, working conditions, and employment standards.

Because of the work of the Joint Committee, many practical nursing programs were strengthened with regard to content. They focused for the first time on the preparation of practical nursing instructors. Up to this point, any graduate nurse was eligible to teach practical nursing. During the 1950s, the number of programs continued to increase, and programs were extended to 9-, 12-, and 18-month programs.

THE KOREAN CONFLICT (also known as United Nations Police Action or the Second Indochina War) 1950—1953

Many in the military believed that women had no place in the military. The term used was *demilitarization*, and it took place rapidly after WWII. Many women lost their jobs in industry. Many reasons were given for sending women back to the kitchen, but one reason not discussed openly was that men would have difficulty taking orders from women if they became officers. It took 3 years for the government to determine that women were an integral part of the military. General Eisenhower finally helped clear up the question by strongly recommending that women become a part of the U.S. military. Several senior officers who had worked with women during WWII had great praise for military women. This led to President Truman signing the Women's Armed Forces Act in 1948. By the time North Korea invaded South Korea, the number of women in the military was at an all-time low.

The United States entered the United Nations Police Action to support their ally South Korea when North Korea crossed the thirty-ninth parallel and invaded the Republic of South Korea. Because of the shortage of nurses in the military, nurses were recruited from civilian hospitals. According to records, 540 Army nurses served in Korea, and none died as a result of enemy action. Of the 3081 active-duty Navy nurses and 1702 reserve Navy nurses, according to records, none were killed or wounded due to enemy action. The Navy nurses served on three troop ships in both U.S. and overseas hospitals. Army nurses cared for wounded in Mobile Army Surgical Hospital units (MASH), prisoner of war camps, makeshift shelters, and hospital trains. Nurses were known for serving in MASH units where their responsibility was beyond that of the usual nurse. The shortage of medical personnel pushed them into doing work past their scope of nursing and into advanced practice. One such task was that of first assistant in surgery, which has now become an accepted part of RN advanced practice (RNFA) nursing (Figure 7-6).

Nurses also worked as flight nurses on evacuation aircraft. One of the women who served was Lillian Kinkela-Keil, a member of the Air Force Nurse Corps and one of the most decorated women in the U.S. military. Captain Kinkela-Keil flew over 200 air evacuation missions during WWII, as well as 25 transatlantic crossings. She went back to civilian flying with United Airlines after the war, but when the Korean Conflict erupted, she donned her uniform once more and flew several hundred more missions as a flight nurse in Korea.

Captain Kinkela-Keil was the inspiration for the 1953 movie *Flight Nurse* and served as technical advisor to the film. Her decorations include the European Theater of Operations with Four Battle Stars, the Air Medal with Three Oak Leaf Clusters, the Presidential Unit Citation with One Oak Leaf Cluster, the Korean Service Medal with Seven Battle Stars, the American Campaign Medal, the United Defense Medal, and the Presidential Citation, Republic of Korea. Captain Kinkel-Keil died in 2005 at age 88 (Wilson, 2011).

FIGURE 7-6 In the Korean conflict, a wounded soldier receives medical attention while lying on a stretcher. A soldier is being helped up the hill by another soldier, while a third soldier looks on.

The Korean War is called "the forgotten war." The men and women who served were forgotten, as was the war itself. Finding records and information about the war is also difficult. Little factual information is available to the public.

RNS REACT

By 1952, nearly 60% of the nursing workforce was made up of practical nurses. In many instances, RNs expressed bitterness because hospitals, clinics, and other agencies were hiring practical nurses for less money and assigning tasks to them beyond their educational level. RNs also expressed concern that the public was unable to differentiate between the levels of nurses. Both wore the same type of white uniforms, caps, and pins. Many practical nurses quickly stopped wearing the practical nursing insignia, which was meant to identify the practical nurse. LPN/LVNs performed tasks belonging to the RN one day and those belonging to nursing aides the next day. Many practical nurses felt trapped in such situations because of their need for employment.

PUBLIC LAW 911

In 1956, Public Law 911 provided for millions of dollars to expand and improve practical nursing programs. By 1975, there were 1337 programs, which graduated a total of 46,080 practical nurses. Approximately two-thirds of the practical nurses were employed in hospitals, 17.3% in nursing homes, 7.5% in private duty, and 6.5% in doctors' offices, clinics, and dental offices. Admission standards in most schools increased, as did the difficulty of the curriculum. Levels of nursing temporarily gained momentum.

THE VIETNAM WAR 1961–1973

The Vietnam War (1961–1973) was the longest war involving U.S. military forces. Numbers vary, but it is thought that about 7484 (79% female, 21% male) nurses served in the war (Martinez, 2010). All of the nurses volunteered and underwent a 6-week basic training course prior to being assigned to a 1-year stint in Vietnam. Assignments were primarily in Vietnamese hospitals, MASH units, as flight nurses, and on board the hospital ships USS *Repose* and *Sanctuary*. Most of the nurses were in their early twenties and recent graduates with less than 6 months of clinical experience.

Some nurses signed up when they learned that if they signed up for 2 years, their schooling would be paid for and they would receive free medical and dental care. Some saw it as an opportunity to travel and get away from their life at home. Some nurses signed up because of patriotism.

Living conditions varied from bug-infested tents to air-conditioned trailers to small, single-occupant rooms. Nurses in field hospitals wore white duty uniforms, and the rest of the medical personnel wore lightweight olive drab made of cotton poplin. It was difficult to keep uniforms clean, and nurses preferred to wear fatigues when available.

Nurses performed duties beyond what they had learned in nursing school. The 6-month basic training did not help the nurses deal physically or emotionally for what they would face. Shifts varied from 12 hours on and 12 hours off, 6 days a week. Days off were often canceled out of necessity when massive casualties arrived. Combat injuries were different in this war. Artillery was specifically designed to inflict massive, multiple injuries. Napalm, white phosphorous, and "antipersonnel" bombs were used as well. Napalm and white phosphorous burned tissue right down to the bone. Nurses described their orientation as being thrown into a "bloody hell" (Carlson, 2010). Nurses treated wounds they had never seen, did tasks beyond their nursing scope of practice, and dealt with illnesses such as typhoid, malaria, dengue fever, and bubonic plague. As in other wars, approximately 69% of admissions were for disease. In this war it was malaria, viral hepatitis, skin diseases, venereal diseases, diarrheal diseases, and diseases of unknown origin. The rest were combat casualties. Assault rifles, rocket-propelled grenades, and booby traps were the major causes of wounds. Infection resulting from animal and human excreta in the paddy fields and waterways created additional problems in treatment.

As the war continued, service personnel were also being treated for drug addiction—especially heroin. Nurses had to deal with soldiers under the influence of illicit drugs. Nurses were told to control their emotions when dealing with severely wounded and dying soldiers but not reassure a soldier that everything would be fine when he was fatally wounded. The hospital mortality rate was 2.6% per thousand in the Vietnam War compared to 4.5% during World War II.

In addition to practicing all the specialties, nurses also voluntarily gave medical assistance to Vietnamese civilians. This included basic care, immunizations, courses in child care, and sick calls at orphanages (Figure 7-7).

Mildred I. Clark, chief of the Army Nurse Corps from 1963 to 1967, and Anna Mae Hays, chief of the Army Nurse Corps from 1967 to 1971, led the Army Nurse Corps during the Vietnam War. On June 11, 1970, Colonel Hays also became a brigadier general, the first woman and the first nurse in American military to attain general officer rank (West, Army Nurse Corps Historian).

Women were treated as second-class citizens both in the military and when they came home. Nurses suffered from posttraumatic stress disorder (PTSD), experiencing feelings of isolation and anger. They had difficulty finding employment and suffered bouts of crying and depression. Vietnam veterans found it

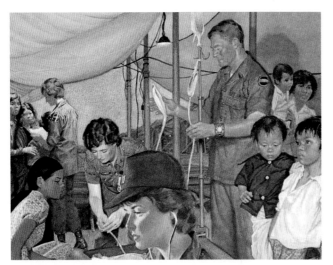

FIGURE 7-7 The American Soldier, 1975. In the foreground, as concerned relatives look on, an Army nurse checks an injured Vietnamese citizen. The scene is typical of many long evenings in tents set up as emergency medical stations on Guam, the first stop for the refugees.

difficult to receive treatment, and both men and women were treated badly by many in the public.

The Vietnam Women's Memorial, designed and sculpted by Glenna Goodacres, is on the National Mall in Washington, D.C. It is located at the south end of the Vietnam Veteran's Memorial and in the vicinity of the Three Servicemen memorial. The Goodacres monument shows three nurses in battle dress. One comforts a wounded or perhaps dying soldier, one is kneeling, and one is looking up in expectation.

? Critical Thinking

Preventing Posttraumatic Stress Disorder

If you were to join the military as a nurse and had to go into a war area, how would you prepare yourself to deal emotionally with the challenges you will face as a military nurse?

AMERICAN NURSES ASSOCIATION MOVEMENT TOWARD TWO LEVELS OF NURSING

In 1965, the American Nurses Association (ANA) presented a position paper outlining how to solve the issues of the levels of nursing. They recommended that all RNs graduate from a 4-year collegiate program and all LPNs graduate from a 2-year technical program. Many hospital-based RN programs closed during that time. In the 1980s, a resurgence of the ANA 1965 movement toward establishing two levels of nursing temporarily gained momentum. Some states worked toward adopting the ANA recommendations. North Dakota made the change to a 2-year practical nursing program and a 4-year BSN professional nursing program. Because a serious nursing shortage developed in the late 1980s, the ANA movement stalled in other states.

AFGHAN WAR (also known as Operation Enduring Freedom) 2001-PRESENT and the IRAQ WAR (also known as Operation Iraqi Freedom, Second Gulf War and more recently Operation New Dawn) 2003—DECEMBER 2011

The wars in Afghanistan and Iraq continue at this writing. The U.S. involvement in the Afghanistan war (2001) was as a result of the attacks on the Twin Towers in New York City on September 11, 2001. The war in Iraq (2003) began as a result of a belief that Iraq had weapons of mass destruction, which it did not. Very little has been written about nurses' experiences in Afghanistan and Iraq.

The Air Force sent 4060 active-duty, guard, and reserve nurses to Afghanistan and Iraq. Since 2003, the U.S. Navy has deployed 1193 nurses to Iraq and 403 nurses to Afghanistan. Since 2007, 114 nurses have been deployed as part of the International Security Assistance Force in Afghanistan (Bolvin, 2010). They quickly helped set up surgical teams and mobile hospitals to receive casualties (Figure 7-8). Issues arose regarding the lack of critical care nursing experience and the lack of experience using some equipment before deployment. Nurses are also assigned to air evacuation units, combat support units in Afghan and Iraqi hospitals, and hospitals for detainees. Living quarters vary from tents to primitive plywood shacks to container housing, depending on where they are sent. A layer of fine sand covers everything, showers are scarce, and feeling dirty all the time is common. Sanitation and sewer systems are scarce, and with the high temperatures, the smell of sewage is often in the air.

FIGURE 7-8 Barbara Smith, U.S. Army Garrison Wiesbaden occupational health nurse, leads a combat lifesaver training course in Afghanistan.

Some nurses described Afghanistan and Iraq as noisy, smelly places. It is not unusual to burn excreta and surgical waste. At the beginning of the war, little food was available, and most meals consisted of ready-to-eat and water stored in containers that tasted like chlorine and was always warm because of the heat. This is a reason soldiers and medical people requested Kool-Aid and Crystal Light packets to add to the water (Desch and Doherty, 2010).

For nurses working in countries beyond our borders, being culturally sensitive when providing care to patients is an even greater issue. Patients' cultural preferences must be integrated into the plan of care. Nursing and medical care extends to America's wounded troops, civilians, National Army soldiers, and other coalition soldiers from around the world (Figure 7-9).

Although it is acceptable in Afghanistan for a male to be a nurse, male nurses may care for males only, and female nurses may care for female patients only. Families, when available, are involved in the care of hospitalized patients. Equipment and medicines are badly needed. Diarrheal illness is always an issue in the civilian community, as are malaria, parasites, polio, and a protozoan illness caused by sand flies (especially in children playing in the sand).

Troops experience severe injuries from mortar fire and roadside explosive devices, as well as gunfire. Approximately 2% to 4% of the troops experience gastrointestinal illness with nausea, vomiting, and diarrhea.

Although many nurses are not directly in harm's way, they are at risk for PTSD because of constant fear, exposure to trauma, and loss, ethical dilemmas, and fatigue (Bolvin, 2010). Each individual undergoes an assessment when he or she returns to this country. Sometimes symptoms do not appear until later, or the individual may have given wrong answers during his or her assessment. They may be concerned about how they will be viewed when they are back home. It is not unusual for a nurse to grieve the person he or she was prior to going to Afghanistan or Iraq. Others appreciate professional growth and all that they learned to do and deal with, and they believe nothing will ever be too challenging again. What seems to stand out for many nurses is the sense of camaraderie and teamwork experienced between the nurses and the doctors while overseas.

 Try This

If you know someone who is serving or has served in the Afghanistan or Iraq war, ask him or her about his/her feelings about nurses serving in the military.

AMERICAN MEDICAL ASSOCIATION MOVES TO EASE NURSING SHORTAGE

With the goal of easing the nursing shortage, in 1989, the American Medical Association (AMA) proposed a new health care worker: the registered care technologist (RCT). The RCT was to be trained in 1- and 2-year programs. Because this new level of health care worker correlated with existing personnel, the practical nurse and the associate degree nurse, the RCT proposal was not successful. This event is a gentle reminder for practical/vocational nurses to be strong, organized, and vigilant as a group. Changes in the health care system are occurring daily, as are opportunities for LPN/LVNs.

UNLICENSED ASSISTIVE PERSONNEL

During the 1990s, unlicensed assistive personnel (UAP) were hired to give patient care. A major concern for LPN/LVNs and RNs was their legal responsibility for the care given by the unlicensed caregivers. Meanwhile, primary employment for nurses, especially for the LPN/LVNs, moved out of hospitals and into the community.

FIRST COMPUTERIZED TESTING: NCLEX-PN®

In 1994, the first computerized adaptive testing (NCLEX-PN® examination) became available for the practical/vocational nursing graduate. The computer format provided an individualized test for each graduate, based on the answer to the previous question. It also excluded questions that were not within the nurse's role, according to their state's Nurse Practice Act.

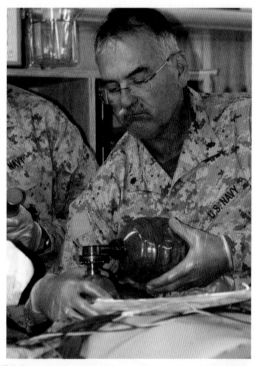

FIGURE 7-9 Commander Paul M. Barfknecht, emergency nurse, Shock Trauma Platoon, Health Service and Support Company, Combat Logistics Battalion 4, simulates pumping air into a patient during a mass casualty training exercise, March 2, 2009, at Camp Baharia, Iraq.

LONG-TERM CARE CERTIFICATION

In 1996, long-term care certification became available to LPN/LVNs in some states. Since that time, other certifications have become available for LPN/LVNs in some states (see Chapter 23).

TWENTY-FIRST CENTURY

Nursing organizations continue to define the responsibilities of the different levels of nursing. More remains to be resolved. Nursing shortages have created changes in nursing programs. Approximately 50 years ago, Associate Degree (AD) nursing programs were set up in technical schools, and they have flourished. Approximately 60% of the current RN workforce consists of AD RNs. The goals of AD programs were to move nursing education out of hospital-based programs and to help ease the shortage by shortening the amount of time required to become an RN. However, the AD graduate, diploma graduate, and baccalaureate graduate all take the same licensing examination to become an RN. It was and continues to be confusing for those doing the hiring at a facility, since all RNs, regardless of their education, can legally assume the same responsibilities. Finances are always a major concern for

health facilities. Years ago, when LPN/LVNs earned much less than RNs, more LPN/LVNs were hired. When salaries were narrowed and the difference in salary was considerably less, more RNs were hired.

Nursing organizations continue to work on resolving the issue of nursing levels and present new recommendations and position papers. Nursing shortages continue periodically. Changes in how health facilities are reimbursed for patient care have had major impacts on patient acuity, staffing ratios, overtime, patient care loads, and patient safety. The average age of the nurse workforce continues to increase.

IMPORTANT INFLUENCES IN NURSING HISTORY

Many RNs influenced the course of nursing and practical nursing history. Table 7-2 identifies some of those registered nurses and events in nursing history.

YOU HAVE COME A LONG WAY!

As a final note, it may be interesting to compare present practical/vocational nursing tasks with those that you would have been expected to perform in 1887. Practical/vocational nursing has indeed come a long way. The job description in Box 7-2 was given to floor nurses by a hospital in 1887 (author unknown).

Table 7-2 People and Events in Nursing History

Mary Robinson	1859	First visiting nurse.
Linda Richards	1873	America's first professionally trained nurse (1-year program); organized other training schools; developed a system of written records and orders.
Euphemia Van Rensselaer	1876	Introduced first uniform—apron and cap (Bellevue Training School for Nurses).
Mary E. P. Mahoney	1879	First African-American graduate nurse.
Clara Barton	1881	Established the American Red Cross.
Elizabeth Weston	1888	First American Indian nurse. Graduate of Training School of the University of Pennsylvania. Came from Lincoln School for Indian girls in Philadelphia. After graduation returned to care for her people on a Sioux reservation in North Dakota.
Emily L. Loveridge	1890	Graduate of Bellevue Training School for Nurses. Went west to establish first school of nursing in the Northwest at Good Samaritan Hospital, Portland, Oregon.
Mabel Staupers	1890-1989	First executive director and last president of the National Association of Colored Graduate Nurses. Credited with integration of African-American nurses into ANA and other nursing organizations. Wrote *No Time for Prejudice*.
Isabel Hampton Robb	1893	Wrote first substantial nursing text: *Nursing: Its Principles and Practice for Hospital and Private Use*. Promoted nurses' rights, 3-year training program, 8-hour day, and licensure.
Lillian Wald and Mary Brewster	1893	First visiting nurse service for the poor: Nurses Settlement House in slum section, Lower East Side, New York City. Later moved to Henry Street and name changed to Henry Street Settlement House.
Lavinia L. Dock	1896	First president of forerunner of ANA (Nurses Associated Alumnae of the United States and Canada). Wrote four-volume *History of Nursing* with Adelaide Nutting. Outlined principles on which ANA was founded.
Dita H. Kinney	1901	First Superintendent of Nurses of the Army Nurse Corps.

Continued

Table 7-2 People and Events in Nursing History—cont'd

Mrs. Bedford Fenwick (Great Britain)	1901	First president of International Council of Nurses. Proposed state registration of nurses.
Adelaide Nutting	1907	First graduate of Johns Hopkins Training School for Nurses. First nurse in the world to hold professorship in a university (Columbia). In 1917, chair of Committee to Develop National Curriculum.
Lillian Wald, Ella Phillips Crandall, Mary Beard, Mary Lent, Edna Foley, Lystra Greiter, Elizabeth G. Fox	1912	Formed National Organization of Public Health Nurses. Lillian Wald, first president.
Margaret Sanger	1916	A public health nurse, she spearheaded the birth control movement as a response to high maternal and child mortality. Opened first birth control clinic in America.
Annie W. Goodrich	1918	President of ANA. Became Chief Inspecting Nurse for army hospitals at home and abroad. Supported formation of Army School of Nursing. Second dean of school.
Lenah S. Higbee	1918	Second Superintendent of Army Nurse Corps from 1911 to 1923. Had destroyer named after her; first fighting ship to be named after a military woman.
	1924	U.S. Indian Bureau Nursing Service founded.
Mary Breckenridge	1925	Organized Frontier Nursing Service of Kentucky.
Sage Memorial Hospital School, Ganado, Arizona	1930	First school of nursing for American Indians.
Captain Lillian Kinkela-Keil		Flew air evacuation missions in WWII and again in Korean Conflict. Inspiration for movie *Flight Nurse*. Received numerous decorations.
Lucile Petry	1943	Director of U.S. Cadet Nurse Corps.
Esther Lucille Brown, a researcher	1948	"Brown" study: Advocated movement of nursing education to collegiate setting.
Mildred L. Montag	1952	Appointed as first associate degree Nursing Program Project Coordinator. Project based on Montag's doctoral thesis "Education of Nursing Technicians." Project located at Queens College, New York.
Vietnam War	1961-1973	Eisenhower recommended women become a part of the U.S. military.
Colonel Linda I. Clark	1963-1967	Chief of Army Nurse Corps.
Colonel Anna Mae Hays	1969-1971	Chief of Army Nurse Corps.
Colonel Anna Mae Hays	1970	Became first woman and nurse to be a brigadier general in the American military.

Box 7-2 Hospital Nursing 1887

In addition to caring for your 50 patients, each nurse will follow these regulations:
- Daily, sweep and mop the floors of your ward, dust the patient's furniture and window sills. Maintain an even temperature in your ward by bringing in a scuttle of coal for the day's business.
- Light is important to observe the patient's condition. Therefore, each day fill kerosene lamps, clean chimneys, and trim wicks. Wash the lamp windows once a week.
- The nurse's notes are important in aiding the physician's work. Make your pens carefully; you may whittle nibs to your individual taste.
- Each nurse on day duty will report every day at 7 AM and leave at 8 PM, except on the Sabbath, on which day you will be off from noon to 2 PM.

- Graduate nurses in good standing with the director of nurses will be given an evening off each week for courting purposes or two evenings a week if you go regularly to church.
- Each nurse should lay aside from each payday a goodly sum of her earnings for her benefits during her declining years so that she will not become a burden. For example, if you earn $30 a month, you should set aside $15.
- Any nurse who smokes, uses liquor in any form, gets her hair done at a beauty shop, or frequents dance halls will give the director of nurses good reason to suspect her worth, intentions, and integrity.
- The nurse who performs her labors and serves her patients and doctors without fault for 5 years will be given an increase of 5 cents a day, providing there are no hospital debts outstanding.

Get Ready for the NCLEX-PN® Examination

Key Points

- Varied and colorful evolution of practical nursing is described with limited reference to roles played by RNs in the course of nursing history.
- Duties have changed according to the needs present at various times in history.
- Currently, practical/vocational nurses are taught basic skills during their educational program.
- According to some states' Nurse Practice Act, LPN/LVNs are allowed to perform complex skills. An RN may teach complex skills, be satisfied with the LPN/LVN's performance, and document this in the LPN/LVN's file.
- Historical figures in nursing include Florence Nightingale, founder of modern nursing; Clara Barton, founder of the American Red Cross; Lillian Wald, founder of public health nursing; and Dorothea Lynde Dix, advocate for the mentally ill.
- Practical nurses have always been in the forefront of doing real, down-to-earth nursing tasks—often what no one else dared or cared to do.
- The quota for black nurses in the military was lifted in 1944 because of negative public opinion.
- Nurses have played a significant role in all wars and continue to do so in Afghanistan and Iraq. Each war has increased nursing knowledge and responsibility.

Additional Learning Resources

evolve Go to your Evolve website (http://evolve.elsevier.com/Hill/Success) for the following FREE learning resources:
- Answers to Critical Thinking Scenarios
- Additional learning activities
- Additional Review Questions for the NCLEX-PN® exam
- Helpful phrases for communicating in Spanish and more!

Review Questions for the NCLEX-PN® Examination

1. Which year did licensing for practical/vocational nursing begin?
   1. 1914
   2. 1919
   3. 1938
   4. 1907

2. Which statement relates to Florence Nightingale's contribution to nursing?
   1. She established the first visiting nurse service for the poor in the Lower East Side slum section of New York.
   2. She wrote the Nightingale Pledge in 1893 to set guidelines and inspire her nurses on graduation.
   3. She wrote the first substantial nursing text and promoted nursing rights, including the 8-hour day.
   4. She stressed environment, the need for careful observation, care of the whole person, and critical thinking.

3. Periodically, various organizations have suggested eliminating practical/vocational programs. Which statement objectively provides a reason for continuing the LPN/LVN programs?
   1. LPN/LVNs possess the same level of skill in patient care as do registered nurses.
   2. RN education is more focused on nursing theory and less on patient bedside care.
   3. LPN/LVN programs evolved to make better use of nursing personnel.
   4. Physicians prefer to work with LPN/LVNs because they follow orders without question.

4. Which statement most closely reflects the experience of nurses in war?
   1. Nursing expectations are according to what their state Nurse Practice Act permits them to do.
   2. The quota for black nurses in the military was dropped during the latter part of World War II.
   3. Nurses receive intensive training prior to deployment regarding expectations at the front.
   4. Nurses are able to keep equipment and surgical tools sterile during surgical procedures.

Alternate Format Item

1. Which experiences are true for military nurses in Afghanistan and Iraq? (Select all that apply.)
   1. Male nurses are assigned to MASH units, and female nurses are assigned to hospitals.
   2. Afghan and Iraqi nurses experience limited responsibility and respect in their facilities.
   3. Extreme heat makes work conditions difficult, and nurses usually experience fatigue.
   4. Cultural sensitivity is a nonissue during care of civilians because of being in the military.

2. Identify possible reasons why a nurse involved in care of soldiers in the war zone may develop PTSD. (Select all that apply.)
   1. Told to do tasks that are out of their scope of practice.
   2. Limited training in what to expect before shipping out.
   3. Faced with caring for patients with gruesome injuries.
   4. Lack of personal amenities available in civilian life.

Critical Thinking Scenarios

Scenario 1

Pamela wants to travel in search of "adventure." She will be graduating from a practical nursing program in July and wants to join the military right away to get started on her dream. Pamela has been doing it her way most of her young life, but you are one of the few people to whom she might listen. Explain your critical thinking to make a plan of what you will suggest to Pamela.

Scenario 2

Jon has been accepted into the practical nursing program. He is intelligent, but he lacks emotional maturity. He lived under strict rules while at home. Now that he is living away from home, he has decided to make up for the "good times I missed." He confides in his sister that this program is a "pussycat," and he will "ace it with no problem." Jon has decided that nothing is going to get in the way of his party time anymore. His sister has a friend who has graduated from the same program and knows it will take a lot of work and study time. Jon will probably flunk out if he does what he says he is going to do. What might his sister say to Jon?

Critical Thinking: A Lifelong Journey

Objectives

On completing this chapter, you will be able to do the following:

1. Discuss the difference between nonfocused and directed thinking.
2. Explain what makes critical thinking an advanced way of thinking.
3. Use techniques that enhance the understanding of information needed to be a practical/vocational nurse.
4. Differentiate among the terms *knowledge, comprehension (understanding), application,* and *analysis.*
5. Evaluate your personal need for help in comprehending information.
6. Identify two new suggestions for increasing reading effectiveness that you will begin to apply immediately.
7. Develop a plan using critical thinking to increase your ability to think critically.

Key Terms

analysis (ă-NĂL-1-sĭs, p. 94)
application (ĂP-lĭ-KĂ-shŭn, p. 94)
attitude (ĂT-ĭ-ood, p. 92)
capability (KĂ-pă-BĬL-ĭ-tē, p. 93)
cognitive levels (KŎG-nĭ-tĭv, p. 94)
comprehension (KŎM-prē-HĔN-shŭn, p. 94)

critical thinking (KRĬT-ĭ-căl, p. 90)
directed (or focused) thinking (dĭ-RĔCT-ĕd, p. 90)
knowledge (NŎL-ĕj, p. 94)
problem-oriented thinking (prŏ-blĕm ŎR-ē-ĕn-tĕd, p. 90)
reflective thinking (rē-FLĔK-tĭv, p. 95)

 Keep in Mind

Become an active learner and critical thinker, and be successful in the practical/vocational nursing program, on NCLEX-PN®, and as a candidate for a job you love as an LPN/LVN.

OVERVIEW OF CRITICAL THINKING

The following are the *Top 10 Reasons to Improve Thinking,* adapted for practical/vocational nurses:*

10. Things are not what they used to be, or what they will be, in this changing health care system.
9. Licensed practical/vocational nurses (LPN/LVNs) frequently care for patients who are not yet stabilized and have multiple problems.
8. More patients and their families are involved in health care decisions.
7. LPN/LVNs must be able to move from one health care setting to another.
6. Rapid change and information explosion requires LPN/LVNs to develop new learning and workplace skills.
5. Patients, families, and insurance companies demand to see evidence of benefits, efficiency, and results of care given.
4. Today's progress often creates new problems that cannot be solved by old ways of thinking (e.g., ethical and legal issues involved in end-of-life decisions, questions regarding stem cell research, who is entitled to receive expensive medical care, and so on).
3. Redesigning care delivery and education programs is useless if students and nurses do not have the thinking skills required to deal with today's world.
2. Learning how to improve your thinking skills does not have to be difficult.
1. Your ability to focus your thinking on how to get the results you need can make the difference between whether you succeed or fail in the fast-paced health care system.

Years ago, nurses saw themselves as doers, not thinkers. Nurses were primarily directed what to do, and they carried out the orders. Certainly there were exceptions, such as Florence Nightingale and Mary Seacole, to name two historical pioneers in nursing. By 1996, the

---

*Adapted with permission from Alfaro-Lefevre R. (2009). *Critical thinking and clinical judgement: a practical approach* (4th ed.). Philadelphia: WB Saunders. (inside cover).

National Council of State Boards of Nursing (NCSBN) included four phases of the nursing process (no nursing diagnosis at this time) in the NCLEX-PN® examination. Nursing diagnosis is discussed in Chapter 9. Questions were at the cognitive level of knowledge, comprehension, and application (NCSBN, 1995). In 1999, the four phases were integrated throughout the test plan (NCSBN, 1998). By 2002, the NCSBN integrated all phases of the nursing process, as well as critical thinking, into the NCLEX-PN® examination. The cognitive level of analysis was added to NCLEX-PN® examination questions (NCSBN, 2001). The expectation was that both the nursing process and critical thinking would be taught to the practical/vocational nursing student (SPN/SVN). Critical thinking is an integral part of the nursing process. To do the nursing process, the work of nursing, is to have to think critically. Today nurses who cannot think critically become one of the problems, rather than the solution, in nursing.

 Professional Pointer

Critical thinking is a lifelong process (Alfaro-Lefevre, 2003).

WAYS OF THINKING

DEFINITION OF APPLIED CRITICAL THINKING

What exactly is *critical thinking*, and how does it relate to the nursing decisions you will make at school and during your career? Alfaro-Lefevre (2003) provides a definition of critical thinking and clinical judgment in nursing. Critical thinking in nursing, adapted for practical/vocational nursing, is defined as the following:*

- Entails purposeful, informed, outcome-focused (results-oriented) thinking that requires careful identification of the problems, issues, and risks involved (e.g., deciding whether a patient needs one or more staff to move from bed to chair in a manner that is safe for both patient and staff).
- Is driven by patient, family, and community needs. The practical/vocational nurse must be able to use knowledge to tailor approaches based on circumstances.
- Is based on the principles of the nursing process and on scientific methods—for example, making judgments based on evidence (facts) rather than guesswork. This is a major difference between LPN/LVNs and unlicensed assistive personnel (UAPs).
- Uses both logic and intuition, based on knowledge, skills, and experience of the LPN/LVN.

- Is guided by professional standards, such as those developed for the LPN/LVN by the National Association for Practical Nurse Education and Service (NAPNES) (see Appendix A), the National Federation of Licensed Practical Nurses (NFLPN) (see Appendix B), and the practical/vocational nursing code of ethics.
- Calls for strategies that make the most of human potential (e.g., using individual strengths) and compensates for problems created by human nature (e.g., overcoming the powerful influence of personal beliefs, values, and prejudices).
- Is constantly reevaluating, self-correcting, and striving to improve (e.g., practicing skills, learning new skills, attending classes, and workshops).

Thinking is divided into nonfocused thinking and directed thinking. At one time or another, most of us have used the following examples of thinking:

- **Nonfocused thinking:** You engaged your brain out of habit without much conscious thought.
- **Habitual thinking:** We get up to go to the bathroom, shower, dress, and so on. This type of thinking involves any routine we do that is important but does not require us to think hard about how to do it (automatic pilot).
- **Random thoughts:** Multiple short scenes and thoughts come and go through the mind and have no particular purpose or goal (mental channel surfing).
- **Ruminative thinking:** The same situation or scene is replayed in the mind over and over, without reaching an outcome (instant replay).
- **All-or-none thinking:** The mind is made up, and no additional facts will be considered (black-and-white thinking with no grays in between).
- **Negative thinking:** The mind is stuck on negative thoughts and blocks worthwhile thinking (emotional sabotage).
- Directed (or focused) thinking: Purposeful and outcome-oriented.
- Problem-oriented thinking: Focus on a particular problem to find a solution (e.g., planning your school, work, and home schedule). This could involve collecting information on school and work schedules and schedules of family members who rely on you. It might include delegating tasks, requesting help, making your goals known, and listening for input from those involved in the immediate situation (see Chapter 2). Once the schedule is developed, no further attention is given to the situation until another problem emerges (problem solving).
- **Critical thinking:** Critical thinking is an advanced way of thinking, a problem-solving method, and more. It is used to resolve problems and to find ways to improve a situation even when no problem exists. It answers the question "How can we do this better?"

*Adapted for practical/vocational nurses with permission from Alfaro-Lefevre R. (2006). *Evidence-based critical thinking indicators.* Available at: www.AlfaroTeachSmart.com.

Try This

Survey of your Current Level of Critical Thinking

Based on a scale of 0 to 10, with 0 as the lowest and 10 as the highest, rate each statement about thinking as it applies to you. Then list the items you rated as lowest.

___I identify the purpose of my thinking.
___My thinking is goal (or outcome) directed.
___I have an organized method of thinking.
___I question what I do not understand.
___I continually question: What does this mean? Is this useful? Is it fact?
___I question the reliability of sources and information available.
___I keep an open mind.
___My judgments are based on fact (evidence).

 Critical Thinking

Make a Personal Plan

1. Prioritize the critical-thinking items you need to work on from the previous learning exercise. Choose the items you think are most important to work on first.
2. Make a schedule and estimate the amount of time it will take to see progress. (We all need to work on critical thinking throughout our lives.)
3. Identify how you will determine what progress is being made.

CRITICAL THINKING AND PRACTICAL/VOCATIONAL NURSING

Critical thinking involves questioning with meaning. This type of thinking involves examining personal thinking and the thinking of others. Judgments are made on facts (evidence), not assumptions. The critical thinker avoids criticizing just for the sake of having his or her own way. Decisions are based on the right thing to do rather than emotions or a need to save face. New ideas and alternatives are offered in a constructive way. The thinker is willing to consider other ideas and recognizes that there may be more than one right way to do something. The thinker realizes that a perfect solution may not be possible.

Critical thinking is at its best when you have your brain purposefully engaged—for example, while you listen to a minilecture, view a video, play a CD-ROM, listen to a podcast, participate in a discussion or study group, or are being tutored. A critical thinker is paying attention to what the speaker is saying.

- Do I understand it?
- What does it all mean?
- Where does it all fit in?

You are examining your thinking and the thinking of others. Critical thinking is based on science and scientific principles. The principles include the following:

- Collecting data in an organized way
- Verifying the data in an organized way
- Arranging the data in an organized way

- Looking for gaps in information
- Analyzing the data
- Testing it out (Is the data purposeful and outcome/goal-oriented?)

These scientific principles align with the nursing process, as you will learn in Chapter 9. A major difference for the scientist is that a problem is identified and then data are collected. The nurse using the nursing process collects data first and then determines the nature of the problem (Ignatavicius and Workman, 2010). The critical thinker should routinely ask the following questions about the subject of the thinking task at hand (adapted from Alfaro-Lefevre, 2009):

1. What major outcomes (observable beneficial results) do you expect to achieve (e.g., when working with the RN to develop a care plan for a newly admitted patient)?
2. What problems, issues, or risks must be addressed to achieve the major outcome (e.g., the hospital unit you are working on is short-staffed)?
3. What is the circumstance or context (e.g., the LPN/LVN is working in the patient's home, where equipment will have to be improvised)?
4. What knowledge is required (e.g., in an area such as mental health, in which you did not have a clinical experience)?
5. How much room is there for error (e.g., the patient is positioned on his back as directed after surgery and begs to be on his side.)?
6. How much time do we have (e.g., the patient who was just admitted is bleeding profusely)?
7. What human and professional resources can help me/us (e.g., the patient is acutely ill and refuses care because of lack of insurance or adequate personal funds)?
8. What perspectives must be considered (e.g., the patient has refused to be examined because of religious beliefs)?
9. What is influencing my thinking (e.g., you are against abortion and do not want to take care of a patient hospitalized because of self-induced abortion)?
10. What must we do to prevent, manage, or eliminate the problems, issues, and risks identified with question 2?

For each element, the thinker—in this case the practical/vocational nurse—must be able to reflect on the 10 key critical-thinking questions that shed light on the effectiveness of his or her thinking. In other words, is the thinking solving the problem or finding the answer you are looking for? Critical thinking is an essential part of nursing. The overall purpose of nursing is to assist people to stay well or regain their maximum state of health as quickly as possible. Both purposes are to be achieved in a cost-effective manner and in a manner that fits with their belief system.

Box 8-1   **Ways to Challenge Yourself to Think Critically**

- Anticipate questions that the patient or instructor might ask.
- Ask for clarification of what you do not understand.
- Ask yourself if there is more that you can do.
- Reword in your own words what you have read or been told (e.g., stating a nursing diagnosis as a nursing problem).
- Make comparisons with something similar to help you understand.
- Organize information in more than one way to see if you have missed anything important. This is to avoid being impressed when the "facts" fall into place but you have missed the obvious.
- Ask your instructor to check out your conclusions.
- Strive for objectivity. Keep an open mind and avoid drawing conclusions in advance.
- Review all your data again, especially after a period of time. It may look different, and you may reach a different conclusion.
- Get used to saying, "I don't know, but I will find out."
- Learn from your mistakes. Fix them if you can. Do not hide an error. Someone's life may be at stake, and others can learn from your error.
- Think about what you are reading about while you are reading it. Ask your instructor or peer to challenge you to think critically while you are on the clinical area.

Nurses make decisions that affect both purposes. Nursing decisions must be accurate and based on sound thinking and data. As a nurse, your critical-thinking skill will vary according to your education and clinical experience. Box 8-1 lists suggestions to increase your critical thinking.

WHAT YOU NEED TO THINK CRITICALLY

For the practical/vocational nurse to think critically, it will be necessary to do the following:

1. Access information.
2. Comprehend (understand) information.
3. Store comprehended information in long-term memory. This includes having strategies to move information to long-term memory.
4. Recall the comprehended information when needed. (You will need to have the most important information in your head for patient care on clinical.)
5. Know what to do when information is not in long-term memory.

As a practical/vocational nursing student, you will be exposed to a great deal of new knowledge during the year in the practical/vocational nursing program. You will gain knowledge, as stated in the course objectives. Your real test as a practical/vocational nurse will be your ability to access information, understand that information, recall it, and use it as the basis for critical thinking in the clinical area.

FACTORS THAT INFLUENCE CRITICAL THINKING

Your current critical-thinking status is influenced by the following personal and situational factors:

- **Upbringing and culture.** Having family and teacher support and opportunities to learn to read well and understand the meaning of what you read; beginning to make simple, limited choices at an early age, which become more complex with consequences as you grow.
- **Motivation.** Whether you learned early to rely on others for motivation or decided you would learn in spite of the lack of external motivators, motivation determines in part the progress you have made in problem solving and critical thinking. You have the ability to think critically if you choose to do so. It is a preference on your part. Remember that the brain is like a muscle: The more you exercise it, the better it works.
- **Attitude influences thinking.** Critical thinkers are humble and recognize that they do not have all the answers and may be influenced by their beliefs and values. While in the process of patient care, it makes a critical difference whether a problem is recognized, missed, or ignored. Take time to collect some data on your attitude by completing the learning exercise in the Try This: Attitude Evaluation—My Attitude box.

⊚ Try This

Attitude Evaluation—My Attitude

Directions: On a scale of 0 to 10 (with 0 as the worst and 10 as the best), rate your attitude.

___I am aware of the limitations of my knowledge.
___I am aware that my dislikes, biases, and prejudices may influence my decisions.
___I try to be fair-minded.
___I am interested in understanding other people's thoughts and feelings.
___I check to find out if my statements are clear.
___I can be influenced by another person's conclusions, if based on fact.
___I question other people's sources of information.
___I acknowledge that what I have been thinking can be incorrect.
___I question the availability of additional alternatives.
___I listen to my intuition and compare it with my reasoning.
___I am aware that perfect solutions are not always available.
___I am willing to work as a team member.
___I try to anticipate problems before they occur.
___I am continually looking for ways to improve my thinking.

These items describe your strong attitudes for the development of critical thinking. The items are attitudes you need to improve to increase critical thinking.

? Critical Thinking

Attitudes to Work On

Prioritize the attitudes you choose to work on first to help increase your critical thinking. How will you recognize improvement in each item you listed?

ADDITIONAL FACTORS THAT INFLUENCE CRITICAL THINKING

Alfaro-Lefevre (2009) discusses the following personal factors that also influence critical thinking. These are summarized with some additional thoughts for practical/vocational nurses.

1. Effective Reading
   a. Effective reading, as you have learned, is more than reading with speed.
   b. It means that you are able to identify the significance and potential application of what you are reading.
   c. An effective learning skill means that you are able to organize the data you have so you can access it efficiently.
   d. Chapter 5 provides suggestions to make studying and comprehending information work for you. Remember that employers need more than someone with random-access memory.
2. Maturity
   a. Maturity most often comes with age.
   b. Maturity provides past opportunities to have worked through problems. It becomes easier to see problems through someone else's eyes.
   c. Do you work to understand others before expecting them to understand you?
3. Problem Solving and the Nursing Process
   a. Knowledge of problem solving and of the nursing process is based on many of the same principles as critical thinking.
   b. Do you use the problem-solving steps to work out problems now? Understanding and applying the problem-solving steps gives you a head start in thinking critically.
4. Communication Skills
   a. Communicating effectively means being aware of the message you are sending verbally, in writing, and through body language. Are you willing to listen and consider ideas and views that are different from your own? Do you express yourself well in writing? Communication is discussed more fully in Chapter 13.
5. Self-Confidence
   a. Self-confidence is often the personal characteristic that is the least available to a student.
   b. Without self-confidence the student is wasting a lot of energy worrying that he or she will not "get it."
   c. It may help to remember that no one can give you self-confidence. You develop self-confidence as you succeed in your endeavors. This is where the saying "Self-confidence is earned, not learned" comes from.
   d. Overconfidence can make people assume they are correct even before data are available to back up what they believe to be correct. Do you acknowledge the limits of your knowledge and skills?
6. Moral Development
   a. Moral development creates fair-mindedness, a strong sense of what is right and wrong and just. Have you examined your values, and can you separate them from the values held by others?
7. Capability in Nursing
   a. Capability in nursing is essential. You must have nursing knowledge and skills to do the work of nursing and know how to access the resources.
   b. Nursing instructors have an enormous amount of factual information that they expect to introduce to their nursing students. The amount is often overwhelming to both the instructor and the student.
   c. Distinguishing what is absolutely necessary to know from what is nice to know is no easy task. The tendency is to hang onto what is fun to know and old information, just in case someone asks or it is in a test somewhere.
   d. With the knowledge explosion, instructors are no longer able to infuse their students with all they need to know.
   e. It is important to have the tools for locating information and comprehending information, storing information in long-term memory, and recalling the comprehended information when needed.
8. Collaboration
   a. A collaborative effort has been shown to promote critical-thinking skills; for example, a small student group could work together on a significant learning project. First, it would entail presenting the instructor with a well-thought-out plan (including observable, project outcomes/goals).
   b. Occasionally we get a student who becomes angry when he or she comes to class and discovers that lecture is not the primary way of teaching. One student who was an auditory learner (learns by listening) explained that in previous classes she never had to read her text and be prepared to participate in a discussion. Being prepared to discuss would have shown that she really understood the information. She had been able to memorize enough to pass her tests just by listening because testing for knowledge, but not critical thinking, was common in the past.

9. Anxiety
   a. When anxiety overwhelms, it effectively stops critical thinking.
   b. The same is true with a high level of fatigue. This is why we are including a chapter on personal health promotion (see Chapter 6).
10. Mentors and Experience in Nursing
   a. Work experience and the guidance of nursing mentors, starting with your instructor, will assist you in learning to identify priorities in nursing care.
   b. Depending on the work area, patients may be there to seek help for only a few hours or days (emergency or treatment) or for the rest of their life (nursing home).

CRITICAL THINKING AND THE NCLEX-PN®

The NCLEX-PN®, the national licensing examination for practical/vocational nurses, includes items that require various levels of thinking to answer a test item. These various levels are called cognitive levels. The cognitive levels used on the NCLEX-PN® examination are knowledge, comprehension, application, and analysis. The following definitions will help you understand the meaning of the words *knowledge* (knowing), *comprehension* (understanding), *application*, and *analysis*.

1. Knowledge refers to the ability to recall and repeat information you have memorized. *Memorizing is not the same as understanding a concept.* Knowledge is the lowest level of learning. Defining a concept as stated in a dictionary is an example of knowledge level.
2. Comprehension refers to the ability to very basically understand information, recall it, and identify examples of that information. To comprehend is to *grasp the meaning* of the material. Comprehension is the lowest level of understanding. An example of the comprehension level is the ability to repeat information in your own words. This indicates that you understand the information.
3. Application means being able to *use learned material in new situations*. For example, you apply what is learned in class to your clinical work. Application involves being able to prioritize or determine what is most important, what comes first. Application is a higher level of understanding. *You must be able to use knowledge to tailor approaches depending on circumstances.*
4. Analysis means to be able to *break down complex information into its basic parts* and relate those parts to the whole picture. An example of analysis is the ability to *organize and prioritize* (what is most important, most urgent) two or more pieces of information in a patient situation to *process a safe response.* Analysis is a higher level of application.

Being able to identify the most important symptoms that a patient with a specific problem presents is an example of analysis.

Comprehension, application, and analysis are what employers expect of a practical/vocational nurse on the job. Your instructors will also expect this level of competence in the clinical area as you continue to develop your critical-thinking skills. Past students with college degrees have told us that the consistent requirement to apply and analyze both prior and newly learned information is the major point about practical/vocational nursing that differs most from their college experience.

The review items for each chapter in this text will include five items. Four items will be in multiple-choice format, the same as in the NCLEX-PN® examination. These multiple-choice items will test you at the knowledge, comprehension, application, and analysis levels. They will help you understand the four cognitive levels and help you prepare for testing. Most important, they will keep your focus on understanding information to be able to continue the development of your critical-thinking skills.

In April 2005, the National Council revised new format items on NCLEX-PN® examinations (first introduced in 2003). Called *alternate format item*, these items may include multiple response, fill-in-the-blank (e.g., calculation, ordered response), and hotspot (e.g., the place on a diagram that answers the question). All format items may have charts, tables, or graphic images. Alternate format items are included at the end of the chapter with review questions. Currently, test items are written at the application and analysis levels (2011 NCLEX-PN® test plan). You have access to more NCLEX-PN®–type questions in Evolve. Your instructor has access to more questions in the *Instructor Resource Manual and Test Bank.* Silvestri's (2010) *Saunders Q&A Review for NCLEX-PN® Examination* has 3200 practice questions, including alternate-format questions and an 85-question comprehensive examination.

Storing information in long-term memory and being able to recall the comprehended information when needed is dealt with in Chapter 5. We stress the importance of learning this information thoroughly. Your effort will make a difference in all of your studies and in being prepared for the NCLEX-PN® examination.

MAKING IT WORK FOR YOU

This is a good time for you to be reminded that we all have special, although different, abilities in the area of thinking. The trick is to discover what those abilities are, embrace them, and make them work for you. You can choose whether to make the most of your abilities. You can also choose to not make a decision about your abilities. However, not deciding is also a decision. There is also the tendency to be impressed by those who begin to speak immediately to an issue as though they have all the facts, when in truth their style of processing is outside of themselves. Perhaps your way is to process internally and not speak out until you have all the words in place. The one who processes externally may ask the questions you wish you had asked. This difference is related to their personality. Their verbalization sounds impressive and tends to frighten the person who processes internally before speaking. Both types can be equally effective in their ability to think critically. Each way is different: A difference in personality is all it has to be unless you allow yourself to begin thinking negatively about your abilities.

WHERE TO GO FROM HERE

This chapter is written as a critical-thinking primer, and it is limited to need-to-know information. The questions and suggestions offered are those that are within the scope of the LPN/LVN and the nursing program. Reflective (critical) thinking will assist you in determining if you need outside assistance from your school's study skills center or the instructor in setting up realistic observable goals/outcomes. You may even decide that the awareness of personal and situational characteristics is enough to get you started on your own. The critical-thinking exercises provide you with a practical framework for increasing your critical-thinking ability.

Get Ready for the NCLEX-PN® Examination

Key Points

- Thinking is divided into nonfocused thinking and directed thinking.
- Critical thinking answers the question "How can we do this better?"
- To think critically, it is necessary to access information, comprehend (understand) information, store comprehended information in long-term memory, and recall the comprehended information when needed.
- Comprehension, application, and analysis are what employers will expect from LPN/LVNs on the job.
- The cognitive levels used in the NCLEX-PN® examination are knowledge, comprehension, application, and analysis. Most questions are written at the application or higher level of cognitive thinking.
- The ability to read with understanding is the cornerstone of critical thinking.
- Both personal and situational factors influence critical thinking.
- The decision is yours whether to use the abilities you already possess to enhance your critical-thinking ability.

Additional Learning Resources

evolve   Go to your Evolve website (http://evolve.elsevier.com/Hill/Success) for the following FREE learning resources:
- Answers to Critical Thinking Scenarios
- Additional learning activities
- Additional Review Questions for the NCLEX-PN® exam
- Helpful phrases for communicating in Spanish and more!

Review Questions for the NCLEX-PN® Examination

1. When was the nursing process and critical thinking mandated as part of SPN/SVN education?
   1. 1990
   2. 1992
   3. 1997
   4. 2002

2. What is a major difference between knowledge, comprehension, application, and analysis?
   1. Knowledge is the ability to understand and give examples of what you have learned.
   2. Comprehension is the ability to explain or summarize information you have read.
   3. Application is the ability to break down information into its component parts.
   4. Analysis is the ability to use principles and general ideas in concrete situations.

3. Which pattern shows the use of critical thinking?
   1. During report, you learned that the new patient is short-tempered. You decide you will humor her, do what is necessary, and give her plenty of space the rest of the time.
   2. Mr. Fodor has to have six small feedings each day, and although he can feed himself, you have decided to increase the intake by sitting on the bed and feeding him.
   3. Mrs. Still is crying when you arrive to give her a bath. She tells you her baby died after birth. You cheer her up by telling her, "That's nothing. I lost two babies."
   4. Charlie was admitted as an emergency admission. You are asked to hold him in position for a spinal tap. You hold him firmly in position and speak softly and reassuringly.

4. Which of the following is a negative example of thinking?
    1. The brain grasps information in phrases.
    2. Negative thinking works as a conscience.
    3. Critical thinking looks beyond the obvious.
    4. Habitual thinking is useful in our life.

Alternate Format Item

1. Which of the following statements do *not* reflect reasons for thinking critically? *(Select all that apply.)*
    1. Time would be better spent on developing an up-to-date curriculum for students.
    2. The way nursing has always been done is the best it can be for nurses and patients.
    3. Rapid change and information explosion create a need for new learning and skills.
    4. Focused thinking in every area may make a difference between success and failure.

2. If you are going to assist someone in learning to think critically, which statements most describe your planning process? *(Select all that apply.)*
    1. When you feel strongly about a situation, you are usually correct.
    2. Remind yourself that you are not always correct in your analysis.
    3. Listen to another opinion even if it contradicts what you believe.
    4. Remember that a patient can provide you with subjective information.

Critical Thinking Scenarios

Scenario 1

Carol, a vocational nursing student, is assigned to Veronica, a patient with the diagnosis of possible depression. The police brought Veronica to the hospital when a neighbor became alarmed by her attempt to cut her wrist. During the past 2 days since Veronica was hospitalized, the staff have seen no behaviors that alarm them. Veronica has showered every morning, fixed her hair, put on makeup, and wears nice clothes brought in by her family. Whenever the staff check on her at night, she appears to be sleeping. She eats modest portions of food at mealtimes and says she wants to keep her weight where it is. She greets staff with a smile and inquires what she can do to be of help.

Today, Veronica will go to court (which is held in the hospital) to determine if she will be committed for care. Carol will accompany her. What is troubling Carol is that Veronica swore her to secrecy and then told her she was using all effort to "hold it together" so she will be discharged after court. Once she gets home, she will kill herself, and this time she has a plan that is "foolproof." Carol feels torn between her promise of secrecy and her concern that Veronica will follow through with her plan for suicide.

As Carol sits in court and listens to Veronica tell her story, what critical-thinking steps will help her reach a decision of what to do?

1. Analyze the situation, as Carol will have to do. Provide a rationale for what she is thinking.
2. Identify the alternatives that Carol is considering. What is the rationale for each of the alternatives?
3. Choose the alternative and provide the rationale for Carol's decision.

Scenario 2

Sarah, age 72, has recently been diagnosed as having a form of chronic leukemia. Her physician has advised treatment, but Sarah always checks out information before making a decision, "I have had a full family life and professional career."

Using critical thinking as described in this chapter, what can Sarah do to arrive at a decision that is right for her?

The Nursing Process: Your Role

Objectives

On completing this chapter, you will be able to do the following:

1. Discuss how the nursing process has evolved from the 1950s to the present.
2. Define your role in the nursing process according to the Nurse Practice Act in your state, territory, or country.
3. Describe assisting with the four steps of the nursing process for the practical/vocational nurse:
   a. Data collection (assessment)
   b. Planning
   c. Implementation
   d. Evaluation
4. Describe nursing diagnosis as the exclusive domain of the registered nurse (RN).
5. Explain why the nursing process and critical thinking are part of the practical/vocational nursing program curriculum.
6. Briefly describe how NANDA-I, NIC, and NOC can be used together to plan patient care.

Key Terms

assisting (p. 98)
data collection (DĀT-ă kŏ-LĔK-shŭn, p. 98)
dependent role (dĕ-PĔN-dĕnt, p. 92)
desired patient outcome (dĕ-ZĪRD PĀ-shŭnt ŎWT-kŭm, p. 104)
evaluation (ĕ-VĂL-ū-Ă-shŭn, p. 98)
goals (p. 98)
implementation (Ĭ-plĕ-mĕn-TĀ-shŭn, p. 98)
independent role (ĬN-dĕ-PĔN-dĕnt, p. 98)
interdependent (ĬN-tĕr-dĕ-PĔN-dĕnt, p. 98)
intervention (p. 98)

North American Nursing Diagnosis Association International (NANDA-I) (p. 99)
Nursing Interventions Classification (NIC) (p. 107)
Nursing Outcomes Classification (NOC) (p. 107)
nursing diagnosis (NŬR-sĭng DĬ-ăg-NŌ-sĭs, p. 99)
nursing process (NŬR-sĭng PRŎ-sĕs, p. 97)
objective information (ŏb-JĔK-tĭv, p. 99)
outcome (ŎWT-kŭm p. 98)
planning (plăn-ĭng, p. 98)
subjective information (sŭb-JĔK-tĭv, p. 99)
taxonomy (tăks-ŎN-ŭ-me, p. 99)
validate information (VĂL-ĭ-dāt p. 99)

 Keep in Mind

The nursing process is the way nurses communicate with one another to identify what the nurse will do to safely help the patient reach desired patient outcomes. It provides for continuity of safe care on every shift.

As a student, you will develop nursing care plans. Nursing care plans are learning tools for practical/vocational nursing students (SPN/SVNs). They are traditionally used in practical/vocational nursing programs to help students learn about patient needs. *A critical-thinking exercise is using your role in the nursing process to devise a care plan as an SPN/SVN in preparation for patient care.* Devising a nursing care plan prior to patient care is necessary to ensure safe patient care.

Currently, unlicensed individuals are doing the tasks and skills that licensed practical/vocational nurses (LPN/LVNs) perform. It is the nursing process and critical thinking that separate the LPN/LVNs from the unlicensed assistive personnel (UAPs). These distinctions make LPN/LVNs attractive to employers. The modern LPN/LVN uses critical thinking and the nursing process to carefully identify patient needs, health issues, expectations, lifestyle, and risks involved through focused thinking. Judgments are based on evidence rather than assumptions and minimal training. The LPN/LVN thinks before acting. The RN uses the nursing process and critical thinking but at a higher skill level based on education and makes final decisions on nursing diagnosis and patient care plans.

THE NURSING PROCESS: THE 1950s

The nursing process originated in the 1950s to provide structure for thinking in nursing. According to Peseit and Herman (1998), "The nursing process was designed to organize thinking so that the problems encountered by patients could be anticipated and solved quickly." The 1950s four-step process was based on a scientific method that included data collection, planning, implementation, and evaluation. A major difference between the scientific method (problem-solving method) and the nursing process is that the scientific method identifies the problem first and then goes on to gather data and other information. The nursing process gathers data first and then identifies the problem (nursing diagnosis). Initially, nursing did not yet see itself as having something unique to contribute to patient care that was separate from and in addition to its dependent role to physicians. Consequently, nursing education programs and textbooks focused on patients' medical problems and associated nursing interventions. To add to the confusion, suggested nursing interventions varied in nursing textbooks and at health care agencies. Although the nursing process had been introduced, it still had a long way to go. The most important outcome of the nursing process for nurses was to provide a structure for thinking before acting.

THE NURSING PROCESS: THE 1970s TO THE 1990s

When the American Nurses Association (ANA) published the standards of nursing practice in 1977, it established a five-step nursing process for the RN: assessment (data collection), nursing diagnosis (a new step for RNs), planning, intervention, and evaluation. The problem-solving format of the original nursing process was replaced with a *reasoning* model. It introduced a way for nurses to identify and respond to patient needs within the scope of nursing. These included the following types of needs:

- Physiologic
- Psychologic
- Social
- Spiritual

It also gave nurses an organized, unique way of contributing to patient care that was separate and additional to its dependent role to physicians. It involved the following roles:

- Collecting data (assessment)
- Nursing diagnosis (RN responsibility)
- Planning
- Implementation
- Evaluating nursing care
- Including the patient in planning
- A way to communicate with other nurses and caregivers

Initially, SPN/SVNs were not taught the steps of the nursing process or how to think critically. Although nursing diagnosis was, and continues to be, within the RN's legal role, it became clear that LPN/LVNs

have an important role in assisting the RN in all the other steps of the nursing process.

 Try This

The Nurse Practice Act

With the assistance of your instructor, review the Nurse Practice Act in your state, territory, or country. Your role in the nursing process is spelled out in this law. There are variations within the states, territories, and countries. It defines your scope of nursing practice.

THE NURSING PROCESS: 2000 AND BEYOND

In 2002, the NCSBN integrated the nursing process into all areas of the NCLEX-PN® examination. By doing so, the council validated the significance of the nursing process and critical thinking for the LPN/LVN as the way to do the work of nursing.

Definitions of the nursing process for the NCLEX-PN® examination (NCSBN, 2001) are as follows:

- Data collection (assessment) is a systematic gathering and review of information about the patient, which is communicated to appropriate members of the health team.
- Planning involves assisting the RN in the development of nursing diagnosis, goals, and interventions for a patient's plan of care and maintaining patient safety.
- Implementation is the provision of required nursing care to accomplish established patient goals.
- Evaluation compares the actual outcomes of nursing care to the expected outcomes, which are then communicated to members of the health care team.
- The definitions of the nursing process remain the same for the 20011 NCLEX-PN® examination.

WHAT DIFFERENTIATES YOUR ROLE FROM THE RN ROLE

Because of the depth of the RN's basic education, the RN functions independently in all five steps of the nursing process (including nursing diagnosis). The nursing actions based on nursing diagnosis do not require a physician's order. Both RNs and LPN/LVNs share an interdependent relationship with other health team members. For example, RNs and LPN/LVNs both carry out orders for treatments and medication written by a medical doctor, podiatrist, or dentist.

The LPN/LVN acts in a more dependent role when participating in the planning and evaluation phase of the nursing process but acts in a more independent role when participating in the data collection and implementation phases of the nursing process. RNs are taught assessment skills as part of their basic education. The skills include patient interview and physical assessment of all body systems. However, practical/vocational nurses learn to gather data about the patient and the environment during every encounter with the patient (as do RNs and UAPs, according to their knowledge and skill level). Data collection for the SPN/SVN includes taking vital signs, checking therapeutic responses to medications and treatments, and collecting data on symptoms of health problems, among other functions. The focus of data collection is based on the current unit of study for the practical/vocational nurse. With each course, SPN/SVNs increase their data collection capabilities. SPN/SVNs continue to hold onto skills they acquire and then add on to these skills as they complete each nursing course. LPN/LVNs may choose to learn more complex skills as part of a postgraduate assessment course.

Some schools offer physical assessment as a course separate from the practical nursing program. Ask your instructor if a physical assessment course is available. It is an excellent way to learn additional interview, observation, and physical assessment skills. Whether you use part or all of these skills at work, the knowledge will improve the care you provide to patients.

The *International Journal of Nursing Terminologies and Classifications* (2008) defines nursing diagnosis as "a clinical judgment about individual, family, or community responses to actual or potential health problems/life processes. A nursing diagnosis provides the basis for selection of nursing interventions to achieve outcomes for which the nurse is accountable." The RN uses an established list of current nursing diagnoses developed by the North American Nursing Diagnosis Association International (NANDA-I). NANDA-I was developed as a standardized, orderly, systematic language (taxonomy) that would provide a common language for nurses to communicate with one another. Nurses are encouraged to use this approved nursing diagnosis list. NANDA-I is periodically updated to meet current changes and needs (see inside back cover of text for 2009-2011 NANDA-I list).

DEVELOPING YOUR PLAN OF CARE FOR ASSIGNED PATIENTS

Patient care for you as a student is a learning experience. It is necessary to plan for patient care assignments. Legally, your Nurse Practice Act will require you to give care at the level of an LPN/LVN. The nursing diagnosis is the problem the patient presented with, and the RN fits this into the categories established by NANDA-I. Because you do not study the NANDA-I diagnostic categories in most practical/vocational nursing programs, it is helpful (i.e., clearer, more objective, more explanatory, makes more sense to you in the learning situation) if you use the original

nursing problem the patient presented with. Turn the nursing diagnosis back to the presenting problem. In this way you clearly understand what you are working with in everyday terms. At this stage you have the benefit of your instructor to help you through the planning process. Planning for patient care becomes easier with each plan. You internalize your role in four steps of the nursing process and are improving your ability to think critically as a practical/vocational nurse.

STEPS OF THE NURSING PROCESS

STEP 1: DATA COLLECTION

Data collection includes many aspects.

Systematic Way of Gathering Data

Data collection begins on admission and continues with each patient encounter. The patient is the primary source of information in data collection. After all, patients know themselves and their body better than anyone else. All patient interview questions should be directed to the patient unless he or she is unable to respond. The RN interviews the patient to obtain the health history and assesses body systems. As part of a practical/vocational nursing program, learning communication skills does not include the formal interview process.

- Subjective information is based on the patient's opinion. Some refer to subjective information as symptoms. This usually includes feelings of physical discomfort, anxiety, and mental stress that are more difficult to measure. The nurse cannot experience subjective symptoms.
- Objective information includes data that the nurse can verify; it is also known as "signs." A physical assessment provides objective data. The terms *check*, *observe*, *monitor*, *weigh*, *measure*, and *smell* are cues that you may be involved in objective data collection. Obtaining initial data, such as vital signs, height, and weight, is often assigned to the LPN/LVN. Objective information helps support or cast doubt on subjective information. For example, a patient's subjective statement about feeling feverish can be verified by measuring his or her temperature (objective).

Verify the Information

Verifying information (validating) is an important step in thinking critically. As an SPN/SVN, it is very important that you seek the assistance of your instructor to discover what resources are available to you for verification of data. Suggestions for verifying information include the following:

- Verify the data and question any information that is not a match to your data collection.

- Differentiate between subjective and objective data. Remember that decisions must be based on evidence, not assumptions.
- Compare findings with the RN and other staff involved with the patient.
- Other staff may help verify when a client has mental limitations.
- Patients or family members may be able to validate information you obtained during data collection (family members with patient permission).
- Document all data and sources, especially when they do not match.
- Compare the data you collected with the medical records.
- Know that what you do for verification will depend on your skill level and whether you are an SPN/SVN or LPN/LVN.
- As a student, ask your instructor for guidance on how to verify data and how to determine if there is a relationship between presenting problems.

Communicate Information to Appropriate Health Care Team Members

- **Emergency data** are reported immediately. For example, suppose you learn that the patient with a fracture has diabetes and fell on his way home from a bar, where he goes daily for "just four beers." If he says, "I pace myself," does that reassure you that this is not an immediate issue? Recall that what you have heard is subjective data, but as a student you will not be in a position to verify it further without direction from the RN. Report what you have heard and any objective data, such as vital signs and observations, to the appropriate person. You have just activated your brain to think critically.
- **Incomplete toolbox:** Subjective data will be charted as "Patient states . . ." Objective data such as temperature, pulse, and respiration (TPR); blood pressure (BP); weight; and skin color will be charted as what you observe and measure without judging or drawing conclusions. Your involvement in this step depends on your place of employment and your experience and skill level. The LPN/LVN usually has more responsibility in the nursing home, where the patient's condition is more stable. At the conclusion of your practical/vocational program, you will have acquired strong, although incomplete, data collection skills: "The toolbox is not complete." An incomplete toolbox is nothing to be ashamed of. For example, you measure the TPR and BP properly. Be proud of your data collection skills. They provide valuable data.

Other Aspects of Data Collection

Data Collection Continues. Data collection starts during the patient's admission. It continues daily at the beginning of the shift for the baseline observations,

---

Box 9-1 Examples of Practical/Vocational Nurse Data Collection

These examples can apply to acute care, nursing home care, long-term care, and so on:

- Observing results of a laxative or enema
- Observing for signs of congestive heart failure for a patient taking furosemide (Lasix) and digoxin (Lanoxin)
- Observing an ulcer on the lower leg of a diabetic: size (measure it), location, appearance, any drainage, and so on
- Observing the ulcer each time the leg is dressed
- Observing behavior for signs of disorientation or confusion
- Observing NPO patient drinking water
- In acute care: observing position in bed. In community: observing gait and posture.
- Observing whether 76-year-old patient is showing signs of ego integrity or despair (Although the patient should be at ego integrity, he is not capable of being there. Because of his cerebrovascular accident [CVA], he has to be washed, fed, and lifted everywhere. He is incontinent. His needs remind you of those of an infant. You will work at establishing trust in the patient instead of ego integrity.)
- Observing family interactions
- Observing the environment for need for safety factors: spills, bed rails, glasses on table, hearing aids, dentures, and so on
- Observing the urine for color, odor, amount, and other characteristics

---

then periodically during the shift, and right before doing your final documentation and reporting off. The practical/vocational nurse is always collecting data on therapeutic responses to treatments, interventions, and medications (Box 9-1).

Accuracy in Data Collection. Florence Nightingale said that if you do not observe your patient, you should not be a nurse. With each contact the LPN/LVN must see, hear, smell, and touch the patient when necessary, and use all the senses to gather data about the patient and the environment. Data collection is vital; the patient condition changes throughout the day. This is why accuracy in measuring vital signs; describing vomitus, bleeding, or a skin lesion; and determining level of consciousness, for example, are so important. Has the patient's skin lesion changed since the last time you checked the lesion? How has it changed? How much has it changed? Sometimes LPN/LVNs do not understand that what they are assigned to do is a vital part of the data collection.

Introduce Yourself. Data collection, whether partial or total, involves courtesy. Introduce yourself to the patient and explain what you are going to do.

- The patient's first impression of you tends to remain. Address the patient as Mr., Mrs., Miss, Ms., or another title, as appropriate. Avoid using a first name unless you have the patient's permission.
- Remind yourself that this is a *professional,* not a personal, relationship that you are building. The most common complaints by patients include "I don't know which one is the nurse"; "I am treated with disrespect"; "I am not their grandma"; and so on. Familiarity—that is, acting toward a patient as though he or she is a family member or friend—does not give the patient a sense of confidence in your nursing skill.
- When in the patient's presence, stand or sit where he or she can see you. Patients often experience fear on being hospitalized or transferred to a new facility.
- Confusion or lack of skills on the nurse's part serves to increase that fear. The focus of the nurse's job is to serve the patient with the greatest skill possible.

Asking Questions. Avoid asking questions that have been asked before unless you are directed to do so or your observation based on critical thinking alerts you to do so.
- Be sure that you have looked at the record before entering the patient's room.
- Explain why you are asking questions and reassure the patient that he or she has the right to not answer questions that cause discomfort.
- Be a good listener. Encourage confidence, but do not promise to keep secrets.
- Request clarification rather than pretending that you understand: "I am not sure that I understand what you mean by that statement." Check out what you think you understand: "Am I correct in saying that you are worried about the kind of care you will receive here?" Avoid using reassuring promises that you cannot deliver, such as "Don't worry; everything will be just fine."
- Also avoid giving approval—for example, "That's right." This statement may make it difficult for a patient to change his or her mind.
- Nursing responsibility does not involve judging the patient's behaviors, values, or decisions.
- Finally, avoid verbalizing disapproval or belittling the patient with statements such as "You know you shouldn't have done that."
- Chapter 13 elaborates on communication techniques that will assist you in making the best use of the limited time you have to obtain needed data from the patient.

Barriers in Data Collection
You must be alert to several possible barriers to data collection:
- Barriers include insufficient time, cultural differences, poor skills in data collection, and communication

failure, such as a comatose patient, a patient who presents a language barrier, the presence of distractions, or a patient who is too sick to speak well.
- If your personal values get in the way, you may label the patient before the interview is complete, instead of basing decisions on facts.
- Respectful distancing is necessary if the nurse is to remain objective and use all senses clearly.

STEP 2: PLANNING
Planning includes assisting the RN to develop nursing diagnoses, outcomes, and interventions.

Assisting the RN to Develop the Nursing Diagnosis
The LPN/LVN assists the RN to collect and group the data that have been collected in a logical order. Only the RN can develop the nursing diagnoses, goals, interventions, and plans of care. It is illegal for the LPN/LVN to write the plan and for the RN to initial it. The LPN/LVN assists in determining a significant relationship between data and patient needs or problems. The focus is on patient functions that will benefit from nursing interventions. After the problems are identified and organized, the RN makes the nursing diagnosis.

 Try This

Assisting During Planning

In the planning phase, the SPN/SVN takes the nursing diagnosis and states it as a nursing problem the patient presented with. SPN/SVNs state the problem, set outcomes, list interventions, and then list data collection for care plans. This process seems to be the opposite of the RN's, but remember that practical/vocational nurses do not have primary responsibility for data collection (phase 1). The SPN/SVN does not study NANDA-I lists in most nursing programs and relies on the RN for the final nursing diagnosis. To demonstrate understanding of the nursing diagnosis, the practical/vocational nurse states the nursing diagnosis in objective and specific terms as a nursing problem (Table 9-1).

Realistic, Useful Nursing Care Plans. For a nursing care plan to be a useful, realistic tool for the nursing staff, priorities must be established:
- A care plan will not include all of the patients' health problems. It is unreasonable to think that nurses will be able to respond to all of the patient's needs and concerns.
- The most important problems, those that are potentially life threatening, must be taken care of immediately.
- Nurses often use Maslow's Hierarchy of Needs (Chapter 10) to assist in prioritizing patient needs.
- The lowest level of needs, according to Maslow, is the physiologic (survival) level of needs. This means that in prioritizing patient needs, attention is paid first to

Table 9-1   **Example of a Student Assignment Sheet and Patient Care Plan**

Student _____

Patient Initials _____ Room _____ Doctor _____ Allergies _____

Age _____ Marital Status _____ Religion _____ Occupation _____

Admission Date _____ Date of Surgery _____ Diet _____

Medical Diagnosis _____ Surgical Procedure _____

Meaning in Own Words _____ Meaning in Own Words _____

Primary Nursing Problem _____

CATEGORIES OF HUMAN FUNCTION	DATA COLLECTION	NURSING PROBLEMS	OUTCOMES	NURSING INTERVENTION	EVALUATION
Protective (e.g., personal care and hygiene, environment, surgery)	You will: Check, observe, monitor, weigh, and measure. Collect data (1) at beginning of shift for baseline, (2) periodically during shift, and (3) right before reporting off duty.	What is the problem, in your own words? Be specific and objective. Could use nursing diagnosis, but . . .	The patient will: (Reverse the problem and state positively what patient will do—realistically, measurably, time-referenced).	The nurse will: (Be objective and specific. Care plans in texts rarely are. What the nurse will do to help patient meet outcomes.)	What progress is patient making toward outcomes? Results of data collection in objective terms.
Sensory-perceptual					
Comfort, rest, activity, and mobility (e.g., sleep and rest, body alignment)					
Nutrition					
Growth and development (e.g., identify Erikson's developmental stage)					
Fluid-gas transport					
Psychosocial cultural (e.g., emotional support, spiritual support, diversion, and recreation)					
Elimination (e.g., urinary and gastrointestinal elimination)					
Need for community resources					

problems related to food, air, water, temperature, elimination, rest, and pain.

- When working on several problems at the same time, you will often find that a relationship exists between problems.
- Priorities may also change rapidly, depending on the patient's condition. The nurse has to remain flexible and recognize the need to shift priorities according to patient needs.
- Patients will be far more cooperative with the care plan if they are included in identifying the priorities of care.
- According to Maslow, regression takes place during illness. The amount of regression depends on the circumstances and severity of the illness. As the patient recovers, he or she advances on Maslow's Hierarchy.
- Ideally the patient is able to regain the former level of functioning. Cooperation is much more likely when the nurse understands this and respects it.
- Whenever a new problem emerges, practical/vocational nurses collect data about the problem because of their data collection skills.
- They collaborate with the RN, and the RN formulates a new nursing diagnosis.

❓ Critical Thinking

The Seven Survival Needs

Write an example of a problem for each survival need.
1. Food _____
2. Air _____
3. Water _____
4. Temperature _____
5. Elimination _____
6. Rest _____
7. Pain _____

Possible answers:
1. Not enough or too much food intake
2. Shortness of breath
3. Dehydration, caused by vomiting
4. Temperature above or below normal
5. Diarrhea
6. Sleeping too much or too little
7. Pain that interferes with functioning

Assisting the RN to Develop Outcomes

Think back to Step 1, data collection, and ask yourself the following questions: What did the patient say on admission about expectations, wants, or needs while a patient? Did you also remember to collect data on patient strengths?

Strengths. Strengths are building blocks in developing a realistic plan. Strengths include whatever the patient and family continue to be able to do that will aid patient care. Patient and family are important partners in attaining the goals/outcomes. Building on patient strengths provides a sense of contribution and some control for the patient. The following are sample questions that may help make the question of strengths patient-focused:

- Can the patient move from the bed to the chair and back alone?
- Does the patient feed himself or herself? Completely? With some assistance?
- Does the patient eat best if someone is present? Alone? During conversation about family?
- Are there any family members who can be instructed in how to act as partners in meeting patient goals?
- Is responsibility for the intervention within the LPN/LVN role?

Goals and Outcomes. Goals state a general intent about what is being accomplished (e.g., "I will learn the medical prefixes, roots, and suffixes by the end of the semester."). Outcome describes a specific result that can be observed at some point (e.g., "I will learn the prefixes, roots, and suffixes well enough by the end of the semester to get an A on the final exam."). The terms are used interchangeably in some agencies, although the ANA prefers the term *outcome*. The focus of the outcome is on the patient, not the nurse. An outcome is thought of as "The patient will..." What is agreed on is that well-written outcomes include patient input, if at all possible, and must have the following characteristics:

- Realistic (attainable, based on the patient's condition and desire)
- Measurable (tells how you will know that the outcome has been reached)
- Time-referenced (an educated guess on the part of the nurse as to how long it will take to attain the outcome)

It may be easier for an SPN/SVN to use the phrase *desired* (or *observable*) *patient outcome*. This focuses directly on what the patient will accomplish rather than on what the nurse will do. For example, the phrase consists of the following characteristics:

- It uses the word *patient* as the subject of the statement.
- It is realistic for the patient and his or her problem.
- It uses a measurable verb: It is specific for the patient and his or her problem.
- It includes a time frame for patient reevaluation.

To state an outcome as a student, reverse the problem and state it in positive terms.

The statement tells what the patient **will** do to overcome the problem rather than what the patient will **not** do. Here are some examples:

- Observable outcome: The patient will eat 1500 calories of ground foods and liquids during each 24-hour period.
- Unclear statement: The patient will not miss any feedings during a 24-hour period.

Assisting the RN to Develop Nursing Interventions

Nursing interventions identify specifically what the nurse will do to assist the patient to reach desired patient outcomes.

- Sometimes this means encouraging the patient to do certain activities, such as self-feeding. (Think back to the patient strengths that were initially identified and additional strengths you have noted since then.)
- Interventions are also called *nursing approach, nursing action,* or *nursing care.* Interventions focus on the "related to" (R/T) portion of the nursing diagnosis. They tell nursing personnel who, what, where, when, and how much.
- When nursing interventions are clearly written, all nursing staffs, according to their skill level and if within their legal role, will be able to carry out the nursing action. *It needs to be identified on the care plan if the RN, LPN/LVN, or UAP will carry out the intervention.*
- Check the nursing interventions: Are they objective and specific as written? Interventions you will develop in your care plan as an SPN/SVN are based on courses you have taken, additional reading, and finding information from alternate sources.
- Interventions do not just come from the top of your head. (See Chapter 5 for information on learning resources.)

Table 9-2 takes you through the process the SPN/SVN can use to plan care for an assigned patient:

- The nursing diagnosis, as written by the RN, is shown.
- The nursing diagnosis is turned back into the problem the patient presented with to make it clearer and more specific.

- The SPN/SVN wrote the outcome by reversing the problem statement; it states clearly what the patient will do and what the observable outcome will be.
- The nursing interventions identify what the SPN/SVN will do to assist the patient in attaining the desired outcome.
- After checking the plan with the instructor, the SPN/SVN is prepared to begin patient care.

Care Plans Vary. Different kinds of care plans are available:

- An individualized written care plan has been demonstrated.
- Some facilities use **standardized care** plans. These plans are based on research of the best possible options for a nursing diagnosis (nursing problem). To individualize a standard plan, cross out interventions that do not apply to the patient and add appropriate interventions that do apply.
- **Computerized care plans** are popular. Individualized plans can be entered into the computer.
- More commonly, standardized care plans are used and then individualized to deal with the nursing problem.
- **Multidisciplinary (collaborative) care plans** work well in settings in which staffs from varied professions and disciplines are involved with the patient. An example is a long-term care or psychiatric setting. More recently, they are being used in medical-surgical and other units. Plans are developed by a multidisciplinary team and reflect specific interventions used by each discipline (e.g., physical therapist, social worker, nutritionist, nurse, and physician). Maintaining a separate plan for each profession is considered repetitious. The plan is developed with an interdisciplinary focus for each professional involved. The language must be common to each discipline involved. Therefore, the medical diagnosis is used rather than a nursing diagnosis. A prioritized problem list is developed based on the medical diagnosis, providing a common language for all health team members involved. The plan identifies shared and specific responsibilities for all professions represented.

Table 9-2 Nursing Diagnosis, Nursing Problem, Outcome, and Interventions

NURSING DIAGNOSIS	NURSING PROBLEM	OUTCOME
Altered nutrition: less than body requirements. Related to (R/T) decreased calorie intake.	Eats only 5% of each meal. R/T loss of appetite and weakness.	The patient will eat 1500 calories of ground foods and drink 2000 ml of liquids during each 24-hour period. (The problem is reversed and stated positively).
INTERVENTIONS		
1. Six small, ground meals at 8 AM, 10 AM, noon, 2 PM, 4 PM, and 6 PM. Patient seated in an easy chair with minimal assistance. Encourage self-feeding. Assist only if needed. 2. Offer 240 ml of liquids at 6 AM, 9 AM, 11 AM, 1 PM, 3 PM, 5 PM, 7 PM, and 9 PM. Vary choices: likes Jell-O, ice cream, 7-Up, chocolate milk, and pineapple juice. Drinks herbal tea with meals.		

- Progress is usually documented on a common form or computer in order to provide easy access for all involved with the plan. A clinical pathway is another type of multidisciplinary plan that schedules clinical interventions over an anticipated time period for a specific type of patient health problem. The clinical pathway is used for high-risk, high-volume, high-cost care. Often, care is documented right onto the clinical pathway. See page 189 for an example of a clinical pathway.
- A concept map, another type of care plan, is a diagram of a patient's condition and treatments. It can help the nurse plan interventions and is also a way to monitor patient progress.

Maintaining Patient Safety. All steps of the nursing process are directed toward patient safety. Remember the patient for whom you were collecting admission data? You discovered that he was diabetic, had four beers at the bar, and fell on his way home, which resulted in a fracture. You reported it immediately to the RN, along with a statement about his vitals. Your critical thinking made you alert the RN to a potentially serious safety issue.

Documenting the Care Plan. Documenting (charting) the plan of care is essential. Legally, if it was not charted, it was not done. In a lawsuit, a lawyer reviewing the chart or computer charting record may interpret sloppy charting as sloppy nursing care. Where the documentation takes place depends on the facility and the type of care plan used. It may be done electronically, in longhand in the nurse's notes, on flow sheets, or on the plan itself. Some agencies have a special care plan Kardex, or clipboard, at the patient's bedside. Eventually these become part of the patient's permanent record. Meanwhile the plan is the recipe for meeting the patient's needs.

STEP 3: IMPLEMENTATION

- The key for all your activity, regardless of your position and the agency involved, is to use the care plan as the basis for your nursing actions and reporting.
- For example, as an SPN/SVN you draw information from the care plan on how to provide individualized patient care.
- While providing care you continue to collect data based on your knowledge of the patient's strengths and disease conditions.
- You chart on flow sheets, nurses' notes, or electronic records, following the priorities indicated by the nursing problem, plus any new observations you have made according to the charting system in the agency.
- You use the care plan as your guideline when reporting to the RN and offer information on any changes you have noted.

Specifically you focus on the nursing interventions outlined in the care plan: Do interventions continue to be appropriate? What patient changes, or lack of changes, have you observed? With this information the RN can update the plan of care and needs only to validate the data. Implementation includes many aspects, which are discussed in the following sections.

Nursing Action

- Follow the established plan of care. Sit with the patient during meals, encourage eating, and assist minimally, if necessary.
- Participate in the patient care conference and offer input. Report specifically on tasks assigned to you, any changes, and progress or lack of progress.
- Review the procedure before preparing the patient. Prepare the patient for the procedure. Ask for help if you are uncertain about what to do.

Maintaining Patient Safety

- Use safe and appropriate techniques during patient care. Check the patient's position before lifting up safety rails to be sure arms do not get caught between the bed and the rail.
- Use precautionary and preventive interventions in providing care to patients. Make sure that wheelchair wheels and bed wheels are locked before moving the patient from the chair to the bed and back again.
- Institute nursing interventions to compensate for adverse responses. If the patient gets weak while standing, assist him or her to lie or sit down and place the patient's head between his or her knees (if not contraindicated by physical condition).
- Initiate life-saving interventions for emergency situations. If the patient begins to choke on food, perform the Heimlich maneuver.
- Monitor care given by unlicensed personnel. As an LPN/LVN charge nurse, you will be involved in this.
- Collect data during every patient contact. Be alert to even minor changes in skin color, breathing, respirations, and so on, even though your contact does not occur at a scheduled time (i.e., perhaps you just brought in the lunch tray).

Initiating Teaching That Is Within Your Role and Supports the RN's Teaching

- Encourage patients to follow their plan of care and treatment regimen. Be alert to any deviations from the care plan. Know all staff persons' roles so that you have a basis for your observations.
- Assist patients to maintain or enhance optimal functioning. Passive range of motion is done every morning as part of basic care for the bedridden patient who has been assigned to you.

- Provide an environment that is conducive to attaining observable patient outcomes. If the room smells of feces, locate the source and deal with it.
- Reinforce teaching of principles, procedures, and techniques for maintenance and promotion of health. For example, if the patient has been newly diagnosed as having type 2 diabetes, reinforce the steps of foot care the RN taught earlier in the morning (you sat in on the session). Be alert to questions that the patient has, based on lack of understanding, and seek answers to the questions as needed. Demonstrate techniques used by the RN, if requested. Check with the instructor if this is something you have not done before.

Reporting and Documenting

- Collect data during every patient contact. If you note the patient is beginning to perspire profusely for no apparent reason, measure vital signs.
- Report observations to relevant members of the health team. Report the aforementioned observation immediately to the RN. Report all daily observations before leaving the unit.
- Document the patient's response to nursing intervention, therapy, or teaching. Document all interventions, responses, and changes. Use the care plan as your guide for documentation and reporting.

 Try This

Implementing the Plan of Care

As an SPN/SVN, the next phase is *implementing* the plan of care that you have developed with your instructor's supervision. Did you remember to include the patient strengths you identified during your data collection? *Which interventions are within the LPN/LVN role?*

The Difference Between LPN/LVN and SPN/SVN Responsibility

As a graduate, your responsibility will vary according to the work area in which you are involved and whether you are functioning in a beginning or expanded role. In an acute care setting, your primary responsibility will be to use the established care plan as a guideline for providing direct patient care, continuing data collection, making verbal reports to the RN, and charting. In nursing homes and extended-care facilities, you may be functioning in the role of an LPN/LVN charge nurse and be responsible for managing patient care under the supervision of the RN.

STEP 4: EVALUATION

The evaluation phase includes assisting in determining patient progress and communicating the findings.

Assist in Determining Patient Progress Toward Meeting Desired Patient Goals/Outcomes

- Collect data during every patient contact. If the patient outcome is written correctly and the data collection list is complete, evaluation will be the result of your daily data collection. The continual data collection helps make daily evaluation part of the natural flow of good nursing care (Table 9-3).
- Compare actual outcomes with desired patient outcomes. If progress is being made toward meeting the outcomes, continue as is.
- Assist in determining the patient's response to nursing care. If the patient is not meeting the outcome, check the way the outcome is written. Is it measurable, realistic, and time-referenced? If you cannot evaluate the outcome, the outcome probably is not measurable or realistic. If necessary, change the portion that needs revision or restate the desired outcome.
- Assist in identifying factors that may interfere with the patient's ability to implement the plan of care. Talk with the patient. He or she may be able to tell you why progress is not being made. Review your daily data collection notes. There may be a pattern that emerges. Have the patient's strengths been considered in the plan of care? Are the stated observable outcomes less than or beyond what the patient can accomplish? Are they realistic? Is the focus on evaluating nursing care, as opposed to evaluating patient progress toward meeting desired outcomes? If necessary, revise nursing interventions that are not working. (Refer to Figure 20-5 Decision Tree for Problem Solving on p. 258.)

Communicate Findings

- Document patient's responses to care, therapy, or teaching.
- Report findings to relevant members of the health care team.

Table 9-3   Data Collection, Outcome, and Evaluation

DATA COLLECTION LIST	OUTCOME	EVALUATION
Check intake: Amount and type of liquid in milliliters Amount of food taken at each meal	The patient will eat 1500 calories of chopped foods and drink 2000 ml of liquids during each 24-hour period	By day 2 the patient was able to consume 1500 calories in ground meals and 1600 ml of liquids during a 24-hour period

Have you noticed how heavily dependent each step of the care plan is on the others and how the steps are often going on simultaneously? Have you noticed that as desired outcomes are met, other problems emerge? Recall that according to Maslow's Hierarchy: Regression occurs with illness. As observable outcomes are achieved at the lower level (patient begins to improve), higher levels of needs begin to emerge. Be aware that the patient may be functioning on more than one level.

 Try This

Evaluating Patient Progress

The time-referenced portion of the desired outcome states the approximate date by which the patient will attain an observable outcome. It is an educated guess on the part of the RN, based on education and experience. The SPN/SVN makes an educated guess on the assignment care plan regarding the time it will take the patient to meet his or her outcome. As an SPN/SVN, your daily data collection assists the RN in evaluating how far the patient has progressed and identifying any difficulties. A complete daily data collection list is essential and, as pointed out, is the basis of your data collection during every patient contact.

WHERE ARE WE NOW IN THE NURSING PROCESS?

Nursing continues to grow as a profession. Nursing research and health industry focus and policy all drive the change from general to specific nursing interventions and measurement of outcomes. Two such well-researched projects are the Nursing Interventions Classification (NIC) and the Nursing Outcomes Classification (NOC) taxonomies. As research has continued on NANDA-I, NIC, and NOC, specific ways have been devised to link the three taxonomies to provide a plan of care for patients. As an SPN/SVN, it is important for you to recognize the terms *NANDA-I*, *NIC*, and *NOC*, even though you probably will not be studying these taxonomies during your basic nursing programs. Your place of employment after graduation may have adopted these taxonomies and will expect you to use them in assisting planning for patient care. Knowing the meaning of the terms will assist you in using the systems.

NURSING INTERVENTIONS CLASSIFICATION

Nursing Interventions Classification (NIC) focuses on intervention—what the nurse does to enhance patient outcomes. Dochterman and Bulechek (2006) of the University of Iowa head a research team who have worked on developing a language that standardizes, defines, and assists in choosing appropriate nursing interventions. Whereas NANDA-I focuses on the patient concerns, NIC is about nurse behaviors (interventions) to support the patient to attain outcomes the patient desires. NIC interventions are both direct and indirect and can be directed at the patient, family, and community. NIC is useful for nurses, student nurses, other health professionals, administrators, and faculty. It includes interventions in the categories of physical and psychosocial; illness treatment and prevention; health promotion; individual, group, family, and community; indirect and direct care; and independent and collaborative. Some nursing programs are planning their curricula around NIC. For example, during the early classroom and clinical experience, patient care planning interventions chosen are basic and related to the course of study. As the nursing program continues and courses are more advanced, so are the interventions.

NURSING OUTCOMES CLASSIFICATION

Johnson, Mass, and Moorehead (2000), also of the University of Iowa, developed Nursing Outcomes Classification (NOC). This taxonomy standardizes the terminology and criteria for measurable or desirable outcomes as a result of nursing interventions. It identifies desired outcomes for individual patients and family caregivers, as well as family- and community-level outcomes. A 5-point Likert scale is used to measure progress and can be done at any time during use of the chosen intervention(s). The Likert scale is as follows:

1. Never demonstrated
2. Rarely demonstrated
3. Sometimes demonstrated
4. Often demonstrated
5. Consistently demonstrated

This scale helps the nursing (or other) staffs to determine if the intervention is working or if changes in interventions need to be made to attain outcomes desired by the patient.

LINKING NORTH AMERICAN NURSING DIAGNOSIS ASSOCIATION INTERNATIONAL, NURSING INTERVENTIONS CLASSIFICATION, AND NURSING OUTCOMES CLASSIFICATION

NANDA-I is a source that helps the RN to determine nursing diagnosis. NANDA-I identified what concerns the patient. NIC is a source for choosing standardized nursing interventions. NOC identifies desired outcomes as a result of nursing interventions and uses a scale to identify if the intervention(s) are producing the desired outcomes. If linked interventions are used in the health care facility where you are working, you will find the information specific and easy to apply. The RN has the final decision on nursing diagnosis, choice of nursing interventions, and measuring desired patient outcomes (Figure 9-1).

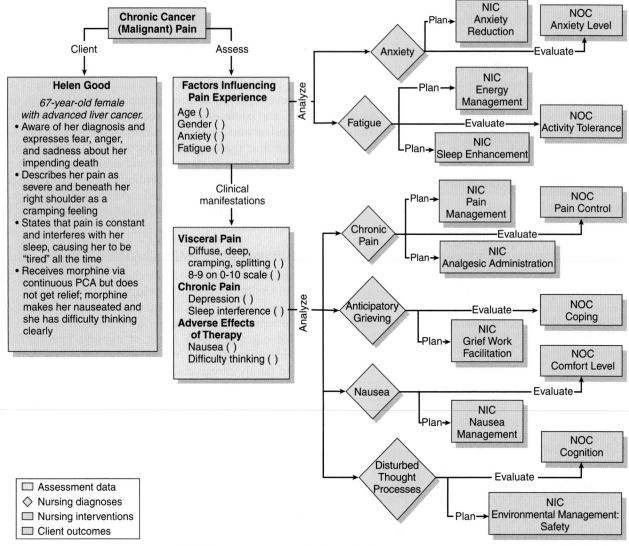

FIGURE 9-1 Concept map of a client with chronic cancer pain.

Get Ready for the NCLEX-PN® Examination

Key Points

- The Nurse Practice Act of your state identifies your legal role in the nursing process as an LPN/LVN. Take time to read it and question what you do not understand.
- The nursing process was originated in the 1950s to provide structure for thinking in nursing. The four-step process included data collection, planning, intervention, and evaluation (problem-solving model).
- The ANA standards of nursing practice, published in 1997, added nursing diagnosis to make a five-step nursing process (reasoning model). Nursing diagnosis is the exclusive responsibility of RNs because of their broad, science-based education.
- In 1996, the nursing process was included in the NCLEX-PN® for the first time. The nursing process and the practical/vocational role became an important part of nursing education for LPN/LVNs.

- In 2002, the nursing process and critical thinking were integrated throughout the NCLEX-PN®. Four steps of the nursing process for LPN/LVNs were redefined. The additional step, nursing diagnosis, is considered the exclusive responsibility of the RN.

Step 1: *Data collection*—patient data are gathered and reported to appropriate personnel.

Step 2: *Planning*—the LPN/LVN assists the RN to develop the nursing diagnosis, outcomes, and interventions for the patient's plan of care. This includes maintaining patient safety.

Step 3: *Implementation*—nursing interventions in the care plan are put into action.

Step 4: *Evaluation*—actual outcomes of the interventions are compared with desired patient outcomes (emphasis is on patient progress toward meeting outcomes). Results are reported and documented.

- Critical thinking and nursing process are mandated for SPN/SVN education.
- NANDA-I is a systemized taxonomy used to determine any patient concerns. NIC is a way of identifying standardized nursing interventions. NOC is a system for measuring patient outcomes. Trial implementation in select hospitals has shown the value of combining NANDA-I, NIC, and NOC.

Additional Learning Resources

evolve Go to your Evolve website (http://evolve.elsevier.com/Hill/Success) for the following FREE learning resources:
- Answers to Critical Thinking Scenarios
- Additional learning activities
- Additional Review Questions for the NCLEX-PN® exam
- Helpful phrases for communicating in Spanish and more!

Review Questions for the NCLEX-PN® Examination

1. How did the origination of the nursing process in the 1950s change the course of nursing?
    1. It provided a reasoning model.
    2. It provided a specificity model.
    3. It provided a problem-solution model.
    4. It provided a critical-thinking model.

2. Some RNs and instructors have questioned the value of teaching SPN/SVNs nursing process and critical thinking. Which statement provides a valid reason for including both in the SPN/SVN curriculum?
    1. Knowledge of the nursing process and critical thinking encourages postgraduate education so that one day the LPN/LVN can be an RN.
    2. LPN/LVNs and RNs both do the work of nursing. A common language provides an organized way of understanding what is to be done.
    3. Learning the nursing process and critical thinking provides the opportunity to be working on both LPN and RN levels of nursing at the same time.
    4. Learning the nursing process and critical thinking provides a cookbook method of learning and provides time to deal with job stresses.

3. Which request by the RN will you refuse to do because it is beyond the LPN/LVN scope of practice?
    1. "Do Mr. Frederic's plan of care, and I will initial it as soon I get back from lunch."
    2. "Catheterize Mrs. Jones as soon as you can and report total output to me STAT."
    3. "Check Mr. Neap's pressure sore on his right hip for changes since his admission."
    4. "Assist Sally (RN) by doing an assessment of our new admission on the south wing."

4. Which action is within the LPN/LVN scope of nursing practice when a patient aspirates a piece of meat and you are sitting opposite the patient in the dining room?
    1. Ask someone to get help as you move quickly toward the patient to perform a Heimlich maneuver.

2. Ask another patient to straighten up the patient while you go to get an RN or other qualified staff member.
3. Immediately call the patient's doctor for permission to perform the Heimlich and mention you are an SPN/SVN.
4. Because you do not know if this patient has a do-not-resuscitate order on the chart, send someone to check.

Alternate Format Item

1. Which of the following is not a reason for verifying data? *(Select all that apply.)*
    1. Patient and family account of what happened differ.
    2. You believe that persons of this culture are dishonest.
    3. Patient complains of fever, but the forehead feels cool.
    4. You note that the patient's body language and words match.

2. A new patient has arrived, and the RN has asked you to begin data collection while she finishes taking doctor's orders. *Prioritize the following steps.*
    1. Ask the patient who accompanied him or her to the hospital.
    2. Measure vital signs.
    3. Introduce yourself to the patient and state what you are going to do.
    4. Ask what is going on with his or her health.
    5. Report information to the RN and ask for further instructions.

Critical Thinking Scenarios

Scenario 1
You have recently read an article in a nursing journal that suggests the nursing process is a waste of time. According to this author, nurses know intuitively what a patient needs because of their love for patients. "After all, this is the reason a person becomes a nurse." You have decided to respond critically to the author's views. What are you going to write to the journal so they will read your response as critically thought out and be willing to print your response?

Scenario 2
Amy wants to improve her grades. She learned about using the nursing process during class a couple of days ago. "If it works for planning patient care, why can it not work for me? I am going to give it a try."

Answer the following questions of what Amy can do for each step of the nursing process to improve her grades:

1. How might Amy **gather data** on her study habits?
2. In the **planning** stage, Amy discovered that she periodically fell asleep while studying (maybe because she was studying in her bed). She was surprised to count that she had a total of 30 cell phone calls or text messages during that time. She spent time talking on the cell or texting in response. She did not even finish the chapter she was trying to concentrate on. What changes could she **implement** to ensure future success?
3. How would Amy **evaluate** her success?

Nursing Theory, Research, and Evidence-Based Practice

Objectives

On completing this chapter, you will be able to do the following:

1. Provide one reason for the development of nursing theories.
2. Briefly describe each of the following theories as they relate to the nursing process:
   - Maslow's Hierarchy of Human Needs Theory
   - Rosenstock's Health Belief Model
   - Orem's Self-Care Deficit Theory
   - Leininger's Culture Care Theory
   - Peplau's Interpersonal Relations Theory
   - Sister Callista Roy's Adaptation Model
   - Nightingale's Environmental Model
   - Jean Watson's Theory of Human Care
3. Briefly explain the importance of nursing research.
4. Compare and contrast quantitative and qualitative research studies.
5. Define evidence-based-practice.
6. Explain the three elements of evidence-based practice (EBP).
7. Briefly describe how best evidence for practice is determined by systematic reviews of research studies.
8. Discuss how your site of clinical experience adopts evidence-based guidelines for nursing interventions.
9. Explain the LPN/LVN's role in nursing research and evidence-based practice.

Key Terms

evidence-based practice (ĔV-ĭ-dĕns bāsd, p. 115)
Leininger's Culture Care Theory (KŬL-chŭr KĀR, p. 112)
Maslow's Human Needs Theory (p. 111)
nursing research (p. 113)
nursing theories (p. 110)
Orem's Self-Care Deficit Theory (SĔLF KĀR DĔF-ĭ-sĭt, p. 111)
Peplau's Interpersonal Relations Theory (ĭn-tĕr-PĔR-sŭn-ăl, p. 112)

qualitative research study (KWĂL-ĭ-tā-tĭv, p. 114)
quantitative research study (KWĂN-tĭ-tā-tĭv, p. 113)
Rosenstock's Health Belief Theory (p. 112)
Sister Callista Roy's Adaptation Model (ă-dăp-TĀ-shŭn, p. 113)
spirit of inquiry (SPĬ-rĭt ĭn-KWĒR-ē, p. 115)
Watson's Theory of Human Care (p. 113)

 Keep in Mind

Becoming acquainted with terminology assists in learning information when it becomes necessary in your career.

NURSING THEORIES

RATIONALE FOR THEORIES

Numerous nursing theories have been developed for nursing, and some of them are the basis for curriculum development. They open possibilities to question and can be used as a basis for research on effectiveness of nursing care. The following three concepts are important to nursing:

1. *Person* (the recipient of care)
2. *Health* (the goal of nursing)
3. *Environment* (the setting where nursing care takes place)

It is important to discuss nursing theories because if you decide to become an RN, you will encounter name recognition when studying theories used as a framework for nursing education and clinical practice. Practical nurses are sometimes asked to gather data for research being done by master's or Ph.D. candidates. Although the LPN/LVN does not evaluate the data for the study, it is important to recognize that the data gathered will influence the outcome of the research.

FLORENCE NIGHTINGALE: THE FIRST NURSING THEORIST

Florence Nightingale was the first to emphasize the environment: ventilation, warmth, noise, light, and cleanliness. Nightingale is considered the first nursing theorist. She strongly believed that environmental issues influenced the course of illness. She also saw the nursing role as separate from the nurse as a "hand-maiden" to the doctor.

ABRAHAM MASLOW'S HUMAN NEEDS THEORY

Although Abraham Maslow is a psychologist, his Human Needs Theory has been adapted by many professional programs, including some nursing programs, as a framework for education. Here is a general description of the theory:

1. Abraham Maslow's theory states that certain internal, external, physical, and psychological needs are common to all people.
2. Common needs are arranged in a hierarchy.
3. Unmet needs create tension, which motivates the person to react to meet the need.
4. When needs are met, the person is no longer aware of the need, and the need (now met) no longer motivates them.
5. Dominant needs that matter to a person can vary in life.

Figure 10-1 provides examples in identifying patient care priorities and responding to the needs according to the patient level of functioning. It is important to remember that a person may be functioning on more than one level of needs at the same time. Read the list on the lowest level of needs again. Individuals go back to the physiologic level periodically to satisfy basic needs—for example, nutrition.

Applying Maslow's Human Needs Theory to the Nursing Process

The first data collection (assessment) of a patient is the lowest level of needs:

- *Physiologic needs:* Oxygen, food, water, elimination, safety, sleep, activity, mental stimulation, sexual procreation (e.g., the nurse collects data on whether the patients are eating enough to maintain their strength and health, if they have relief from pain, and if interventions are planned with the patients to meet the need). Once physiologic needs are met, data can be collected on safety and security needs.
- *Safety needs:* Security, freedom from harm, protection (e.g., data are collected on real or imagined safety needs—for example, do you need more

than one nurse to move the patient safely from the bed to the toilet?). The primary areas that involve hospital nursing care are the first two levels: physiologic and safety needs.

- *Love and belonging needs:* Love, affection, and companionship (e.g., data are collected on whether the patient has a support system to assist with care once hospitalization is over). This is a part of discharge planning to be sure the patient has support meeting needs posthospitalization. The nurse may be involved in doing follow-up care in the home after hospitalization (home health, visiting nurse service, etc.).
- *Esteem needs:* Respect and recognition (e.g., data are collected on what the patient is doing or can do that will assist in earning a positive sense of self). Is the person able to do volunteer work or join a Senior Center that has activities, provides an opportunity to help others, and offers meals at a reasonable price)? Once esteem needs are met, the individual may be ready to focus on self-actualization. A parish nurse, for example, may be providing care at this level.
- *Self-actualization:* This is the highest level of needs, and not everyone attains this level. This involves maximum realization and fulfillment of the individual's potential.

OREM'S SELF-CARE DEFICIT THEORY

Dorothea Orem's Self-Care Deficit Theory is a general theory that consists of three subtheories:

1. *Self-care:* This involves a goal that is directed toward a safer environment for life, health, and well-being. (Ideally, individuals learn to respond to health cues in themselves or the environment as a way to maintain personal health.)
2. *Self-care deficit:* Personal care does not meet therapeutic self-care demands. (The individual does not recognize or know what to do in regard to personal health situations.)

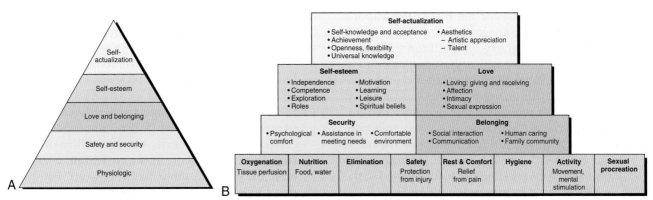

FIGURE 10-1 **A.** Maslow's Hierarchy of Human Needs. **B.** Evolving Hierarchy of Needs adapted by nursing.

3. *Nursing system:* Nurses empower the patient through their interpersonal relationship to help meet their self-care demands. (Nursing responds to the person's care needs totally, partially, or in a supportive role according to the need.)

Orem's theory is concerned with growth and development needs, as well as physiologic and psychosocial needs. Nurses can use the data collection step of the nursing process to identify specific self-care deficits. By working with the patient, nurses can then choose interventions that will have the desired outcomes for the patient.

MADELINE LEININGER'S CULTURE CARE THEORY

Leininger's interest in cultural care and how nursing responds to people of different cultures began when she was working with disturbed children. She recognized a link to understanding care based on their cultural background. When developing her Culture Care Theory, Leininger identified two kinds of care in every culture: *generic,* meaning home remedies used in care, and *professional,* which is provided by people who are specifically trained to provide care.

Leininger proposed three modes to guide nursing decisions when providing care:

1. *Cultural care preservation or maintenance.* This means assisting persons of particular cultures to maintain care values that help them to maintain health or restore health. As an example, some cultures use periodic "cupping" (bloodletting) as a way to relieve symptoms of hemochromatosis (excess iron deposits throughout the body). A method in other cultures is to periodically give blood at a blood blank to reduce the hematocrit (the percentage of your blood that is made up of red blood cells).
2. *Cultural care accommodation or negotiation.* In some cultures, Vicks VapoRub is placed in the nostrils, which can potentially be aspirated and lead to pneumonia. The visiting nurse demonstrated placing the Vicks on the chest and neck and rubbing it in a soothing manner. A warm cloth was placed on the chest for the night. The vapor's fumes relieved the congestion.
3. *Culture care repatterning or restructuring.* Leininger's theory is concerned with respecting cultural differences and yet providing a safe and protective environment (e.g., in some cultures, mud is placed on the infant's umbilicus after delivery). Because of concern for local and systemic infection, the visiting nurse provided clean pads. The nurse demonstrated their use, how to clean the area, and how to leave the area uncovered for a period so the umbilicus could be exposed to the air.

HILDEGARD PEPLAU'S INTERPERSONAL RELATIONS THEORY

Nurses who work with adult or child psychiatric patients are more likely to use Peplau's Interpersonal Relations Theory as a basis for developing a therapeutic relationship with the patient. The relationship that is developed has certain parameters and is the major part of the treatment.

Peplau describes four overlapping phases:
- *Orientation:* The patient seeks assistance because of a felt need. A problem has been identified, and the nurse works with the patient to help him or her recognize the problem. The process is often complex, but personal and social growth can develop during this step.
- *Identification:* During this phase, the patient understands the situation and responds to the nurse who supplies the needed help.
- *Exploitation:* During this phase, the patient begins to depend on the nurse and uses the help offered, exploring all possibilities.
- *Resolution:* The dependent behavior that developed must now be given up as the therapeutic relationship comes to an end. How the nurse handles this phase is crucial because faulty resolution can possibly end with vague physical symptoms.

During the therapeutic relationship, the nurse fulfills the roles of resource person, teacher, leader, surrogate, and counselor.

ROSENSTOCK'S HEALTH BELIEF THEORY

Irwin Rosenstock developed the Health Belief Theory that tries to explain why or why not a person will take action to prevent or detect illness. According to this theory:

1. *Perceptions vary and may have no basis in reality.* For example, Marta came to the emergency room because she was no longer able to sit down. Upon examination, it was determined that she had advanced cancer of the vulva. Marta was very shy, and even though she was aware of changes, she just hoped that whatever it was would just go away. Even Marta's sister, with whom she lived, was unaware that there was any disease process going on. She explained, "We have never seen each other naked." The thought of being examined embarrassed Marta: "No one has ever looked at me down there."
2. *Beliefs are connected to existing barriers* (e.g., may see the preventive or treatment activity as expensive, painful, or inconvenient). If there are fewer perceived negative aspects, the possibility of doing something is higher: If more negative aspects exist, the person is more likely not to act. For example, Cora, age 82, began to have gastrointestinal

symptoms and asked her son to make a doctor's appointment for her. He did so and drove 8 hours to take her to the appointment. When he arrived, she refused to go in, explaining, "I've changed my mind. It's nothing." This went on several more times over a period of years before she was so uncomfortable that she finally kept the appointment. Cora was diagnosed with advanced cancer of the colon. Cora explained that she had already had seven surgeries and did not want to put up with another uncomfortable healing process. Because of the pain she was having now, Cora agreed to surgery. The surgery was palliative, which gave her relief from pain, but she was told she probably had only 6 months to live.

3. *A cue to action is seen as necessary* (e.g., pain, a news story, a reminder call from the doctor's office). The cue (finally) for Cora was the pain she began to experience.

This theory can be useful when using the nursing process to promote health. It can be used to promote yearly examinations, vaccinations, wellness classes, and so forth. It is also helpful to the nurse and patient when developing interventions and outcomes to deal with a disease process or health problem that has been identified.

SISTER CALLISTA ROY'S ADAPTATION MODEL

Sister Roy describes the recipient of care (the patient) as a "holistic adaptive system" in her Adaptation Model. Both internal (from inside the patient) and external (from outside the patient) stimuli affect the system. She identifies the following types of stimuli:

- *Focal*—meaning something direct, such as a patient experiencing pain
- *Contextual*—meaning other factors that affect the focal stimuli, such as being examined in the area of pain
- *Residual*—meaning both internal and external factors that may not always be evident, such as a memory of previous pain and the effect it had on the patient

Coping methods are known as *regulator* and *cognator* subsystems:

- A *regulator* subsystem refers to the internal effects that take place in response to what is happening internally. These include neural, chemical, and endocrine processes. The body automatically attempts to regulate the system when it is being affected negatively.
- A *cognator* subsystem refers to learning, processing, judging, and emotion that the patient uses to cope with what has happened.

Two adaptive modes are available to help the patient deal with the situation:

1. *Physiologic*, which includes the senses, fluids, electrolytes, neurologic, and endocrine systems
2. *Self-concepts, role functions, and interdependence*

- Self-concepts are related to psychological and spiritual aspects of the patient.
- Role functions are related to the patient's role in society.
- Interdependence is related to love, respect, and values and can include the patient's support system.

The response is either:

- *Adaptation:* The patient reaches his or her goal of recovery.
- *Ineffective:* The patient does not survive or has a poor outcome.

JEAN WATSON'S THEORY OF HUMAN CARE

According to Watson's Theory of Human Care, health is harmony between the body, mind, and spirit. It also involves self-perception and how the self is experienced. Illness is a lack of harmony within the self and the soul. The nursing role is a caring process to help the patient regain harmony and health. Through the caring, the patient develops self-knowledge and self-healing. The enabling actions allow the patient to solve problems and grow. Both the patient and the nurse grow through this process.

Many other theories are used in nursing. If you want to learn more about theories, most nursing fundamental and foundations texts have a chapter devoted to theories and models.

NURSING RESEARCH

Research in any profession supports existing knowledge and develops new knowledge based on observation and experimentation. Starting with Nightingale's study of soldier morbidity and mortality data during the Crimean War through today's emphasis on evidence-based practice, nursing research has improved existing nursing knowledge and generated new knowledge that influences nursing practice. Research studies in nursing are important because they do the following:

- Identify specific nursing interventions that are proven effective and not merely based on tradition.
- Provide evidence that supports the quality and cost-effectiveness of what nurses do.
- Generate knowledge for clinical practice, nursing education, and delivery of nursing services.

Nurses of all educational levels are encouraged to participate in and promote nursing research in varying degrees (Cherry and Jacob, 2011). These are the two main types of research studies done in nursing:

- Quantitative research study, which is objective study. A *variable* is the event the researcher is trying to measure. There are two types of variables; one variable is the group receiving the intervention and the other variable is the group that does not receive the intervention. Numeric data are collected and measured using statistics to describe variables, examine relationships among variables or determine cause-and-effect interactions between variables.

- Qualitative research study, which is subjective study. Data are gathered by interviews, and study is a narrative description of the "lived experience" of individuals—for example, living with chronic pain. *Phenomenology* is a type of qualitative study. *Grounded theory* studies describe a process that people use to deal with problem areas of their lives—for example, coping with a diagnosis of cancer.

See Evolve for a Quantitative Research Study of Practical Nursing Students and a List of Terms used in Quantitative Research.

EVIDENCE-BASED PRACTICE

BACKGROUND OF THE EVIDENCE-BASED PRACTICE MOVEMENT

- Dr. Archie Cochrane (1901-1988), a British epidemiologist, challenged the public to pay only for medical care that was proven to be effective and advocated the use of randomized, controlled trials (RCTs) as a means of reliably informing health care practices. In 1993, the Cochrane Collaboration, an independent, not-for-profit organization, was established to prepare and promote the accessibility of *Cochrane Reviews*, a collection of evidence-based health care interventions obtained by systematic reviews of research.
- In 1999, the Institute of Medicine (IOM) issued the report *To Err Is Human: Building a Safer Health System*, which discussed the incidence of medical errors in health care and the need for reform.
- In 2001, the IOM issued *Crossing the Quality Chasm: A New Health System for the 21st Century*, calling for consistent, high-quality health care for all people. Included in the 10 rules or general principles issued by the IOM was "Patients should receive care based on the best available scientific knowledge."
- Insurance companies are beginning to pay for health care practices only if their effectiveness is supported by scientific evidence.
- Hospitals are denied payment when complications in a Medicare patient develop if evidence-based guidelines are not followed.
- Patients and families are seeking the latest evidence on websites about the most effective treatment for illnesses and diseases.

HOW BEST EVIDENCE FOR PRACTICE GUIDELINES IS DETERMINED

Best evidence is determined through a complex, rigorous process:

- The clinical question being investigated is formulated in an objective, concise manner.
- Using professional resources, the latest, most relevant research evidence that pertains to the clinical question is located (Box 10-1).
- An expert or panel of experts conducts a systematic review, which is a summary of the results of selected studies.
- Guidelines are determined. These are specific practice recommendations derived from the summary of research articles.

Box 10-1   Systematic Reviews Used to Develop EBP Guidelines

PUBMED (http://pubmed.gov)
The U.S. National Library of Medicine (NLM) database of biomedical citations and abstracts.
- **MEDLINE** is the largest component of PubMed and is freely accessible. (Fact Sheet@http://www.nlm.nih.gov/pubs/factsheets/dif_med_pub.html).

CUMULATIVE INDEX OF NURSING AND ALLIED HEALTH LITERATURE (CINAHL)
- A source for practical/vocational nurses for EBP interventions.

COCHRANE REVIEWS (http://www.cochrane.org/cochrane-reviews)
- Each review addresses a clearly formulated question. All of the existing research on a topic that meets certain criteria is searched for and collated and then assessed using stringent guidelines to establish whether or not there is conclusive evidence about a specific treatment. The reviews are updated regularly, ensuring that treatment decisions can be based on the most up-to-date and reliable evidence.

AGENCY FOR HEALTHCARE RESEARCH AND QUALITY (AHRQ) (http://www.ahrq.gov/)
- An agency of the U.S. Department of Health and Human Services.
- The National Guideline Clearinghouse™ (NGC) (http://www.guideline.gov) is an initiative of AHRQ. Provides a comprehensive database of evidence-based clinical practice guidelines and related documents with syntheses and comparisons. It provides Internet users with free online access.

THE JOANNA BRIGGS INSTITUTE (JBI) (http://www.joannabriggs.edu.au/)
- An international not-for-profit membership-based organization in the Faculty of Health Sciences at the University of Adelaide, Australia. The Institute develops methods to appraise and synthesize evidence, conducting systematic reviews and analyses of the research literature to provide the best available evidence to inform clinical decision making.

- Using critical-thinking skills, the gathered evidence is combined with clinical experience and the patient's preferences and values for use in a specific clinical situation.

 Try This

How do agencies where you have clinical rotations obtain their guidelines for evidence-based nursing interventions?

EVIDENCE-BASED PRACTICE (EBP) IN NURSING

Nursing care that is based on comments such as "This is how we do that procedure here"; "This is how I was taught to do this nursing intervention 20 years ago"; or "We always do things this way" is not sufficient in today's health care environment. Nursing interventions such as cleansing wounds with Betadine or hydrogen peroxide and massaging over bony prominences are examples of common nursing interventions in past years that have been proven through research to be potentially harmful (Ackley, 2008). The clinical practice of nurses needs to be based on scientific knowledge with proof that the knowledge is effective. Research provides the foundation for evidence-based nursing practice.

ELEMENTS OF EVIDENCE-BASED PRACTICE

The elements of evidence-based practice are like a triangle with the following three areas (Figure 10-2):
- Best research evidence
- Nurse's clinical expertise
- Patient preferences

THE NURSE'S ROLE

In 2010, the National League for Nursing (NLN) established competencies of nursing graduates at all levels. The competency that addresses nursing research and evidence-based practice is spirit of inquiry. A nurse with a spirit of inquiry is one who "will raise questions, challenge traditional and existing practices, and seek creative approaches to problems." The following describes what the NLN expects of all levels of nurses in regard to research and evidence-based practice:
- Nurses with a *research doctorate* design and implement research studies and publish findings.
- Nurses with a *practice doctorate* review present research and formulate evidence-based protocols.
- Nurses at the *master's level* formulate research questions and evaluate the effect of evidence-based solutions on nursing problems.

FIGURE 10-2 The triangle of evidence-based practice.

- Nurses with a *bachelor's degree* identify questions needed to be studied, critique published research, and use evidence as solutions to nursing problems.
- *Associate degree/diploma* nurses challenge the status quo, question assumptions, and offer new insights to improve the quality of care.
- *Practical/vocational nurses* question the basis for nursing actions by considering research, evidence, tradition, and patient preference (Outcomes and Competencies for Graduates of Practical/Vocational, Diploma, Associate Degree, Baccalaureate, Master's, Practice Doctorate, and Research Doctorate Programs in Nursing, 2010).

The Practical/Vocational Nurse's Role in Evidence-Based Practice

Practical/vocational nursing students participate in the nursing research process by reviewing current articles in professional sources as part of their student learning experience and support nursing interventions on care plans and in practice with evidence-based nursing practices. As students and graduates, they need to follow protocols and procedures for nursing interventions of the agency in which they practice. Protocols are the general outlines used to manage a clinical situation—for example, a care plan. Procedures include the detailed steps of nursing interventions for implementing the protocol. Objective data gathering is essential for evaluation of the effectiveness of selected evidence-based practices.

Get Ready for the NCLEX-PN® Examination

Key Points

- Nursing involves many different theories. Choosing the appropriate theory for a nursing curriculum can be used as a guide to improve the course of study.
- Maslow's Human Needs Theory is based on Maslow's Hierarchy of Needs, which says that as needs on one level are met, others emerge.
- Rosenstock's Health Belief Theory tries to understand why people do or do not take action to prevent or detect disease.
- Orem's Self-Care Deficit Theory looks at why some individuals are goal-oriented toward taking care of their health and well-being, why some do not meet their self-care demands, and how the nurse, through an interpersonal relationship with the patient, can assist the patient with a self-care deficit to meet his or her self-care demands.
- Nursing research is a scientific process that validates and refines existing knowledge and generates new knowledge that influences nursing practice.
- The clinical practice of nurses needs to be based on scientific knowledge with proof that the knowledge is effective.
- Research provides the foundation for evidence-based practice in nursing.
- The elements of evidence-based practice are best research evidence, nurse's clinical expertise, and patient preferences.
- Spirit of inquiry for a practical/vocational nurse means a nurse who "will raise questions, challenge traditional and existing practices, and seek creative approaches to problems."
- Practical/vocational nurses participate in the nursing research process by reviewing current articles in professional sources; supporting clinical interventions on care plans and in practice with evidence-based nursing practices; collecting data for research studies as requested by the registered nurse; following protocols and procedures of the agency in which they are employed; and providing objective data gathering to evaluate the effectiveness of selected evidence-based practices.

Additional Learning Resources

evolve Go to your Evolve website(http://evolve.elsevier.com/Hill/Success) for the following FREE learning resources:
- Answers to Critical Thinking Scenario
- Additional learning activities
- Additional Review Questions for the NCLEX-PN® exam
- Helpful phrases for communicating in Spanish and more!

Review Questions for the NCLEX-PN® Examination

1. Elements of evidence-based practice in nursing do not include:
   1. Best research evidence.
   2. Nurse's clinical expertise.
   3. Patient preferences.
   4. Tradition in agency.

2. An abstract found on a database or at the beginning of a research study is:
   1. Something difficult to understand.
   2. Something designed to distract you.
   3. A summary of the research performed.
   4. A complete account of the research study.

3. Which of the following statements is accurate regarding theories useful to nursing?
   1. Orem's interpersonal theory defines roles and steps in developing a therapeutic relationship.
   2. Maslow's culture care theory is concerned with how to meet cultural needs through nursing care.
   3. Rosenstock's needs theory focused on meeting patient needs that may have no basis in fact.
   4. Maslow's theory is often used because it works well using nursing process steps in patient care.

4. Crystal is explaining qualitative research to a classmate. What response does not apply to qualitative research?
   1. A cause/effect relationship of variables is confirmed.
   2. Interviews are used to gather data.
   3. Lived experiences—for example, pain—are studied.
   4. Problem areas of participants' lives are studied.

Alternate Format Item

1. List in order the steps taken to find best practices in nursing.
   1. Find the latest, most relevant research evidence.
   2. Formulate the clinical question being investigated.
   3. Using critical thinking skills, combine the gathered evidence with clinical experience and the patient's preferences and values.
   4. Evaluate the validity, relevance, and how you can apply the evidence to the clinical situation selected.

2. Select the items that describe the LPN/LVN's role in nursing research and evidence-based practice. (Select all that apply. No partial credit is given for correct selections.)
   1. Collect data for research studies as requested by the registered nurse.
   2. Formulate clinical questions that need to be investigated for validity.
   3. Follow protocols and procedures of the agency in which they are employed.
   4. Gather data for evaluation of the effectiveness of evidence-based practices.
   5. Support clinical interventions in practice with evidence-based nursing practices.

Critical Thinking Scenario

Corey, an SPN, has his medical/surgical clinical experience in a hospital that uses evidence-based practice when selecting nursing interventions to implement. During preconference, Corey's clinical instructor notes on his care plan that he will instill five cc's of air into the patient's gastric feeding tube while auscultating over the epigastric area for a "swooshing" sound to ascertain proper tube placement. The patient is receiving an intermittent tube feeding. The instructor questions Corey's source of information, and Corey states that he found the information on the Internet. What did Corey do wrong for obtaining information and what should he have done to obtain proper tube placement?

Ethics Applied to Nursing: Personal Versus Professional Ethics

Objectives

On completing this chapter, you will be able to do the following:

1. List four current ethical issues of concern in twenty-first-century health care.
2. Explain the differences among ethics, morals, and values.
3. Differentiate between personal and professional ethics.
4. Identify ethical elements in your state's Nurse Practice Act.
5. Describe how the role of nursing has changed since the introduction of the nursing process and critical thinking into nursing curricula.
6. Discuss how nonmaleficence is more complex than the definition of "do no harm."
7. Differentiate between beneficence and paternal beneficence.
8. Explain the steps for an autonomous decision.
9. Describe how fidelity affects nursing care.
10. Discuss how a nurse applies the principle of justice to nursing.
11. Discuss the role of beneficent paternalism.
12. Differentiate between ethical and legal responsibility in nursing.

Key Terms

autonomy (Ăw-TŎN-ŏ-mē, p. 124)
beneficence (bĕ-NĚF-ĭ-sĕns, p. 123)
beneficent paternalism (bĕ-NĚF-ĭ-sĕnt-pă-TŬR-nă-lĭz-ŭm, p. 126)
ethics (ĕ-THĬKS, p. 118)
fidelity (fĭ-DĚL-ĭ-tē, p. 125)
justice (JŬS-tĭs, p. 125)

morals (MŎR-ăls, p. 119)
nonmaleficence (nŏn-mă-LĚF-ĭ-sĕns, p. 122)
nursing ethics (NŬR-sĭng ĕ-THĬKS, p. 119)
personal ethics (PĚR-sŭn-ăl ĕ-THĬKS, p. 120)
privacy (PRĪ-vă-sē, p. 124)
values (VĂL-ū p. 119)

 Keep in Mind

Nurses make decisions daily about right, wrong, good, bad, ought, and duty.

The twenty-first century presents numerous ethical issues in health care, as reflected in agency policies and medical procedures that create life, prolong life, cure chronic diseases, ensure a peaceful death, and end life. Additional ethical issues will arise as scientific research continues to explore possibilities, the procedures are discussed, and, if procedures are legalized, people press for their right to make autonomous decisions. Students in personal/vocational nursing classes identified the following current ethical issues in health care: in vitro fertilization, artificial insemination, surrogate motherhood, cloning, organ donation (including cadaver donations), child organ donors, procedures that use fetal tissues (stem cells) or organs from aborted fetuses, conceiving a child to produce tissue for a sibling, abortion, experiments that destroy a human embryo, euthanasia, assisted suicide, advance directives

(including living wills and durable power of attorney), and insertion and/or withdrawal of feeding tubes. An example is when the patient has verbalized to the physician the wish to avoid further heroic means to stay alive. Two adult children have arrived and insist that all means be used to maintain life, but the three children already at the bedside do not agree. The patient lacks a living will and durable power of attorney and is unconscious at this point. As you progress in your nursing program, add additional areas of ethical issues to this list started by your peers.

 Critical Thinking

Where do nurses get their ethics and morals in terms of self-analysis?

DESCRIPTION AND SCOPE OF ETHICS

Ethics is a system of standards or moral principles that direct actions as being right or wrong. Ethics is concerned with the meaning of words such as *right, wrong, good, bad, ought,* and *duty*. Ethics is concerned with the ways people, either individually or as a group, decide the following:

- What actions are right or wrong
- If one *ought* to do something
- If one has the *right* to do something
- If one has the *duty* to do something

This basic definition is somewhat of an oversimplification. Ethics sounds like the words *morals* and *values*, but there are differences among them.

 Critical Thinking

How does the nurse avoid imposing his or her morals and ethics in a working situation?

MORALS AND VALUES

Morals are concerned with dealing with right or wrong behavior (conduct) and character. The terms *ethics* and *morals* are difficult to define separately. *Morals* come from a Latin root, and *ethics* comes from a Greek root. Both words mean "customs" or "habits" and refer to the general area of rights and wrongs. The words are often substituted for each other. We will use *ethics* and *morals* in the same way in this chapter.

Values involve the *worth* you assign to an idea or an action. Values are freely chosen and are affected by age, experience, and maturity. A child usually embraces family values during childhood. The teen years are a time of trying out family values and either incorporating them or rejecting and replacing them with new values. Values continue to be modified throughout your lifetime as you acquire new knowledge and experience. Based on changes in values, one's code of ethics/morals can be shifted (e.g., organ transplants after you have learned about or cared for a patient who receives a transplant).

Law is thought of as a minimum ethic that is written and enforced. As a licensed practical/vocational nurse (LPN/LVN), the Nurse Practice Act in your state is your final authority on what you are legally obligated to do as a nurse regardless of where you are employed (see Chapter 12 for more about nursing and the law).

Have a thorough knowledge of the Nurse Practice Act in the state in which you are employed.

COMPARISON OF LEGAL ASPECTS OF NURSING AND ETHICS

Nursing ethics are similar to, but also different from, the legal aspects that regulate your nursing practice. Table 11-1 presents a comparison of legal aspects and nursing ethics.

NURSING ETHICS

According to the *Miller-Keane Encyclopedia & Dictionary of Medicine, Nursing & Allied Health*, nursing ethics are "the values and ethical principles governing nursing practice, conduct, and relationships." Nursing ethics deals with the relationship of a nurse to the patient, the patient's family, associates and fellow nurses, and society at large. Nursing ethics attempts to look for underlying patterns or order in a large number of ethical decisions and practices of nurses, individually or as a group. Codes provide a guideline for what the LPN/LVN ought to do. However, codes do not carry the weight of law. It is interesting to note how many ethical items are actually found in the law, such as your Nurse Practice Act. When ethical items are included in a legal document, it places emphasis on the importance of these items. It also gives the LPN/LVN a source to fall back on to defend the choices in behavior they make in regard to patients and families; it is then a matter of law.

ETHICAL CODES OF THE NATIONAL ASSOCIATION FOR PRACTICAL NURSE EDUCATION AND THE SERVICE AND NATIONAL FEDERATION OF LICENSED PRACTICAL NURSES

Ethics that are adopted by nursing groups are in their codes of behavior. Both the National Association for Practical Nurse Education and Service (NAPNES) and the National Federation of Licensed Practical Nurses (NFLPN) have ethical codes for LPN/LVNs (see Appendixes B and C).

Table 11-1 Comparison of Legal Aspects and Nursing Ethics

	LEGAL ASPECTS	NURSING ETHICS
Definition	The state statutes that apply to licensed persons and the situations in patient care that could result in legal action	Set of rules of conduct
Focus	Rules and regulations	Ideal behavior of a group of licensed people
	Obligations under the law	Morality
		Higher standards
Applies to	Member of a professional/career group	Member of a nursing group
Participation	Mandatory	Voluntary
Source	Your state's Nurse Practice Act	NFLPN and NAPNES codes, Florence Nightingale Pledge, PN Pledge

Try This

Ethical Issues and Your Nurse Practice Act

Discover how your state includes ethical issues (what you ought to do as an LPN/LVN) in the law, which is your Nurse Practice Act (what you must do as a licensed person).

- Read the ethical codes of the NAPNES and NFLPN.
- Use the NFLPN code as an example.
- Search for the elements of this ethical code in your Nurse Practice Act. Fill out the following worksheet.
- Summarize the ethical elements found in the Nurse Practice Act.

Ethical Area	Is this ethical area addressed in your state's Nurse Practice Act?	If "yes," cite section
1. Know the scope of maximum utilization of the LPN/LVN, as specified by the Nurse Practice Act, and the function within this scope.		
2. Safeguard the confidential information acquired from any source about the patient.		
3. Provide health care to all patients, regardless of race, creed, cultural background, disease, or lifestyle (e.g., single parent, sexual orientation).		
4. Refuse to give endorsement to the sale or promotion of commercial products or services.		
5. Uphold the highest standards in personal appearance, language, dress, and demeanor.		
6. Stay informed about issues affecting the practice of nursing and the delivery of health care, and, where appropriate, participate in government and policy decisions.		
7. Accept the responsibility for safe nursing practice by keeping mentally and physically fit and educationally prepared to practice.		
8. Accept the responsibility for membership in NFLPN or the LPN/LVN organization of your choice, and participate in its efforts to maintain the established standards of nursing practice and employment policies that lead to quality patient care.		

YOUR PERSONAL CODE OF ETHICS

Practical/vocational nursing students and LPN/LVNs also have personal ethics that provide personal guidelines for living. You ultimately chose what your personal code of ethics would include. Your personal code of ethics will influence your nursing ethics. Sometimes personal ethics conflict with the law (state's Nurse Practice Act). When this occurs, you have an obligation to follow the law. If you object to a medical procedure on religious or moral grounds, state this objection in writing. Present the statement to the employer *before* starting employment. The employing agency and *you* need to be clear in advance about your objection to procedures because of religious or moral reasons. For example, you may be ethically opposed to abortion. Abortion in the United States is permitted under certain circumstances. You may ethically refuse to assist with the abortion procedure (and have stated this in writing at the time of employment), but postprocedure you cannot refuse to give nursing care to the woman involved. In the words of Sister M. Antoinette, former Director of Nursing at Sacred Heart Hospital in Allentown, Pennsylvania, "You may not abandon your patient." Abandonment is a legal matter, and your license may be at stake. The best strategy is to seek employment in a health agency that does not participate in procedures or nursing care of which you do not ethically approve.

Some nurses have tried to opt out of caring for patients who have an illness that may be related to a lifestyle of which they do not approve. A nurse needs to separate personal ethics from nursing ethics. You are legally expected to care for a patient regardless of his or her lifestyle. For example, when caring for an AIDS patient, use proper technique during care as you would with any patient with an infectious disease. You may not refuse to care for this patient. Ethically and legally this patient must receive the same level of care, with dignity and respect, that other patients do. *Nursing is not about giving care selectively to those patients you approve of and refusing care to others you see as less deserving.*

Critical Thinking

Personal Values

Write your personal value system regarding health and illness. Be concerned with content, not form. What you write will be an ethical code in progress. You may want to add or subtract statements after you have completed this chapter. It will also be a code you can modify as your experience with patients increases.

ROOTS OF NURSING ETHICS

Years ago, nurses saw themselves as doers, not thinkers. Nurses worked only to serve the physicians' wishes. Before the nursing process and critical thinking were added to nursing curricula, those in the nursing profession did not see themselves as having something separate to contribute to patient care (in addition to the nurses' dependent role to physicians). Nursing ethics was primarily a modification of medical ethics and ethics of other professions at that time.

WHAT CHANGED?

Nursing education was initially disease-oriented. Nursing textbooks focused on the disease process, including cause, signs, symptoms, treatment, prognosis, and nursing care related to the treatment. Physicians did the medical assessment and wrote orders for the nurse to carry out. The nurse reported on patient progress, based on physicians' orders. Nursing assessments did not exist. Additional concerns the patient might have had (e.g., spiritual, cultural, emotional, sexual) were not routinely assessed. Patients were expected to follow physicians' orders without question. The nurse's job was to see that the orders were carried out. The early nursing role was limited to the dependent relationship with the physician.

As nursing theories emerged, so did the nursing process and critical thinking, and nursing textbooks began to include these topics. Nurses discovered that in addition to their dependent role to physicians, they had something special to contribute to the patient. Finally, it was understood that the patient was a person, not just a disease. With the help of the nursing process, nurses had a way to identify additional needs that could be responded to through nursing care. Rather than expecting patients to blindly follow orders because "we know what is wrong with you and we can fix it" (benevolent paternalism), patients were encouraged to be an active part in planning and implementing their own nursing care plan (support of patient **autonomy**).

Changes in nursing did not happen easily. Many nurses were entrenched in their dependent role to physicians, and they believed that nursing was being ruined by the changes that were taking place. Nursing textbooks and curricula, however, both had to change to reflect the nursing process, critical thinking, and a focus on the total patient (not just the physically diseased or injured portion of the patient). Adding the nursing process and critical thinking changed the nursing role and changed nursing philosophy. This in turn influenced a change in nursing ethics.

Ethical principles in this chapter are about application of nursing ethics to nursing decisions and action. You are encouraged to look at both sides of an ethical principle. Recognize that no principle applies in the same way to all patients and their unique situation. No principle is absolute.

Critical thinking (see Chapter 8) plays a major role in sorting out ethical choices and legal responsibilities in regard to the patient. The patient's knowledge of choices regarding care also affects ethical decision making.

ETHICAL DECISIONS IN HEALTH CARE

ETHICS COMMITTEES

Health agencies such as hospitals have a medical ethics committee. This multidisciplinary team assists with difficult ethical decisions. Usually the discussions relate to new or unusual ethical questions. However, if you think the ethics committee makes all the medical ethical decisions, you are only partially right. Patients arrive with their culture- and/or religion-based ethics, which were often established long before they were born. What the person can and cannot do in regard to health care has already been established by the culture of which they are a part. See Chapter 17 for a discussion of spiritual needs, spiritual caring, and religious differences.

WESTERN SECULAR BELIEF SYSTEM

In the Western secular belief system, the emphasis is shifted from duties to the rights of the individual. This system has the following characteristics:

1. *Individual autonomy* means "self-rule." Individuals have the capacity to think and, based on these thoughts, to make the decision freely whether or not to seek health care (the freedom to choose).
2. *Individual rights* mean the ability to assert one's rights. The extent to which a patient can exert his or her rights is restricted (i.e., their rights cannot restrict the rights of others). For example, the patient's right to refuse treatment can be at odds with the health professional's perceived duty to act always in a way that will benefit the patient (do good and prevent harm). The individual's right has become a central theme of health care.
   a. Right to consent to care
   b. Right to choose between alternative treatments
   c. Women's rights over their own bodies
   d. Right to consent or refuse treatment

Numerous bills of rights have been written, and fierce debates have taken place at both state and national levels. The question of individual autonomy and individual rights is far from being settled. At the time of this writing, some laws based on individual autonomy and rights have been passed (e.g., Oregon, Washington, and Montana assisted suicide laws; *Roe v. Wade*). However, attempts to rescind laws that have been passed continue. The question is, to what extent do one's individual moral decisions (rights) get in the way of another's moral autonomy?

? Critical Thinking

Personal Beliefs That May Affect Medical Decisions

What cultural or religious values do you hold that may affect personal health care decisions? Use your response to this Critical Thinking Exercise to get started.

ETHICAL RESPONSIBILITIES OF NURSES

Sometimes a problem arises that appears to be an ethical problem, but it may actually be a problem of communication, trust, or insufficient information (Soglin, 2005). Adding the nursing process and critical thinking to nursing curricula changed the nursing focus to the whole patient. The dependent role to the physician remains, and responsibilities that are unique to nursing were added. The following responsibilities are both ethical and legal:

1. *Patient advocacy:* For example, the patient needs to be informed of what you will be doing to him or her (e.g., steps of a procedure). Find out what your role is in keeping the patient informed. In most states the LPN/LVN's role is to support teaching done by the registered nurse (RN) or the physician. If the patient has questions, and you are unsure about whether you should provide an answer, ask the RN. When the patient does make a decision, be supportive even though you might not agree with the decision.

2. *Accountability:* The word *accountability* means that you are answerable to yourself, to your assigned patient, to the team leader, to the physician, and to your instructor who evaluates your work. As an LPN/LVN, accountability to the instructor is replaced by accountability to the employing agency. You are held accountable for all the nursing actions that you perform or are assigned to perform. The measures of accountability are the nursing standards of practice—that is, what a nurse with your education would do in a similar situation (see Chapter 12).

3. *Peer reporting:* Report peers for behaviors that are potentially harmful to patients (e.g., impaired at work because of alcohol and/or other drug use, stealing patient's medication, substituting water or normal saline for injectable narcotics, giving patients a cold shower).

PRINCIPLES OF ETHICS

As a nurse of the twenty-first century, you recognize there is something unique that a nurse has to offer patients beyond the dependent role to physicians. This realization places greater responsibility on practical/vocational nursing students (SPN/SVNs) to learn all they can during the nursing program of study. For example, now you can add knowledge of basic ethics to critical thinking as you assist the RN with the nursing process. The data you collect will have an added dimension of ethics. It will make a difference in developing a quality care plan that considers the patient as a whole person and not just the part of his or her body that is sick.

At this level you incorporate a basic understanding of how SPN/SVNs and LPN/LVNs practice nursing according to nursing codes. Learning about ethics is more than being able to recite the definition to pass a test; it means being able to help make ethical decisions when ethical dilemmas arise.

The following ethical principles are discussed in this chapter:

1. Nonmaleficence (do no harm)
2. Beneficence (do good)
3. Autonomy (free to choose)
4. Fidelity (be true)
5. Justice (fair to all)

NONMALEFICENCE (DO NO HARM)

In her book *Leadership and Management According to Florence Nightingale,* Nightingale said the following:

> It may seem a strange principle to enunciate as the very first requirement in a hospital that it should do the sick no harm. It is quite necessary nevertheless to lay down such a principle.

Nightingale is referring to the ethical principle nonmaleficence, which comes from the Latin *primum non nocere,* meaning "first do no harm." Nonmaleficence is the basis of many of the "rules" promoted by your instructors, such as the following:

- "Rule of 5" for giving medications
- Checking the temperature of bath or shower water
- Checking the temperature of formula before feeding the patient
- Returning the bed to its lowest position after completing a treatment or preparing to leave the room
- Raising side rails after nursing care if it is in the plan of care
- Providing care for your patients when their ethical principles conflict with yours
- Performing only necessary procedures on patients, instead of unnecessary procedures just to gain additional experience
- Protecting those who cannot protect themselves—for example, mentally challenged, unconscious, weak, or debilitated patients

If the principle of nonmaleficence is taken to the extreme, however, SPN/SVNs and LPN/LVNs would not be able to perform many nursing duties. Few beneficial treatments are entirely without harm, including the following:

- Anytime you puncture the patient's skin with a needle, there is some tissue damage, a risk of infection, and the possibility of an untoward reaction to a solution if administered. All drugs have side effects: rare, serious, and not so serious.
- Anytime you put a tube into a bodily opening (e.g., catheterization, irrigating a colostomy),

there is some trauma to surrounding tissue. There is the possibility of introducing infection and penetrating the tissue wall.

- Many procedures hurt physically in the process of performing them (e.g., positioning a patient properly after surgery, cleansing the mouth of an elderly patient who has not had proper mouth care for a period, irrigating a pressure ulcer, moving a patient with osteoporosis from bed to chair to toilet and back).

- Giving a vaccination carries the risk of the patient experiencing a side effect, but the overall effect for most people is the prevention of serious diseases.

- When you monitor an IV, one thing to check is that the solution and additive, if any, are infusing, as compared to what the physician ordered. A common additive is KCl (potassium chloride). KCl within a narrow blood level range is necessary for proper heart functioning. If too little or too much is administered, it can result in heart dysfunction, sometimes resulting in death. (Jack Kevorkian, a physician who participated in several assisted suicides, used KCl as one of the drugs in his suicide machine.) KCl can save lives, but it can also kill.

Each of the preceding procedures has the potential for doing good and doing harm. The question always is how to do the least amount of harm when doing something that is expected to result in good. The obvious answer is to never knowingly participate in any action that will deliberately harm the patient. The patient must also have agreed to the procedure verbally or in writing, depending on the procedure (autonomy). This is a reason for practicing procedures in the nursing lab; preparing for nursing care; reviewing your nursing care plan with the instructor; and reviewing action, side effects, and dosage with the instructor before giving a medication.

The following are negative examples of nursing actions that were meant to do no harm but resulted in injury:

- Putting down a patient's side rail without first checking that the patient's arm is not hanging between the rail and the bed. The patient who immediately comes to mind is a woman in her eighties whose arm was fractured and who received several skin tears and bruises. The staff person who put the rail down was irritated because of "a bad night shift" and was hurrying to get off duty.

- Rapidly feeding large spoonfuls of food to a patient who has a dry mouth as a side effect of medication. Because of the lack of liquid before beginning to eat, large spoonfuls of food, lack of adequate time to chew, and lack of additional liquid before the next bite, the patient aspirated some of the food that accumulated in his mouth.

The patient survived but refused future attempts to eat when he saw the same nurse come in with his food tray.

- Placing a lap restraint incorrectly (the physician's order was for the patient to be restrained when up in a wheelchair). Because of improper placement of the restraint and lack of monitoring, the patient slid down and died as a result of hanging by the neck.

◎ Try This

Procedures and Their Effects

Think about procedures with which you are familiar. Review the procedure. List two procedures that "do good" but also have the potential to do harm. State both the good and potential harmful effects of each procedure.

BENEFICENCE (DO GOOD)

Beneficence means to "do good" with your nursing actions and is the basis of trust in nursing. It also involves preventing harm and removing harm. You have read how nonmaleficence and beneficence are often difficult to separate and may go hand in hand. The following major nursing duties to the patient are associated with beneficence:

1. Put the patient's interests first—for example:
   - You do not go off duty until you hand over the care of the patient to equally skilled nursing staff to continue the nursing care. You are obligated to report to the nurse taking over the next shift what has transpired during the time you have been responsible for nursing care.
   - If you give the wrong medication, report it as soon as you recognize the error. Your ethical concern is to "do good" and "prevent harm." Beneficence is a greater good than concern for self in regard to the error.
   - You go to work even though you are tempted to call in sick because you want to go out of town for the weekend.

2. *Place the good of patients before your needs.* This is where interpretation of duty gets more complex. Does this mean that duty to the patient means utmost sacrifice? No, it does not, but it does mean that you sacrifice something. Here are some examples:
   - Patient needs are above organizational needs. You may have administrative responsibility (perhaps as a charge nurse) that must be completed by the end of the day or meetings you are expected to attend that day. If a patient needs your skill and expertise, as in an emergency situation, your first duty is to the patient.
   - Placing the good of patients before your needs does *not* mean that you begin to behave as though no one in the world can assume the nursing care you give to a patient. Do not stay past your

scheduled hours when there is someone ready to assume responsibility for nursing care. This also means that you do not call the patient from home, accept calls in your home from the patient, or visit the patient after hours. If you are doing any of this, you have just entered an unhealthy codependent relationship with the patient.

? Critical Thinking

Ethical Obligations

When a patient is demanding, angry, or uncooperative and threatens to become violent, is the nurse obligated to put herself or himself in danger of serious harm? Are nurses ethically obligated to perform heroic acts of self-sacrifice?

Volunteer (pro bono) work is a professional obligation of beneficence for nurses. For example, a nurse may decide to volunteer some hours a week at a free clinic or children's center.

AUTONOMY (FREE TO CHOOSE)

Autonomy does not mean that patients can do whatever they want. Autonomy means the following:

- *Thinking* through all the facts
- *Deciding* on the basis of an independent thinking process
- *Acting* based on a personal decision
- *Undertaking a decision voluntarily* without pressure, direct or subtle, from anyone else

However, this does not mean that patients can do whatever they want. Rumbold (2002) states the following:

> Autonomy does not mean freedom to do as one wants or to act in accordance with one's desires. Autonomous action is based on rational thought or reason. It embodies the notion of freedom and liberty, but only within the constraints of reason.

We expect people to respect our rights, and we respect their rights as long as their rights do not interfere with someone else's rights.

For patients to make an autonomous decision, they must have all the facts without leaving out information in order to influence the decision in a particular way. For example, the nurse may unintentionally (sometimes intentionally) influence the patient's decision by repeating what the physician has suggested is best for the patient ("The doctor would not have suggested the treatment if he/she did not think it best for you.").

There is also a fine line between autonomy and abandonment. Excessive control means interfering too much in a patient's life. Not interfering enough results in neglect of the patient. Here are some examples:

- The right of the elderly to make decisions about their treatment.
- A patient's right to be left alone or not treated.

More information is needed in both situations to determine if more or less interference is recommended.

Role of Privacy in Autonomy

Privacy is both an ethical and a legal issue. Autonomy includes a patient's right to privacy. This is the reason your instructor asks a patient directly for permission to allow SPN/SVNs to observe a particular treatment or to do a procedure. Similarly, the instructor checks with the patient before assigning a student to give nursing care. Privacy includes the right to choose care based on personal beliefs, feelings, or attitudes. It includes the patients' right to decide what is done to their body (accepting or rejecting treatment or exposure of the body). As an SPN/SVN, you respect the patient's decision. When giving care, avoid exposing the patient needlessly in the course of care. *This is an invasion of privacy.*

Role of Culture, Religion, and Personal Values in Autonomy

Culture or a religion-based belief system may be contrary to the accepted medical ethics. Examples of decisions based on religion and culture include the following:

- The patient, a Jehovah's Witness, could benefit from a blood transfusion for severe blood loss. The adult patient has refused because a blood transfusion is forbidden by his religion (religion based).
- If the patient had been an underage child whose parents forbade the blood transfusion on religious grounds, the physician might decide to go to court to ask the court to overrule the parents' decision. The physician can do this because parents cannot give *informed consent* for the treatment of underage children. An underage child is too young to understand all the facts to make a decision required for informed consent. Parents can *authorize treatment* for what is appropriate for their children up to a certain age. In this case the physician has decided that the value of beneficence is greater than the value of respect for the parents' autonomy. The court is the greater authority and will decide if the physician can transfuse the child.
- A young woman is diagnosed with breast cancer. Her husband has received a complete explanation from the physician about her illness, alternatives for each treatment, anticipated effects, possible side effects, and prognosis with each treatment. Her husband will not permit any treatment to take place (culture based).

The patient's personal values may also be opposed to accepted medical ethics. The following is an example of a personal value–based decision:

- A man in his late sixties is diagnosed with advanced cancer of the colon. He has refused to have treatment, even though he understands that while not curative, the surgery could result in less discomfort for a period and more time to live (personal value based).

FIDELITY (BE TRUE)

Fidelity challenges each practical/vocational nurse to be faithful to the charge of acting in the patient's best interest when the capacity to make free choice is no longer available to the patient. This does not include rescuing behaviors and becoming paternalistic in making decisions for vulnerable patients (legal competency will be described in Chapter 12). As a nurse, you must *differentiate* between your feelings and choices regarding an issue and the feelings and wishes of the patient. These points are foremost in making a decision. Charting the patient's feelings and wishes as expressed, without your personal interpretation, provides information for the physician when important decisions need to be considered. Examples of breaching fidelity include the following:

- Discussing a patient in a public area such as the cafeteria, an elevator, at home, or when you are out with friends breaches fidelity. Never mention a patient by name. Fidelity and confidentiality (a legal term) have both been compromised, as has the patient's dignity. The action says the patient has limited worth in the eyes of the nurse and chips away at the patient's dignity.
- You overhear LPN/LVNs speaking disrespectfully about an obese patient and complaining about how difficult it is to move her. What will you do in response to this discussion? Explain why you will take the action you have chosen. Is it an ethical response?
- A student practical nurse shared a personal experience that sharpened her awareness of the meaning of fidelity. During her first day of the mental health rotation, she spotted her neighbor, now a patient, in the day room. The SPN's husband worked with the patient. One day the patient did not come to work. The boss offered no information about what happened. Being a close-knit neighborhood, the SPN's husband, other workers, and neighbors speculated with great concern about the missing worker. Seeing him on the psychiatric unit was a shock, and the SPN did not know how to approach him. The SPN asked her instructor for assistance. The instructor suggested that the SPN approach the patient and let him know that she recognized him but reassure him that she would not tell anyone he was hospitalized. The SPN was also to tell the patient that not telling anyone outside of the hospital was part of her nursing education and duty. That took care of the discomfort for both the SPN and the patient regarding his hospitalization. The class after the clinical day was about fidelity and confidentiality (a legal concern). The SPN was sure she would never breach her promise not to talk about patients, except to the health care team and her instructor. That evening at dinner with her husband, she decided he should know because of his concern for his coworker. The SPN made her husband promise not to tell anyone about the patient, and the husband agreed. Later that evening, while they were grocery shopping, the SPN was in another aisle, and she heard her husband say to someone, "My wife ran into Joe at the psych hospital this morning. He's a patient, but don't tell anyone." The SPN breached confidentiality, an ethical and legal matter. She also started a chain reaction of "I'll tell you, but you can't tell anyone."

You alone make the decisions regarding what you do when you are away from the clinical area and the immediate support and supervision of the instructor. In a sense, fidelity sits on your shoulder—to ignore or to embrace.

JUSTICE (FAIR TO ALL)

Justice means that SPN/SVNs and LPN/LVNs must give patients their due and treat each patient fairly. For example, each patient with the same diagnosis should receive the same level of care. Being fair does not mean giving every patient the same things. It means treating them all the same (i.e., with dignity and respect). As a nurse, you make daily decisions in order to give patients their "due." For example, say the patients on your floor in the hospital represent different levels of wealth, social status, culture, religion, and moral and value systems, but all of them are acutely ill. The newest patient has Kaposi's sarcoma, a defining component of acquired immune deficiency syndrome (AIDS). Do you classify AIDS as a life-threatening illness or as a retribution for behaviors you consider immoral? If your personal ethics interfere with the care you give, you may find yourself giving this patient more time than needed and doing less than needed for other acutely ill patients or providing minimal care for the patient and lavishing attention on those who "deserve the care."

It is within your power to make decisions about daily issues related to justice. Listen to your inner voice: "He's so young—so much living left to do"; "She's had a full life already"; "She's an alcoholic—never took care of her kids"; and so on.

> **? Critical Thinking**
>
> At the end of your next clinical day, take time to reflect on your reaction to patients and how it affected your patient care. Did the word *deserve* enter into your thoughts, or did you provide justice for all?

As an SPN/SVN, you report patients' comments regarding ethical matters to the RN. Final ethical decisions are not within the LPN/LVN scope of nursing practice. Recall also that ethics is what you *ought* to do; law is what you *have* to do.

ROLE OF BENEFICENT PATERNALISM

We are including beneficent paternalism because it continues to be confused with the ethic of beneficence (do no harm). **Beneficent paternalism** is a disrespectful *attitude* toward the patient and what the patient has to contribute to personal care and recovery. It is an "I know what's best for you" attitude that discounts the patient's knowledge of self. The following are examples of beneficent paternalism:

- When assisting to collect data, it is important to really *hear* what the patient is trying to tell you. If you have determined in advance that this patient fits into a "specific category," you will discount what the patient wants you to know.
- Assisting with developing the care plan without patient input will reflect the nurse's needs, not the patient's. Later on you will complain that the patient is noncompliant and will not cooperate with the plan of care. Ask yourself: Did the patient know what the alternatives were for treatment? Did the patient have the opportunity to offer input into the plan and agree to what the care plan would be? It is difficult for patients to cooperate when the staff have bruised their sense of autonomy.
- If the patient has agreed to the patient care plan, then coaxing the patient to do what has been agreed upon is beneficence. However, if you are influencing the patient into choosing one alternative treatment over another, it is paternalistic beneficence. If you find yourself saying, "I overheard the doctor saying he thinks you should choose this treatment" or "My husband chose the treatment and he is doing great," you are actively influencing the patient's decision (paternalism).
- Perhaps the patient asks your opinion for the choice, and you respond with your choice ("Well, if I were you, I would . . .") instead of saying, "The doctor explained the alternatives for treatment and the possible side effects of each, and it is for you to decide what is best for you."

Beneficent paternalism is justified only in extreme circumstances and is most often a medical decision (e.g., a physician approaching the court to be allowed to do a potentially lifesaving procedure when parents have refused to sign an authorized treatment form for the child).

To avoid paternalism with new mothers, a lactation counselor at a public health nursing seminar presented the following method: "I wish all women would breastfeed their babies. The value to both mother and child is a scientific fact. I present the facts and respond to their questions, but the final decision belongs to the mother. I respectfully support their decision."

PATERNALISM AND WOMEN'S HEALTH

The issue of paternalism toward women in medical research and receiving health care is slowly changing through the efforts of women themselves and the advocacy of nurses. The term *paternalism* is derived from a Latin word that means "father" (i.e., father knows best). In the health system, it is interpreted as "doctors know best because of their superior knowledge." Because the word is derived from the Latin word *pater*, they believe that men know better than women. Physicians define what is considered ill health for women. Anything that is normally different from men is considered an illness and requires the physician's intervention. Because women are different from men biologically, medicine has defined what is normal for women as being abnormal. For example, menstruation, pregnancy, and menopause are defined as ill health instead of normal, healthy processes. Many of these same attitudes toward women continue in the health care system. Women are seen as victims of their own bodies who cannot help being sick. This sometimes leads to a patting-on-the-head approach: "You can't help it, but I can help you" is implied and is often followed by "Just take these pills." Male physicians are just mirroring the attitudes of males toward females in society (Rumbold, 2002).

Your responsibility is to advocate for your female patient. Speak up when you see decisions being made based on incomplete information (e.g., the physician or other health care worker did not really listen to the female patient). Review Chapter 14 regarding assertiveness and your responsibility. It reminds you that an aggressive, rude approach does not gain you anything except a bad reputation among your peers and patients. Practice assertiveness, and remember that change will occur slowly. Many female patients are already experiencing a change and assertively state their needs. Nurses who advocate for their female patients assist in this process of reducing a paternalistic attitude toward women—one patient at a time as the need arises.

? Critical Thinking

Do I Respond Differently to Male and Female Patients?

Keep track of the differences in your responses to male and female patients for 2 or 3 days. Record your response to the male or female patient and what the patient said.

When you think you have enough examples, review the data you collected. Use critical thinking to determine what differences you noted in your response to male and female patients. Because this is for your eyes only, be candid. Are there any changes that you recommend for yourself? If so, write them down.

Get Ready for the NCLEX-PN® Examination

Key Points

- Ethics is concerned with the meaning of words such as *right, wrong, good, bad, ought,* and *duty.*
- Nursing ethics provide guidelines for making ethical decisions in nursing.
- Practical/vocational nurses need to be aware of the contents of their state's Nurse Practice Act regarding ethical issues.
- Ethics is something an SPN/SVN *should/ought* to do. However, ethics themselves do not carry the weight of law.
- Content of the law (state's Nurse Practice Act) is something the SPN/SVN has to do.
- Both NAPNES and NFLPN provide an ethical code for SPN/SVNs and LPN/LVNs.
- SPN/SVNs and LPN/LVNs must know the nursing code of ethics and not confuse it with their personal code of ethics.
- The nursing role includes a dependent role to physicians and has progressed to include providing nursing care to the whole patient and being a patient advocate.
- Cultural and religious backgrounds and personal values may influence ethical decisions of patients seeking health care.
- Nonmaleficence means "do no harm." Few treatments are entirely without harm.
- Beneficence means to do good with your nursing actions and is the basis of trust in nursing.
- Autonomy means respect for a patient's right to choose, as long as the patient's rights do not interfere with the rights of others.
- Fidelity means to be true. It challenges SPN/SVNs and LPN/LVNs to be faithful to the charge of acting in the patient's best interests, even when the capacity of free choice is not available to the patient because of his or her condition.
- Justice means that the SPN/SVN and the LPN/LVN must give the same level of care to all patients, with dignity and respect.
- If the LPN/LVN has ethical objections to procedures being done, a statement should be made in writing before beginning employment.
- Beneficent paternalism is justified only in extreme circumstances and is most often a medical decision.
- Paternalism in women's health care is changing slowly. Nurses' advocacy for women helps promote this change, one patient at a time.

Additional Learning Resources

evolve Go to your Evolve website (http://evolve.elsevier.com/Hill/ Success) for the following FREE learning resources:
- Answers to Critical Thinking Scenarios
- Additional learning activities
- Additional Review Questions for the NCLEX-PN® exam
- Helpful phrases for communicating in Spanish and more!

Review Questions for the NCLEX-PN® Examination

1. Which of the following defines *ethics*?
   1. Concern with practical issues of habits and conduct of persons or groups.
   2. The worth assigned to an idea or an action, freely chosen, affected by maturity.
   3. Concern with the meanings of words such as *right, wrong, good, bad, ought,* and *duty.*
   4. Customs, habits, and behaviors in a society that are approved by that society.

2. Select the statement that **best** describes how nursing has evolved.
   1. Nursing discovered its unique role in nursing the whole patient, not just the diseased part.
   2. Nurses became upset by their dependent role to physicians and forced changes in the medical system.
   3. The nursing process and critical thinking promoted an easy change in how nursing is taught in schools.
   4. Nurses discovered that curricula and textbooks changed but not the work on patient care units.

3. How will you respond to the mother who has refused a blood transfusion for her 2-year-old son, but the doctor has asked the court to overrule her refusal?
   1. "In your son's case, beneficent paternalism overrules respect for your autonomy."
   2. "In this hospital, the doctor knows best because of his/ her superior knowledge."
   3. "We have saved many children by ignoring parents' religious beliefs and doing what is best."
   4. "He is too young to understand and make his own choice in something this serious."

4. After seemingly successful treatment for depression and a serious suicide attempt, a patient will be in court this morning to find out if she will be released. The patient tells the SPN/SVN, "As soon as I get out, I am going to kill myself. Promise me you won't tell anyone." What course of ethical action should the SPN/SVN take?
   1. The SPN/SVN promises not to tell anyone. His personal ethic is to never break a promise when one is made.
   2. Both psychiatric and nursing testimony are favorable to the patient. The SPN/SVN reports the patient's comment to the judge.
   3. The SPN/SVN believes in waiting to see what will happen. He plans to do the same during the court hearing.
   4. The SPN/SVN keeps the promise made to the patient but convinces himself he is not meant to be a nurse.

Alternate Format Item

1. Which statements **best** describe steps in making an autonomous decision? *(Select all that apply.)*
   1. Voluntary without pressure
   2. Fair to all parties involved
   3. Doctor suggests solution
   4. Ability to consider all facts

2. Which statements best describe the difference between personal and professional ethics? (*Select all that apply.*)

1. Personal ethics means the same as beneficent paternalism.
2. Professional ethics sometimes conflict with the law.
3. Personal ethics provide guidelines for one's life.
4. Professional ethics means you cannot abandon the patient.

Critical Thinking Scenarios

Scenario 1

You are currently at the Good Haven Nursing Home 3 days a week on a geriatric nursing clinical rotation. The instructor has talked to the class about being aware of sounds when walking in the halls. You see Mrs. Garnet being pushed to the shower room in a wheelchair by one of the nursing aides.

On the way back down the hall, you hear a sound from the shower room and decide to open the door to the shower room. Much to your surprise, you see the aide putting a washcloth into the resident's mouth. The muffled sound from Mrs. Garnet is barely audible. The aide does not notice you and turns on the shower—cold water. What will you do?

Scenario 2

The instructor asked Shawn, a staff LVN, and the patient permission to have Kathy, an SVN, observe Shawn insert a urinary catheter. Permission was granted (Kathy had already watched a catheter insertion and given a successful return demonstration in class).

Kathy watched Shawn open the "catheteriztion tray" and noted a couple of breaks in technique. Shawn contaminated her gloves when cleansing the patient's perineal area. Shawn then began to reach for the sterile catheter. What did Kathy do?

Nursing and the Law: What Are the Rules?

Objectives

On completing this chapter, you will be able to do the following:

1. Discuss the content of your state's Nurse Practice Act.
2. Describe the responsibilities of your state's board of nursing (or nursing regulatory board).
3. Explain the limits of nursing licensure within your state.
4. Define the nursing standard of care.
5. Differentiate between common law and statutory law.
6. Explain the difference between criminal and civil action.
7. Discuss the difference between intentional and unintentional torts.
8. List the four elements needed for negligence.
9. Review the steps for bringing legal action.
10. Differentiate between practical/vocational nursing student (SPN/SVN) and instructor liability in preventing a lawsuit.
11. Summarize the American Hospital Association's publication *The Patient Care Partnership: Understanding Expectations, Rights, and Responsibilities*.
12. Describe the major focus of the Health Insurance Portability and Accountability Act.
13. Discuss the differences among general consent, informed consent, and authorized consent.
14. Differentiate between the living will and durable power of attorney.
15. Explain the difference between physician-assisted suicide and euthanasia.
16. Discuss the difference between a multistate compact and a border agreement.
17. Explain how you would legally deal with two difficult situations that might occur in a clinical setting.

Key Terms

accountability (ă-kŏwn-tă-BĬL-ĭ-tē, p. 138)

advance directives (ăd-VĂNS dĭ-RĔCT-ĭvs p. 143)

assault (ă-SŎLT, p. 134)

authorized consent (ĂW-thŏr-izd kŏn-SĔNT, p. 143)

basic patient situation (p. 130)

battery (BĂT-ĕr-ē, p. 134)

border recognition agreement (BŎR-dĕr rĕk-og-NĬ-shŭn, p. 132)

breach of duty (brēch, p. 136)

civil action (sĭ-vŭl ĂK-shŭn, p. 134)

common law (KŎM-mŏn, p. 133)

complex nursing situation (KŎM-plĕks NŬR-sēng sĭt-u-Ā-shŭn, p. 130)

confidentiality (kŏn-fĭ-dĕn-chē-ĂL-ĭ-tē, p. 139)

criminal action (KRĬM-ĭn-ăl ĂK-shŭn, p. 133)

damages (DĂM-ăj-ĕs, p. 136)

defamation (dĕf-ă-MĀ-shŭn, p. 134)

delegated medical act (dĕl-ĕ-GĀ-tĕd, p. 130)

depositions (dĕp-ō-ZĬSH-ŏn, p. 137)

direct supervision (dĭ-RĔCT soo-pŭr-VĬ-shŭn, p. 130)

do-not-resuscitate (DNR) (rĭ-SŬS-ĭ-tāt, p. 144)

durable medical power of attorney (p. 144)

duty (DOO-tē, p. 134)

end-of-life principles (EOL) (p. 146)

euthanasia (ū-thă -NĀ-zhē-ă, p. 144)

felony (FĔL-ō-nē, p. 134)

general (implied) consent (JĔN-ĕr-ăl kŏn-SĔNT, p. 142)

general supervision (JĔN-ĕr-ăl soo-pŭr-VĬ-shŭn, p. 130)

Good Samaritan Act (p. 146)

Health Insurance Portability and Accountability Act (HIPAA) (p. 140)

informed consent (ĭn-FŎRMD kŏn-SĔNT, p. 133)

institutional liability (ĭn-stĭ-TOO-shŭn-ăl lī-ă-BĬL-ĭ-tē, p. 138)

intentional tort (ĭn-TĔN-shŭn-ăl tŏrts, p. 134)

interstate endorsement (ĭn-tĕr-STĀT ĭn-DŎRS-mĕnt, p. 132)

law (p. 130)

liability (lī-ă-BĬL-ĭ-tē, p. 136)

libel (LĪ-bĕl, p. 135)

living will (lĭ-VĬNG wĭl, p. 143)

malpractice (professional negligence) (măl-PRĂK-tĭs, p. 136)

misdemeanor (mĭs-dĭ-MĒ-nŏr, p. 133)

multistate licensure (Nurse Licensure Compact) (LĪ-sĕn-shŭr, p. 132)

negligence (NĔG-lĭ-jĕns, p. 135)

Nurse Practice Act (nŭrs PRĂK-tĭs ăkt, p. 130)

nursing standard of care (NURS-ĭng STĂN-dĕrd, p. 133)

Oregon Death With Dignity Act (p. 145)

patient competency (PĀ-shĕnt KŎM-pĕ-tĕn-sē, p. 142)

Patient Self-Determination Act (PSDA) (p. 143)

personal liability (PĔR-sŭn-ăl lī-ă-BĬL-ĭ-tē, p. 137)

physician-assisted suicide (PAS) (fĭ-ZĬ-shŭn ă-SĬS-tĕd
   SOO-ĭ-sīd, p. 144)
preponderance (prĭ-PŎN-dĕr-ănts, p. 134)
proximate cause (PRŎKS-ĭ-mĕt căws, p. 136)
slander (SLĂN-dĕr, p. 135)
statutory law (STĂ-chū-TŏR-ē, p. 133)

The Joint Commission (TJC) (p. 133)
*The Patient Care Partnership: Understanding
   Expectations, Rights, and Responsibilities* (p. 140)
unintentional tort (ŭn-ĭn-TĔN-shŭn-ăl tŏrts p. 134)
vicarious liability (vĭ-KĂR-ē-ŭs, p. 137)

 Keep in Mind

Ethics and law drive the practice of nursing. When there is a dispute, law—the Nurse Practice Act in your state—is the final authority. According to Elizabeth Johnson, a lead instructor at Northeast Wisconsin Technical Institute, "No employer/health care agency can give you permission to do something that your license/state's Nurse Practice Act does not allow you to do."

Ethics in nursing deals with rules of conduct—what is right and what you should do in a particular situation. Ethical values, in turn, are the *basis* of nursing law. Law has to do with regulations that control the practice of nursing. Your state's Nurse Practice Act, discussed following, is your *legal* guideline in nursing.

Knowledge of your state's Nurse Practice Act will be valuable to you in making nursing decisions. Such knowledge also will help you to protect yourself against acts and decisions that could involve you in lawsuits and criminal prosecution.

NURSE PRACTICE ACT

The state Nurse Practice Act defines nursing practice and establishes standards for nurses in your state. Ignorance of your state's Nurse Practice Act is never a valid defense against any legal proceeding regarding your license.

BASIC TERMINOLOGY

Basic terminology in a Nurse Practice Act remains standard in many states. As you study the scope of practice for licensed (or trained) practical/vocational nurses (LPNs/LVNs) in your state, an understanding of the following terms is necessary.

- **Basic nursing care.** Nursing care that can be performed safely by the LPN/LVN, based on knowledge and skills gained during the educational program. Modifications of care are unnecessary, and patient response is predictable.
- **Basic patient situation.** The patient's clinical condition is predictable. Medical and nursing orders are not changing continuously. These orders do not contain complex modifications. The patient's clinical condition requires only basic nursing care. The professional nurse assesses whether the situation is a basic patient situation.
- **Complex nursing situation.** The patient's clinical condition is not predictable. Medical orders or

nursing interventions are likely to involve continuous changes or complex modifications. Nursing care expectations are beyond those learned by the LPN/LVN during the educational program. The professional nurse assesses whether the situation is a complex nursing situation.

- **Delegated medical act.** During a delegated medical act, a physician's order is given to a registered nurse (RN), an LPN, or an LVN by a physician, dentist, or podiatrist.
- **Delegated nursing act.** In a delegated nursing act, an RN gives nursing orders to an RN, LPN, or LVN.
- **Direct supervision.** With direct supervision, the supervisor is continuously present to coordinate, direct, or inspect nursing care. The supervisor is in the building.
- **General supervision.** Under general supervision, a supervisor regularly coordinates, directs, or inspects nursing care and is within reach either in the building or by telephone.

CONTENT OF NURSE PRACTICE ACTS

The Nurse Practice Act of each state commonly includes the following content:
- Definition of nursing
- Definition of LPN/LVN
- Use of the title of LPN or LVN
- Scope of practice
- Elements of unprofessional conduct
- Functions of the state's board of nursing

 Try This

Get Familiar with Your Scope of Practice in the State's Nurse Practice Act

Obtain a copy of your state's Nurse Practice Act (or occupational title act). What does it state about the following topics?
1. Definition of licensed practical/vocational nursing in your state
2. Use of the titles *licensed practical nurse* and *licensed vocational nurse*
3. Specific functions of the LPN/LVN
4. Elements of unprofessional conduct

STATE BOARD OF NURSING

All states and provinces have examining councils that provide nursing examinations for licensure and review complaints that can lead to revocation of a license.

FUNCTIONS OF THE BOARD

State boards of nursing (sometimes called nurse regulatory boards) have committees or councils that decide whether specific activities are within the scope of LPN/LVN practice in their state. An activity that is legal in one state may not be legal in another state. See Box 12-1 for common board of nursing functions.

Some state nursing boards have developed a website and may offer a variety of services (e.g., license renewal, application for licensure by examination, verification of licensure status of a state nurse, change of address/phone number/email address, downloadable forms, links to continuing education courses,

the state's Nurse Practice Act). It is important as a practical/vocational nurse to understand that you must limit your work to the area of nursing defined in the state's Nurse Practice Act.

In 2003, the National Association for Practical Nurse Education and Service Inc. (NAPNES) issued a professional guideline for LPNs/LVNs titled "The LPN/LVN Fulfills the Professional Responsibilities of the Practical/Vocational Nurse" (see Appendix B). This is an example of a statement from an official nursing organization, but it does not carry the weight of law. These statements are useful as *guides* for behavior and may be used in a court of law as a point of reference. *The Nurse Practice Act in your state is always your final authority.*

DISCIPLINARY RESPONSIBILITY OF THE BOARD

Each state's Nurse Practice Act lists specific reasons for which they seek to discipline a nurse. Eight general categories of disciplinary actions can be taken against nurses. Brent (2001) lists them as "fraud and deceit; criminal activity; negligence; risk to patients because of physical or mental incapacity; violation of the Nurse Practice Act or rules; disciplinary action by another board; incompetence; unethical conduct; and drug and/or alcohol use." See Box 12-2 for the eight categories of disciplinary action.

Box 12-1   Common Board of Nursing Functions

- Licensing and certifying nurses
- Setting fees
- Establishing standards for educational programs
- Determining duration and renewal of licenses (some boards require continuing education credits for renewal of license)
- Maintaining inactive status lists
- Carrying out disciplinary action for violators
- Developing programs for impaired nurses
- Suspending and revoking licenses and dealing with the appeal process

---

Box 12-2   Eight Categories of Disciplinary Actions Taken Against Nurses

1. **Fraud and deceit:** Most often, fraud and deceit involve a person using fake means to get a nursing license (e.g., forging documents).
2. **Criminal activity:** This includes conviction of a felony, such as murder; or conviction for gross immorality, such as theft, fraud, personal misrepresentation, or embezzlement.
3. **Negligence:** The nurse does not do what a reasonable, prudent nurse would do in a similar situation. Negligence includes serious risk to the health, safety, or physical or mental health of a patient. (This may include patient injury.)
4. **Violation of the Nurse Practice Act:** Some states' Nurse Practice Acts list specific violations (e.g., unprofessional conduct, such as becoming personally involved with a patient).
5. **Discipline by another jurisdiction:** In the past, it was difficult to find out if a nurse had been disciplined in another state. Now there are two national data banks that make it easier to track disciplinary action of LPNs/LVNs in other states. However, it is not mandatory for the disciplining authority to notify a data bank. The data banks are as follows:
   a. *National Practitioner Data Bank* (NPDB). Established by federal law, it has been in operation since 1999. It contains information on final actions when guilt of a professional violation has been established or admitted. The NPDB primarily contains disciplinary actions taken against dentists and other health practitioners, including nurses. The purpose of the data bank is to

restrict the ability of incompetent professionals to move from state to state without disclosure of previous incompetence.
   b. The *National Council of State Boards of Nursing Disciplinary Data Bank* (NCSBNDB) was established in 1990. It collects disciplinary information about nurses from all state boards of nursing, and distributes it to all state boards of nursing. The state boards of nursing use this information for disciplinary and licensing purposes. Action by the Board can affect your license or certificate to practice in another state.
6. **Incompetence:** Examples include failure to meet generally accepted standards of nursing practice; negligence; and a nurse's mental disability that would interfere with patient safety.
7. **Unethical conduct:** Examples include a breach of nurse-patient confidentiality; refusal to provide nursing care for someone because of race, creed, color, national origin, disease, or sexual orientation; violation of the ethical code for LPNs/LVNs; and failure to maintain nursing competence.
8. **Alcohol and/or other drug abuse:** Alcohol and other drug abuse by a nurse (e.g., diversion of drugs, often controlled substances, for personal use) is a threat to patient safety. Some nurses steal and sell diverted substances and equipment such as syringes and IV tubing, falsify patient records, and deprive patients of their medication. The number of nurses disciplined for alcohol and/or other drug abuse is increasing.

DISCIPLINARY PROCESS AND ACTION

The disciplinary process is based on law and follows the rules of law. See Box 12-3 for the steps of a disciplinary process.

NURSING LICENSURE

It is nursing licensure that defines and protects the title of LPN or LVN. Some states (e.g., Minnesota) have amended their Nurse Practice Act to include the provision that only licensed practical or registered nurses may use the professional title "nurse."

On completion of a state-approved practical/vocational nursing education program, a graduate is eligible to apply for the national licensing examination in practical/vocational nursing (NCLEX-PN® examination). While awaiting examination results, the graduate may apply for a temporary permit to practice nursing. On successful completion of the examination, the graduate receives a nursing license. If the graduate nurse fails the NCLEX-PN® examination, the temporary permit is revoked. The graduate has an opportunity to retest at a later date for an additional fee. Until successful completion of the NCLEX-PN® examination, the temporary permit remains revoked and the graduate can work only as a nursing assistant.

WORKING IN OTHER STATES

States have arrangements for interstate endorsements for nurses who choose to work in other states. This means that it is possible to work in another state without repeating the NCLEX-PN® examination, after you meet that state's criteria for licensure by endorsement.

Some states are involved in multistate licensure: a mutual recognition model for nursing regulation. The NCSBN adopted the Nurse Multistate Licensure Mutual Recognition Model in 1997. Utah was the first state to adopt the NCSBN compact language that took effect in 2000. The mutual recognition model allows a nurse to have one license in his or her state of residency and practice in other states, depending on each state's Nurse Practice Act and legislation. To become law, each state must pass the law as part of their state Nurse Practice Act. As of 2012, 24 states had mutual recognition compacts. Check the Nurse Practice Act of the state in which you will be working to find out if it is a compact state.

 Try This

Compact States and the Nurse Practice Act

Obtain and read the Nurse Practice Act of a compact state by contacting that state's board of nursing. Addresses are available online. If approved to work in a compact state, the LPN/LVN must know the contents of the NPA of the compact state.

The mutual recognition model is not the same as Minnesota's border recognition agreement (effective January 1, 2003), which allows nurses who have a license in the border states of Iowa, North Dakota, South Dakota, or Wisconsin to practice nursing in Minnesota. All of these states are compact states. The Minnesota Board of Nursing has endorsed the compact, but it has not become law because the Minnesota Nurses Association and the National Nurses United oppose it. The issue has gone before the Minnesota Legislature in 2003, 2008, 2009, 2010, and 2011. At this time, nurses who reside in Minnesota are not permitted to practice nursing in other states without obtaining a license in that state.

 Try This

Interstate Agreement

Contact the board of nursing in the state in which you will be employed. Inquire if they have multistate licensure or a border recognition agreement. If the state involved does not have such an agreement with other states, inquire what is needed for interstate endorsement.

VERIFICATION OF LICENSURE

Some boards of nursing are instituting online verification of nursing licensure. The board provides public information about nurses who have current licensure. The verification system enables potential employers to call and obtain a nurse's license number, registration

---

Box 12-3   Steps for Disciplinary Action

- **Sworn complaint:** Filed against the LPN/LVN by a person, health care agency, or professional organization.
- **Complaint is reviewed:** The LPN/LVN receives a notice of the hearing, which will be before the state board of nursing or a state officer. Evidence of wrongdoing is presented to the nurse and board. The nurse and the nurse's attorney (who is familiar with nursing) present witnesses. The board makes a decision on findings.
- **Finding of not guilty:** No action is taken.
- **Finding of guilty of misconduct:** The board may issue a public or private reprimand, such as:
  - Continuing education
  - Probation
  - Nonrenewal of license
  - Suspension of license
  - Revocation of license
  - If nurse is involved in alcohol or drug abuse, a diversion program may be an alternative. "Many states have developed Alternative to Discipline Programs for nurses with drug or alcohol dependencies that also meet certain requirements. These programs promote early intervention; support the treatment and recovery, and most important, monitoring when the nurse returns to work."

Source: the National Council of State Boards of Nursing at http://www.ncsbn.org/163.htm.

expiration date, and whether any board action has taken place. The service is available 24 hours a day, 7 days a week. Check your state's board of nursing site to find out if this service is available.

Employers are able to use this option to comply with requirements for written verification of a nurse's registration by The Joint Commission (TJC).

UNLICENSED ASSISTIVE PERSONNEL

The use of unlicensed assistive personnel (UAP) to provide patient care has grown dramatically in recent years. It is expected that the trend will continue. These unlicensed persons are trained to perform a variety of nursing tasks. Licensed nurses need to be aware of specific training that UAPs have had and facility job descriptions so they can safely make assignments. Supervision of UAPs by the RN and the LPN/LVN charge nurse in long-term care to ensure safety of patient care is a major concern. There is concern that because of the lack of licensed nurses in an agency, duties might be delegated and/or assigned inappropriately to UAPs. It is the RNs and LPNs/LVNs who stand to lose their jobs and licenses if the care provided by UAPs does not meet the standards of safety and effectiveness. The training program for UAPs does not provide the same in-depth education and experience that programs for student nurses provide. Licensed nurses are also accountable to both their employers and their state nursing boards (see Chapter 21).

NURSING STANDARD OF CARE

The nursing standard of care is your guideline for good nursing care. The phrase "You are held to the nursing standard of care" has important legal implications. The standard is based on what an ordinary, prudent nurse with similar education and nursing experience would do in similar circumstances. Resources for the nursing standard of care are found in Box 12-4. Note that unit routine ("I know you studied how to do this in nursing school, but this is how we do it here.") is not on the list.

 Keep in Mind

Accurate documentation is an important part of nursing care. In the eyes of the law, if it was not documented, it was not done.

HOW THE LAW AFFECTS LICENSED PRACTICAL NURSES AND LICENSED VOCATIONAL NURSES

COMMON LAW VERSUS STATUTORY LAW

The legal system in both the United States and Canada originates from English common law. Common law is called *judge-made law* because it originates in the courts. Common law is one way of establishing standards of legal conduct and is useful in settling disputes. Once

---

| Box 12-4 | Resources for the Nursing Standard of Care |

- **Nurse Practice Act:** Identifies the minimum level of competency necessary for a person to function as an LPN or LVN in a particular state.
- **Nursing licensure examination** (NCLEX-PN® examination): Tests for minimum competence.
- **Practical/vocational nursing programs:** Based on guidelines provided by the board of nursing, these programs guarantee a minimum knowledge base and the clinical practice necessary to provide safe nursing care.
- Curricula, textbooks, and instructors are resources for information about the standard of care.
- **Written policies and procedures:** The agency that employs the individual provides a standard of nursing care that must be followed. It is important to read the policies of the agency to find out whether verbal directions are supported by written policies. If a question about care ever comes up in court, a lawyer will use the agency's policy and procedure manual as one guide to expected behavior. Remember that policies and procedures do not overrule the state's Nurse Practice Act and educational preparation. However, institutional policies may be stricter than state law.
- **Custom:** An unwritten, usually acceptable way of giving nursing care. Expert witnesses, not coworkers, would be called to testify to "the acceptable way."
- **Law:** Decisions that have been arrived at in similar cases brought up before a court (judge-made law).
- Statements from the NAPNES and NFLPN. See Appendixes A and B.
- Nursing texts and journals.
- Administrative rules of the board of nursing.

---

the judge has made a decision, this decision *sets the precedent* for a ruling on a case with similar facts in the future. Informed consent and a patient's right to refuse treatment are examples of common law.

Statutory law is law developed by the legislative branch of the state and the U.S. Congress of the federal government. The Nurse Practice Act, which governs the practice of nursing, is an example of a statutory law. State boards of nursing can make nursing laws as long as the items in their laws do not conflict with any federal statutes.

CRIMINAL VERSUS CIVIL ACTION

The two classifications of legal action are criminal action and civil action. A criminal action involves people and society as a whole. It involves relationships between individuals and the government. A criminal action is classified as follows:

- **Misdemeanor:** A misdemeanor is the least serious charge and can result in a fine or prison sentence of no more than 1 year. This criminal act might include taking a narcotic intended for the patient's pain relief and giving the patient another substance in its place.

- **Felony:** A felony is a serious offense with a penalty that ranges from more than 1 year in prison to death—for example, when the nurse injects a patient with a lethal drug to hasten death or removes life support before the patient has been pronounced dead by the physician.

Guilt on the part of the nurse needs to be established by producing proof *beyond a reasonable doubt*. Regardless of the outcome of the criminal case, when a criminal case is completed, it is possible to be sued in a civil court.

A civil action protects individual rights and *results in payment of money* to the injured person (e.g., a back injury was sustained during a fall because spilled urine was not wiped up. This injury caused the patient additional treatment time, including physical therapy, pain, suffering, and loss of time from work). A civil action involves a relationship between individuals and the violation of those rights. A *tort* is a civil wrong. The two kinds of torts are intentional and unintentional, which are described as follows:

- **Intentional:** An intentional tort is intended to cause harm to the patient (e.g., threat or actual physical harm).
- **Unintentional:** An unintentional tort did not mean to harm the patient. "I did not mean to hurt the patient" is no defense when you did not use the "Rule of 5" and gave the patient an incorrect medication, which caused injury.

Guilt on the part of the nurse can be established by a preponderance (majority) of the evidence. Table 12-1 provides a comparison of criminal and civil law.

INTENTIONAL TORTS

Tort law is based on the premise that in the course of relationships with one another there is a general duty to avoid injuring one another. A tort is a wrong or injury done to someone that violates his or her rights.

Intentional torts require a specific state of mind—that is, that the nurse intended to do the wrongful act. Assault and battery, false imprisonment and use of restraints, defamation that includes both libel and slander (discussed later), and physical and emotional abuse are examples of intentional torts. Not all insurance companies cover intentional torts in their malpractice insurance policies, so you should check your policy.

Assault and Battery

Assault is an unjustified attempt or threat to touch someone. Battery means to cause physical harm to someone. When a patient refuses a treatment or medication, forcing the patient to take medication could result in an assault and battery charge against you. The patient gives *implied consent* (permission) for certain routine treatments when entering the institution. Patients retain the right to refuse any treatment verbally and may leave the institution when they choose, unless they are there for court-ordered treatment. Nurses can also protect themselves from assault by a patient but can use only as much force as is considered reasonable for self-protection.

Treating a patient without consent is battery even if the treatment is medically beneficial. A physician might go to the court to attempt to get a court order to allow a blood transfusion for someone who opposes it on religious grounds. If the patient is fully

Table 12-1 Comparison of Two Basic Classifications of Law

	CIVIL LAW	CRIMINAL LAW
Who law generally applies to	Relationships between private individuals and infringements on individual rights	Relationships between individuals and the government (state) Society as a whole
Sources of law	U.S. Constitution, state and federal legislatures	U.S. Constitution, state and federal legislatures
Punishment for breaking law	Payment of a monetary compensation	Death, imprisonment, fines, restrictions
How guilt is established	Proof by a preponderance of the evidence	Proof beyond a reasonable doubt
Examples of nursing liability	Contract Tort Unintentional Intentional Negligence	Murder, rape, larceny, homicide, manslaughter, assault and battery, embezzlement Felony/misdemeanor

Basic sources of law:
Common law—judge-made law. A trial judge's ruling lays down a legal principle and sets a precedent. These principles are used to decide future cases. This type of law is continually adapted and expanded.
Statutory law—formal legislative enactment. Law passed by Congress or enacted by state government. May be amended, repealed, or expanded by the legislature. The Nurse Practice Act is an example of statutory law.

competent, is not pregnant, and has no children, the court is likely to rule for the patient even if a blood transfusion would save his or her life. When faced with a similar situation, the practical/vocational nurse respects the patient's belief system and notifies the supervisor for further advice or interpretation.

False Imprisonment and Use of Restraints

False imprisonment is keeping someone detained against his or her will. It can include the use of restraints or seclusion in a room without cause and without a physician's order. Restraint by verbal threats of physical harm is also included in this category. Chemical restraint (with medication) is defined as administering a PRN medication with a sedating side effect every 4 hours to keep the patient tired and in his or her room. In this situation, the intent is to keep the patient quiet and out of the way. The intended use of the medication has been circumvented to meet the nurse's need.

Defamation

Defamation means damage to someone's reputation through false communication or communication without their permission. Libel and slander are included in this category and are described as follows:

- Libel is defamation through *written* communication or pictures.
- Slander is defamation by *verbalizing* untrue or private information (gossip) to a third party.

The patient has the right to expect you to speak the truth. Additional unnecessary conversation with coworkers and those outside the agency can result in a charge of defamation. The same is true for taking unwanted photographs or showing a patient's injury, cancerous growth, gunshot wound, and so forth to others, students included, without the patient's permission.

Consider also that you often are privy to information about the personal lives of other nurses, physicians, and other coworkers, and they are privy to information about you. Although the desire to repeat the information you hear may be tempting, it is best left unsaid. Later in the chapter, you will learn about HIPAA and how that law defines privacy.

Physical and Emotional Abuse

Physical abuse is generally easier to identify, although the victim may find creative ways to hide the injuries for a period of time. Emotional abuse is more difficult to identify. The person doing the abusing may be very personable and attentive to the victim when out in public. A former student described how everyone thought her husband loved her and how fortunate she was. When they were alone, he would tell her she was ugly, worthless, and no one else would ever want her or love her. When she became pregnant, he would always take her to her doctor appointment. He would answer the doctor's and nurse's questions for her, and when she tried to speak, he would take over in gentle terms, doing the explaining. At no time was she alone with a doctor or nurse.

In the course of your career in practical/vocational nursing, you will probably suspect or actually see the results of some types of abuse. As a practical/vocational nurse, you have a legal responsibility to report your suspicions or observations of abuse by following your facility's abuse policy. Note that a "suspicion" is a nagging doubt. Refer to your state's abuse laws for specific rules that govern your responsibility for reporting abuse. It is important to be empathetic (as opposed to sympathetic) so that your observations or reporting will be as objective as possible. Becoming a part of the patient's emotions may lead you to jump to conclusions or accept a particularly convincing but untrue explanation. Whether the patient is a child, woman, man, or elder, reputations are at stake. Once an accusation has been made, it is difficult to be truly free from it, even when it is proved groundless.

Follow your facility's policy for reporting abuse. The social services department can help you report abuse. Offer concrete, specific observations. Quote the statements made, and avoid offering a personal interpretation. Let the facts speak for themselves.

UNINTENTIONAL TORTS

An unintentional tort holds that the nurse did not intend to injure the patient. However, the nurse did not maintain the nursing standard of care and did not do what a prudent nurse with comparable education and skills would do in a similar situation. Negligence and malpractice (professional negligence) are examples of unintentional torts.

NEGLIGENCE

Brent (2001) defines negligence as "conduct that falls below the standards established by the law for the protection of others against the unreasonable risk of harm." A common type of negligence is personal injury. For example, say your town has a law that sidewalks must be shoveled within 24 hours after a snowstorm. Your sidewalk has not been shoveled within the 24 hours, and your neighbor falls in front of your house and breaks her arm. The neighbor sues you for negligence. It is important to remember that in negligence the property owner did not intend to cause the injury to the neighbor, but knowing the risks and the law, he or she should have guarded against the injury. Good intentions do not enter in. It is your conduct, not your intent, that is the issue.

MALPRACTICE (PROFESSIONAL NEGLIGENCE)

Malpractice, the legal name for professional negligence, means negligence by a professional—in this case, an LPN/LVN. The most common type of negligence in practical/vocational nursing relates to action or lack of action, not what you intended to do. Box 12-5 lists the most common sources of malpractice, according to O'Keefe (2001). All the charges of professional negligence (malpractice) listed could be avoided by good nursing practice (i.e., what a reasonable, prudent nurse would do in a similar situation). **The student practical/vocational nurse is held to the level of a licensed practical/vocational nurse's performance. Know your state's Nurse Practice Act.**

There are occasions when the evidence is overwhelming and indicates the accused nurse is responsible for the patient injury. Such an occasion is called *res ipsa loquitur*, meaning "the evidence speaks for itself." For example, a patient develops a drop in blood pressure immediately after the nurse administered an injection improperly.

MALPRACTICE INSURANCE FOR NURSES

More nurses are being named in lawsuits. Nurses assume liability for their own acts. Although the employing agency may assume responsibility for the nurse during a lawsuit, the agency can then turn around and sue the nurse. You can also be held responsible for the "neighborhood advice" you give—for example, telling a neighbor how to care for her sick child.

Each nurse must carefully consider whether it is necessary to purchase a malpractice insurance policy. Incidents of suing for malpractice continue, although your chances of being sued as an LPN/LVN are statistically small. Look carefully at the policy of the agency of which you are an employee. Some reasons for having your own malpractice insurance are found in Box 12-6.

◎ Try This

Malpractice Coverage

If you are currently assigned to a clinical area, find out what the agency policy is on malpractice coverage for practical/vocational nurses.

Box 12-5   Some Common Sources of Malpractice

- Medication and treatment errors
- Lack of observation and timely reporting about the patient
- Defective technologies or equipment
- Infections caused or worsened by poor nursing care
- Poor communication of important information, including change of condition
- Failure to intervene to protect the patient from poor medical care

Box 12-6   Reasons for Your Own Malpractice Insurance

- The jury's award could exceed the limits of your agency's coverage.
- Your *employing agency* could pay out an award to a plaintiff and then countersue you.
- You acted outside the scope of employment, and the agency argues it is not liable.
- Your employer's policy covers you only on the job.
- An agency might carry a policy that covers you only while you are employed by that institution. A suit may come up years after you have stopped working for the employer. It is suggested that nurses purchase occurrence coverage if malpractice coverage is desired and not claims coverage. For this reason, occurrence coverage protects the nurse for each incident regardless of the present employer.
- The agency may decide to settle out of court. The plaintiff could pursue a case against the nurse.
- Has your employer paid the insurance premium?
- After a settlement, *insurers* could turn around and sue the nurse.
- If you have your own coverage, you will have your own lawyers, not the lawyers who are also defending the agency.

FOUR ELEMENTS NEEDED TO PROVE NEGLIGENCE

Duty, breach of duty, damages, and proximate cause are the four elements that must be present to cause an action for negligence against the nurse. Each of the four elements must be proved by the patient to receive compensation. Box 12-7 lists the four elements needed to prove negligence.

❓ Critical Thinking

Develop a scenario of an LPN/LVN who is being sued. Use the four elements needed to prove negligence as the basis for the suit.

Box 12-7   Four Elements Needed to Prove Negligence

1. Duty refers to the nurse's responsibility to provide care in an acceptable way. The nurse has a duty based on education, as well as the policies and standards of the place of employment.
2. Breach of duty means that the nurse did not adhere to the nursing standard of care. What was expected of the nurse was not done (omission) or was not done correctly (commission). An expert nurse witness establishes the standard of care.
3. Damages mean that the patient must be able to show that the nurse's negligent act injured him or her in some way. The patient must prove actual damage.
4. Proximate cause means that a reasonable cause-and-effect relationship can be shown between the omission or commission of the nursing act and the harm to the patient. Did the nurse's negligent act cause the injury in question?

STEPS FOR BRINGING LEGAL ACTION

Legal actions follow an orderly process. Remember that the nurse also has rights and is not considered guilty simply because someone filed a complaint. Steps for bringing a legal action by a patient are found in Box 12-8.

DEPOSITIONS

Depositions are used to gather information under oath (fact finding). Once the deposition is scheduled, provide information on where and how you can be reached. The depositions usually take place in an attorney's office. You may be able to request that it be in your attorney's office. (It will be helpful to have an attorney who understands nursing and is familiar with legal action against a nurse). Opponents' attorneys may also be present. However, only one of the opponent's attorneys should be permitted to ask questions so as not to "tag team"—that is, multiple attorneys firing questions at the nurse. A court reporter or stenographer will record your testimony.

Dress professionally, as you would for a job interview (see Chapter 22). Do your utmost to be calm and polite no matter how rude others, including the opposing attorney, seem to you.

ATTORNEY PROCEDURES

In preparation for a deposition, your attorney will do the following:
- Provide a checklist of basic instructions for the deposition.

| Box 12-8 | Steps for Bringing a Legal Action by a Patient |

- The patient believes that the nurse has violated his or her legal rights.
- The patient seeks the advice of an attorney.
- The attorney has a nurse expert review the patient's chart to see whether the nurse has violated the nursing standard of care. If it is determined that a standard of care has been violated, a lawsuit is filed.
- The patient (the plaintiff) files a complaint that documents the grievance (violation of rules). This is served to the defendant (the nurse).
- The defendant responds in writing.
- The discovery period (pretrial activity) begins. Statements are taken from the defendant nurse, witnesses, nurse expert, patient (plaintiff), and other caregivers. Policies and procedures of the health care facilities are reviewed.
- During the trial, important information is presented to the judge or jury. A verdict (decision) is reached. The plaintiff (the patient) has the burden of proof (evidence of wrongdoing) during the trial.
- An appeal (request for another trial) can be made if either the plaintiff or the defendant does not consider the verdict acceptable.

- Practice likely questions that may be asked and critique your responses.
- Prepare you for types of questions that may slant your testimony.
- Suggest appropriate ways to respond, but not tell you what to answer.
- Use a practice deposition video (usually, not always).
- Meet with you in advance the day of the deposition to answer any last-minute questions.

GIVING TESTIMONY

Here are some basics to keep in mind during a deposition:
- It is important to tell the truth—*always*. Avoid trying to be clever.
- A court reporter or stenographer can only record words, so questions must be answered verbally.
- Listen carefully to the question. If you do not understand the question, ask that the question be repeated or rephrased.
- Before answering, pause. This will give you an opportunity to consider the question. Think about what is being asked and how you will answer.
- Be specific in answering a question: If it is a "yes" or "no" question, then answer it that way. *Resist the urge to say more.* If you do not know the answer to a question, say so, and do not speculate. If you do not remember, say, "I do not remember."
- If your attorney instructs you to not answer a question, do not answer. Instruction to not answer a question is permitted under certain circumstances.
- Be careful not to reveal the content of any conversation with your attorney.
- Ask for a break, especially if you are tired or not thinking clearly. If there is a question pending, you will be expected to answer it before taking a break.
- You will not be permitted to take any notes during the deposition, nor will you be able to bring in notes, files, a calendar, notepad, or pen (Main and Todd, 2005).
- A few weeks after the deposition, you and your attorney may be able to review the testimony and make corrections. You may be asked about the corrections during the trial.

LIABILITY

KINDS OF LIABILITY

Personal liability holds us responsible for our own behavior, including negligent behavior. This rule makes it impossible to completely shift responsibility onto someone else. Vicarious liability means responsibility for actions of another because of a special relationship with the other. The term *respondeat superior*, Latin for "let the master speak," is based on vicarious liability. It is applied in the following two ways:

1. *Borrowed servant doctrine* (e.g., the master/servant relationship between an employer [hospital] and an employee [nurse]). The employer (master) is assumed to be better able to pay for the injuries than the employee (servant). The employer may also be held responsible in a suit for the negligent acts of the employee performed during the time of employment. This provides incentive for health care agencies to hire carefully, as well as orient and supervise the work of the employee.

2. *Captain of the ship doctrine* (e.g., in an operating room). A nurse becomes the temporary employee of the physician doing the surgery. This doctrine assumes that in this situation the surgeon exerts control of the nurse in relation to specific conduct that caused patient injury in the operating room.

Institutional liability is vicarious liability. It assumes that the health facility provides certain safeguards to keep the patient from harm. This includes a safe facility to prevent physical harm (e.g., adequate supervision of staff, adequate staffing, and safe equipment).

COMMON CAUSES OF NURSING LIABILITY

Many of the errors leading to common nursing liabilities can be avoided by following the guidelines you learned in nursing school. The major areas of liability (responsibility/accountability) can be categorized as lack of safety, knowledge, skill, observation and reporting, documentation, and acceptance of responsibility for nursing actions—all of which are part of the usual clinical evaluation. The most common errors are drug errors, most of which can be avoided if you follow the guidelines you learn in basic nursing and practice in the clinical areas. One of the best defenses for prevention of legal liability is development of rapport with the patient. If you treat patients with courtesy and respect, they are less likely to sue (unless you provide care below the nursing standard of care). The very best defense is not to err in the first place.

 Professional Pointer

Ignorance of nursing law is no excuse.

RESPONSIBILITY AND ACCOUNTABILITY IN NURSING

Nursing demands that you be responsible. This means being reliable and trustworthy. At no time can you expect a peer, supervisor, or patient to say to you, "It's okay that you didn't come to work today because your car wouldn't start"; "It's okay if we talk about just your problems today instead of the patients'"; or "It's okay that you didn't do the work you were assigned because you're having a bad day." Nursing says, "I'm sorry that you have personal problems that are distracting you, but you have to deal with them because your priority in this vocation is the patient."

The word *accountability* means that you are answerable. As a nursing student, you are answerable to yourself, to your assigned patient, to the team leader, to the physician, and to your instructor who constantly evaluates your work. As an LPN/LVN, accountability to the instructor is replaced by accountability to the employing agency. You are held accountable for all the nursing actions that you perform or are assigned to perform. The measures of accountability are the following nursing standards of practice:

- Nurse Practice Act of the state
- NAPNES Standards and Educational Competencies of Graduates of Practical/Vocational Nursing Programs (see Appendix A)
- NFLPN Nursing Practice Standards for the Licensed Practical/Vocational Nurse (see Appendix B)

They recommend minimal acceptable standards of nursing behavior for the SPN/SVN and the LPN/LVN.

LIABILITY OF STUDENT NURSES AND INSTRUCTORS

Student nurses are held accountable for the nursing care they give. They are held to the standards of a licensed practical/vocational nurse. This emphasizes *the necessity to prepare for providing care for assigned patients in the clinical area*. The instructor has the responsibility to make patient assignments based on the student's knowledge base and ability to give safe nursing care. The instructor is also expected to provide reasonable supervision for the care given by a student. A list of your responsibilities is found in Box 12-9.

Box 12-9   SPN/SVN Responsibilities for Patient Care

- Prepare by reading the assigned patient's chart, patient profile, and established plan of care, and develop your own plan of care for the patient to whom you are assigned.
- Look up action, safety of ordered dose, side effects, and nursing considerations for the assigned patient's routine, PRN medications, and IV additives.
- Review how to perform ordered treatments.
- Compose a time sequence for care during your time with the patient.
- When you arrive on the clinical unit, review your plan of care with the instructor before you begin your nursing care.
- Identify a need for and request additional help or supervision.
- Comply with agency and school of nursing policies.

FUNCTIONING BEYOND THE SCOPE OF PRACTICE AND EXPERIENCE

As an LPN/LVN, you might be asked by an RN or physician to perform nursing duties that are beyond your scope of practice or experience. It is up to you to speak up. Box 12-10 contains examples of responses when asked to perform beyond your scope of practice. When seeking employment, check out the philosophy, mission statement, and policies of your potential place of employment. Ask what is included in your job, the period of orientation you will receive, what the orientation will cover, and who will do the orientation. If you discover during your inquiry that your work will cover more than you have learned or tasks that are beyond the scope of practice, say so. Listen also to your affective response: What is your intuition saying? Getting a job just to get a job may result in your being fired or losing your license. You may end up losing your job for something that was not your fault. The ideal is that everyone around you shares your ethics and demonstrates fairness, but the reality of ethics is sometimes quite different.

SPECIFIC PATIENT SITUATIONS

A professional relationship between the nurse and the patient is essential for the provision of nursing care. Legal precedent has established that the health care agency also has a responsibility to the patient. Patients have become increasingly concerned and vocal about the quality of care they expect to receive. Many of the issues are directly related to privacy, confidentiality, and safety. These are also concerns of health agencies and health care workers, including nurses.

Box 12-10   Possible Responses When Asked to Perform Beyond Your Scope of Practice

- "I am not legally able to do something beyond the LPN/LVN Nurse Practice Act."
- "I have never done this before. I will be glad to learn if you teach me, watch me demonstrate in return, and write a memo for my file that you have taught me to do this and watched a satisfactory return demonstration."
- "I was taught to do this while in school but did not have a chance to catheterize a real person. Please demonstrate and then watch me do a catheterization before I catheterize a patient on my own."
- "My orientation here did not include how to make daily assignments according to skill level of staff. I need to be shown. Will you show me how to make assignments? I learn quickly, so it will be time well spent."
- "You have provided a detailed orientation, but I do not feel ready (or qualified) to assume a charge nurse position. I think I need more experience as a staff nurse so I can function effectively and within my Nurse Practice Act."

PRIVACY AND CONFIDENTIALITY

Privacy in health care means the right to be left alone and free from intrusion, including the right to choose care based on personal beliefs, feelings, or attitudes; the right to govern bodily integrity (accepting or rejecting treatment or exposure of the body); and the right to control when and how sensitive information is shared. Confidentiality in health care refers to the nondisclosure of information regarding patients.

INFORMATION THAT MUST BE REVEALED

Some laws require that certain patient information must be reported without the patient's consent. The purpose is to protect the public. Patient information that must be revealed is listed in Box 12-11.

PATIENTS' RIGHTS

Patients' rights in all types of institutions are mandated by the U.S. Constitution and by state and federal laws. Legal rights vary depending on the health care agency

---

Box 12-11   Patient Information That Must Be Revealed

In all situations the supervisor, director of nursing, and policy set by the facility are resources.

- **Communicable disease:** To the local health department or the Centers for Disease Control and Prevention. This includes AIDS, but the nature of the disclosure varies according to state law.
- **Vaccine-related adverse reactions:** To the Department of Health and Human Services. (Reporting of some reactions is mandatory; for others it is voluntary. Call (800) 822-7967 for the Food and Drug Administration's reportable events table.)
- **Criminal acts:** All states mandate reporting of rape cases. Some mandate reporting of injuries by gunshot or sharp instruments. Some states require reporting of blood alcohol levels (BAL) beyond the legal limit. Clarify your state's specific mandates. The local police department is a good place to clarify what is reportable *before* an incident occurs.
- **Equipment-related injuries:** When use of a medical device results in injury or death, it is reported immediately to your supervisor and physician. If emergency first aid is called for, follow the procedure you have been taught.
- **When there is a clear and present danger:** HIPAA laws, for example, mandate reporting of patient mistreatment or professional misconduct. Report immediately to your supervisor or follow the policy manual for an emergency course of action.
- **Abuse and neglect of a patient or elderly person:** Report the incident immediately to your supervisor or director of nursing. He or she will usually follow up by reporting to police or social services.
- **Incompetence or unprofessional acts:** As defined by state law. Facilities have policies for how to report and to whom. Report immediately to your supervisor, your director of nursing, or as directed in the facility's policy manual. Violation of nursing law will be reported to the state board of nursing.

Box 12-12	*The Patient Care Partnership* Recommendations: What to Expect During a Hospital Stay

- High-quality hospital care
- A clean and safe environment
- Involvement in your own care
  a. Discussing your medical condition and information about medically appropriate treatment choices
  b. Discussing your treatment plan
  c. Getting information from you
  d. Understanding your health care goals and values
  e. Understanding who should make decisions when you cannot
- Protection of your privacy
- Preparing you and your family for when you leave the hospital
- Help with your billing and filing insurance claims (AHA, 2011)

Box 12-13	Basic Health Insurance Portability and Accountability Act Terminology

- **HIPAA:** Passed in 1996. Enforcement began April 14, 2003.
- **Portability:** Original intent of HIPAA (see Chapter 17) was portability of health insurance for employees from one job to the next.
- **Protection of patient privacy:** Main focus of HIPAA is protection of patient health information.
- **Covered entity:** Health facilities that provide, bill, or receive payment for health care as a normal part of business.
- **Health care:** Any care, services, or supplies related to the care of a patient.
- **Privacy officer:** HIPAA requirement that all covered entities designate a privacy officer.
- **Notice of privacy practices:** Each covered entity must develop a document, written in plain language, that explains the facility's privacy practices. It is distributed to all patients. The notice is also posted in a prominent place to be read by all interested parties.
- **Department of Health and Human Services (DHHS):** The federal agency that oversees HIPAA.
- **Mandatory law:** Law that must be followed, or penalties will be involved.

and the patient's competency. The American Hospital Association (AHA) developed *The Patient's Bill of Rights* in 1972. It was revised in 2003 and renamed *The Patient Care Partnership: Understanding Expectations, Rights, and Responsibilities*. This is an ethical, not legal, document for hospitals recommending ways to guarantee patient rights. It is intended as a model for states to develop rights statements. Some state legislatures have adopted patient rights statements. Additional bills of rights have been developed for pregnant patients, nursing home residents, and mental health patients. The document is reviewed and revised yearly as needed. Box 12-12 provides *The Patient Care Partnership* recommendations.

 Try This

Patients' Rights

Obtain a copy of your state's or health facility's patient rights statement. Briefly explain what is meant by each of the main topics. Identify the topics that are a part of what you have already learned in nursing.

HEALTH INSURANCE PORTABILITY AND ACCOUNTABILITY ACT

The U.S. Health Insurance Portability and Accountability Act (HIPAA) rules took effect on April 14, 2003, for health insurance companies, hospitals, clinics, doctors, pharmacies, and other health groups throughout the United States. The original intent of HIPAA was portability of insurance for employees from one job to the next. Portability is addressed in the law, but the main focus of the law is privacy. Changes to modify HIPAA privacy, security, and enforcement of rules are being considered. The law gives patients rights over their health information. Basic HIPAA terminology is provided in Box 12-13.

Basics of the Health Insurance Portability and Accountability Act

The following are the three basic parts of HIPAA:

1. **Protection of privacy.** HIPAA provides a guide for health-related facilities and individuals to establish privacy standards based on the HIPAA model. This is intended as a national privacy standard throughout the United States. When discussing privacy, HIPAA uses the term *protected health information* (PHI) when referring to patient information that should not be revealed. Proposed are rules to increase efficiency of the health care system by creating standards for use and disseminating of health care information.

2. **Administrative simplification.** The overall goal of administrative simplification is to reduce paperwork related to health care reimbursement (e.g., a goal is to develop a universal insurance claim form).

3. **Security standards.** The overall goal is to establish security standards for the protection of electronic (computer and fax) transmission of PHI (e.g., password protection when using a computer is a HIPAA requirement). Confidentiality and complete security requirements have increased since February 2010, including having a small health plan use a single national provider identifier.

The Department of Health and Human Services is the federal agency that oversees HIPAA. It has emphasized reasonableness as a guide to applying HIPAA regulations. Depending on the facility with which you are involved, interpretation of HIPAA ranges from reasonable to very strict. HIPAA rules and regulations have been reviewed and updated yearly since 2003.

? Critical Thinking

Patient Privacy

List examples of patient information that can compromise patient privacy if revealed.

_____

_____

_____

The Notice of Privacy Practices

The main focus of HIPAA is protection of privacy. Each covered entity (health facility) must develop a written "Notice of Privacy Practices." The notice is made available to all patients, employees, and health-related companies with whom the facility does business (e.g., health insurance companies, medical equipment companies). The patient receives a personal copy to read and sign. Signing the copy denotes understanding of and agreement with the use and disclosure of PHI for treatment, payment, and facility operation. This is not the same as consent for treatment. If the patient is incompetent, state laws are followed. This usually means that the patient's health proxy is treated as though he or she is the patient.

What the Notice of Privacy Practices Addresses

The Notice of Privacy Practices must address the following in plain language:

1. **Access to medical records.** Patients have a right to a copy of their medical records and to review the records upon request. The facility determines under what conditions the records can be reviewed. Generally this means reviewing the records with an RN or a physician present to translate medical terminology and answer questions. At no time does an SPN/SVN or LPN/LVN provide the records, or any part of them, to the patient. The request must follow the protocol set up by the facility. The Notice of Privacy Practices must clearly state how to access the record. HIPAA provides up to 30 days for a facility to provide a medical record for a patient. However, Medicare regulations require that the record be made available to a Medicare patient within 24 hours. Proposed rules include that the patient may be charged for being provided PHI on electronic media—for example: the cost of a CD or flash drive.
2. **Amendments to the medical record.** According to HIPAA, patients have the right to request changes in their medical records. All covered entities must appoint privacy officers. It is the job of the privacy officer to process a request for change in a patient's medical records. The facility is obligated to consider the request and then notify the patient of the final decision.

3. **Restrictions on the use of protected health information.** Patients can restrict use of their PHI as long as the requested information does not interfere with activities related to treatment, payment, or facility operation. The privacy officer usually makes the final decision. Proposed rules include prohibition of the sale of PHI (without authorization) for use in marketing and fund raising.
4. **Access to an accounting.** Patients can request a list of the people, companies, or agencies that have received their PHI. The Notice of Privacy Practices lists steps for requesting an accounting on written request from a patient. Proposed are rules on restricting certain types of information to health plans.
5. **Confidential communications.** Patients may request that PHI be delivered in such a way that the sender cannot be identified. For example, the patient may request that blood test results be mailed in a plain envelope without the agency's return address. Proposed are provisions to strengthen and expand HIPAA's enforcement rule.
6. **Complaints about violations of privacy.** Patients can file a complaint if they think their privacy has been violated. The Notice of Privacy Practices tells them how to contact the privacy officer, as well as how to file the complaint. The Notice also provides information on how to contact the Department of Health and Human Services (DHHS), the federal oversight agency for HIPAA. If a patient is not satisfied with the outcome of filing a complaint with the facility's privacy officer, he or she may choose to contact DHHS. If DHHS determines there is reason to investigate, it will do so and impose a fine on the covered entity if it has violated HIPAA law.
7. **Minimum necessary rule.** This rule assists you in making an on-the-spot decision about how much patient PHI you need to divulge. For example, if you are ordering a special bed for a patient, you will need to include the patient's height and weight. You will usually have no reason to include diagnosis, among other information.
8. **Telephone requests for PHI.** Nurses are often faced with telephone inquiries about a patient. It is difficult to identify who is really making the inquiry and for what purpose. Ecker (2003) states the following:

   HIPAA suggests that whenever a caller asks for a patient, the provider can verify whether that person is in the hospital, but only if the caller asks for the patient by name. If the caller asks for specific information about the patient, the new guidelines recommend that only minimal information about general status be communicated. The caller should be directed to speak to the patient or family for further details.

Exceptions to this rule include clergy who ask for all people of a certain faith or a patient who requests anonymity on admission. A parent, for example, may request anonymity regarding his or her child's hospitalization when there is concern of the child being abducted by the other parent.

9. **Email and faxes.** To reduce the possibility of error during electronic transfer of information, the "minimum necessary" rule applies. Perhaps you have experienced sending an email or fax to the wrong person. Think about the possible consequences of this happening with PHI. One safety feature is a disclaimer on an email or fax that identifies the mail as confidential and explains how to notify the sender in case of error.

? Critical Thinking

Medical Records

Think of one or more reasons why if a patient removes or changes information in a medical record, it can affect a pending legal case.

Concerns That the Health Insurance Portability and Accountability Act Does Not Address

Additional concerns that the HIPAA does not address include discarding PHI that is not meant for the patient's chart and hallway conversations (Box 12-14).

 Try This

Maintain Patient Confidentiality

Keep confidential the conversations you overhear in the clinical area that include personal information about a patient and those that include more than the "minimum necessary" about a patient. List one time that you were trapped into providing confidential information to an unauthorized person about a patient.

Box 12-14	**Additional Concerns Not Addressed by HIPAA***

- PHI not meant for the chart includes daily patient assignments, nurse's personal notes about the patient (used as the basis for charting), and anything else that could identify the patient that is crumpled up and thrown in the wastebasket at the end of the shift. Many facilities are already dealing with this by identifying a specific disposal area where the notes ultimately get shredded.
- Hallway conversation remains a problem. For example, a conversation about a patient might not be overheard by the patient involved but is often overheard by other patients or visitors. The same is true with conversation in lunchrooms, nursing desk areas, waiting rooms, and elevators.

*Adapted from Ecker M. (2003) Protecting patient privacy: understanding the new federal HIPAA standards. Midwest/Heartland Nurse Week. pp. 20–21.
Anderson F. (2007) Finding HIPPA in your soup. AJN, 107(2) 66–72.

Expect to find differences in interpretation of the HIPAA law. Find a copy of the facility privacy policy during each clinical rotation, and do the same with each job you have after graduation. Note the differences and adjust to them.

PATIENT COMPETENCY

You can expect to hear increased use of the term *competency* in both a legal and a clinical sense. The following details provide a brief framework to help you use this term correctly.

Patient competency has both a legal meaning and a clinical meaning. Some patients' rights issues are based on proof of competence or incompetence within the court system. *Legal* competency refers to a patient who is:

- Eighteen years old or older
- A pregnant or married woman
- A self-supporting minor (referred to as a legally emancipated minor)
- Competent in the eyes of the law (incompetence is determined by the court)

Clinical competency refers to a patient who is able to do the following:

- Identify the problem for which he or she is seeing the physician
- Understand the options for care and the possible consequences
- Make a decision
- Provide sound reasons for the option he or she chooses

PATIENT'S RIGHT TO CONSENT

The patient's right to consent to or refuse treatment is a significant example of patient autonomy (right to choose). It is advisable for a patient to be accompanied by someone he or she trusts whenever he or she goes to a health agency for care. Patients are often stressed to the point that they do not "hear" what is being said to them. Words such as "cancer" and "heart attack" can cause sheer terror. Furthermore, some patients still are afraid to question the physician and therefore agree to procedures that they do not understand: "Whatever you think is best" is a frequent answer.

General (Implied) Consent

General (implied) consent for treatment is obtained on admission. It may be obtained by the LPN/LVN or by an admission clerk during a routine admission. The fact that a person has voluntarily sought admission to a health care agency and willingly signs a general admission form is an example of general consent. A patient may revoke this permission verbally or in writing (e.g., you walk into patient's room with a syringe and explain that the doctor has ordered Demerol for pain relief; the patient might say, "I don't want a shot; I'm going home").

Critical Thinking

Resolve Consent Issues

What steps will you take in the case of the patient refusing Demerol?

Informed Consent

Informed consent must be obtained for invasive procedures ordered for therapeutic or diagnostic purposes (e.g., surgery). Informed consent means that the patient is told the following in nonmedical language:

1. Diagnosis or suspected diagnosis
2. Purpose and description of treatment (some surgeons are sending the patient home with a video that shows the surgery being performed before asking them to sign a consent form)
3. Expected outcome, expected benefits, and possible side effects or complications
4. Explanation of alternative treatments and their benefits, possible side effects, or complications
5. Names and qualifications of the people who will perform the procedure (treatment)
6. Prognosis if treatment is not done (when known)
7. Answers to questions patient wants clarified
8. Explanation that the patient has the right to revoke written permission at any time

The patient must indicate comprehension (understanding) of the information. This means considerably more than just nodding the head. For example, have the patient explain in his or her own words what he or she thinks is going to happen and the benefits and risks involved. Document the patient's understanding of the information.

Informed consent is the responsibility of the physician because he or she must explain the implications and complications of the procedure to the patient before written permission is obtained. *It is never the responsibility of the LPN/LVN.* If you are in the room when the physician is obtaining informed consent, you might be asked to witness the signing. Sullivan (1998) explains:

> Being asked to witness a patient's signature on a consent form is no small responsibility. Your signature attests to three things: that the patient gave his consent voluntarily, that his signature is authentic, and that he appears to be competent to give consent.

If the LPN/LVN is present when the treatment is being explained and the informed consent signed, in most states the LPN/LVN may support the teaching that has taken place by the physician. Be sure to check your state's Nurse Practice Act.

Authorized Consent

Parents cannot give informed consent for the treatment of their children, but they can authorize treatment for their children up to a certain age; this is called authorized consent. Courts of law recognize that parents generally authorize what is appropriate for their children. In most states, "minor" is defined as younger than age 18. Some states allow minors to give their own consent for treatment of substance abuse, mental health problems, and sexually transmitted diseases (STDs). Emancipated minors are defined as those living on their own and managing their own finances or who are married and have children. They are competent to give their consent.

END-OF-LIFE ISSUES

PATIENT SELF-DETERMINATION ACT

The Patient Self-Determination Act (PSDA) is an amendment to the Omnibus Budget Reconciliation Act (a federal law). The PSDA requires many Medicare and Medicaid providers (e.g., hospitals, nursing homes, hospice programs, home health agencies, and HMOs) to give adult individuals, at the time of inpatient admission, certain information about their rights under state laws governing advance directives, including the following:

- The right to participate in and direct their own health care decisions
- The right to accept or refuse medical or surgical treatment
- The right to prepare an advance directive
- Information on the provider's policies that govern the utilization of these rights

Source: The Patient Self-Determination Act available at http://www.ascenionhealth.org/ethics/public/issues/patient_self.asp.

ADVANCE DIRECTIVES

Two types of written advance directives are available to patients giving direction to health care providers about treatment choices in certain circumstances. The two types of advance directives are a living will and a durable power of attorney for health care. A good advance directive describes the kind of treatment that is desired by the person depending on how sick he or she is. Usually the advance directive indicates what type of treatment is not desired. However, it can indicate that the person wants all possible measures used to prolong life. Information on advance directives can be found by Googling "advance directives" and clicking on "familydoctor.org."

Living Will

A living will is a legal document that describes the kind of medical treatments or life-sustaining treatments the person would want if seriously or terminally ill. There are many issues that can be addressed, including the following:

- Transfusion of blood or blood products
- CPR
- Diagnostic tests
- Administration of drugs

- Tissue or organ donations
- Dialysis
- Use of respirator
- Tube feeding
- Surgery
- Hydration, pain medication, food, and other comfort measures

A living will does not let the person select someone to make decisions for them. An attorney is not required to draft a living will. The living will is filled out by the individual and witnessed by a person who will not benefit by the death of that individual.

Living wills are recognized as legal documents in most states in the United States, the District of Columbia, and Guam. California does not recognize a living will as binding. Living wills are not recognized as legal documents in Canada. The individual generally is advised to give a witnessed copy to the health care provider and a trusted friend or relation and to keep one copy in a location that is easily accessible. If a person is moving to or spending time in another state, he or she is advised to determine whether the living will is considered legal in that state. Otherwise, the person may discover too late that the written directive may not be honored. Blank forms are available from hospitals, other health care agencies, age-related organizations such as the American Association of Retired Persons (AARP), and attorneys' offices. Living wills can be revoked in writing or orally.

Durable Medical Power of Attorney (Advanced Health Care Directive)

A durable medical power of attorney (DPOA) is a legal document that is valid in all 50 states. It names a health care proxy (anyone at least 18 years old) to make medical decisions if that person is no longer able to speak for himself or herself. The DPOA is generally more useful than a living will. It becomes active anytime the person is unconscious or unable to make a medical decision. The DPOA may not be a good choice if the person has no one he or she trusts to make these decisions. There are some differences in various states; for example, the title of the document.

 Try This

Legal Directives

Discuss the difference between a durable medical power of attorney and a living will.

DO-NOT-RESUSCITATE ORDER

A do-not-resuscitate (DNR) order is an advance directive based on the Patient Self-Determination Act that gives a physician legal permission to write such an order. The physician may also write a DNR order for a patient who no longer has decision-making ability but does not have personal advance directives written

and signed. Commonly called a "no-code" order, it is a legal order to not resuscitate a patient. The DNR order does not have to be updated unless the patient changes her or his mind. If a written DNR order does not exist and the nurse does not try to resuscitate the patient, the nurse is in effect making a medical decision. The nurse is essentially practicing medicine without a license and may be subject to a lawsuit. There is no such thing as a partial or slow code. All caregivers must know when a written DNR order exists. Check your state and agency policies regarding DNR orders because they vary considerably among states.

The role of the next of kin in making decisions about care for the patient differs from state to state. In the article "End of Life Issues," Hanawalt (2001) addresses this problem:

> The biggest challenge: no advance directive and family opposition. Only about 15% to 20% of patients have advance directives in the form of a living will or health care proxy. Although patients often express a preference to die at home, statistics show that 76% to 80% of people die in the hospital, 15% in hospice care, and 5% to 9% in nursing homes.

Sometimes providers ignore patient advance directives. The patient's instructions may be too vague, or the physician might assume that the patient did not know about an available treatment or simply defers to the wishes of family members. Sometimes patients have not discussed advance directives with their physician, or a facility has a policy that a written physician's order of DNR must be in the chart to comply with the patient's wish. For your legal protection, find out about your state's and facility's policies and if the patient has a written advance directive of which the physician is aware. Do-not-hospitalize (DNH) orders may be more effective than DNR orders in limiting treatment and preventing unnecessary or unwanted patient transfer *from* a long-term care *to* an acute treatment facility. Most important for you, as an LPN/LVN, is to know your agency's policy.

REMOVAL OF LIFE SUPPORT SYSTEMS

The physician must pronounce the patient dead and document this status before the nurse turns off a ventilator. If the nurse removes a life support system before the physician pronounces the patient dead, it can be considered an act of murder.

PHYSICIAN-ASSISTED SUICIDE AND EUTHANASIA

Physician-assisted suicide (PAS) and euthanasia are not the same. "Physician-assisted suicide refers to a physician providing the means for death, most often with a prescription. The patient, not the physician, will ultimately administer the lethal medication. Euthanasia generally means that the physician would act

Table 12-2	Active and Passive Euthanasia	
ACTIVE (actions that speed the process of dying)	**PASSIVE** (do nothing to preserve life)
Actively end person's life	Avoid prolonging person's life
Initiate the dying process	Allow to continue a process that causes death
Morally wrong	Morally permissible
Legally not allowed	Legally allowed
Forbidden by professional organizations	Approved by professional organizations

directly—for instance, by giving a lethal injection—to end a patient's life." Source: http://depts.washington.edu/bioethx/topics/pas.html.

Both are different from the DNR order that a physician writes based on an agreement the physician makes with the patient or the patient's family. A DNR order is a passive action, with the goal of avoiding prolonging life unnecessarily, not actively ending it. Table 12-2 provides a comparison of active and passive euthanasia.

The following practices are also different from PAS:

- Terminal sedation that refers to sedating terminally ill persons to the point of unconsciousness and allowing them to die. If the person has made the decision to refuse further treatment, the law and medical profession respect this.
- The practice of administering pain medication that may hasten death and relieve suffering for a terminally ill person has been held justifiable by courts (as long as the intent is to relieve suffering).
- In their article "Assisted Suicide," Daly and colleagues (1997) state, "The American Nurses Association (ANA) as well as the American Medical Association (AMA) and the National Hospice Association have issued position statements expressly declaring opposition to nurse or physician participation in assisted suicide."

Oregon Death With Dignity Act

The Oregon Death With Dignity Act allows terminally ill Oregonians to end their lives through the voluntary self-administration of lethal medications that are expressly prescribed by a physician for that purpose. Death With Dignity Act information is available at http://www.Oregon.gov/DHS/ph/pas/faqs.shml. The Death With Dignity Act legalizes physician-assisted suicide but specifically prohibits euthanasia. Only six places in the world openly and legally authorize active assistance in dying patients:

- Oregon (since 1997, physician-assisted suicide only)
- Washington State (since 2009)
- Montana (since 2009)
- Switzerland (1941, physician- and non-physician-assisted suicide only)
- Belgium (2002, permits "euthanasia" but does not define the method)
- Netherlands (voluntary euthanasia and physician-assisted suicide since April 2002, but permitted by the courts since 1984)

According to McNeil's (2003) article "First Study on Patients Who Fast to End Their Lives," doctors note that one option is always legal: A sane, alert person can simply refuse to eat or drink. It is an option rarely taken, but now the first survey of nurses whose patients took the option to fast to end their lives has contradicted the popular assumption that such a death is painful and gruesome. Almost all of the 102 nurses surveyed said their patients who refused water and food had died "good deaths," with little pain or suffering, generally within 2 weeks. McNeil was hesitant to publish the article because of the number of vulnerable patients, many of whom suffered with depression. The LPN/LVN should not inform patients about this study and its results.

Try This

Terminally Ill Patients

With the permission of the instructor, divide into three groups. Choose a viewpoint about the terminally ill from the following descriptions. Be prepared to present reasons for the viewpoint. Choose a spokesperson to summarize the group's views.

- Group 1: Terminally ill patients have the right to choose death by physician-assisted suicide.
- Group 2: Terminally ill patients must wait to die of natural causes.
- Group 3: The nurse's personal ethics conflicts with the decision of groups 1 and 2. Discuss the nurse's rights, roles, and responsibilities to the patient.

Refer to the critical-thinking steps in Chapter 8 to assist you in making your decision.

ORGAN DONATION

Organ donations are voluntary. At this time organs cannot be bought or sold. Although many patients and families give permission for organ donation after death, the demand for organs far exceeds the supply. You may have been asked to agree to personal organ donation when you got your driver's license. Many states participate in this effort. To increase the number of donors, it has been suggested that money be allocated to cover the donor's funeral expenses.

Body tissues that can be donated include skin, corneas, bone, heart valves, and blood. One example of a successful body tissue transplant was the transplantation of umbilical cord blood for a rare genetic bone disease at the University of Minnesota in Duluth in 1995. Approximately one cup of blood, taken from a newborn's discarded umbilical cord and placenta, was donated. Donated body organs include the heart, liver, kidneys, lungs, and pancreas. Organ donation has raised both ethical and legal questions in some instances—for example, having a baby so that select organs or body tissues can be used to save a sibling.

END-OF-LIFE CARE

Many organizations and projects are devoted to establishing end-of-life (EOL) principles. Numerous medical specialties, including the American Medical Association and TJC, have adopted or support core principles for end-of-life care. They use the term "palliative care" to identify the wide range of clinical services available for patients whose disease is not responsive to curative treatment.

An end-of-life movement article by Cox and Parkman (2002) notes that the end-of-life movement "is not about relearning death and dying, it is about being proactive by increasing conversations and actions toward the preparation for better end-of-life journeys." A list of the principles for care of end-of-life patients is available at www.milbank.org/endoflife/index.html.

In 2001, Partnership for Caring: America's Voices for the Dying replaced the 62-year-old organization Choices in Dying. The best-known achievement of Choices in Dying was the development of advance directives, introducing the living will, in 1967. Partnership for Caring describes itself as "a national nonprofit organization devoted to raising consumer expectations for excellent end-of-life care and increasing demand for such care. It is the only end-of-life organization that partners individuals and organizations—consumers and professionals." Last Acts is a national coalition and campaign to improve the quality of life. Former first lady Rosalynn Carter is honorary chair. Information and articles on palliative, end-of-life-care, advance directives, and links to other resources are available at http://www.lastacts.org.

GOOD SAMARITAN ACT

The Good Samaritan Act stipulates that a person who renders emergency care in good faith at the scene of an accident is immune from civil liability for his or her action while providing the care. All 50 states and the District of Columbia have enacted Good Samaritan laws (Brown, 1999). The state statutes are of special concern to nurses and physicians who provide emergency care outside of the agency that employs them. The statutes vary, so check with your state's board of nursing or agency risk manager for information about your state's Good Samaritan laws. For example, in some states a nurse has a choice of whether to give aid to someone during an emergency outside of a health care setting. A few states obligate health care professionals to assist at a scene of an accident requiring medical help. If, for example, you provide pressure to stop severe bleeding and the patient develops complications, you will not be held responsible as long as you acted without gross negligence. The laws also permit the nurse to give aid to a minor at a sports event or accident scene before getting authorized consent from the parents. The LPN must have permission to treat the person, and verbal permission must be obtained from the victim. The person has the right to refuse. Once first aid is initiated, the nurse is obligated to continue until the victim can be turned over to someone with comparable or better training (Christensen and Kockrow, 2011).

 Try This

Good Samaritan Act

Explain the protection that your state's Good Samaritan Act provides for the LPN/LVN.

Get Ready for the NCLEX-PN® Examination

Key Points

- The state's Nurse Practice Act is the most definitive legal statute or legislative act regulating nursing practice. It governs what you can and cannot do as a nurse.
- Student nurses are held to the standard of an LPN/LVN.
- Basic terminology in the Nurse Practice Act is standard in many states.
- Eight general categories of disciplinary action by the board of nursing include fraud and deceit, criminal activity, negligence, incompetence, violation of the Nurse Practice Act or rules, disciplinary action by another board, unethical conduct, and alcohol and/or other drug use.
- Disciplinary action is based on rules of law. If guilty, the board may issue a public or private reprimand, such as probation, nonrenewal of license, suspension of license, revocation of license, or instruction to enter into a voluntary diversion rehabilitation program if the issue is alcohol and/or other drugs.
- After successful completion of the NCLEX-PN® examination, the LPN/LVN may practice in the state of licensure. Some other states accept licensure through interstate endorsement, a multistate licensure compact, or a border recognition agreement.
- The nursing standard of care is what an ordinary, prudent nurse with similar education and experience would do in a similar situation.
- Ethics deals with rules of conduct; law provides regulations that control the practice of nursing.
- Common law is judge-made law that is useful in settling disputes.
- The legislative branch of the state and federal government develops statutory law: The Nurse Practice Act is a statutory law.

- Civil action is related to individual rights; criminal action involves persons and society as a whole.
- Tort law has to do with a wrong or injury to someone that violates his or her rights.
- Intentional torts involve intended harm by the nurse, such as assault and battery; false imprisonment and use of restraints; defamation; and physical and emotional abuse.
- Unintentional torts mean no harm was intended by the nurse (e.g., professional negligence [malpractice]).
- Elements necessary for negligence are duty, breach of duty, damages, and proximate cause.
- Personal liability holds us responsible for our behavior, including negligent behavior.
- Depositions are used to gather information under oath.
- When giving testimony, take your time; say "yes" or "no" when possible, *without adding details*; stick to the facts; and correct mistakes and misconceptions.
- Documentation is a legal expectation in nursing regardless of the method used. If it was not charted, it was not done or it did not happen.
- Medication errors are among the most common errors related to nursing liability.
- Patient competency has both a legal and a clinical definition.
- Patient's right to consent is general, informed, or authorized, depending on the situation.
- Patient rights include *The Patient Care Partnership: Understanding Expectations, Rights, and Responsibilities*; the HIPAA Privacy Rule; and the Patient Self-Determination Act.
- The Patient Self-Determination Act includes advance directives (living will and durable power of medical attorney), written and signed by a patient to state his or her wishes for end-of-life care.
- DNR orders written by a physician are legal orders to not resuscitate a patient and are made possible because of the Patient Self-Determination Act.
- Nurses may not remove a life-support system until a patient is declared dead by the physician.
- Physician-assisted suicide involves a patient voluntarily ending his or her life by self-administering lethal medication prescribed by a physician, especially for that purpose. In the United States this is legal in Oregon, Washington State, and Montana.
- Active euthanasia entails physicians directly administering a lethal medication to end a patient's life. This is not legal in the United States or Canada.
- The ANA and AMA oppose nurse or physician participation in assisted suicide.
- Organ donation has cultural, religious, legal, and ethical constraints. In the United States, you can note on your driver's license if you wish to donate your organs.
- Good Samaritan Acts hold that a person who gives emergency care in good faith at the scene of an accident is immune from being sued. Some states have laws that make it mandatory to assist at the scene of an accident. A victim has the right to refuse aid.
- Incident reports should be legible, factual, specific, objective, and not worded to place blame.

Review Questions for the NCLEX-PN® Examination

1. Which of the following is your legal guideline for all you can do as an LPN/LVN?
   1. NFLPN and NAPNES
   2. State board of nursing
   3. Employee handbook
   4. School of nursing

2. Which situation most clearly illustrates negligence?
   1. The nurse became angry when the patient would not stop screaming and slapped the patient's face.
   2. The nurse inserted the urinary catheter even though the patient said she just voided a large amount.
   3. The nurse decided to restrain an elderly female patient to prevent her from falling out of bed.
   4. The nurse forgot to lower the patient's bed after completing colostomy care, and the patient fell when he tried to get out of bed.

3. How do you best respond to a teenage neighbor who is thinking about becoming an LPN/LVN "because it only takes a year and isn't hard like real nursing"?
   1. "Surprise! Surprise! An LPN (or LVN) is a different level of nursing. You will have to learn a great deal of medical information and nursing care skills in a short period of time. Even as a student you will be held to the legal standard of a licensed nurse."
   2. "You win the jackpot! Practical/vocational nursing is quicker and easier than becoming a registered nurse. Instructor expectations are not very high, and they are quick to forgive mistakes. The national examination at the end is a joke—so easy."
   3. "It is, and it isn't! The trick at the end is to locate the state that has the fewest restrictions for what you can do. I've heard that some LPNs work as RNs, and the doctors don't know the difference! They start IVs and stuff right out of school."
   4. "What an idea! They have already scared us with what the state board of nursing will do if we don't toe the line. Instructors make us learn a lot of extra stuff just in case the RN or doctor isn't available to answer patient questions and do their procedures."

4. How will you answer the lawyer's questions when asked to give testimony during a legal action?

1. Offer to tell what really happened when the wrong medication was given.
2. Avoid referring to any documents to show how well you recall the incident.
3. Fill in silences with information about the physician who ordered the medication.
4. Be specific, answering "yes" or "no" whenever possible, without adding details.

Alternate Format Item

1. Which of the following are legal patients' rights? *(Select all that apply.)*

1. The right to revoke a signed informed consent verbally on the way to surgery.
2. The right to take their medical records with them when they leave the hospital.
3. The right to designate who will make decisions for them should they become incapable.
4. The right to ask their physician to inject them with lethal drugs that will end life.
5. The right to file a suit for injury that they see as being the result of carelessness.

2. Which of the following are needed to prove negligence? *(Select all that apply.)*

1. Deposition
2. Nurse Practice Act
3. Duty
4. Proximate cause

3. If a nurse faces disciplinary action, what possible consequences could there be?

1. Probation
2. Suspension of license
3. Revocation of license
4. Nonrenewal of license

Critical Thinking Scenarios

Scenario 1

You volunteer to be on a planning task force for a new nursing home. The committee you are assigned to work on is writing policies to meet state nursing home regulations. Each month you report progress at the task force meeting. During one of the meetings, a member who is also a chaplain at a local church offers to be chaplain for the new home. You are surprised by the offer because the nursing home will not be faith based, but you avoid saying anything until you check this further. You have studied hospital HIPAA law, but you are uncertain if the same applies to nursing homes. You are especially concerned about resident privacy. After completing your research on the Internet, you write a sample policy for your committee. What will your policy say?

Scenario 2

Julia, an RN, works nights on the neurology unit in a small private hospital. During the night, George, a patient who had cranial surgery, began to have a great deal of pain. Julia called George's physician and gave her a brief review about George, his surgery, and his recent medications. Julia asked the physician if she could come to the unit to evaluate George's condition. The physician told Julia to give George morphine sulphate. The dose was large, and Julia repeated the order and asked if she really meant the amount she stated. The physician became angry, insisted that Julia immediately give George the dosage instructed and to repeat the dose in an hour, and threatened to lodge a complaint against Julia if she did not follow instructions. Julia gave George the morphine as directed, and George died. Julia was charged with negligence, and at the trial, the physician testified that Julia had never called. Julia was given a prison sentence of 20 years for murder. What could Julia have done to protect both George and herself?

Straightforward Communication: Instructors, Coworkers, and Patients

Objectives

On completing this chapter, you will be able to do the following:

1. Explain the sender-receiver process in:
   a. One-way communication
   b. Two-way communication
2. Discuss how nonverbal and affective communication can support or cancel the meaning of verbal communication.
3. Provide an example of how you use communication strategies in nursing.
4. Give an example of blocking therapeutic communication.
5. List two common differences in male/female communication that have biologic roots.
6. Give an example of a cultural communication difference in the area in which you live.
7. List two common factors related to role change for a hospitalized patient that can create distress.
8. Identify a communication difference for patients in two separate age groups.
9. Explain how common characteristics apply to straightforward communication with all people.
10. Identify the four steps of SBAR and give an example of how it can be used for nurse–physician communication.
11. Discuss ways to resolve conflict between you and another staff member.

Key Terms

active listening (ĂK-tĭv, p. 151)
affective communication (ă-FĔK-tĭv, p. 150)
belittling (bĕ-LĬT-lĭng, p. 153)
chiding (chĭd-ĭng, p. 153)
closed-ended questions (KLOZD-ĔN-dĕd, p. 152)
commitment (kŏ-MĬT-mĕnt, p. 156)
communication blocks (kŏm-U-nĭ-kā-shŭn blŏks, p. 153)
empathy (ĔM-pă-thē, p. 155)
false reassurance (RĒ-ă-shŭr-ĕns, p. 153)
feedback (FĒD-băk, p. 150)
focused questions (FO-kŭsd, p. 152)
giving advice (GĬV-ĭng ăd-VĪS, p. 153)
honesty (ŎN-ĕs-tē, p. 155)
humor (HU-mŏr, p. 155)
knowledge (NŎL-ĕj, p. 156)
message (MĔS-ĕj, p. 150)
nonverbal communication (nŏn-VĔR-băl, p. 150)

one-way communication (wŏn-wăy, p. 150)
open-ended questions (O-pĕn ĕn-dĕd, p. 152)
pat answers (păt ĂN-sĕrs, p. 153)
patience (PĀ-shĕnts, p. 155)
probing (PRO-bĭng, p. 153)
purpose (PĔR-pŭs, p. 151)
receiver (rĕ-SĒ-vĕr, p. 150)
respect (rē-SPĔKT, p. 155)
SBAR (156)
self-esteem (SĔLF-ă-STĒM, p. 156)
sender (SĔN-dĕr, p. 150)
sensitivity (SĔN-sĭ-TĬV-ĭ-tē, p. 155)
therapeutic communication (THĔR-ă-pū-tĭk, p. 151)
trust (trŭst, p. 155)
two-way communication (TOO-wăy, p. 150)
verbal communication (VĔR-băl, p. 150)

Keep in Mind

Purposeful communication is an integral part of your personal and professional world. Take time to learn, and know that language is never innocent.

COMMUNICATION PROCESS

Sara walked into the patient's room without knocking on the door. "I'm going to measure your blood pressure. Give me your arm," she said. The patient gave her a quizzical look, but he put out his arm. This was Sara's first contact with a patient. When she finally got the cuff on, her face was flushed, and her own heart was beating so hard that she could not hear the patient's heartbeat.

Try This

Communicating with Your Patient

1. What kind of communication did Sara engage in with the patient?
2. Who was Sara's focus?
3. What steps did Sara skip that resulted in showing disrespect for the patient?

Sara engaged in one-way communication, in which the sender (Sara) controlled the situation by telling the receiver (patient) what she was going to do (the message). Sara offered no opportunity for feedback (response) from the patient. Feedback would have provided the patient an opportunity to question, agree, or refuse the procedure. Sara was so focused on herself that she omitted common courtesies: a knock on the door, addressing the patient by name, and introducing herself, her position, and reason for being there. The patient's unspoken response may have increased Sara's discomfort.

ONE-WAY VERSUS TWO-WAY COMMUNICATION

One-way communication is used to give a command, as in military service, or information with no expectation of feedback. Sometimes one-way communication must be changed to two-way communication, in which there is feedback or discussion. During an emergency a doctor may give an order. Take a few seconds to change the order to two-way communication by repeating the order to the doctor so it is verified for accuracy. Two-way communication is the usual form of conversation. Each person contributes equally, and feedback is both expected and respected.

FACTORS THAT AFFECT COMMUNICATION

Some common factors that can influence communication include the following:

1. Personal characteristics of both the sender and receiver
2. Cultural characteristics
3. Situational influences
4. Context in which the message is sent and received

Personal characteristics can include such things as age, gender, income, and marital status. Life experiences, attitude, and personal opinions are other personal characteristics. *Cultural characteristics* can involve space and distance, language and dialect, use and meaning of touch, bad or good manners, meaning of gestures, and time of day. *Situational influences* can include the physical and emotional state of the patient and nurse, the room temperature, interruptions, background noises, and body odor. *Context* can include the

appropriateness or inappropriateness of the communication. "What can I do to make you more comfortable?" is an appropriate question directed to a dying patient. Discussion by the family about who gets what after the patient dies, within earshot of the patient, is inappropriate communication.

TYPES OF COMMUNICATION

The three types of communication are verbal (spoken or written word), nonverbal (body language), and affective (feeling tone). They may or may not all occur at the same time. When they do occur together, all three must mirror one another (be congruent) for the communication to be honest (Figure 13-1).

VERBAL COMMUNICATION

The spoken word is powerful. A patient may accept what you say as completely as though the team leader or doctor had spoken. Know in advance what you can or cannot discuss with a patient. Sometimes your response will be "I do not know, but I will find someone who does."

Speak as clearly as possible, using proper grammar. Slang is usually not appropriate and may have a different meaning. Depending on age and culture, the patient may not understand slang. Using out-of-date slang also can make you come across as unprofessional or silly.

Medical jargon is rarely helpful. If you truly understand the medical terms, you can translate the words into everyday language. The use of colloquial (common) expressions will be appropriate with some patients. For example, the word "urinate" may be understood by some as pass water, tinkle, or pee-pee. Use the word that the patient understands. Remember that the patient needs a professional he or she can look up to and one who will respect his or her individual differences; the patient does not need the nurse to be a buddy.

Maintain professional boundaries. Interestingly, a patient will respect you and is more likely to follow the directions you are giving than if you are trying to be "familiar" with him or her. When a nurse at a nursing home was asked why she continued to wear her white uniform and cap instead of wearing scrub-type

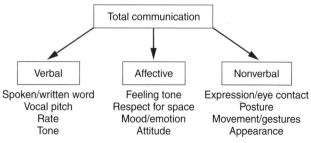

FIGURE 13-1 Communication.

clothes like the rest of the staff, she responded, "The residents take the medications I give them and will follow directions I offer them. They also ask for me by name if they are worried about something or do not understand what is happening to them. They know that they can trust me. Sometimes residents want to know who all these other people are who come into their room! I know that wearing my uniform plays a big part of the rapport I have with the residents."

Some illnesses also affect a patient's interpretation of verbalization. Patients diagnosed with schizophrenia interpret words concretely (literally). They experience difficulty with abstract (inferred) meanings. For example, after using a stationary bicycle, a patient was asked by the nurse, "How do you feel now?" He grabbed his buttocks and responded, "My butt is numb; that's how." The nurse had been trying to determine change in his stress level. Instead, his response was based on literal interpretation of the question.

NONVERBAL COMMUNICATION

Commonly known as body language, nonverbal communication either supports or cancels out verbal communication. Expressions, posture, movements, and gestures, whether they are your own or the patient's, give important clues to the truth of the verbalization. Careful observation of body language may clue you in to patient discomfort, even though pain has been denied verbally. Gathering additional data will help clarify the real issue creating the discomfort.

Verbal communication works both ways. Patients tend to observe you closely, as well, looking for clues regarding the seriousness of their illness. For example, your distressed look may be interpreted as disapproval or serious concern about their health. How are they to know that you brought your personal life worries to work?

Physical appearance is a part of nonverbal communication. The patient's appearance on admission provides signs of personal care plus important clues about the illness. Patients also quickly evaluate you and, based on what you project and even before you speak, will draw conclusions about your competence as a nurse. Arnold and Boggs (2003) explain, "Clothing communicates a nonverbal message about competence and professionalism to a patient, which can influence the nurse-patient relationship." This is a major reason why most nursing schools continue to have a dress code. It is also the reason why your instructors model appropriate dress and behavior for their students.

 Try This

Appropriate Dress Code and Behavior

What kind of statement are you making by the way you dress and behave at the patient's bedside?

AFFECTIVE COMMUNICATION

"Affect" refers to mood or emotion. The feeling tone that you pick up on as you approach a person or step into a room is real. For every thought you have, there is a physiologic response in your body. The same is true for the patient and others you encounter. We are made up of energy, so we emit energy. The tendency may be to ignore this level of communication because we cannot see, hear, or read it. Affective communication is as significant as verbal and nonverbal communication. Truly honest communication integrates verbal, nonverbal, and affective communications so they all express the same message.

 Critical Thinking

Affective Communication

1. Give an example of a time that you stepped into a room or approached a person and, before anyone spoke a word, experienced a feeling of excitement, happiness, sadness, anger, or some other emotion. What was the outcome?
2. Think of a time when you were angry and tried to hide the feeling. Did anyone pick up on your feeling tone and ask you if you were angry? How did you deal with the question?
3. Give examples of how you try to be congruent (together) verbally, nonverbally, and affectively in your communication.

COMMUNICATION STRATEGIES

Please do not interpret the term *strategies* (hints) to mean predetermined script, as in telemarketing. In real life this would be awkward, and even boring. You might even lose track of where you are in your conversation because of the focus on strategies. Work to understand the meaning of active listening, active listening behaviors, and types of questions discussed.

ACTIVE LISTENING

Active listening is probably the most important part of any therapeutic (health-related) communication. Key factors in active listening include purpose, disciplined attention, and focus. Purpose refers to the health-related reason for gathering data or giving information. *Disciplined attention* means that you do not assume accuracy of information without checking it out. Clarify what you think you understand the patient to say and ask further questions as needed. This applies both to gathering data and giving health-related information. *Focus* means that all your senses are alert to clues that the patient may be communicating. A common mistake in listening is to listen to the words but not really hear the words (i.e., comprehend [understand] the meaning).

ACTIVE LISTENING BEHAVIORS

The most commonly used active listening behaviors include restating, clarifying, reflecting, paraphrasing, minimal encouraging, remaining silent, summarizing, and validating.

- **Restating** refers to repeating in a slightly different way what the patient has said—for example:

  Patient: "My chest hurts. I can't sleep at night."

  Nurse: "You've been unable to sleep at night because of chest pain."

- **Clarifying** is asking a closed-ended question in response to a patient's statement to be sure you understand—for example:

  Patient: "My chest hurts."

  Nurse: "Exactly where does your chest hurt?"

- **Reflecting** is putting into words the information you are receiving from the patient at an affective communication level—for example:

  Patient: "I'm sick of seeing doctors and not getting answers."

  Nurse: "You are upset with the lack of answers to your health problems."

- **Paraphrasing** refers to expressing in your own words what you think the patient means—for example:

  Patient: "I don't think I'm being told the truth about my condition."

  Nurse: "You think you may be more ill than what the doctor is telling you."

- **Minimal encouraging** involves using sounds, words, or short phrases to encourage the patient to continue—for example:

  Patient: "It just happened so fast. . . ."

  Nurse: "Yes . . . go on . . . and then what . . . hmmm . . . uh huh. . . ."

- **Remaining silent** involves using pauses effectively. The normal tendency is to fill silence with chatter or your speculation. This may cause the patient to "turn off" or change the story. Maintaining disciplined attention and focus during silence lets patients tell the story in their own way. Avoid making interruptions and doing busywork while the patient is speaking.

- **Summarizing** means briefly stating the main data you have gathered—for example:

  Nurse: "This is what I heard you say. Is that correct?"

- **Validating** provides the patient with an opportunity to correct information, if necessary, at the time of summary—for example:

  Patient: "That is correct" or "No, you got this part wrong. . . ." (This allows the patient to correct the information.)

TYPES OF QUESTIONS

The three types of questions that are commonly used in therapeutic communication are open-ended, closed-ended, and focused questions. **Open-ended questions** permit the patient to respond in a way that is most meaningful to him or her. The questions often begin with what, where, when, how, or why. For example, the nurse might ask, "What happened to your leg?" **Closed-ended questions** require a specific answer. For example, the nurse might ask, "When did you first notice the pain?" **Focused questions** provide even more definitive information. For example, the nurse might ask, "On a scale of 1 to 10, with 10 as the worst possible pain, how do you rate your pain right now?"

NURSE–PATIENT COMMUNICATION EVALUATION

Communication is far more complex than just talking. Some of the many contributing characteristics are listed in this section, with a brief description in the following learning exercise. Evaluate the characteristics of your communication that are working for you and those you need to work on.

◎ Try This

Self-Evaluation of Personal Characteristics

Characteristic	Desirable	Self-Evaluation
Eye contact	Usually 3-5 seconds. Cultural variations.	_____
Respect for personal space	Approximately 1.5 feet, except for personal care. Cultural variations.	_____
Appropriate touch	Gentle, but firm. Cultural variations.	_____
Attitude	Nonjudgmental. Practices unconditional love.	_____
Voice/tone	Moderate or according to growth and development needs. Example: Newborns	_____
Rate	Paced according to patient's ability to comprehend.	_____
Appearance	Models positive nursing image. Looks healthy.	_____
Posture	Open, without folded arms or hands on hips. Stands or sits upright.	_____
Gestures	Moderate to enhance conversation.	_____
Language	Speaks effectively and at patient's level of understanding. Correct grammar.	_____
Expression	Congruent with topic. Nonjudgmental.	_____

❓ Critical Thinking

A Plan for Change

List the personal characteristics that are not working for you. Develop a plan for change and measuring improvement, using the phases of the nursing process.

BLOCKS TO COMMUNICATION

It is sometimes easy to slip into communication styles that block communication. Perhaps the patient reminds you of someone you know, or you have had personal dealings with the patient in the past. Sometimes you do not like the patient or are just plain tired. Whatever the reason, it is worth thinking about the possibility in advance. As a nurse you want to continue to give every patient the best care possible, regardless of your personal response. Common communication blocks involve false reassuring, probing, chiding, belittling, giving advice, and providing pat answers.

AVOIDING BLOCKS

- "Why" questions put the patient on the defensive.
- False reassurance involves making statements to the patient such as "Everything will be okay," "You'll be just fine," "Don't worry about anything," "We'll make sure you get well," "This experience will make you stronger," or "You'll see the good in this someday." There is no way you can guarantee what you just told the patient.
- Probing means pushing for information beyond what is medically necessary to know. Curiosity takes over, and the patient's privacy is no longer respected. Ask yourself about the value of the information and how you will use the information once you have it. Think twice before continuing with statements such as "Let's get to the bottom of this once and for all."
- Chiding (scolding) for behavior such as smoking is of limited value to the patient with severe emphysema or lung cancer (or perhaps the patient never smoked). Your information is hardly an "alert." You can be sure that she or he has heard the message over and over. Without supporting the behavior you can continue to be therapeutic to the patient.
- Belittling involves mimicking or making fun of the patient in some way. It may include downplaying the importance of the symptoms—for example, "You could be having heart surgery! This is just wart removal." As a physician pointed out, "If you have a tonsillectomy, it's minor surgery; if I have a tonsillectomy, it's major surgery." It is all a matter of perspective.
- Giving advice when you know what someone else should do is very tempting. Unsolicited advice is rarely beneficial and closes the door to having the patient solve the problem herself. A more beneficial response, even when the patient asks what you would (or he or she should) do, is "What ideas do *you* have? I'm sure you've thought of ways you might solve this problem." Listen carefully, summarize what the patient has said, and then ask, "Which one of your ideas do you want to begin with?" After

the patient's response, you could say, "When do you think you'll start?"

- Pat answers such as "Everyone feels this way" come so easily, but they make patients feel dismissed and misunderstood. Patients do not really care if everyone else feels this way. As far as they are concerned, these feelings are theirs, they are different from everybody else's, and they need a comforting touch or reassuring words. If you can, offer something you know you can deliver, such as "I'll be with you the entire time you are having your bone marrow drawn" or "I'll be in the room when you return."

MALE/FEMALE DIFFERENCES

Being equal does not mean being the same. Men and women communicate differently for biologic reasons. Although there are examples of similarities between the sexes, most males and females follow certain patterns. According to Sieh and Brentin (1997), four areas that relate to nursing communication are conversation patterns, head movements, smiling, and posture.

CONVERSATION

Men tend to approach a conversation with an eye to maintaining status and independence, to report or to get information, and to solve problems. They express their ideas more assertively; women do so with less certainty. Therefore, male opinions are often valued more highly without validation. Women seek to establish intimacy and develop rapport, share feelings, and establish relationships. Men ask fewer questions, but they readily interrupt during conversations without apology. Women use questions to encourage conversation. They wait for a pause to seek clarification and apologize for the interruption. Men apologize for a wrong, whereas women say "I'm sorry" to indicate regret, sympathy, or concern. Men rarely say, "I don't know"; women often phrase ideas as questions, such as "Have you thought of ... ?" Men make decisions, but women look for agreement. Men make demands more often, whereas women express preferences with reasons. Men's sentences are shorter and fewer; women create longer, more complex sentences, linking more ideas together. Men make declarations, whereas women often end a statement with a question, such as "Don't you think so?" (Tannen, 1990).

HEAD MOVEMENTS

Men nod if they are in agreement. Women nod to show they are listening. A man may be surprised to discover that a woman does not agree at all with what he said. Men hold their heads erect while speaking; women frequently assume a lower status position by tilting their head to the side or placing their chin down with eyes gazing upward (Sieh and Brentin, 1997).

SMILING

If a woman is smiling, it may or may not denote happiness. A smile is also used to mask unhappiness and other emotions. Reactions by others to her smiles may leave her feeling unheard. Others may acknowledge her nonverbal communication but be unable to interpret that she is feeling sad, angry, or afraid. Sometimes men will mask their emotion with a smile. Usually men tend not to show an outward reaction when criticized, making them seem strong and in control.

POSTURE

A rounded posture with the chest in and chin down gives an appearance of being threatened. Standing tall, with shoulders back and head held high, speaks of confidence and control. Looking at differences in the way men and women communicate has important implications in working with patients, staff, and instructors. Smiling and nodding by a woman does not have to mean she understands the instructions. A lack of questions from a male patient may not mean he knows what the surgery entails. Gather all three types of communication data. Ask the patient to tell you what he or she understands, then summarize and validate. *Use the skills you are learning.*

CULTURAL DIFFERENCES

Members of diverse cultures within our dominant culture embrace and value their beliefs and practices. You need to be respectful of these beliefs and practices and respond therapeutically. Know about cultural differences in communication. Individual patient differences need to be identified. Be sure to read Chapter 16 for a more complete understanding of cultural diversity. Mark the chapter and use it as a reference for the Learning Exercise.

◎ Try This

Cultural Differences

List two cultural differences of someone in the area in which you live.
1. _____
2. _____

Communication patterns change with time, vary with the situation, and differ in public or private settings. It is important to learn as much as possible about the cultures frequently served where you work. Remember also that just because you can identify someone's ethnic background, the families may have been in this country for generations, and differences may be nonexistent.

ROLE CHANGES FOR THE PATIENT

What happens to patients who find themselves in a dependent position after having always been in charge of their lives? The concerns they have go beyond the physical realities into areas we consider in the next section.

❓ Critical Thinking

Immediate Concerns upon Hospitalization

Imagine yourself being hospitalized. List four immediate concerns you would probably have.
1. _____
2. _____
3. _____
4. _____

Professional Pointer

"Err on the side of politeness and use Mr., Mrs., or Ms. until you have established respect" (Pagana, 2008).

IT BEGINS WITH "HELLO, MY NAME IS . . . ."

Whatever you communicate verbally, nonverbally, and affectively sets the tone for rapport with the patient. You have some preliminary information (a name), even if the patient is just being admitted. Knock on the door or the door frame; pause briefly to collect data *before* walking in. You begin to pick up nonverbal and affective communication clues. Address the patient as Mr., Mrs., Miss, or Ms., or by a professional title if it applies. Extend your hand (unless culturally improper). Give your name; identify yourself as a student practical/vocational nurse, plus the name of the school and your purpose for being in the room.

It may sound something like this: "Mrs. Hill, my name is Mr. Fry. I am a student practical nurse from the Middle American Technical College. I am here to measure your blood pressure, pulse, and respiration. It is a part of the admission procedure." The patient may request that you address her by her first name, but do not assume this without permission. Some hospitals and other health agencies limit use of the employees' names to first name only. This will dictate how you introduce yourself.

NURSING JARGON

Remember how time-consuming it was to learn all those medical terms? Using the terms may sound impressive to you now and involve a feeling of having arrived, but using unfamiliar terminology can increase patient fears and cause misunderstandings: "What does it mean that I will have an IV started, have a WBC stat, and you'll be doing vitals q2h for now?"

When you really know something, you can explain words and symbols in terms the average layperson can understand. Now *that's* impressive!

FEAR OF THE UNKNOWN

Patients often have numerous unspoken fears about tests, procedures, and possible outcomes. These include, but are not limited to, pain, sleep, needle sticks, thirst, hunger, and being treated respectfully. A pat answer of "Everything will be fine" displays a lack of understanding of the depth of the fears. Patients may not ask questions because they think it might sound silly or that they are bothering the staff. An open-ended question from you, such as "What questions do you have? If I don't know the answer, I'll try to find out for you," can open the way for expression of fears.

PERSONAL FACTORS

A patient's illness rarely affects the patient alone. Thoughts and concerns may extend to family, work, finances, and so on. For example, the mother of a newly hospitalized child was irritable and inattentive when the nurse was explaining the unit rules. Finally the nurse stopped midsentence and said to the mother, "Tell me what is troubling you." The mother looked at her and then blurted out that she had a sick child at home, her husband worked nights and slept days, and she had been up most of the last three nights. "Where should I be? Both kids need me, and my neighbor can only come in for two hours a day. I'm at my wits' end!" The mother could not begin to focus on the unit rules until there were solutions to the problems at home. You may not have a solution, but you can be a catalyst to make needs known to the instructor or team leader. They are aware of additional resources.

ENVIRONMENTAL FACTORS

Health care settings—whether a clinic, hospital, rehabilitation center, or nursing home—are very different from home. There is no true opportunity for privacy. A variety of staff show up at different times throughout a 24-hour period; lights are on day and night; the staff make more noise than they realize; machinery is humming, buzzing, or beeping; staff check out different parts of your body, picking and poking—you get the picture. The patient may have put the light on because of a need to go to the bathroom *now*. By the time someone arrives, it may be too late, much to the patient's embarrassment.

Advance communication and planning does not take as long as it sounds. You may find out that the patient always has a snack of toast and tea at 9 PM, always gets up to go to the bathroom at 11 PM, always has bran cereal and a banana at 6 AM, and so on. Notes of this nature in the patient's care plan assist in the continuity of communication and care.

COMMUNICATING WITH INSTRUCTORS AND STAFF

Communication characteristics involve respect, trust, honesty, empathy, sensitivity, humor, knowledge, patience, commitment, and self-esteem. These characteristics are equally important in communicating with patients, instructors, and staff.

RESPECT

Respect involves both self-respect and respect for others. You communicate self-respect by doing your best each day. When you treat yourself with self-respect, it becomes easy to extend respect to your instructors, staff, and patients. Patients quickly pick up on whether they are being respected during conversation and physical care (e.g., verbal and nonverbal communication, such as eye signals between staff).

TRUST

Trust begins with confidence in your ability to make decisions. You communicate this to instructors and staff by consistently doing the required preliminary preparation for assignments.

HONESTY

Honesty implies that you will not deliberately deceive in order to present yourself in a more favorable light. Arranging a time with the instructor for you to repeat a procedure for more practice is an example of this characteristic in communication.

EMPATHY

Empathy is the ability to understand and appreciate what someone else is feeling without experiencing the emotion itself. When you are sympathetic, as you would be with a family member or dear friend, you actually experience the emotion. Being empathetic permits you to understand how someone is feeling and why he or she feels that way, to maintain control of your emotions, and to think clearly. For example, you might offer to help a staff member who is having a bad day do patient care (a practical intervention), instead of getting pulled into an "Isn't it awful?" conversation.

SENSITIVITY

Tuning in on nonverbal and affective communication helps you to verify verbalization or a lack thereof. Picking up at nonverbal and affective levels permits you to check them out with the staff or instructor: "Is there something else I need to know?"

HUMOR

Healthy humor at the patient's level of appreciation can help "lighten up" a situation. Offensive humor and poking fun at the patient or at other cultures or races is unacceptable. The staff sometimes privately gets involved in "gallows humor," which is laughing at something very serious or medically gross. Look for examples in movies and television programs with medical themes.

KNOWLEDGE

The cornerstone of gathering data and other health-related communication is knowledge. Instructors and staff quickly determine your level of knowledge. Instructors communicate the significance of this characteristic by making assignments early enough for you to research the information. You communicate back to the instructor (and staff) by preparing for patient care.

PATIENCE

In this modern world we are often accustomed to instant results and gratification. It is sometimes difficult to provide the time needed to learn, receive explanations from instructors, or follow staff orders. This extends to our work with patients, in whom illness and growth and development levels dictate the need to slow down or repeat directions. The patient (or you) may be tempted to say "I know" when such is not the case. The characteristic of patience takes time to perfect. You may initially feel like you are moving backward in your communication attempts with patients.

COMMITMENT

Commitment means incorporating all the previous characteristics as a part of your nursing communication. Decide that you are in nursing because you really want to be here. Then do the work that needs to be done. It shows, and it pays off. Take time to appreciate the uniqueness of each patient (see Chapter 16).

SELF-ESTEEM, THOUGHTS, AND STRAIGHTFORWARD COMMUNICATION

Self-esteem is earned, not learned. No one can give it to you or take it away! It is that special sense that it is okay to receive credit for something you did well. Self-esteem also gives you permission to recognize that you have something very special to offer in nursing communication—such as being able to communicate effectively with patients and other health workers.

What kinds of thoughts do you have?

- Are they positive or negative when you think about yourself?
- The two basic types of thought are random and active. Random thoughts just show up, but you initiate active thoughts. Random thoughts usually pass through, unless you pick a thought and change it into an active thought.
- What do your active thoughts say about you and the person you are? Do they support your sense of self, or do the thoughts tear you down?
- If your thoughts are not serving you, change them. If you have made a mistake, learn from it and let it go. Do not continue to punish yourself.

- Every day, look for what you have done well and give yourself a cheer for a job well done!
- Thoughts also set the feeling tone for how you communicate with patients and other staff. How you feel about something creates actions that bring about results.
- Actions are the bridge from the inner world to your outer world. Start by changing your inner world (Fuimano, 2004).

Practice makes your conversation meaningful. Make peace with silence. If you find yourself talking just to fill in the silence, *stop!* Learn to say what you mean. Be direct in your conversation, remembering that language is never innocent. When you give patients information or directions, avoid medical jargon. Being long-winded just means that you do not know how to express yourself clearly. Ask the patient what they think you said as a way to avoid misunderstanding. If you are on the receiving end of a lengthy conversation, remember that you can take control. Check out what it is the person really wants you to know and set a time limit if needed: "I have to go in __ minutes."

Remembering the affective component of conversation helps you to be aware of your and the other person's feelings. It is not unusual if after a conversation the other person's feelings mirror what you were experiencing. Fuimano (2004) said the following:

> If you take care of the words you chose, if you take the time to be purposeful and intentional, if you practice, knowing that it takes time to become an effective communicator—you'll become more effective in every area of your life: You'll experience more joy and satisfaction, and you'll achieve the results you want.

SITUATION, BACKGROUND, ASSESSMENT, RECOMMENDATION

Nurses are taught to be objective and detailed when providing information. Physicians generally are brief and to the point: They are more interested in the "bottom line." The situation, background, assessment, and recommendation called SBAR, was first developed in the military and has been adopted by some hospitals to facilitate clear communication. For example, if you are calling a physician because of concern about a patient, SBAR can be useful following these guidelines:

- **S** – Situation (about 10 seconds). Identify the following:
  1. The situation
  2. Who you are
  3. Your unit
  4. Patient name and room number
  5. What the problem is (briefly), when it started, and how severe it is

- **B** – Background
  1. Patient's admitting diagnosis
  2. Date of admission
  3. Information related to current status, such as:
     a. Recent mental status
     b. Vital signs
     c. Oximetry
     d. Oxygen device and flow rate
     e. Current medication
     f. Allergies
     g. IV fluids, lab results
     h. Code status
- **A** – Assessment (data gathered) includes the following:
  1. What you think is going on
  2. If appropriate, if, based on the signs and symptoms, you believe the problem is life threatening
- **R** – Recommendation involves what you need from the physician. Terms like "could be" and "might be" are usually effective—for example:
  1. Do you want the physician to come and see the patient?
  2. Do you want the physician to give an order for a medication?
  3. Do you want to transfer the patient to a higher level of care?

SBAR FOR THE SHIFT REPORT

SBAR is also a useful tool for the shift report, reporting off when you leave the clinical unit, or transferring a patient to another unit. The process will have some differences, such as the following:

Situation: Include the admission date, chief complaint, and diagnosis.

Background:
1. Patient's medical history
2. Allergy status
3. Code status
4. If patient is in isolation
5. Pain management strategies and response to interventions
6. Imaging studies
7. Lab results or glucometry readings
8. Location of peripheral or central venous line access devices

Assessment (data gathered): Provide relevant information in a systematic manner using a systems approach.
1. Vital signs and range of vital signs since admission
2. Pain assessment and patient's pain goal
3. If patient has diabetes, how frequently monitored and readings since admission
4. Diagnostic studies and results
5. If patient needs turning, how often and whether patient can turn self

6. Fall risk if it applies and any other precautions specific to this patient

Recommendations:
1. The patient's goals of care
2. What needs to be done on the next shift
3. Any procedures that must be done
4. Patient's education and discharge needs

Both the Joint Commission and the Institute for Healthcare Improvement support the use of SBAR in health care facilities.

 Try This

Using the SBAR Method

Write an example of how you will have used the SBAR method with a patient you are assigned to when you are on clinical. Identify differences compared to the way you made reports in the past.

LIFE SPAN COMMUNICATION

Growth and development levels, male/female differences, and medical conditions all affect communication with patients. Each age group—whether infant, preschool, school age, teenage, adult, or elderly—has somewhat different communication needs.

INFANT

Infants' communication includes crying, cooing, and body language. They act out their feelings with total body language. As their recognition of words grows, certain words act to soothe or trigger a reaction. Up to that time, infants are most influenced by the sound of voices. As one father pointed out, "I used to put my baby to sleep each night by rocking her and reading *USA Today* aloud in a soothing voice." Newborns respond favorably to a high-pitched voice, but that changes by the end of the first month. After that, calm, low tones are more soothing.

Parents (caretakers) are the best source for learning the meaning of different cries. They learn quickly to differentiate among wet, hungry, and uncomfortable. Rely on them for specific information on communication style.

PRESCHOOL

We are including toddlers in this category as early preschoolers. They are usually known for magnificent tantrums, and it is no wonder: They have learned some words, but when frustrated, they may not be able to put them together effectively. Thus, the body acts out what the words cannot tell. Laughing at or trying to reason with the preschooler is counterproductive.

When a child has a tantrum, he or she should be removed from the immediate situation and audience. Once preschoolers are more composed, they can communicate by pointing or by showing on their bodies or in a picture what they are upset about. During procedures, explain briefly and simply what is going to happen. Tell them what they can do to help. For example, preschoolers will often assist and cooperate with receiving injections if they are patiently coached on exactly what to do (e.g., position, what to do with their feet and hands, how long they need to stay still, what to expect during the injection).

SCHOOL AGE

The vocabulary of school-age children has increased considerably. They are ready to be a part of most (but not all) discussions with their parents. Drawings or pictures can be used to explain an illness or procedure. Ask for feedback to avoid misconceptions: "Tell me in your own words what...." The child may not be privy to all information. In that case, go with the parent to a separate area so the child will not overhear the conversation or parts of it. Whispering and misinterpretation can evoke new problems. Remember that younger children think well in the afternoon.

TEENAGE

Teenagers are the easiest or the most difficult to communicate with, depending on your perspective. When ill, they need to believe that someone knows more than they do and that someone is in charge. Deal with them with the same courtesy that you extend to adults. Have similar expectations of them. Encourage expression of feelings, fears, and concerns. Their sense that nothing will happen to them has been shaken. Answer questions within your role. Seek out answers as appropriate. Avoid hiding behind nursing jargon. Using teen slang generally does not work out. Without real knowledge of the meaning, you may end up looking foolish instead of "cool."

ADULT

Many of the issues discussed in this chapter apply to adult communication. Collecting data at all three levels of communication is essential. Remember to limit your questions to areas that are medically related. Pushing and probing based on curiosity may open a Pandora's box (i.e., painful issues that have been suppressed). It does not work to probe and then leave the patient to pick up the pieces of what he revealed to you under pressure.

Patients with diminishing memory seem to have a relatively preserved reading ability. Visual information seems to be more permanent. Verbal information is so transient that the person may not have time to process it completely before it is gone (Banotai, 2007). The health care worker or family member can try writing the information in a size that is easy for the patient to read. Written information seems to be more neutral and does not evoke the emotional reaction that words would have.

ELDERLY

How do you picture elderly people in your mind? Unresolved parental issues, for example, can get in the way of quality care. If you can see aging as just another part of the life cycle, you may be able to work effectively with elderly patients. Gurian (1997) states, "Boys and men take in less sensory or proximal data than girls and women. They smell less, taste less, get less soothing and input from tactile information, hear less, and see less." Most elderly people think more clearly in the morning.

When hearing begins to diminish, it is easier for both men and women to hear lower-frequency sounds. As with younger men, check elderly men to determine which ear has better hearing. Remember that the left eye, even without loss of vision, has more acuity for a man. It works best for explanations and table games to be focused on the left side.

Women see and hear equally well with both eyes and ears. Women can also differentiate sounds from background noises easier. There is some evidence that both men and women recall emotional words better when spoken into their left ear. The elderly man may not hear you if you call when the TV is on. The male brain shuts on and off according to load. Part of it must remain active to continue vital functions. Men may continue to have reading problems, so it is a good idea to read directions aloud to older male patients. You will continue to find that many female patients are orderly and satisfied with a smaller amount of space. The male patient is generally the opposite, and you may have to seek additional space for games and puzzles in the dayroom.

Preparing for discharge begins after admission. The nurse takes advantage of teachable moments to interject information, demonstrate techniques, and have the patient repeat the demonstrations. This includes the patient and any family members or friends who are planning to assist posthospitalization. Listen carefully when the patient describes what is waiting at home. Will adaptive equipment be necessary? Will other health providers have to be involved in making the transition between this facility and home? The best part of being a student in this situation is that the instructor and RN assigned to the patient are available to assist you.

CONFLICT RESOLUTION

In the health setting, conflict can be related to diversity, English as a second language, and differences in gender, generation, and personality. Doctors and nurses often provide information in different formats. According to Federwische (2007), "Nurses are taught to communicate through narrative, through a story, to give a lot of background. Physicians are trained to communicate in bullet points. So they have two totally different styles." Differences can be magnified in high-stress situations. It is thought that only about 2% to 3% of physicians and nurses are truly disruptive, but that still creates problems for the rest of the staff. Problems can translate into medication errors, patient safety, and even patient mortality. Some health facilities have set up major programs to teach their staff how to communicate with one another. Keep the following basic steps in mind, and try to focus on a mutually beneficial solution based on shared interests.

1. Accept conflict as a natural part of life. Different points of view, needs, and beliefs are often involved.
2. Temper your own attitude and behaviors. Be aware of your initial reaction, and take a deep breath. (Your automatic defense system wants to dig right in and fight.)
3. Take time to think critically before reacting. For example, did you think through beforehand what you were going to report, or did you come off as rambling?
4. Treat conflict as an opportunity to voice your own opinion and listen to the other side of the story. Know that you may have to take the initiative to approach the physician or nurse (or other person) regarding what you are seeing as a conflict. They may not be aware of how you are being affected, and ultimately feelings may escalate and patient care will suffer.
5. Choose your approach. The winner takes all: A winlose approach will only escalate the intensity of the feelings involved. The best choice for a solution depends on the situation. There is no "blanket" correct way.
6. Listen and learn. Conflicts are often based on assumptions and a lack of information. If you did happen to be entirely wrong, apologize, and find out how to correct your mistake in future incidences. Take your lumps and get on with it!
7. Discover what is important—that is, the core issue. It can range from hurt feelings to unmet needs. Getting to the root of the problem gets you closer to resolving the conflict.
8. Respect one another. Conflict can be very emotional. Show respect despite the angry and hurt feelings. Stay away from name calling and blaming. Using "I" statements—for example, "I don't understand what you mean"—lets you own your own statements.
9. Find common ground to create the highest common denominator. In this case, it is generally for the patient's highest good (see Chapter 21).

Try This

Resolving Conflicts

Think of a time recently when you experienced a conflict with someone. What was the outcome? Are you still upset with the other person, or was the issue resolved in a mutually beneficial way? What part of your behavior are you especially pleased with? What, if anything, would you do differently the next time?

ELECTRONIC COMMUNICATION

Faxes, electronic documentation, and email are all valuable modern methods of communication when used effectively and appropriately. Fax machines, for example, often shorten the time in which information can be sent between agencies and departments. Electronic documentation ideally provides a location where all agency professionals involved in patient care enter the most recent information. Electronic documentation may be part of your basic education for learning to document medications and treatments. Each facility may have slightly different protocols. Email is a popular way of communicating with administration, within departments, and with other departments. Before getting involved in sending email, it is important to review the basics of email etiquette. Some people email things they would never write in a memo or say directly to someone. Box 13-1 lists some email essentials suggested by Lauchman (1999) and Pagana (2008).

CELL PHONES AND TEXT MESSAGING

You are sitting in class or watching a demonstration on clinical, when someone's cell phone rings. It certainly disturbs the chain of thought for both the students and the instructor. Although the phone can be set to vibrate, the shuffle to see who called is annoying. Who knows—you may have missed something essential for the care of a future patient.

Box 13-1   Email Etiquette

- Consider the content of the email message and to whom you are sending it.
- To emphasize a point, let the sentence stand alone. Special effects, such as boldface, may not show up on someone else's screen.
- Keep your sentences and paragraphs short.
- Skip a line to separate topics.
- Send your message to the right person.
- Be especially careful filling in the "subject" line. People read this first to decide whether the message is worth opening.
- Be specific. Avoid useless information.
- Avoid using inappropriate language.
- Determine whether email is the best way to send your message.
- Be cautious with humor. The person sees only the written word.
- Check your spelling and punctuation. Proofread all messages before sending them.
- Avoid typing an entire email in uppercase. The message "screams" at the recipient.
- Don't use lowercase letters. They make you look sloppy and lazy.
- Avoid sending confidential information.

Text messaging has been integrated into student life with astonishing momentum. Some students continue to text during class, often by holding the phone under the desk or in a backpack. An additional concern is not only the distraction but that some students are using it as a way to cheat on exams.

Many programs have adopted a rule of shutting off cell phones during class and clinical. No text messaging is permitted during class either. As a matter of etiquette, it is just plain rude to behave in ways that are disruptive to the instructor and other students.

Get Ready for the NCLEX-PN® Examination

Key Points

- Communication can be one-sided or two-sided. Both forms involve a sender, a receiver, and a message. In one-sided communication, the receiver does not have the opportunity to provide feedback. During two-sided communication, feedback is an expectation.
- Communication involves verbal, nonverbal, and affective communication.
- The most important part of therapeutic communication is active listening. It involves purpose, focus, and disciplined attention.
- Common active listening behaviors involve restating, clarifying, reflecting, paraphrasing, minimal encouraging, remaining silent, summarizing, and validating.
- Common blocks to communication involve false reassuring, probing, chiding, belittling, giving advice, and pat answers.
- Male/female differences do exist. Some differences are "hardwired" biologically. Characteristics can be modified, if desired.
- Cultural differences in communication exist, especially with individuals who are new to the country and/or continue to have strong cultural ties.
- Role changes for the patient during an illness experience can be distressing. Staff attitude, nursing jargon, fear of the unknown, and personal and environmental factors are all involved.
- Communicating with the instructor and staff involves the same characteristics as communicating with a patient. They include trust, honesty, empathy, respect, sensitivity, humor, knowledge, patience, and commitment. Self-worth is earned as your knowledge and skill in application grow.
- SBAR is a way to give precise information when contacting a physician or providing shift report.
- Life span communication differences are related to growth and other issues, male/female differences, and medical problems.
- Be alert to what your thoughts are saying and if they help you or hinder you.
- Take your conversation seriously: Practice saying what you mean, and know that your thinking affects your feelings and the way you communicate with patients and staff.
- Successful conflict management is based on a mutually beneficial solution.
- Email etiquette is essential for effective and efficient electronic communication.
- Many programs have adopted a no private cell phone or text messaging policy during class or clinical.

Additional Learning Resources

evolve Go to your Evolve website (http://evolve.elsevier.com/Hill/Success) for the following FREE learning resources:
- Answers to Critical Thinking Scenarios
- Additional learning activities
- Additional Review Questions for the NCLEX-PN® exam
- Helpful phrases for communicating in Spanish and more!

Review Questions for the NCLEX-PN® Examination

1. What accounts for basic male/female differences in communication?
   1. Socialization
   2. Environment
   3. Acculturation
   4. Biology

2. What is the sender-receiver-feedback process in one-way communication?
   1. It concludes when the message reaches the receiver.
   2. It uses verbal, nonverbal, and affective communication.
   3. Once feedback has been provided, the message is final.
   4. It is useful, shorthand communication in close friendships.

3. Which is an appropriate response to the patient when you pick up affectively and nonverbally on the patient's anger?
   1. Leave the room and report your observations to the team leader immediately.
   2. Lighten up the situation by sharing some funny email jokes with the patient.
   3. Provide observations of nonverbal behavior and ask the patient what is going on.
   4. Continue what you came in to do silently and leave as soon as you are through.

4. Which statement most accurately reflects a communication difference that is age related?
   1. Speaking in a loud, high voice makes it easier for the elderly patient to hear you.
   2. School-age patients are ready to be included in discussions about their illness.
   3. Distract the toddler having a tantrum by offering a special treat if he or she cooperates.
   4. Using medical jargon and current slang helps the teenager to see you as human.

Alternate Format Item

1. Marty has arrived for her first clinical experience in the nursing home. She wants to do everything right and feels she is ready because she has an elderly grandmother. What tips will you give her for getting acquainted with the resident? (Select all that apply.)

   1. Walk in with great enthusiasm and say, "Hi, Grandma, how are you doing?"
   2. Talk loudly in the resident's left ear to be sure the resident can hear her.
   3. Say, "Good morning, Mrs. Wayne. My name is Latoya. I am a student nurse from the college."
   4. Knock on the door before entering. Take time before moving into personal space.

2. A physician has reprimanded you at the patient's bedside. You feel an instant flash of anger, but you say nothing. When the physician leaves the room, you follow quickly to catch up before he moves on to another room. What will you say? (Select all that apply.)

   1. "Dr. Jones, I wish to speak with you privately."
   2. "How dare you shame me in front of the patient?"
   3. "Please explain what you wanted me to know."
   4. "In the future, talk to me privately, not at the bedside."

Critical Thinking Scenarios

Scenario 1

The instructor has discussed using SBAR when reporting off clinical. You have had a chance to practice this in class using a case study provided by the instructor. The case study indicates that Mrs. Dithers is 78 years old and has a diagnosis of dementia due to delayed diagnosis and poor control of her hypothyroid medication. She seems upset when you arrive. Discuss your approach to Mrs. Dithers.

Scenario 2

Mrs. Rotherham is used to having things her own way and is critical of everything the staff are doing to deal with her illness. Neil, a student nurse, has been assigned to give her medication this morning. When Neil enters the room, Mrs. Rotherham demands to know what he is doing there. What might Neil say?

14

Assertiveness: Your Responsibility

Objectives

On completing this chapter, you will be able to do the following:

1. Explain why assertiveness is a nursing responsibility.
2. Differentiate among assertive, aggressive, and nonassertive (passive) behavior.
3. Describe three negative interactions in which nurses can get involved.
4. Maintain a daily journal that reflects your personal interactions and responses.
5. Explain the use of the problem-solving process to make a personal plan for change toward assertive behavior.
6. Discuss positive manipulation as a cultural choice.

7. Discuss codependency as an attempt to find relief from unresolved feelings.
8. Differentiate between lateral violence, bullying, and vertical violence in nursing.
9. Discuss dealing with sexual harassment in nursing.
10. Explain why insidious aggression is difficult to deal with.
11. List two to three behavioral changes in an individual that may clue you in to possible employee violence.
12. Identify steps you can personally take to make your workplace a happier and safer environment.

Key Terms

aggressive (ă-GRĔS-ĭv, p. 163)
assault (ă-SŎLT, p. 171)
assertiveness (ă-SŬR-tĭv-nĕs, p. 164)
automatic responses (ĂW-tŏ-MĂT-ĭk, pp. 162–163)
bullying (p. 175)
choice (chŏys, p. 162)
compensation (KŎM-pĕn-SĂ-shŭn, p. 167)
denial (dē-NĪ-ăl, p. 167)
insidious aggression (ĭn-SĬD-ē-ŭs ă-GRĔ-shŭn, p. 175)

lateral violence (p. 175)
manipulation (mă-NĬP-ū-LĀ-shŭn, p. 171)
nonassertive (passive) (nŏn-ă-SŬR-tĭv, p. 163)
problem solving (prŏ-blem sol-ving, p. 167)
projection (prŏ-JĔK-shŭn, p. 165)
rationalization (RĂSH-ăn-ă-lĭ-ZĀ-shŭn, p. 166)
sexual harassment (HĂR-ăs-mĕnt, p. 174)
vertical violence (horizontal hostility) (p. 175)

 Keep in Mind

Assertiveness is an expectation in nursing—a responsibility for you as a patient advocate.

 Critical Thinking

Personal Expectations

Imagine for the next few minutes that the nurse-patient roles are reversed and that you are the patient. What are your expectations of the nurse assigned to you? List the rationale for each expectation you identify.

Expectations	Rationale
_____	_____
_____	_____
_____	_____

The exercise in the Critical Thinking: Personal Expectations box should give you some insights into why a nurse must have assertiveness. At the end of this chapter you are encouraged to do this exercise again. Evaluate any changes in your expectations.

Verbal, nonverbal, and affective communication translates into three major behavior patterns. You will *hear*, *see*, and *feel* the message acted out. The most effective communication style is open and honest. It promotes positive relationships and a healthy sense of self. Ineffective communication or behavior is hurtful. It blames, attacks, or denies and is harmful to the self as well.

An *assertive* style separates the person from the issue. Most important, you speak out of choice. An emotional hook catches you when you use either an *aggressive* or a *nonassertive* (passive) style of communication. Both types of responses are automatic responses. You no longer respond from choice. The three major behavior styles are nonassertive (passive), aggressive, and assertive.

NONASSERTIVE (PASSIVE) BEHAVIOR

Nonassertive (passive), fear-based behavior is an emotionally dishonest, self-defeating type of behavior. Nonassertive nurses attempt to look the other way, avoid conflict, and take what seems to be the easiest way out; they are never full participants on the nursing team. Nonassertive individuals do not express feelings, needs, and ideas when their rights are infringed on, deliberately or accidentally. There may be a lack of eye contact, swaying and shifting from one foot to the other, and whining and hesitancy when speaking. The overall message is "I do not count. *You* count." This personal pattern of behavior is reflected in their nursing as well. Consequently, they are unable to recognize and meet patient needs. Some examples of nonassertive behavior, with the type of behavior in parentheses, that were observed in one nurse follow:

- Tells another nurse how "stupid" the doctor is for ordering a certain type of treatment (indirect, nonassertive behavior).
- Limits contact with a patient he or she is uncomfortable with to required care only (indirect nonassertive behavior).
- Routinely tells patients who ask questions about their illness, test, medications, or treatment to "ask the doctor" or "ask the RN." Although this answer is advisable some of the time, it certainly is a form of brush-off. Part of nursing responsibility is to seek answers for the patient (takes the easy way out).
- Experiences inability to continue with a necessary, uncomfortable treatment ordered for the patient (interprets patient's expression of discomfort personally: "The patient will not like me if I do this").
- May assume, without checking, that the patient wants to skip daily personal care when a visitor drops in (avoids conflict).
- Experiences a feeling of being "devastated" when a patient, doctor, nurse, or other staff person criticizes his or her work (interprets criticism of work as criticism of self).
- Responds to patient's questions about own personal life and that of other staff (afraid of not being liked).
- Patient asks nurse to pick up some personal items on the way home. Nurse frowns but agrees to do so (communicates real message nonverbally).
- Becomes angry with the team leader and drops hints to others about own feelings (communicates real message indirectly).
- When asked by another nurse to assist with the care of assigned patients, responds by saying, "Well, uh, I guess I could," although already too busy (hesitate, repressing own wishes).

- Needs help with assignment but says nothing (refrains from expressing own needs).
- After making an error, overexplains and overapologizes (is unaware of the right to make a mistake; should take responsibility for it, learn from the error, and go on).
- Plans on finding a new job because of fear of approaching supervisor to tell own side of what has happened (avoids conflict).
- When "chewed out" by the doctor in front of a patient, gets angry but says nothing (refrains from expressing own opinion—internalizes anger).

 Try This

Nonassertive Behavior

Identify nonassertive behaviors in which you have been involved. Describe how each behavior worked or did not work for you.

By not taking risks and not being honest, nonassertive nurses typically feel hurt, misunderstood, anxious, and disappointed and often feel angry and resentful later. Because they do not allow their needs to be known, they are the ones who lose out.

 Critical Thinking

Nonassertive Behavior

Develop a plan for change for each one of the nonassertive behaviors that you identified as having unsatisfactory outcomes.

AGGRESSIVE BEHAVIOR

Outspoken people are often automatically considered assertive, when in reality their lack of consideration for others may be a sign of aggressive behavior. Aggressive (anger-based) behavior violates the rights of others. It is an attack on the person rather than on the person's behavior. The purpose of aggressive behavior is to dominate or put the other person down. This behavior, while expressive, is self-defeating because it quickly distances the aggressor from other staff and patients. Examples of aggressive body language include leaning forward with glaring eyes; pointing a finger at a person to whom you are speaking; shouting; clenching fists; putting hands on hips; and shaking the head. The overall message is *"You do not count. I count."* The following examples show how aggressive behavior can be recognized. An explanation of the rationale is included in parentheses.

- You have asked to go to a workshop, and the supervisor says, "Why should you go? Everyone else has worked here longer than you have" (attempts to make you feel guilty for making a request).
- Another nurse points out your error in front of other staff and adds, "Where did you say you graduated from?" (attempts to humiliate as a way of controlling).

- A peer approaches you with a problem. You don't want to listen and say, "If it isn't one thing, it's another for you. Why don't you get your act together?" (disregards others' feelings).
- A new rule is instituted without requesting input from or informing those it will involve. You protest but are told, "That's tough; this is the way it's going to be from now on" (disregards others' feelings and rights).
- The patient has had his call light on frequently throughout the morning. You walk in and say, "I have had it. You have had your light on continuously for nothing all morning. Do not put your light on again unless you are dying, or I will take it away" (hostile overreaction out of proportion to the issue at hand).
- You attempted to express your feelings to a peer about his or her behavior toward you. Today the peer greets you with an icy stare when you say hello (hostile overreaction).
- The patient tells you, "I thought this was a pretty good hospital, but none of you seem to know what you are doing" (sarcastic, hostile).
- You push yourself in front of others in the cafeteria line (rudeness).
- You ask the nurse manager a question. Instead of answering, he just stares at you with lips curled slightly upward (attempt to make you uncomfortable, a put-down).

 Try This

Aggressive Behavior

Circle the aggressive behaviors in the previous example that are similar to behaviors you have experienced.

 Critical Thinking

Aggressive Behavior

Develop a plan for dealing with the aggressive behaviors you identified in the previous learning exercise.

Aggressive behavior certainly is a way of saying what you mean at the moment, and it does produce temporary relief from anxiety. The feeling, however, does not last. Very often the aggressive person is left with residual angry feelings that simmer until the next stressful situation or person comes along. It is interesting to note that sometimes an aggressive person was once passive and made a decision that "no one will ever step on me again." However, instead of practicing assertiveness, such a person practiced and became involved in another form of destructive, self-defeating behavior. Aggressive nurses, like nonaggressive nurses, are unable to function as true advocates for the patient because they are too busy taking care of what they perceive to be their personal needs.

ASSERTIVE BEHAVIOR

Assertiveness is another name for "honesty"—that is, it is a way to live the truth from your innermost being and to express this truth in thought, word, and deed. The concept seems simple enough, but it is another thing to be truthful all the time. According to *Webster's Dictionary, assertiveness* means "taking a positive stand, being confident in your statement, or being positive in a persistent way." You, the nurse, work in a setting that requires speaking frankly and openly to others in such a way that their rights are not violated. *Assertiveness is a tool, not a weapon.* As with any new behavior (or skill), becoming truly assertive will take practice and time. Avoid being harsh with yourself or giving up just because old behaviors emerge when you are under pressure. Resolve to try again until assertive behavior is integrated as a part of your being. Although it is not the nurse's right to hurt others deliberately, it is unrealistic to be inhibited to the point of never hurting anyone. Some people are hurt because they are unreasonably sensitive, and some people use their sensitivity to manipulate others. Assertiveness is not only what you say but how you say it. Examples of assertive body language include standing straight, steady, and directly facing the people to whom you are speaking while maintaining eye contact; speaking in a clear voice, loud enough so the people to whom you are speaking can hear you; and speaking fluently without hesitation and with assurance and confidence.

Nurses have a right to express their own thoughts and feelings. To do otherwise would be insincere. It would also deny patients and other staff the opportunity to learn to deal with their feelings. Assertiveness, then, is a way of expressing oneself without insulting others. It communicates respect for the other person, although not necessarily for the other person's behavior. The overall message is *"I count, and you count, too."* Being assertive does not guarantee that you will get your way. What it does guarantee is that you will experience a sense of being in control of your emotions and your responses. Win or lose, you gave it your best shot. The real bonus is freedom from residual feelings of fear and anger. Later in this chapter, we will deal with exceptions when you are faced with a potentially violent situation.

The following examples, with the rationale in parentheses, are expressions of assertive behavior. As an assertive nurse, you claim responsibility for your own feelings, thoughts, and actions. Using "I" in your statements shows acceptance of responsibility for your thinking, feeling, and doing.

- The doctor orders a medication or treatment that seems inappropriate. You request to talk to the doctor privately and ask about expected outcomes. You present any new information you have that may potentially affect the decision to continue with the order (direct statement of information).

- The patient has been giving you a bad time. Pulling up a chair and sitting down, you say, "Mr. Smith, I would be interested in knowing what is going on with you. I have noticed that whatever I do, you are critical of my work." Then you listen attentively and with understanding (comprehension) and respond nondefensively (direct statement of feelings; does not interpret patient's criticism as a personal attack).
- When the patient requests information you are unfamiliar with regarding the illness and treatment, you say, "I do not know, but I will find out for you." You follow through by checking with appropriate staff. You determine who is to inform the patient (respects the patient's right to know).
- The doctor has ordered the patient to walk for 10 minutes out of each hour. The patient complains that it hurts and asks to not be required to walk. You respond by saying, "I know it is uncomfortable, but I will walk along beside you. We can stop briefly any time you like. I will also teach you how to do a brief relaxation technique [see Chapter 6] that you can use while you are walking." If pain medication is available, you will also make sure that this is given before walking and in enough time for the medication to take effect (respects patient's feelings but supports the need to carry out doctor's orders).
- Unexpected visitors arrive when it is time for you to help the patient with personal care. You ask the patient directly if care should be done now or postponed briefly. You state the time that you will be available to assist with care (respects the patient's right to choose, as long as it does not compromise the care).
- You have just been criticized for your work. You respond by saying, "Please clarify. I want to be sure I understand." If the error is yours, ask for suggestions to correct it or offer alternatives of your own (separates criticism of performance from criticism of self).
- The patient asks for personal information about you (or another staff member). You respond by saying, "That information is personal, and I do not choose to discuss it" (stands up for rights without violating rights of others).
- Your patient asks you to pick up some personal items from the store. This would mean doing it on your own time, which is already very full. You respond by saying, "I will not be able to do the errand for you" (direct statement without excuses).
- The team leader has been "on your case" constantly and, you think, unfairly. You approach the team leader and say, "I would like to speak with you privately today before 3 PM. What time is convenient for you?" (direct statement of wishes).
- You are being pressed by other staff members to help with their assignments but are too busy to do

so. You say, "No, I do not have the time to help today, but try me again on some other day" (direct refusal without feeling guilty; leaves the door open to help at a future date).
- Your day is overwhelming. You approach your team leader and say, "I know you would like all of this done today. There is no way I can get it all done. What are your priorities?" (direct statement of information and request for clarification).
- The doctor has criticized your work in front of the patient. You feel embarrassed and angry. You approach the doctor and ask to speak privately. Using "I-centered" statements, you begin by saying, "I feel both embarrassed and angry because you criticized me in front of the patient. Next time, ask to talk to me privately. I will listen to what you have to say" (stands up for your rights without violating the rights of others).
- You are ready to leave work, when a peer approaches you about a personal problem. You respond by saying, "I have to leave now, but I'll be glad to listen to you during our lunch break tomorrow" (compromise).
- Another staff person moves into the cafeteria line ahead of you with a nod and a smile. You are in a hurry, too, and feel this is an imposition. You say firmly, "I do not like it when you cut in line ahead of me. Please go back to the end of the line" (stands up for your rights).

Now complete the exercise in the Try This: Identify Assertiveness box.

◉ Try This

Identify Assertiveness

List examples of assertiveness you can identify in your own behavior or in people around you.

The following three rules are helpful overall in being assertive:

1. Own your feelings. Do not blame others for the way you feel.
2. Make your feelings known by being direct. Begin your statements with "I."
3. Be sure that your nonverbal communication matches your verbal message.

NEGATIVE INTERACTIONS: USING COPING MECHANISMS

With the availability of so many types of preparation for nurses and the lack of differentiation in roles based on preparation, nurses sometimes experience insecurity in their role and the worth of the role as they understand it. **Projection** is a coping mechanism during which individuals attribute their own weaknesses to others. The interaction can be characterized as "my education is better than yours" or "I'm more competent than you are" or "You're only a practical nurse," and so on. Unfortunately, this negative, aggressive interaction wastes energy that could be used to provide the patient with the care that is being alluded to. Nurses who are confident and assertive enhance one another's knowledge base and legal responsibility. The patient benefits from the assertiveness.

Another negative interaction is based on a previous unresolved incident between the patient and the nurse. The nurse uses the coping or mental mechanism of rationalization, in which a logical but untrue reason is offered as an excuse for the behavior. The nurse quickly informs others that this patient is a "troublemaker" or a "manipulator" or "uncooperative." This is a nonassertive, indirect type of behavior on the part of the nurse. Obviously, if other nurses incorporate this information into their transactions with patients, patients will never be seen as their true selves. Anything the patient does can be interpreted within the context of the label given by the nurses. A vicious circle can ensue. If the patient's needs are not met because of this labeling, this increases his or her frustration. This in turn is a threat to self, resulting in anxiety. Depending on the patient's personal strength at this time, the situation can lead to problem solving, the use of coping/mental mechanisms, or symptom formation (Figure 14-1).

An honest, assertive response on the part of the original nurse involved would consist of dealing with the patient directly in regard to the previous situation.

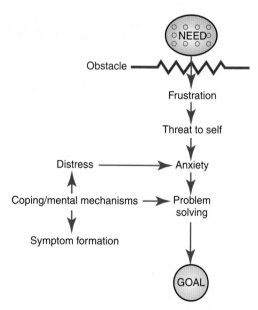

If patient feels overwhelmed by anxiety and stress (distress), coping/mental mechanisms may be resorted to in order to deal with the distress. If coping/mental mechanisms fail, the result will be mental or physical symptom formation. Unmet needs are a threat to self, resulting in stress and anxiety. If the patient has the personal strength to problem-solve, needs can be met.

FIGURE 14-1 A vicious circle showing a negative interaction from an unresolved incident between the patient and the nurse.

It would not involve other nurses as allies in "getting this patient." An example of an extreme situation resulting from just such a seemingly innocent rationalization occurred at a nursing home. A young man who was paralyzed from the waist down as a result of a car accident was being transferred from one nursing home to another. A transfer form arrived before he did. The information on the form created immediate anxiety for the nurses involved before they had even met the man. The form labeled the man as "manipulative." It stated, "He will be pleasant and polite at first, but watch out because it is a trick. When he has won you over, you will see his 'true colors.'" The nurses discussed the prospective admission. They expressed gratitude that their colleagues in the other nursing home had warned them. After all, that is what colleagues are for. They felt, "Forewarned is forearmed."

When the patient arrived and attempted to get acquainted, he was dealt with coldly and abruptly and made to wait. The nurses intended to show him that he could not manipulate them. As his frustration and discomfort increased, he began to demand that his treatments be done on time. He shouted angry comments at the nurses when they finally arrived to assume his care. The nurses called him "demanding" and "hostile." The original label of "manipulative" was supported when the patient asked his roommate to put on the call light to get help to take him to the bathroom. Each day seemed worse than the day before. The showdown finally came when a longtime nurse employee left, saying that she would not come back until the patient was transferred to another facility. She would even volunteer to do the transfer note. Other nursing staff threatened to follow suit. Finally, the administrator gave in. The patient was transferred, and the nurses congratulated one another for having worked together! Complete the exercise in the Critical Thinking: Negative Interactions box.

? Critical Thinking

Negative Interactions

1. What factors contributed to the patient's behavior?
2. What factors contributed to the nurses' response to the patient?
3. How could this situation have been handled differently?
4. Was the behavior of the nurses passive, aggressive, or assertive? Explain your answer.

Another negative transaction involves the patient's right to know (for example, a patient being transferred from a skilled nursing home facility to an intermediate nursing home facility). This transaction can be known by many titles, depending on the issue. It can be called "I've got a secret"; "It is not my responsibility"; "She will be upset"; or "She is too weak to figure out what is going on." The responsibility of informing the patient about his or her condition or transfer plans is not carried out just so the present staff does not have to deal with the full impact of the patient's reaction to the information. The coping or mental mechanism used by the nurses is denial. The nurse refuses to recognize the existence and significance of the patient's personal concerns. The nurse also uses denial as a way of excusing personal responsibility: "The doctor should tell him" or "It's the team leader's responsibility." Although the decision may not be entirely yours, it is clearly your responsibility to check out what portion of the information is yours to give. You also have the responsibility to check out who is going to present the information and when. Complete the exercise in the Try This: Identify If Behavior Is Passive, Aggressive, or Assertive box.

 Try This

Identify If Behavior Is Passive, Aggressive, or Assertive

Is the nurse's refusal to take responsibility to seek out the information the patient needs to know a passive, aggressive, or assertive transaction? Explain your answer.

GOSSIP HURTS

Although it has many possible negative interactions, certainly the passive or aggressive game of gossip—for example, "Did I tell you?" or "I just found out"—is a destructive interaction that has the potential to ruin the reputations of both patients and personnel. The coping or mental mechanism is compensation. The nurse is covering for real or imagined inadequacies in his or her work by developing what he or she considers desirable traits of observation, listening, and reporting. The energy is misguided because reputations are at stake, and time spent socializing while at work is time away from providing quality patient care. A listener can squelch this game by saying assertively, "I will work on a good relationship between you and me, but I would prefer you do not talk to me about others." Instead, if the listener, while calling the other nurse a gossip, listens with interest, continuation of this behavior is supported. Complete the exercise in the Critical Thinking: More Damaging Interactions box.

? **Critical Thinking**

More Damaging Interactions

1. What other damaging interactions among staff or between patients and staff do you know about?
2. Provide examples of how continuation of this type of interaction is supported by others.
3. What can you do or say to avoid being drawn into these interactions?

GUIDELINES FOR MOVING TOWARD ASSERTIVENESS

Read the poem "Myself" in Box 14-1. It captures the reason for working toward assertiveness and being able to feel good about yourself as you continue to grow as a person. Changing behavior is difficult. After all, the behaviors have been practiced and perfected for years. It is so much easier to tell others what *they* should do to change. The decision to change must come from inside you so it becomes yours alone.

PROBLEM-SOLVING PROCESS

The problem-solving process is a series of steps used to solve problems long before the nursing process was developed. You will note similarities between problem-solving and nursing processes. The nursing process is a more focused method of using the problem-solving steps. We reintroduce you to problem solving in this chapter because of its continued usefulness in dealing with self.

It is easier to begin the problem-solving process before feelings and behaviors about a troublesome problem become deeply rooted. A common response to unresolved problems is the cycle of worry → fear → anger → rage. This cycle can be interrupted and resolved at any stage, but it requires different levels of nursing skill. When dealing with the underlying problem, ask the person, "What do you want?" Putting the problem-solving steps into action is work! Without resolution the cycle continues and intensifies with time. This behavior, for example, can be seen in the nursing home patient who strikes out, seems calm for a period, gets irritable, and eventually strikes out again. If the underlying problem is not resolved, the cycle continues. The person gets labeled as one who strikes out without warning, so "Watch out." Ask a more skilled staff member to do the behavioral intervention if you are uncomfortable. You must not set yourself up for injury (Figure 14-2).

| Box 14-1 | Myself |

I have to live with myself and so,
I want to be fit for myself to know.
I don't want to stand with the setting sun
And hate myself for the things I've done.
I want to go out with head erect.
I want to deserve all men's respect.
But here in this struggle for fame and self,
I want to be able to like myself.
I don't want to look at myself and know
That I'm bluster and bluff and empty show.
I never can fool myself, and so
Whatever happens, I want to grow
More able to be more proud of me,
Self-respecting and conscience free.

Author: Unknown

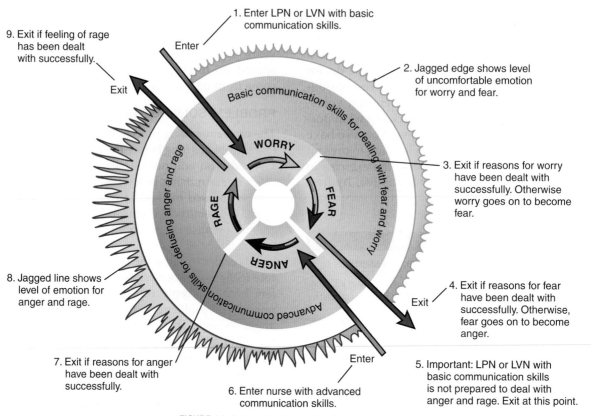

10. Cycle continues until patient acts out with rage. Emotion temporarily calms down after release, but builds up again if reason(s) for emotion have not been resolved.

1. Enter LPN or LVN with basic communication skills.

9. Exit if feeling of rage has been dealt with successfully.

2. Jagged edge shows level of uncomfortable emotion for worry and fear.

3. Exit if reasons for worry have been dealt with successfully. Otherwise worry goes on to become fear.

8. Jagged line shows level of emotion for anger and rage.

4. Exit if reasons for fear have been dealt with successfully. Otherwise, fear goes on to become anger.

7. Exit if reasons for anger have been dealt with successfully.

6. Enter nurse with advanced communication skills.

5. Important: LPN or LVN with basic communication skills is not prepared to deal with anger and rage. Exit at this point.

FIGURE 14-2 A cycle of unresolved patient issues.

The self tries to find relief of unresolved feelings through behavior such as codependency, self-medicating with alcohol and/or other drugs (or food), and projecting the anger toward patients (burnout). Prolonged, unresolved negative emotions such as worry, fear, and anger create changes in the body at a cellular level and can result in physical illness. We first get clues in our thoughts of how we will become ill. Listen to your self-talk: "I'm sick of this!"; "I feel like I have the weight of the world on my shoulders"; "He's a pain in the neck (or butt)"; "Oh, my aching back!"; "I'm so upset I can't speak"; "I can't take this much longer"; and so on. If your self-talk is negative, pay attention. These statements give clues to potential areas of physical involvement. We also read or hear news almost daily of mild-mannered, nice people who suddenly acted out because of rage. No one wants to get there. Rage can be turned against others (including homicide), or it can be turned against oneself. Passive means of rage turned against oneself include adopting personal habits that are damaging to one's health. Active rage against self includes the extreme act of suicide. The risk of suicide for nurses is real, and according to Belanger (2000), it ranks "among the top five causes of death in nurses, and all nurses—from students to retirees—have higher rates of suicide than the general population."

The problem-solving process is a conscious growth-producing method of dealing with challenges in your life. It is important to note that problem solving is an active process and is more than simply developing an intellectual awareness of the challenge at hand.

PROBLEM-SOLVING STEPS

Step 1: Define the Problem
Sometimes what is perceived as the problem is not really the problem. For example, you may have been blaming another individual for talking you into behaviors of which you do not approve. Before making a commitment to change, it is important to look objectively at the gains and losses associated with the

present behavior. For example, blaming someone else for your behavior may get you sympathy and concern from your friends. However, you lose by not taking responsibility for your own behavior and dealing with it in a growth-producing way. Your present way of responding to others developed as a response to anxiety-producing situations in life. The behavior usually has its roots in childhood. Complete the exercise about gains and losses in the Critical Thinking: Gains and Losses box.

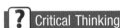 **Critical Thinking**

Gains and Losses

Answer the following questions in your confidential journal: What are you gaining from staying nonassertive/aggressive? What are you losing from staying nonassertive/aggressive?

Another consideration is that when you change the way you act toward others, you change the way they act toward you. What has been a predictable reaction will no longer be predictable. Initially the "others" will test you. They will increase their old way of behaving as a way of getting you to give up the new behavior. If you persist with your new way of dealing with and responding to situations, their behavior toward you will gradually change. *This is the only way to influence change in anyone's behavior.* No amount of "telling" or "scolding" makes a difference as long as others can count on you to continue behaving in the old, predictable way.

Defining the problem depends on collecting data for 2 or 3 days and writing your problem statement based on this information. Collecting data needs to be done in an objective manner, as though you were observing someone else.

 Try This

Keep a Daily Journal

Maintain a daily confidential journal to help pinpoint specific situations that create worry, fear, anger, and rage in you. Track the following:
1. What happened
2. When it happened
3. How you felt physically
4. The emotion you felt
5. What you would have liked to have done instead
6. What kept you from doing it

Step 2: Decide on a Goal

Review the problem statement and write it out, applying the nursing process. Ask yourself what you want to do differently. This can be stated as a single goal. Often it is more useful to break the goal down into a long-term goal (what change or outcome you want) and several short-term goals (steps needed to attain the desired

 Critical Thinking

Defining the Problem

Review the data you have collected for 2 or 3 days in your daily journal. It will give you insight into the pros and cons of your current behavior. Develop a problem statement that is personal and specific for you. Before writing the problem statement, read the following sample:

Sample

I am afraid to say what I mean for fear that others will get angry with me.

This behavior is characterized by the following situations:
- Saying "yes" to requests to babysit when I need the time for homework.
- Not asking for help with household chores, even though I am a full-time student plus a homemaker.
- Saying "yes" to added requests not related to responsibilities for school that I must complete on my own time.
- Feeling tired and resentful much of the time and eventually blowing up over something insignificant.

long-term goal). All goals must be realistic (attainable), measurable (tells how you will know the goal has been attained), and time-referenced (an educated guess on when you will see results). Before you read further, complete the exercise in the Critical Thinking: Deciding on a Goal box.

Critical Thinking

Deciding on a Goal

Write a goal about assertiveness for yourself. Before you write the goal, read the sample that follows.

Sample

Long-Term Goal	Short-Term Goal
Within 6 months I will say what I mean without fear that others will be angry with me (give actual date—this is your best "guesstimate").	Within 2 weeks I will say "no" to babysitting requests when I need the time to do homework (give actual date—this is your best "guesstimate").

As you read each of the goals you have written, ask yourself whether they are realistic. Are they reasonable to attain? Next, review each goal and ask whether it is measurable. Are they so specific that you can use the senses to detect the change? Note that each goal begins with the phrase "I will." This phrase signals a personal commitment to work on the goal. Note that the goals are to be attained within a designated period—that is, they are time-referenced. This is also the only way to give yourself a push to get started.

All the changes are not going to occur exactly by the projected date. You will have to revise the goal dates from time to time. Most important, they provide target dates to strive for. As you accomplish each short-term goal, cross it out and go on to the next one. Do not be alarmed if you find yourself working on more than one goal at a time. This is possible and even desirable when the opportunity presents itself. It is important to continue recording your progress in the confidential journal that you began initially to obtain data. Its value now lies in keeping a record of the process you are going through and seeing the changes taking place. Unless you do this, you may not fully appreciate your work and its progress. Many changes will be subtle and will not be accompanied by bells and claps of thunder.

Step 3: Choose Alternatives

Alternatives are the approaches that you will be using to attain each of the established goals. When you make a list of alternatives in your journal, let your imagination run wild. Consider all the possible solutions, from serious to humorous. This may even provide some comic relief from the serious challenge with which you are dealing. Remember to include "do nothing" in the list of alternatives. Doing nothing is a *choice* and therefore an alternative. Look at each of the goals and think of specific things you can do or say to help support the goal. Complete the exercise in the Critical Thinking: Personal Alternatives box.

 Critical Thinking

Personal Alternatives

Write alternatives to support the short-term goal(s) you chose in the Deciding on a Goal exercise. Before you write in your journal, read the sample that follows.

Sample

Approach: Practice in front of a mirror. In an even tone of voice, say, "No, I will not be able to babysit tonight, but try again another time." If the person persists, say, "No, I do not have the time tonight." Repeat as needed until heard. Compliment yourself for not giving in.

How does the approach (alternative) correspond specifically to the short-term goal from the assertiveness exercise?

Step 4: Try Out the Alternatives

The initial plan has been made. It is now time to put the plan into action. For many of you, the paperwork is far easier than taking the first step to make the "paper trip" a reality. You may also have discovered that it is far easier to offer ideas to peers than to take the first step into action with your own plan.

It is a good idea to build in an incentive to continue using the new assertive approaches. Promise yourself something that is worthy of you (a worthy goal). As you go along, you will sometimes slip back into old familiar ways of behaving. Do not be dismayed. This is normal. Simply reinstitute the newly planned approaches immediately and continue. The more you

practice the new approaches, the more they will become part of you. Ultimately, new assertive behaviors will replace old nonassertive or aggressive behaviors.

 Try This

Celebrate Attaining Your Goals

Identify a worthy incentive to celebrate attaining your goal. To make it work, the goal must be within your budget and not create a new problem for you to solve!

Step 5: Evaluate the Effectiveness of Your Approach

The evaluation mechanism is built into the overall plan for change by making the goals time-limited. This tells you that each goal, along with the alternatives you have chosen, will be evaluated at the time indicated. Do not change a goal or approach too quickly. Give it at least 2 to 3 weeks. You need to do this for two reasons: The negative behaviors of other individuals toward you will increase initially as they attempt to resist the change created by the change in you, and it takes a minimum of 3 weeks for the new behavior to catch on. (It takes approximately a year for a new behavior to become part of you.)

Try This

Review Your Journal

As a part of the evaluation process, review your entire confidential journal. This is an excellent source of information for what happened, how you dealt with it, and whether the present course is effective.

Step 6: Repeat the Process If the Solution Is Not Effective

Step 5 gave you information about whether to pursue the established course of action. If changes are needed, go back to step 3, identify additional alternatives, or perhaps choose alternatives that you originally identified but did not use. Then go through the rest of the steps as before.

As you pursue an assertive way of behaving, monitor your nonverbal messages. The nonverbal communication you provide is even more powerful than your words. It is possible to have the words just right but to sabotage the words by hesitation, a sarcastic tone of voice, or emphasis on certain words. Practice in front of a mirror. If you feel like you don't have the time, do it while taking your shower. Listen to the way you sound. A video is helpful, as is speaking into an empty corner and hearing your words bounce back. Try lowering your tone of voice. Be sure that the last word of a sentence is no higher than the one before it. Listen for this in others. It makes a statement sound like a question.

Posture plays an important role. Sit up straight; walk with the shoulders back and a confident stride. Make eye contact when speaking. If this is new and difficult for you, look at the area between the eyes of the person you are addressing. This provides an illusion of eye contact. Periodically look away so that it does not look as though you are staring. Avoid annoying characteristics such as staring, nail biting, finger or foot tapping or jiggling, playing with your hair, chewing on a pencil or glasses, nervous laughter, putting hands in and out of pockets, and so on.

When someone asks you what you think of an issue or what you would like to do, answer the person. Instead of saying, "I really do not know" or "Whatever you like" or "It does not matter," take the risk and express your opinion. Life is an adventure. Your ideas count, and the more you express your opinion, the easier it becomes.

CULTURAL DIFFERENCES: MANIPULATION

With feedback from valued teachers, students, and reviewers, we have learned that it is not safe to assume that all cultures are focused on moving toward assertive behavior. In some cultures, manipulation is an accepted norm. Although the term *manipulation* has a negative connotation in our society, manipulation in itself is not a maladaptive behavior. In some cultures it is taught and accepted as a purposeful way of meeting one's needs. Skillful manipulation is especially applauded in some cultures. People are taught to be indirect in their comments, to be polite, and to avoid confrontation or direct expression of disagreement so as not to give offense and cause loss of face (Lipson and Dibble, 2006).

It is easy to jump to the conclusion that a manipulative person is trying to "trick" you when you do not share the same cultural background. Make time to talk. The differences will be interesting and revealing for both of you.

NEGATIVE MANIPULATIVE INTERACTIONS

Manipulation is considered maladaptive if the feelings and needs of others are disregarded or other people are treated as objects to fulfill the needs of the manipulator. The following examples of negative manipulative interactions show a lack of consideration for others' feelings and needs:

- The *seducer* initiates a relationship with someone (e.g., a nurse with a supervisor). They share what seem to be common goals and insights. Ultimately, the seducer asks for special favors or privileges. If denied, the seducer pushes the guilt button, saying, "I thought you liked me" or "I thought we understood each other." The other person is left feeling guilty, angry, or both.

- The *passive-aggressive* manipulator focuses on the other person's weaknesses. He or she uses this knowledge to exploit or create anxiety for the victim. For example, a physician might point out a nurse's errors or personal or professional problems in front of a patient or other staff. The nurse is left feeling guilty, angry, embarrassed, or all of these emotions.

- The *divide-and-conquer* manipulator "confides" half-truths, rumors, gossip, and innuendo. A skilled manipulator can sever work relationships by sowing seeds of distrust. As the staff squabbles, there is less energy to unite and focus on common patient issues. For example, a divide-and-conquer manipulator who is an established member of the community might "confide" to another department head that a newer employee cannot be trusted. By the time this information proves to be untrue, valuable time has been lost in patient planning and care. Meanwhile, the divide-and-conquer manipulator has continued to tell the same story to other listeners. Because the feelings and needs of others are not considered, they are left with anger and seeds of distrust.

Dealing with a negative manipulator is difficult. An assertive approach is the best recourse. This will, however, be met with resistance and resentment. You may end up backing off if the problem cannot be worked out. Set limits on any inappropriate manipulative behavior toward you. Refuse to play the game anymore.

As a nurse, you must learn to take care of yourself. In turn, you will be more effective in meeting patients' nursing needs. In taking care of yourself assertively, you serve as a positive role model for your coworkers, those you lead and manage, and your patients. How you view and deal with an event determines the outcome for you.

AGGRESSIVENESS AND WORK-RELATED ISSUES

ASSAULT

Workplace violence has always existed in nursing facilities. It is the increase in violence, however, that is making nurses take notice. Nurses are frequently targets of violence, hostility, sexual harassment, and discrimination. It has been shown that health care workers, especially nurses, are the victims of physical assault at their place of employment even more often than prison guards and police. (Taken from www. nurseweek.com/news/features/).

The U.S. Department of Labor's Occupational Safety and Health Administration (OSHA) guidelines for security in health care facilities report that in general hospitals 41% of assaults occur in psychiatric units; 18% in medical units; 13% in surgical units;

Box 14-2	OSHA National Guidelines for Deterring Violence

- Safer nurses' stations: bullet-resistant glass
- Unit arrangement with staff safety in mind
- No toleration of violence policy
- At least two exits in rooms to prevent entrapment of staff
- Adequate, qualified staff coverage at all times
- Policies and procedures for protecting home care providers
- Prompt medical evaluation and treatment regardless of severity of incident
- Victims' right to prosecute perpetrators
- Investigation of all incidents and installation of corrective action
- Alarm systems: security devices such as panic buttons and cell phones
- Metal detectors
- Closed-circuit televisions
- Curved mirrors in hallway intersections
- Time-out rooms for upset patients
- Bright lights

and 7% in pediatric units. Patients do most of the assaults, and almost three-fourths of those assaulted are staff nurses. In March 1996, OSHA released its first *Act of Violence Prevention Guidelines* (1996) geared toward protecting health care and social service workers on the job. The national guidelines are designed to protect employers and employees with a framework for deterring violence and increasing safety (Box 14-2).

Not all agencies have complied with the OSHA guidelines, but some state nurses associations are working toward increased penalties against those guilty of assaulting a health care worker or to establish task forces to study workplace violence.

 Try This

The American Nurses Association Bill of Rights

The ANA *Bill of Rights for Registered Nurses* states, "Nurses have the right to a work environment that is safe for themselves and their patients." Research what your state practical/vocational nurses association is doing to minimize risks of violence in the workplace.

CONTRIBUTING FACTORS

Many of the findings regarding factors contributing to violence apply to all of nursing.

Personal Factors

Personal factors include verbal, nonverbal, and affective communication, including nurses' attitudes and behaviors. Attitude and body language are considered more significant than the sex and age of the nurse. The manner of approaching a patient, such as with respect and confidence, emerged as important.

Workplace Practices

A shortage of staff and a reduction in trained, regular staff contribute to incidences of assault on staff. Assaults are often associated with mealtimes, visiting times, and times of increased staff responsibilities at night when staffing is reduced (OSHA, 2004).

The quality, performance, and availability of security personnel are important. Nurses believe they are safer when security officers wear police-type uniforms. Officers convey authority in uniform more so than when they wear a customer-friendly jacket and tie—a nonverbal form of communication. Incidents are also more common when nurses and security personnel lack aggression management skills. Finally, not all administrators back nurses on reporting incidents of physical and verbal abuse, including those involving supervisors and physicians.

Environmental Factors

The type of patient seen and the location of the care facility (for example, high–crime risk area) determine the type of patient admitted to a hospital. An important risk factor at hospitals and psychiatric facilities is the carrying of guns by patients, family, or friends of the patient. Other issues include early release of acute or chronic mentally ill, the right to refuse psychotropic medication, the inability to voluntarily hospitalize mentally ill persons unless of immediate danger to self or others, and the use of hospitals for criminals instead of incarceration.

Risk Diagnosis

The majority of all assaults are perpetrated by a minority of persons. A history of previous violence is the best indicator, but sometimes this information is not available to the staff. Mentally ill persons commit a small percentage of assaults. More common are gang members, drug users, social deviants, distraught relatives, and those who feel threatened.

Nurses need to learn how to read cues for potential risk of violence in the patients (and others) with whom they are dealing. Some diagnoses that can cue you to possible risk include affective disorders, paranoid delusions, chemical abuse/dependency, dementia, impulse control disorders, and personality disorders.

If you find yourself in potential danger, take the following immediate steps:

- Have an escape route in mind.
- Stand at the side of the door; do not block a door.
- Maintain an open position: hands out of pockets, uncrossed arms and legs, hands visible.
- Call the person by name.
- If the person's voice is raised, speak softly and maintain a quiet, controlled voice.
- Remain calm; sit or stand still; do not fidget.
- Keep 5 to 7 feet of distance between you and the person.

- Do not touch, point, order, challenge, argue, plead, belittle, threaten, or intimidate the person.
- Never turn your back on the person.
- Match eye contact.
- If overtly threatening, some people will respond to being told firmly, "You may not harm me" or "You do not want to harm me" or "It's against the rules."
- If the behavior continues to escalate, throw something like a blanket or coat over the patient's head and run to get help.

Many other practical suggestions are available from experienced nurses like your instructor. This is a time to keep a cool, calculating head (function now, and shake later). Complete the exercise in the Try This: Evaluate Protection Against Potential Dangers box.

 Try This

Evaluate Protection Against Potential Dangers

Do the health care agencies where you receive your clinical experience train their employees in management of assault behavior and/or gentle self-defense? Are assaults at this facility reported to the police? Under what circumstances are charges pressed against the perpetrator?

Investigate where in your nursing program you learn about identifying signs of possible danger to you and techniques of gentle self-defense to protect yourself.

? **Critical Thinking**

Preventing Possible Assault

Depending on what you discovered in the previous learning exercise, make a plan for learning what you need to know to better protect yourself from possible assault.

Professional Pointer

If you feel unsafe, follow your intuition and remove yourself from the situation (Pagana, 2008).

EMPLOYEE VIOLENCE

Workplace violence is classified according to the following four categories:

1. Employee: Violence is directed toward supervisors or management.
2. Domestic: The issue is personal, but the violent act takes place in the workplace.
3. Property: Violence is directed against the employee or employer's property.
4. Commercial: The employee engages in activities such as stealing from employers. Violence may ensue as a result of the activity.

Signs of Workplace Violence

Be alert to signs of violence. Early signs of workplace violence might include the following:

- Unusual behavioral change
- Lack of cooperation with nursing supervisors
- Cursing and other hostile forms of communication
- Short fuse and frequent arguments
- Spreading gossip or rumors to harm others deliberately
- Uninvited sexual remarks
- Hostile responses to other nurses, patients, or family members
- Sleep disturbances mentioned at work
- Increased irritability and anxiety

The next stage of violence might include the following signs:

- Conversation focused on "poor me, the victim"
- Notes with threats or violent or sexual content
- Verbalization that includes plans or a desire to harm someone
- Stealing workplace property
- Less interested in work and workplace assignments
- Increased arguments
- Increased physical accidents or injuries

As the anger intensifies, and if conflicts remain unresolved, the result can be violence against oneself or others:

- Behaviors directed toward oneself might include depression or suicidal threats.
- Behaviors directed toward others might include physical fighting, property destruction, or use of a weapon to harm others.

Prevention of Workplace Violence

Prevention entails management commitment and employee involvement.

- Prevention begins when each nurse makes a personal commitment to practice prevention guidelines.
- Participate in the training and refresher courses offered by the health care agency.
- Take advantage of programs offered by your police department or other agency.
- Remember that your focus is on *gentle self-defense*, not offense.
- Be prepared before workplace violence becomes an issue.
- There are policies in every workplace that cover forms of violence, as well as harassment. Check them out.
- Be alert to warning signs. Think through what you can do.
- **Take all threats seriously.** Report them to management.
- Advocate assertively for implementing prevention guidelines in the facility (Box 14-3).

Box 14-3 Some General Safeguards for Preventing Workplace Violence

- Do your part to promote a supportive, congenial, yet professional work environment.
- Whenever possible, resolve conflicts as they arise. Know that there are times when you have to back off. However, most of the time people want to have their point of view heard. A technique called *creative communication* encourages you to do the following:
  - Listen carefully to the other person's point of view.
  - Ask questions to clarify what you do not understand. (Remember that this step is not a sneaky way to argue or interject your own opinion!)
- Tell the person what you think he or she said and what you think he or she is feeling. If your version is inaccurate, have the person repeat the explanation. When you can repeat back accurately what the person thinks and feels, then it is your turn to present your view.
- Use these steps as well when you present your point of view.
- Deal directly with unwanted or unwelcome behavior, including uninvited sexual advances. Review your own behavior to determine whether:

- A clarification of the person's signals is in order.
- Limits must be stated clearly and firmly on what you consider unacceptable behavior.
- Supervisor or management intervention may be needed.
- Get to know your fellow workers, and look out for one another.
- Promote workplace integrity. Treat one another, your patients, and their families with respect, courtesy, and professionalism. Negative comments by patients and relatives usually are a response to their fear of the unknown. Rarely are the comments meant to be personal. Check out the fear. What are the questions? What can you do to help find answers?
- Be alert to changes in behavior that may signal violence.
- Avoid putting yourself in obvious danger. Make use of security guards for escorts to parking lots and out-of-the-way areas. Listen to your intuition. This is making conscious use of affective communication.

 Critical Thinking

Personal Violence Prevention Plan

What additional ideas do you have to put into action to defuse or prevent violence of any kind in the workplace? Create an assertive approach.

SEXUAL HARASSMENT

Sexual harassment is about abuse of power. It is not about sex or passion. More than 50% of female nurses report that they have been sexually harassed. However, it is not limited to female nurses. Nearly a third of male nurses and nursing administrators believe that they too have been sexually harassed (Kurz, 2002). Most nurses do not report the incidents, mostly from fear of losing their job, embarrassment, or fear that he or she will not be believed. According to the Equal Employment Opportunity Commission (EEOC), sexual harassment includes unwanted sexual advances or other verbal or physical conduct of a sexual nature, such as a condition of employment or advancement or a hostile environment, where the advances intimidate, offend, or interfere with the nurses' ability to do their work. The key word is "unwanted." A distinct difference is made between consent and unwanted.

If you are the target, confront the person who is harassing you. Your assertive response is to tell the person clearly what he or she is doing—that this behavior is offensive to you and is unwanted. Be sure that your response is firmly assertive. Your message must be congruent so that the verbalization, body language (nonverbal), and affective communication all say the same thing. Mere words do not justify a physical response on your part. Document for yourself what happened, as well as what you said and did. Employers have the responsibility to correct unwanted (unwelcome) behavior that they know about or should know about in the workplace. If the unwanted behavior does not cease, report it to the supervisor, union representative, or department head, as needed, until you are heard. Take along your documentation. If the employer is convinced that someone is harassing you, they can reprimand, require counseling, demote, transfer, deny a promotion or raise, or dismiss the harasser. The seriousness of sexual harassment can no longer be ignored. The nurse's work is usually affected, and some will even leave their jobs to get away from it. For others, their emotional and/or physical health is affected, sometimes with long-term consequences. Complete the exercises in the Try This: Sexual Harassment Policy, and Critical Thinking: Personal Plans for Safety boxes.

 Try This

Sexual Harassment Policy

Locate your school policy regarding sexual harassment.

 Critical Thinking

Personal Plans for Safety

Make a plan for yourself on how you will deal with any harassment attempts during future employment.

COUNSELING AND FILING CHARGES

Levine and colleagues (1998) concluded that assault-related injuries are preventable. Only physical injuries are treated; all employees who have been verbally or physically assaulted should be referred for postincident debriefing. Hospital managers should implement violence prevention programs. If you are harmed or threatened by a patient or a patient's family member, you have the option to file charges. Some agencies will do this for you after a review board hearing, or they will support you if you file charges yourself. Legal redress becomes an assertive stance for you and your fellow nurses (Carrol, 1997).

LATERAL VIOLENCE

Some of the worst attacks on nurses are from within their own medical community. The attacks range from nasty words and vicious threats to physical assaults. Many nurses accept the violence as the norm and do not report an attack to their supervisor.

Lateral violence occurs between nursing colleagues. It includes both overt and covert physical, verbal, and emotional abuse by one nurse against another. These are the most common forms of lateral violence:

* Nonverbal innuendo such as eye rolling or eyebrow raising intended to belittle another nurse
* Verbal affronts
* Undermining activities
* Withholding information
* Sabotage
* Infighting
* Scapegoating
* Backstabbing
* Failure to respect privacy
* Broken confidences (Jahner, 2011)

Bullying is described as acts perpetrated by one in a higher level of authority. It includes behaviors such as the following:

* Intimidation, malice, or insults
* Abuse of power by an individual or group against others

The behaviors are humiliating and threatening, and they can undermine self-confidence.

Vertical violence (horizontal hostility) occurs between persons of unequal power. For example, it might occur between a staff nurse and a student; a nurse manager and a student; an instructor and a student; or a new nurse and a seasoned staff nurse. The behavior humiliates and undermines confidence. The person who is bullied ends up feeling fearful and unsafe.

INSIDIOUS AGGRESSION

Insidious aggression, which is aggressive behavior in the workplace, is more harmful than sexual harassment. A study presented March 2008 at the International Conference on Work Stress and Health (Health Day, 2008) had reviewed 110 case studies over 21 years. According to the study:

* Agencies are more aware of sexual harassment, and it is lessening.
* Measures are being taken to recognize and prevent sexual harassment.
* Victims of sexual harassment find it easier to report incidences.
* Help is available to victims of sexual harassment.
* Insidious aggression is not against the law.

Issues of insidious aggression involve incivility, interpersonal issues, and hostile acts that are not obvious to others. For example, nurses do not generally report that they are not being invited to lunch by other staff or that a staff member is not speaking to them. This can result in more job stress, less job satisfaction, less job commitment, less satisfying relationships, higher levels of anger and anxiety, and lower levels of overall well-being. Individuals who are subjected to insidious aggression are more likely to quit their job.

A lack of action on the part of the nurse gives approval and permission for the perpetrator to continue the behavior. As a nurse, you have the responsibility to act assertively, with the cooperation of other nurses, to advocate for a safe workplace.

 Critical Thinking

Think of a time that you might have experienced insidious aggression. What were your feelings during that time? Did your quality of work suffer? Did the experience make a change in your health? How did you ultimately resolve the situation?

Get Ready for the NCLEX-PN® Examination

Key Points

* Communication translates into behavior.
* Assertiveness is honest and open behavior. It considers others' feelings and needs. It is based on choice.
* Nonassertive (passive) and aggressive behaviors are based on emotional hooks. These styles are ultimately damaging to both parties involved. Be alert to unresolved feelings leading to a cycle of worry → fear → anger → rage.
* Using the steps of the problem-solving process can change undesirable behaviors and interactions. Verbal, nonverbal, and affective interactions must be dealt with during this change.
* Some cultures value skillful positive manipulation. Positive manipulation involves consideration of others' needs and feelings. Other individuals are treated with respect rather than as objects to be used for personal gain.

- Violence in the workplace has always been there, but it is on the increase in some areas.
- OSHA has established national guidelines to deter violence toward health care workers.
- Nurses are physically assaulted more often than are police and prison guards.
- Violent incidents are more common when nurses and security lack assertive management skills.
- Some patient diagnoses provide clues to potential violence.
- Legal redress is available to nurses who are injured during physical violence.
- Both female and male nurses report sexual harassment as a condition for employment or advancement.
- Insidious aggression on the job includes incivility, interpersonal conflict, and bullying.
- Focusing on learning to be assertive in nursing benefits both you and the patient.
- According to Canadian researchers, insidious aggression on the job is more harmful than sexual harassment.

Additional Learning Resources

evolve   Go to your Evolve website (http://evolve.elsevier.com/Hill/Success) for the following FREE learning resources:
- Answers to Critical Thinking Scenarios
- Additional learning activities
- Additional Review Questions for the NCLEX-PN® exam
- Helpful phrases for communicating in Spanish and more!

Review Questions for the NCLEX-PN® Examination

1. What is assertiveness?
    1. A level of communication that few nurses attain.
    2. Outspoken, anger-based, honest communication.
    3. Indirect method of getting others to do what you wish.
    4. Taking a positive stand without violating others' rights.

2. Which of the following best describes sexual harassment?
    1. A coworker and you have been sharing sexual jokes since you started working.
    2. The immediate supervisor has asked you to spend a weekend together.
    3. A patient asks you if you are willing to go out on a date after he is discharged.
    4. Your coworker calls you at home after you have firmly refused to date him.

3. What is an assertive response to a boss who is beginning to talk to you about problems with another nurse on the unit?
    1. I am honored that you trust me to try to resolve this issue with you.
    2. Maybe you and I can meet over coffee after the shift so it will be more private.
    3. I'll talk to you about problems we have, but I won't discuss other persons with you.
    4. If you don't tell anyone of our conversation, I'll tell you what I know.

4. Which of the following recommendations will you offer the committee to promote unit safety?
    1. We need to look at staff attitude and body language in dealing with patients and visitors.
    2. Safety is an issue that must be placed in the hands of nonuniformed, outside security staff.
    3. It is necessary to go back to the strict visiting rules and limit hours and visitors to family.
    4. Violence is a part of our current culture, and there is very little you can do to effect change.

Alternate Format Item

1. Which of the following is not an example of an "I"-centered statement? *(Select all that apply.)*
    1. I feel you are not quite working up to your potential.
    2. I think that you could do your work a lot more carefully.
    3. I saw that you had a problem getting the patient in the chair.
    4. I will watch you demonstrate putting in a catheter today.

2. Which of the following are examples of insidious on-the-job aggression? *(Select all that apply.)*
    1. Another nurse interrupted me to tell the physician about my patient.
    2. I am assigned the heaviest patient on the unit for morning care.
    3. It seems no one has time to help me when I request help with a transfer.
    4. When I am asked to go to lunch with someone, I refuse and go off by myself.

Critical Thinking Scenarios

Scenario 1
Pat is an AD RN who had recently been appointed as unit manager in the Susan Nursing Home. The staff thought they had a winner: He is smart and outwardly charming to visitors and physicians. One day, Sara, an LPN, opened a door to a resident's room and heard Pat telling Mrs. B. in a sharp voice, "You are so stupid, and either you do as you're told or I will see to it that you are put out of the home." Neither Mrs. B. nor Pat heard her open the door, so Sara backed out quietly, unsure of what she should do. What are your options and the rationale for each option?

Scenario 2
Caroline is a newly licensed LPN. She is eager to do well in her new job at Dr. Smith's Medical Clinic. She is also trying hard to fit in with the rest of the staff: an APRN and a medical technologist. Caroline is responsible for greeting the patients, getting a brief statement of why they came in, measuring vitals and weight, and remembering to place the chart in the slot outside the door. What suggestions do you have as a former office nurse to help Caroline get started?

The Health Care Team: Where the Practical/Vocational Nurse Fits In

Objectives

On completing this chapter, you will be able to do the following:

1. Explain in your own words the goal of the health care team.
2. List 10 members of the health care team. (All levels of nurses count for only one member on your list.)
3. Identify the nursing personnel who are part of the health care team, according to the following criteria:
   a. Education
   b. Role and responsibilities
   c. Licensing
   d. Sites of employment
4. Define *nursing*.
5. Describe in your own words the following methods used to deliver nursing service:

   a. Case method
   b. Functional method
   c. Team method
   d. Primary care
   e. Case management method
6. Describe the practical/vocational nurse's role in the methods used to deliver the nursing services listed in objective number 5.
7. Describe how the philosophy of patient-centered care impacts nursing care.
8. Discuss how the hidden nursing shortage impacts jobs for the LPN/LVN.

Key Terms

advanced practice (ăd-VĂNSD PRĂK-tĭs, p. 183)
associate degree nursing (ă-SŌ-sē-ăt dĕ-GRE, p. 181)
bachelor's nursing program (p. 182)
case management method (kās MĂN-ăj-mĕnt, p. 188)
case method (kās, p. 187)
certification (SŬR-tĭ-fĭ-KĀ-shŭn, p. 183)
clerk receptionist (rĕ-SĔP-shŭ-nĭst, p. 186)
clinical pathway (care maps) (KLĬN-ĭ-kăl PĂTH-wāy, p. 188)
diploma program (dĭ-PLŌ-mă, p. 182)
functional method (FŬNK-shŭn-ăl, p. 187)
general supervision (p. 184)
independent (ĬN-dĕ-PĕN-dĕnt, p. 182)
interdependent (ĬN-tĕr-dĕ-PĕN-dĕnt, p. 182)
nurse manager (p. 179)

nursing assistant (NŬR-sĭng ă-SĬS-tĕnt, p. 186)
nursing case management (p. 188)
patient-centered care (PĀ-shĕnt SĔN-tĕrd, p. 190)
practical/vocational nurse (PRĂK-tĭ-kăl/vo-KĀ-shŭn-ăl, p. 179)
primary care method (PRĪ-măr-ē, p. 188)
registered nurse (RĔJ-ĭ-stĕrd, p. 181)
skill mix (skĭl mĭks, p. 188)
standards of care (STĂN-dĕrds, p. 182)
student nurse (STOO-dĕnt, p. 185)
team leader (p. 179)
team method (tēm, p. 187)
unit manager (YOO-nĭt MĂN-ăj-ĕr, p. 187)
unlicensed assistive personnel (UAP) (ŭn-LĬ-sĕnsd, p. 186)

 Keep in Mind

You can't tell the players without a program. Chapter 15 is your program to identify players on the health care team.

WHO IS RESPONSIBLE FOR MRS. BROWN'S DISCHARGE?

Mrs. Amelia Brown, age 75, lives with her daughter on a 200-acre farm in rural Wisconsin. While working in the barn, Mrs. Brown fell and broke her right hip. She required surgery to repair the hip. Under general

anesthesia during surgery, Mrs. Brown's blood pressure reached dangerously high levels, but it quickly stabilized under the anesthesiologist's interventions. Despite this setback, Mrs. Brown was discharged after 3 days in the hospital. She and her family agreed that she was not ready to return home at that point in her recovery, so she was discharged to an extended-care facility, where she was given physical therapy to learn how to function at home with her restrictions in ambulation. Two weeks later, Mrs. Brown was discharged from the extended-care facility to her home.

This sounds like just another success story for nursing, doesn't it? We will follow Mrs. Brown as she progresses through the health care system and then decide who should get credit for Mrs. Brown's discharge back to the farm.

MRS. BROWN'S EMERGENCY CARE

After Mrs. Brown falls, her daughter calls the emergency squad to transport her mother to the nearest hospital. The hospital is located 20 miles away in a city with a population of 98,000. The three people manning the emergency squad are *emergency medical technicians* (EMTs). Each EMT has taken an approximately 150-hour course in basic life support skills and has been certified as an EMT after passing a national test. The EMTs are currently taking an 18- to 24-month paramedic course, which is preparing them to provide more advanced life support skills. On the way to the hospital, the EMTs monitor Mrs. Brown's blood pressure, pulse, respirations, and level of consciousness. They keep her right leg immobilized. The EMTs maintain contact with the hospital emergency room by means of a two-way radio.

On arriving at the *emergency room* (ER), the EMTs provide the *registered nurse* (RN) with verbal and written reports of Mrs. Brown's status. The emergency room doctor examines Mrs. Brown and orders an x-ray film of her right hip. The *x-ray technician* brings the x-ray equipment to the ER and takes an x-ray film of Mrs. Brown's right hip. This x-ray technician has taken a 2-year program conducted by a hospital or technical college to prepare her to perform diagnostic measures involving radiant energy. The *radiologist* on duty reads the x-ray film of Mrs. Brown's right hip. On the basis of the physical examination and the results of the x-ray, the ER physician diagnoses a fracture of Mrs. Brown's right proximal femur. The ER physician notifies Mrs. Brown's *family physician* and contacts the *orthopedic surgeon* whom Mrs. Brown requests.

The RN receives Mrs. Brown in the ER, assesses her, and provides care until she is admitted to the hospital. The RN is a graduate of a diploma or 3-year program in nursing. This nurse has passed a national examination to become an RN. RNs who work in the ER participate regularly in continuing education courses at the hospital and at seminars given regionally and nationally for ER nurses. Mrs. Brown's RN prepares her for surgery.

To be qualified to be in charge of the medical care of Mrs. Brown, the family physician has attended 4 years of college, 4 years of medical school, 1 year of internship, and approximately a 3-year residency program. Medical school consists of a program that provides the basic knowledge and skills needed to be a medical doctor. Internship involves a program of clinical experiences designed to complete the requirements for licensure as a practicing physician. The residency program prepares physicians for practice in a specialty. The specialty in this situation is family practice. The ER physician, the radiologist, and the orthopedic surgeon

have had the same education as the family physician, up to the residency experience. The ER physician has completed a residency program in emergency or trauma medicine. The radiologist has completed a residency program in the reading and interpretation of x-ray films. The orthopedic surgeon has completed a 3- to 5-year residency in performing surgery for problems of bones and joints. Each of these physicians has passed the board examinations, which licenses them as physicians and allows them to practice under the state medical practice act. Each physician in this scenario is board certified in his or her specialty area.

Laboratory studies are ordered preoperatively. *Lab personnel* draw blood for these studies. Lab personnel have varied educational backgrounds. Some have on-the-job training to obtain blood samples. A medical lab technician has 2 years of education. A medical technologist (MT) has more than 4 years of education and can be certified by a national examination. Lab personnel are responsible for collecting the specimens needed for lab tests, performing the tests, and reporting the results to physicians and staff.

The family members request that their parish *priest* be contacted to give Mrs. Brown the sacrament of the sick (see Chapter 17). Because surgery is imminent, the pastoral care department is notified. A Roman Catholic priest, a member of the pastoral care team, anoints Mrs. Brown with holy oils, prays with her, and gives her Holy Communion. To be able to meet Mrs. Brown's spiritual needs, the priest has had 4 years of college and 4 years of theological school before being ordained.

THE SURGICAL EXPERIENCE

In the ER the *anesthetist* prepares Mrs. Brown and her family for the anesthesia part of the surgical experience. This health care worker is an RN with a bachelor of science in nursing (BSN). This nurse has studied an additional 2 to 3 years in an approved school of anesthesiology after the 4-year BSN program. The anesthetist provides anesthesia to patients undergoing surgery. Mrs. Brown is transferred to the surgical suite, where she undergoes a right hip pinning procedure under general anesthesia. This type of anesthesia will put Mrs. Brown in a state of unconsciousness. During surgery, the anesthetist monitors Mrs. Brown's vital signs continuously while she is unconscious. The *surgical technician* assists the orthopedic surgeon. The surgical technician sets up the sterile environment in the operating room. This health care worker makes sure the surgeon's instruments and supplies are available when he requests them for the pinning of Mrs. Brown's right hip. The surgical technician is a graduate of a 1-year *diploma program* at a local technical college. The professional nurse, who has a minimum qualification of a BSN, coordinates the overall functioning of the surgical team.

During surgery, the anesthetist notes that Mrs. Brown's blood pressure is rising to a dangerous level. She contacts the anesthesiologist STAT (i.e., immediately!). The *anesthesiologist*, a medical doctor with a residency in anesthesiology, orders antihypertensive drugs (i.e., drugs that lower the blood pressure). The situation is quickly brought under control. Surgery is completed, and Mrs. Brown is sent to the postanesthesia care unit (PACU).

POSTANESTHESIA CARE UNIT

The purpose of the PACU is to monitor the patient's vital signs, level of consciousness, movement, and any special equipment required by patients after surgery. When patients' conditions are stable, they are transferred to their hospital room. A PACU registered nurse, who is a graduate of a 3-year school of nursing program, assesses Mrs. Brown. After 1.5 hours, Mrs. Brown is assessed as being ready to leave the PACU. Because of the episode involving high blood pressure during surgery, Mrs. Brown's surgeon orders her to go to the intensive care unit (ICU) overnight for closer observation instead of to the postoperative surgical floor. A *transport aide*, who is trained on the job, and a *staff nurse* from the PACU take Mrs. Brown to the ICU.

INTENSIVE CARE: A TIME FOR CLOSE OBSERVATION

The ICU is staffed by RNs who went to school for 2 years (associate degree nurses), 3 years (diploma nurses), or 4 years (bachelor's degree nurses). Each nurse has taken the same national examination to become an RN. None of these nurses are qualified to work in the ICU immediately after graduation from their nursing programs. Most institutions prepare a nurse for the responsibilities of this unit through in-service classes after a minimum amount of experience or through a postgraduate or continuing education course. Mrs. Brown's nurse, a *2-year graduate*, is responsible for the care and observation of two patients.

The family is unable to answer some additional questions about Mrs. Brown's medical history. The family physician asks the *clerk receptionist* (*ward clerk*) to obtain Mrs. Brown's medical records from the medical records department. The clerk receptionist assumes the responsibility for many of the clerical duties that are a necessary part of any patient care area. The clerk receptionist learns these skills by taking a course that varies in length, depending on the area of the country. The course averages approximately one semester of theory and clinical experience. The *medical records department* is staffed by personnel who have gone to school for 2 to 6 years to learn the skills required for indexing, recording, and storing patient records, which are legal documents. Thanks to Mrs. Brown's old records, which are sent to the ICU, the family physician receives answers to his medical questions.

The surgeon writes postoperative orders for Mrs. Brown, including an order for patient-controlled analgesia (PCA) to control postoperative pain. The hospital *pharmacist* has studied for a minimum of 8 years to become licensed to prepare, compound, and dispense drugs prescribed by a physician or dentist. The pharmacist fills the order for Mrs. Brown's drugs and intravenous solutions.

The *respiratory therapy department* is contacted to evaluate Mrs. Brown's respiratory status and suggest treatment to prevent respiratory problems. Certified respiratory therapists (CRTs) are graduates of 2-year programs in respiratory therapy and have passed a certifying examination. Registered respiratory therapists (RRTs) are graduates of associate degree or 4-year college programs in respiratory therapy and have taken three examinations to register. Within 24 hours of admission to the ICU, Mrs. Brown is judged to be in stable condition. A *transport aide* and an *ICU staff member* transfer her to the surgical floor.

SURGICAL FLOOR: AN EYE TO DISCHARGE

The nurse manager on the surgical floor at this hospital is an RN who has graduated from a 4-year nursing program. As manager of the unit, this nurse is responsible for all the care given to patients. Mrs. Brown's team leader is an RN from a 2-year nursing program. This nurse is responsible for formulating a plan of care for each of the assigned patients and modifying these plans as needed.

The team leader receives a verbal report and the current care plan for Mrs. Brown from the ICU personnel. The team leader begins assessment of her new admission. The practical/vocational nurse (LPN/LVN) helps put Mrs. Brown to bed and immediately takes her vital signs. The LPN/LVN is a graduate of a 1-year vocational program in nursing. The LPN/LVN has taken a national examination to become licensed as a practical/vocational nurse. The practical/vocational nurse is assigned to give Mrs. Brown bedside care.

A referral is sent to the physical therapy department. The *physical therapist* (PT) assesses the strength of Mrs. Brown's unaffected extremities. The PT sets up a program of exercises and ambulation with no weight bearing on the right extremity. The goal of treatment is to restore function and prevent the development of complications. Physical therapy keeps up the strength of Mrs. Brown's unaffected extremity until she is able to bear weight fully on the right side. The PT has been educated in a 4- or 5-year college program. Some PTs have a master's degree in physical therapy. The *physical therapy assistant* (PTA) has been educated in a 2-year community college or technical school setting. The PTA carries out the plan of care developed by the PT.

Soon after the patient is transferred to the surgical floor, the *social worker* visits Mrs. Brown and her family to discuss discharge plans. The social worker suggests that Mrs. Brown stay in an extended-care facility for 2 weeks to participate in extensive physical therapy before returning to the farm. Social workers help patients and families solve problems with the financial concerns of hospitalization. They arrange for community agencies to provide appropriate care and services needed by patients after discharge from the hospital. Social workers also help the family communicate their health care needs more clearly. Social workers obtain a bachelor's degree in social work in 4 years and a master's degree in 1 additional year of college. Mrs. Brown's social worker talks to the PT and the family. All agree that with exercise and skills teaching, the family eventually will be able to care for Mrs. Brown at home.

As the time for discharge to the extended-care facility gets closer, a *patient care technologist* (PCT) is assigned to take Mrs. Brown's vital signs. PCTs perform treatments and skills assigned to them by the RN or the LPN/LVN. PCTs are trained by the hospital for the specific duties they are to perform. Training involves classes (sometimes autotutorial or self-study classes) and a clinical component. The training a PCT gets is short and varies among facilities. The job titles **unlicensed assistive personnel** (UAP), *nurse's aide, nursing assistant,* and *patient care assistant* are used in some facilities. The responsibilities of the LPN/LVN in relation to PCTs are discussed in Chapters 20 and 21.

Because Mrs. Brown is 50 pounds overweight, her physician orders a weight-reduction diet. The *dietitian* teaches Mrs. Brown and her daughter the elements of weight reduction that will be carried out when Mrs. Brown returns to the farm. A hospital's dietitian is responsible for planning the meals and supplementary feedings for patients and the cafeteria meals for staff. The dietitian also supervises the preparation of food and counsels patients and their families about nutritional problems and therapeutic diets. This health professional is educated in a 4- to 5-year college program, followed by a year of internship in a health care agency.

The *housekeeper* cleans Mrs. Brown's room and bathroom every day of her stay. Maintaining cleanliness is an effort to maintain medical asepsis (absence of germs) and to provide a pleasant environment. The housekeeper receives training in the needed skills by the employing institution or through a short course in a technical school.

Finally, Mrs. Brown is discharged from the hospital. She leaves by *Medi-Van* and is transported to the extended-care facility.

EXTENDED-CARE UNIT: ON THE ROAD TO REHABILITATION

Mrs. Brown's roommate in the extended-care facility is an 80-year-old woman who has had a stroke. The roommate is also preparing to go home after additional physical therapy. The *PT* conducts an initial assessment of Mrs. Brown and incorporates the hospital physical therapy plan of care with her findings. The *PTA* helps Mrs. Brown daily with exercises and ambulation, using a walker, and minimum weight bearing on her right leg. A *nursing assistant* (NA) is assigned to assist Mrs. Brown with her personal care. NAs are educated to give bedside care through courses of a minimum of 75 hours. Successful completion of this course of study makes the NA eligible to be placed on the state registry as a certified nursing assistant (CNA).

A referral is sent to the occupational therapy department. The *occupational therapist* (OT) completes an assessment of Mrs. Brown. The *occupational therapy assistant* (OTA) carries out the plan of care. The goal for Mrs. Brown is to be as *independent* as possible when she returns to the farm, despite her physical limitations. Occupational therapy helps patients restore body function through specific tasks and skills. Educational requirements include a 4-year occupational therapy program. Some 4-year graduates pursue a master's degree in their field. A 2-year program prepares OTAs for their roles.

Mrs. Brown receives her newly prescribed blood pressure medication from the *practical/vocational nurse,* who also is functioning in her expanded role as charge nurse in this facility. The *day supervisor,* an RN with a BSN, checks Mrs. Brown daily to monitor her progress. Ten days later, Mrs. Brown excitedly waits for her family to take her back to the farm. She is pleased with her progress and is confident about going back to her home. She knows that at this time she is unable to gather the eggs each day, but she is anxious to get back in the kitchen.

? Critical Thinking

Who Is Responsible for Mrs. Brown's Recovery?

Who is responsible for Mrs. Brown's return to the farm?

HEALTH CARE TEAM

A primary goal of health care is to restore optimal physical, emotional, and spiritual health to patients. This goal is accomplished by promoting health, preventing further illness, and restoring health when illness or accident has occurred. Health care includes a large number of specialized services. It is necessary for these health care workers to work together to integrate care that will provide patients with all the services they need to maintain safe, quality, comprehensive health care. These groups of health care workers are called the *health care team.*

For Mrs. Brown to be rehabilitated after her fall, it took a minimum of 127 years of education for all the health care workers in this scenario to learn how to perform their respective jobs. The x-ray technician's x-ray film confirmed the presence of a hip fracture. The pharmacist supplied the narcotic pain reliever that relieved pain after the surgical procedure, allowing Mrs. Brown to move more freely and avoid complications. The treatment by the RRT helped prevent pneumonia. The PTs, OTs, and nursing staff all helped restore Mrs. Brown's health and prevent further illness by avoiding complications. The dietitian's expertise allowed Mrs. Brown to receive the basic nutrients she needed to maintain her health, heal her fracture, and lose weight. Teaching about weight-reduction diets promoted health by pointing out the importance of keeping Mrs. Brown's weight within acceptable limits.

As you can see from Mrs. Brown's case, each member of the health care team, because of his or her specific preparation in a field of study, can increase the quality of health care for a patient. It is impossible for one person to provide the knowledge, expertise, and skills that the health care team as a whole can provide. Everyone needs to work together. It is a team effort.

The members of the health care team are generally on duty in acute or residential health care organizations 24 hours a day, 7 days a week. Some members of the health care team may not be scheduled at night or on weekends or holidays, and some of these persons are available on an on-call basis. In the community, health care workers' hours vary depending on the site of employment. Some sites are open Monday through Friday, during day hours only, whereas others also offer services in the evening. Other sites are open 7 days a week and sometimes 24 hours a day.

Each member of the health care team needs to have good communication skills. Good communication ensures that care is coordinated for the patient's benefit (see Chapter 13). Fragmentation of care can be avoided. Each health care team member has to be able to anticipate problems and avoid them when possible. This is accomplished by using critical-thinking skills. When problems do occur, the health care team needs to use problem-solving skills to find solutions in the process of delivering care. In this way the quality of patient care is continuously improved. The team must strive continually to keep its care patient-centered. The team needs to realize that a cooperative effort is needed to reach patient goals.

WHAT IS *NURSING*?

Virginia Henderson (1966), a nursing theorist, stated, "The unique function of the nurse is to assist the individual, sick or well, in the performance of those activities contributing to health or its recovery (or to peaceful death) that he would perform if he had the necessary strength, will, or knowledge." Henderson refers to nursing's interest in illness and wellness. The direction of practical/vocational nursing has

been channeled by this definition. For a definition of nursing Google *Nursing's Social Policy Statement of the American Nurses Association* @ ANA.org.

It is necessary for practical/vocational nurses to understand their role in Mrs. Brown's care. An understanding of the education, licensure, roles, and responsibilities of the varied members of the health care team is also necessary

NURSING'S PLACE ON THE HEALTH CARE TEAM

Nursing staff on the health care team includes *unit managers, RNs, LPNs/LVNs, student nurses, NAs,* and *cross-trained staff.* UAPs assist the nursing staff. Clerk receptionists, although not nurses, are an important part of the unit staff. Most people are unaware of the different types of nurses on the health care team. Sadly, some RNs do not know the educational requirements for LPNs/LVNs, and some LPNs/LVNs do not know what education professional nursing entails. A common question from the public is "What is the difference between a registered nurse and a licensed practical/vocational nurse?" Members of the health care team generally, and nursing specifically, need to know about one another. For this reason, general information about the education for and the many roles of registered nursing is provided in this section, which describes the members of the nursing team.

DIVERSITY IN EDUCATIONAL PREPARATION OF NURSES

REGISTERED NURSES

Education

Registered nurses (RNs) are the largest group of health care workers in the United States. About 3.1 million RNs work in the United States, and approximately 5.8% of them are men (HHS, 2004). The graduates of the three types of educational programs for professional nurses—2-, 3-, and 4-year programs—currently take the same licensing examination. On successful completion of this examination, all these graduates hold the title of registered nurse.

Associate Degree Nursing Program
- An associate degree nursing (ADN) program is a 2-year educational program that can be found in community colleges, junior colleges, and technical schools.
- The ADN program includes general education courses (e.g., courses in the biologic, behavioral, and social sciences), nursing courses, and clinical practice.
- On graduation, the 2-year graduate receives an associate degree in nursing and is eligible to take the NCLEX-RN® examination to become a registered nurse.

Diploma Program

- A **diploma program** is a 3-year educational program conducted by a hospital-based school of nursing.
- The diploma program comprises the same general education courses as 2-year programs, with nursing courses and clinical practice. Diploma programs traditionally have emphasized clinical experience.
- On graduation, the 3-year nursing graduate receives a diploma in nursing and is eligible to take the NCLEX-RN® examination to become a registered nurse.

Bachelor's Nursing Program

- A **bachelor's nursing program** is a 4-year nursing program that can be found in public and private colleges and universities.
- The bachelor's program emphasizes course work in the liberal arts, sciences, and nursing theory, including public health. Clinical practice is included.
- On graduation, the 4-year nurse receives a BSN and is eligible to take the NCLEX-RN® examination to become a registered nurse.

Role of Registered Nurses

Graduates of all three nursing programs are prepared for general duty staff nursing in a hospital or nursing home. Nursing education programs also prepare graduates of all three programs to function in a community-based, community-focused health care system. Although you may find 2- and 3-year RNs in supervisory and administrative positions, only bachelor's graduates have been prepared in their nursing education programs for advancement to these positions. Bachelor's graduates are also prepared for beginning positions in public health agencies.

Approximately 3% of new nurses graduate from diploma programs, 60% of new nurses graduate from associate degree programs, and 36% are graduates of bachelor's programs (Aiken, 2010). This education mix is expected to continue.

All RNs function under the Nurse Practice Act of the state in which they are working. RNs use the nursing process to identify patient problems, formulate nursing diagnoses, and plan and evaluate care. Standards of care are used instead of care plans in some acute care agencies. These standards include the priority nursing diagnosis for each patient, with appropriate assessments, nursing interventions, and expected outcomes (goals). Standards provide minimum guidelines for a consistent approach to delivering patient care. The RN uses standards as a reference when individualizing patient care.

Registered nurses assign routine care and the care of stable patients to assistive personnel. This allows RNs to do the following:

1. Plan care.
2. Coordinate all the activities of care.
3. Provide care that requires more specialized knowledge and judgment.
4. Teach patients, families, and other members of the health care team.
5. Act as a patient advocate.

Independent Role of the Registered Nurse. Registered nurses function independently in nursing, initiating and carrying out nursing activities. For example, to prevent complications in the respiratory and circulatory systems, RNs assess the patient on bed rest. They identify the need for a turning routine, deep breathing, leg exercises, and range-of-motion exercises. If not contraindicated by the patient's diagnosis and/or treatment, RNs add these nursing interventions to ordered care. Because of their level of education, RNs can identify which patients can and cannot receive these nursing interventions. In the community, RNs will initiate dietitian and social worker referrals. *It is the **independent** role in decision making that distinguishes RNs from LPNs/LVNs.* Registered nurses have the ultimate responsibility for the care given to patients.

Interdependent Role of the Registered Nurse. When RNs carry out the legal orders of another health professional (e.g., the physician or physical therapist), they are functioning in an interdependent role. Often, RNs function interdependently (collaboratively) when carrying out decisions about patient care that are made jointly by members of the health care team.

Education In Addition to the Basic Nursing Programs for Registered Nurses

The postgraduate educational opportunities available to RNs are presented here to explain the various RNs found on the health care team.

BSN Completion Program. After passing the NCLEX-RN® examination, associate degree and diploma graduates can enroll in a program that will grant a BSN. Programs vary in length, content, and mode of delivery, including online programs.

Accelerated BSN Program. Individuals with an undergraduate degree in another discipline can earn a bachelor of science degree in nursing in approximately 15 months. The 15-month program is very intensive, and when completed, the student is eligible to take the NCLEX-RN® examination.

Master of Nursing Programs. Master's of science in nursing programs prepare registered nurses for a specialty area in nursing, such as medical-surgical, pediatrics, management, nursing education, psychiatric/mental health, and geriatrics. The MSN is a requirement for teaching in associate degree programs. Generally, nurses with BSN degrees are the only nursing graduates who may elect to do graduate work in nursing at the master's and doctoral levels. However, MSN programs exist that offer an MSN degree to nurses with an undergraduate degree in an area other than nursing. The MSN then becomes the entry degree into nursing.

Certification. Passing the NCLEX-RN® examination provides initial licensure in nursing and ensures basic competence for entry into nursing practice. After gaining work experience, RNs can receive certification from numerous professional nursing groups. The certificate that is awarded after passing a comprehensive examination indicates that the nurse has demonstrated competence in a select area of practice. The American Nurses Credentialing Center (ANCC), a subsidiary of the American Nurses Association (ANA), makes certification available to all RNs. There is no difference in credentials based on type of RN educational program from which one is a graduate for basic specialty certification. All basic specialty-certified nurses are board certified (AACN Nurse Certification, 2011). The requirement of a master's degree in nursing remains for certification as an advanced practice registered nurse. Because certification needs to be renewed periodically, certification through ANCC allows the registered nurse to demonstrate ongoing competence in a selected area of nursing. A move in nursing is currently underway to shift the standard for qualification to be an APRN to that of a doctorate in nursing practice (DNP) by 2015 (ANA, 2011).

Advanced Practice Registered Nurse. With an additional degree, RNs can pursue expanded roles, called *advanced practice.* These nurses acquire specialized nursing knowledge and skills and demonstrate a greater depth and breadth of nursing knowledge and an increased complexity of skills and interventions. The term *advanced practice registered nurse* (APRN) identifies the advanced practice roles of a clinical nurse specialist, a nurse practitioner, a nurse anesthetist, and a certified nurse-midwife. Each of these nurses has a minimum of a master's of science degree in nursing (MSN), obtained in a 1- to 2-year program of study.

- **Clinical nurse specialist (CNS).** This registered nurse has a minimum of an MSN in a specialty area (e.g., medical-surgical nursing). The CNS is a clinical expert in nursing practice based on the latest research and has certification as a clinical nurse specialist. When employed by acute care organizations, the CNS serves as a mentor, role model, and resource person for staff by setting standards for nursing care. The CNS provides direct care in challenging patient situations and shares knowledge, experiences, and resources with staff. The CNS also is employed by clinics, nursing homes, nursing schools as instructors, and in other community settings. In all sites of employment the CNS also serves as an educator, consultant, researcher, and administrator.

- **Nurse practitioner (NP).** This registered nurse has a minimum of an MSN and certification by a national body. There are many areas of specialization for nurse practitioners, such as family (FNP), geriatrics, pediatrics (PNP), primary, or acute care. Some NPs provide primary care in the community in physicians' clinics or in their own offices. Others provide acute care services in hospitals and nursing homes. NPs order and interpret lab and diagnostic tests, develop diagnoses, and prescribe treatments, including drugs, for acute and chronic diseases. Their care differs from medical care because of their interest in and awareness of psychosocial aspects of illness.

- **Certified nurse-midwife (CNM).** This registered nurse has a minimum of an MSN and certification as a nurse-midwife. The CNM provides holistic maternal/family-centered health care in the area of prenatal low-risk pregnancy, childbirth, the postpartum period, care of the newborn, and family planning at home, in hospitals, and birthing centers and in the gynecologic care of women. They diagnose and treat illness, including prescribing drugs.

- **Certified registered nurse anesthetist (CRNA).** This registered nurse has a minimum of an MSN, is a graduate of an accredited nurse anesthesia educational program, and has certification as a nurse anesthetist. CRNAs work in every setting where anesthesia is given: operating rooms, clinics, and outpatient surgical centers. They prepare patients for anesthesia; induce and maintain local, regional, and general anesthesia; provide postanesthesia care, including pain management; and provide emergency resuscitation.

The American Association of Colleges of Nursing (AACN) developed a clinical nurse leader (CNL) role that requires a master's or postmaster's CNL program of study that makes one eligible for the AACN CNL certification exam. This evolving advanced generalist role was developed to educate clinicians as leaders. The CNL oversees the care coordination of a distinct group of patients and actively provides direct patient care in complex situations (see AACN.org).

Doctoral Nursing Education. There are two types of doctoral programs in nursing:

- Research-focused: These programs lead to an academic doctorate (Ph.D.) or professional doctorate (DNS or DNSc). Graduates are prepared as a scientist and do rigorous investigation into, for example, clinical or educational issues, to help build the science of nursing (NLN, 2010).

- Practice-focused (DNP): These evolving programs graduate nurses who are considered nursing's expert clinicians (nurses working in health care agencies) and most effective practice leaders who will promote and facilitate changes in practice that enhance quality care (NLN, 2010).

Nursing Management, Leadership, and Executive Roles

The twenty-first-century health care system requires nursing managers who also possess leadership skills. These nurses possess the ability to develop a shared vision with nursing staff of quality, safety, and cost control that will help improve outcomes in patient care. The four levels of nursing management are supervisor, nurse manager, director, and chief nursing officer (CNO) (Box 15-1). The practical/vocational nurse's role as charge nurse is discussed in Chapters 20 and 21.

 Try This

Get to Know the Nursing Team

During an unhurried moment in the clinical area, ask the RN with whom you are working about the educational requirements to be employed for his or her position. If there are initials behind his or her name, ask for them to be explained.

PRACTICAL/VOCATIONAL NURSES

Background

Since little information about the exact number of licensed practical/vocational nurses can be found in the literature, information needs to be extracted from other information. Licensed practical/vocational nurses held about 753,600 jobs in 2008 (Bureau of Labor Statistics, 2010-11) and are the second-largest group of licensed health care workers in the United States. In 2009, 12.1% of newly licensed LPNs/LVNs were males (National Council of State Boards of Nursing, 2009).

Box 15-1   Nursing Management and Executive Roles

Supervisor: BSN preferred; deals with specific problems with nursing personnel; makes rounds to all nursing units on assigned shift to ensure patients' needs are met according to organization's procedures; clinical resource.

Nurse manager: Middle management position; MSN preferred; leader of a specific clinical department—for example, medical services; responsible for personnel, quality of care, safety, and cost of running department.

Director: Entry level of executive role; MSN or master's degree in business or health-related field required; coordinates the development and implementation of strategies to initiate new programs and improve current services of several departments.

Chief nursing officer (CNO): Highest-ranking administrative nurse in a health care organization; MSN, master's in business or health-related field required; doctorate may be required in larger organizations; organizes and coordinates the nursing department; responsible for excellence in nursing that is consistent with the mission, vision, and values of the organization.

Source: Hader R. (2009). Is being a chief nursing officer in your future? NSNA imprint. Retrieved on July 24, 2011, from www.nsna.org.

Education

The educational program for practical/vocational nurses varies from 9 to 18 months. The practical/vocational nursing program is found in trade, technical, and vocational schools, as well as community colleges. These institutions are usually public, tax-supported institutions. Practical/vocational nursing programs are also found in private schools.

Practical/vocational nurse education concentrates on clinical care at the bedside, based on fundamentals of biologic sciences. Courses in basic nursing care, the behavioral sciences, and the biologic sciences are included. Basic nursing care includes the administration of medications. Critical thinking is stressed, and the practical/vocational nurse's assisting role in the nursing process is included in all phases of the nursing program, as determined by each state's Nurse Practice Act. Clinical experience in acute care facilities, extended care facilities, and the community is included. On graduation, the practical/vocational nurse receives a diploma in practical nursing and is eligible to take the NCLEX-PN® examination to become an LPN/LVN.

Role of Practical/Vocational Nurses

Practical/vocational nurses must be aware of the content of the Nurse Practice Act of the state in which they are employed. The LPN/LVN's role and scope of practice is found in this law, and the law differs from state to state. Administrative rules and regulations and interpretations of the state's Board of Nursing provide more *specific* details and clarification. Some NPAs list specifically what LPNs/LVNs can do, but others are written more broadly to allow for changes in the evolving role of the LPN/LVN. This eliminates the need for state legislatures to reopen the act and revise it each time a change is required. It is your responsibility to be aware of the law of the state in which you are employed. Generally, the role of the LPN/LVN includes the following:

- Cares for patients within the scope of the state's NPA while upholding clinical standards.
- Regardless of the site of employment, provides care in basic and complex patient situations under the general supervision of an RN, physician, podiatrist, or dentist, as determined by the state Nurse Practice Act.
- Provides safe patient care, serves as a patient advocate, teaches patients, and communicates effectively, all while functioning as a collaborative member of the health care team.

Employers expect practical/vocational nurses to think critically and solve problems in patient care situations. Practical/vocational nurses function interdependently when they offer input to the RN about the effectiveness of patient care or offer suggestions to improve care. When practical/vocational nurses provide actual care at the bedside in acute care situations, their collection of data while engaged in giving care is valuable in determining whether progress is being made to meet patient outcomes.

A major criterion in differentiating between the roles of the registered and practical/vocational nurse is that the practical/vocational nurse does not function independently. Practical/vocational nurses must function safely and are accountable for their actions. They function interdependently (collaboratively) with other members of the health care team, but the LPN/LVN role is basically a dependent role. They should assume responsibility only for nursing actions that are within their legal role and that they feel competent in carrying out. Table 15-1 identifies the differences between the LPN/LVN and the RN roles.

 Critical Thinking

The LPN/LVN Role in Assisting with the Nursing Process

Identify the major difference between the RN's and LPN/LVN's roles in the nursing process. How is the LPN/LVN's role in the nursing process determined?

Expanded Role of Practical/Vocational Nurses

In some settings practical/vocational nurses are being used in their expanded role. An example of the expanded role of the practical/vocational nurse is the charge nurse position in nursing homes/long-term care facilities. During implementation of care by the LPN/LVN, the RN is available to help in decision making when questions arise, either on-site (direct supervision) or by phone (general supervision). See Chapters 20 and 21 for further discussion of the expanded role of the LPN/LVN.

 Critical Thinking

Expanded Role of the LPN/LVN

Refer to your state's Nurse Practice Act. List the circumstances under which you may function with the direct or general supervision of an RN and in your expanded role.

STUDENT NURSES

Student professional and practical/vocational nurses come to the clinical area under the supervision of clinical instructors. The clinical area is an extension of the classroom. It provides an opportunity to apply theory to practice. When assigned to patients, these student nurses have a responsibility to give safe care and function responsibly under the supervision of the instructor. Students are in the clinical area to learn, not to give service. It is possible that a clinical instructor can remove students from the assigned clinical site at any time for additional learning experiences.

Table 15-1   Differences Between the Roles of RNs and LPNs/LVNs

FIVE NURSING ROLES	ROLES OF RN AND LPN/LVN
1. PROFESSIONAL	
RN	Belongs to and is actively involved in ANA at state and local levels.
LPN/LVN	Belongs to and is involved in NFLPN and/or NAPNES at state and local levels (see Chapter 24).
2. PROVIDER OF CARE	
RN	This is an independent role. Initiates all phases of nursing process; formulates nursing diagnoses.
LPN/LVN	This is a dependent and interdependent role. Assists with all phases of the nursing process. Works with established nursing diagnoses. Identifies possible new nursing problems and reports same to RN.
3. MANAGER OF CARE	
RN	Controls decisions regarding staff and care of patients.
LPN/LVN	First-line manager in nursing home/extended care. Responsible to RN nurse manager.
4. TEACHER	
RN	Initiates all health teaching.
LPN/LVN	Initiates health teaching for basic health habits (e.g., nutrition and cleanliness). Reinforces health teaching of RN in other areas.
5. RESEARCHER	
RN	Theory included in 4-year program. All levels interpret and implement evidence-based practice guidelines. Participates in the research process.
LPN/LVN	Assists in implementing evidence-based practice guidelines. Collects data, as instructed, for research studies.

Students are members of the health care team. They are expected to assist other team members in addition to performing their patient assignment. Examples of such assistance include passing trays, answering call lights in acute care and long-term care situations, and assisting patients and staff in the community. These activities help students learn how to get along in a team situation.

Student practical/vocational nurses are responsible for giving the same safe nursing care that licensed practical/vocational nurses provide. This is a legal matter. Therefore, the student role demands preparation and supervision.

NURSING ASSISTANTS

Nursing assistants (NAs) are trained for their positions by combining federally mandated classroom instruction with close supervision by RNs while in the clinical area. Vocational schools offer programs that last a minimum of 75 hours and are up to 12 weeks in length. These programs combine classroom or autotutorial instruction with clinical practice. During the course, testing for competence occurs to meet federal Omnibus Budget Reconciliation Act (OBRA) requirements. When test results are satisfactory, the names of NAs are placed in a registry.

NAs function under the direction of registered or practical/vocational nurses. NAs who work in hospitals, nursing homes, extended care units, or psychiatric hospitals assist in providing personal and comfort needs for stable patients. They are assigned routine tasks, sometimes involving housekeeping chores. A large number of NAs are employed by nursing homes. The supply of NAs does not meet the demands of employers. People in some areas of the country refer to male NAs as orderlies.

Some states offer an advanced NA course that teaches more complex skills. These skills include many that are performed by the practical/vocational nurse. The demand for home health care workers continues to increase. NAs are allowed to perform a wider variety of skills in the home as home health care workers. Some states offer a postgraduate course for NAs to prepare them for the transition to home care. The comprehensive home care program may also be available to individuals without NA experience.

 Keep in Mind

Diversity of Age for Coworkers on the Nursing Team

In addition to a diversity of educational preparation, the nursing team needs to contend with four generations of its members. Four generations of personnel on the nursing team can have different goals, priorities, and work preferences (Yoder-Wise, 2011). Awareness and understanding of these differences is necessary for successful communication and working as a team. Box 15-2 lists the worker characteristics of these team members.

Box 15-2   The Four Generations of Nursing Teams

MATURES
- Are team players.
- Have years of knowledge to share.
- Work hard and are stoic (patient and enduring) when faced with higher workloads.
- Are loyal to the organization.

BOOMERS—77 MILLION IN THE WORKFORCE
- Are team workers.
- Have years of knowledge to share; hold most nursing leadership positions.
- Are highly motivated and driven; willing to work long hours to get the job done no matter what (workaholics).
- Work takes priority over family; may experience physical stress and family–work conflict (may need to care for aging parents).

GENERATION X—44 MILLION IN THE WORKFORCE
- Prefer working independently (value self-reliance).
- Seek balance among work, family, and leisure; avoid overtime ("My kids have a soccer game").
- Do not have as much emphasis on career and employer loyalty.
- Stay in job as long as something benefits them.

GENERATION Y—70 MILLION IN THE WORKFORCE
- Have a team orientation.
- Like excitement in work and to have fun at work; dress more casually.
- Choose where and when to work; life/work balance.
- Want input about decisions that affect them.

Data from Halfer D, Saver C. Bridging the generation gaps. *Nursing Spectrum/Nurse Week.* Retrieved June 8, 2008, from http://www.nurse.com/ce/print.html?CCID=4533; Hartner K. Generational diversity. *ADVANCE Newsmagazines for LPNs.* Retrieved September 20, 2007, from http://lpn.advanceweb.com/Common/Editorial/PrintFriendly.aspx; Olson M. The Millennials: first year in practice. *Nursing Outlook* (57)1: 10-17; Billings D, Halstead J. (2009). *Teaching in nursing: a guide for faculty.* St Louis: Elsevier; Yoder-Wise P. (2011). *Leading and managing in nursing.* St Louis: Elsevier.

UNLICENSED ASSISTIVE PERSONNEL

In an effort to use health care workers more efficiently and effectively, health care organizations have added another level of worker to the health care team. Unlicensed assistive personnel (UAP) are trained by health care organizations to function in an assistive role to RNs and LPNs/LVNs. Some health care organizations require applicants for UAP positions to be registered as NAs. These workers learn selected skills, sometimes by the autotutorial method or module method, combined with some clinical teaching. Actual skills learned depend on which skills are needed in specific patient care units. UAPs are also known by the terms *patient care technician, patient care associate, care pair, nurse extender,* and *multiskilled worker.*

CLERK RECEPTIONISTS

The job of the clerk receptionist is mainly secretarial in nature, but the duties vary from site to site. With the clerk performing this job, nurses are freed from much of the paperwork involved in patient care. Clerk receptionists are trained on the job or in programs of several months' duration in technical schools. Clerks prepare, compile, and maintain patient records on a nursing unit. Duties include transcribing physicians' orders; scheduling lab tests, x-ray procedures, and surgeries; scheduling other appointments for services; routing charts on patient transfers or discharges; compiling the patient census; answering the telephone; maintaining established inventories of supplies; distributing mail to patients; and generally ensuring that the unit functions smoothly.

UNIT MANAGERS

Some large health care organizations have unit managers to supervise and coordinate management functions for patient units. A college background and supervisory experience are desirable for this position. This job is combined with on-the-job training for specific duties. Responsibilities include budgeting, supervision of ward clerks, assignment and evaluation of clerical personnel, inventory of patient's valuables, coordination with housekeeping and maintenance, and clarification of hospital compliance with Medicare requirements. If a health care organization does not have unit managers, the clerk receptionist and the nurse manager assume these duties.

 Critical Thinking

Know Your Health Care Team

When on the clinical area, list the various members of the health care team with whom you have contact. Draw a concept map describing their role on the team and education required for their job.

DELIVERY OF NURSING CARE IN ACUTE CARE SETTINGS

With the goal of providing optimal care, the nursing team uses different methods to assign patients to staff. The methods evolved as a response to changing needs of the health care system, including staffing. Each of the methods is discussed in its general form as it was intended to function. Health care organizations modify these methods to fit their individual needs.

CASE METHOD

At the turn of the twentieth century, families hired nurses to meet a patient's special needs in the home. By the 1920s, private-duty nursing was popular. This case method of patient care continued in various degrees into the 1960s. Vestiges of the case method, or a one-to-one relationship with a patient, are found today in acute care situations as total care nursing (comprehensive care). In the case method, one nurse is assigned to one or two patients and is responsible

for planning, organizing, and carrying out the care for these patients. Today, total care nursing occurs in intensive care or special care units, as Mrs. Brown experienced in the ICU after she left the PACU. Nursing instructors frequently use the total patient care method when assigning beginning students to the acute care clinical area.

FUNCTIONAL NURSING

During World War II, the functional method was a popular method of patient assignment. Registered nurses were in scarce supply because of the war. Hospitals increased the number of LPNs/LVNs and NAs to provide care for patients. The functional method of patient care is task-oriented. The tasks that have to be done for patients are divided among the staff. For example, one person might measure all vital signs, another might do all treatments, and still another might make all the beds. This method's emphasis on efficiency and division of labor is based on the assembly line production concept found in industry.

The nursing home nearest Mrs. Brown's home schedules resident assignments by the functional method. An NA helped Mrs. Brown with her physical care. An LPN/LVN gave her medications and did her treatments. In addition to assuming responsibility for all care given to residents, the charge nurse, a practical/vocational nurse, would be kept busy with managerial (e.g., staff evaluations) and nonnursing duties (e.g., inventory of supplies).

Functional nursing can easily overlook holistic care, especially in the area of psychosocial needs. This results in fragmentation of care. Although this method is efficient and appears to be less costly to implement, it can discourage patient and staff satisfaction. The functional method, however, may work well in times of critical shortages or need of large numbers of personnel, such as disaster situations and emergencies.

TEAM NURSING

After World War II, the shortage of registered nurses continued. The team method of patient care was introduced, aided by the increasing number of LPNs/LVNs and NAs. The team method is based on the belief that goals can be achieved through group action. The patients on a unit are divided into small groups. Small teams are assigned to care for the patients in each group. Assignments are based on the needs of each patient and the skills of the team members. The team leader, the RN, leads the team. The RN continues to have the final responsibility of planning, coordinating, and evaluating the implementation of care for each patient and supervising the personnel giving the care.

In team nursing the capabilities of each team member are used effectively. This increases the quality of care for the patient and the satisfaction of the team member. An integral part of the team method is the team conference. During this conference, which should be held daily, team members share information about specific patients. Patient problems are identified and solved, and plans of care are developed and revised. The team method is rarely carried out in this manner. When busy, the team leader may administer medications and perform treatments. Team conferences are often postponed. The team method then becomes a functional method of assigning care. Several years ago, the nurses on the medical floor where Mrs. Brown was a patient used the team method, but often the team leader functioned as the medication nurse.

Modular nursing is a method of delivering nursing care that modifies team nursing by arranging the physical layout of units so nurses can stay near the bedside of assigned patients for convenient patient access and record keeping. For consistency, the same group of caregivers is assigned to a specific patient area.

PRIMARY NURSING

The hospital in which Mrs. Brown was a patient adopted the primary care method several years ago to replace the team method of assigning care. The intention was to increase the quality of care for patients. This method was instituted in the 1970s as a result of the dissatisfaction of professional nurses with their lack of direct patient contact and the fragmentation of care that resulted from functional and team nursing. In primary nursing, RNs individualize patient care and accept responsibility and accountability for total patient care, generally eliminating the need to delegate to other licensed staff persons. Ideally, staffing for this method requires a nursing staff composed entirely of RNs. Each nurse is assigned a maximum of six patients. There are no team leaders in this method. Each primary nurse is a bedside nurse, who has received the assignment from and in turn reports to the nurse manager.

The major characteristic of this method is the responsibility and accountability of the primary nurse. The primary nurse is assigned to a patient on admission, develops the nursing diagnoses after the admission interview, develops a plan of care, and is responsible for the care of that patient 24 hours a day until he or she is discharged. When the primary nurse is off duty, an associate RN continues care as planned by the primary nurse. If any changes are contemplated in patient care, the primary nurse must be contacted.

Primary nursing facilitates continuity of care but has advantages and disadvantages. Positive aspects of the primary method include shorter hospital stays for patients, improved communication among staff, and a more holistic focus of care. The difficulty of recruiting a sufficient number of RNs is one negative aspect, but the greatest drawback is the cost of a staff composed entirely of RNs. Practical/vocational nurses are used as assistive nurses in primary care situations and have performed safely and effectively.

NURSING CASE MANAGEMENT

In acute care, nursing case management focuses on achieving patient outcomes within a specified time frame. Clinical pathways or critical paths are used as a tool by all health care workers involved with the patient's care to identify incidents that must occur at specific times to achieve patient outcomes within an appropriate length of stay. These pathways provide a blueprint for care that includes a time frame of significant events that are expected to occur each day a patient with a specific diagnosis is in the hospital. Figure 15-1 is an example of a clinical pathway.

Nursing case management became popular in the 1980s in response to the increasing complexity of patient care, the need to use scarce nursing resources, and meeting patient needs in a *cost-effective* manner in acute care. Depending on patient needs, this method uses bachelor degree registered nurses, diploma and associate degree registered nurses, licensed practical/vocational nurses, nursing assistants, and unlicensed assistive personnel in varying ratios to deliver nursing service.

Some institutions use care maps, which are a combination of care plans and critical paths. The case manager keeps an eye on timely discharge and continuity of care in the community by planning, directing, and evaluating care throughout the patient's stay in acute care. The strength of the case management method of delivering nursing services is its focus of delivering cost-effective, quality care to patients with complex needs. Quality, service, and cost are timely considerations for health care in the twenty-first century.

SKILL MIX

Skill mix refers to the different levels of educational preparation of members used to staff the nursing team. The skill mix on the nursing team can be varied. Some hospitals are converting to all-RN staffs. Some hospitals utilize LPNs/LVNs, nursing assistants, and unlicensed assistive personnel to deliver patient care.

Research and data are needed to evaluate the quality of care provided by variously composed teams of RNs, LPNs/LVNs, and nursing assistants in a variety of health care settings. Investigate the skill mix of nursing staff in health care agencies at which you have clinical experiences.

PATIENT-CENTERED CARE—A PHILOSOPHY

Nursing has always been concerned with total patient care, focusing on the patient's physical and emotional needs, preferences, and values when giving care. The Institute of Medicine (IOM), an independent organization that advises the nation about health care, focuses on safety and quality in health care. You can find information about the IOM and its role in health care at http://www.iom.edu/About-IOM.aspx.

Clinical Pathway | **Postanesthesia Care Unit Coordinated Care Track**

Patient classification: III
Date:

Patient imprint

Time frame	Time of admission: 0-30 minutes	30-90 minutes	90-180 minutes	Time of transfer: 3-6 hours
Patient satisfaction	Pediatric support person at bedside		What can we do to enhance your stay with us?	
Discharge planning	Identify risk factors for prolonged recovery		Plan for bed availability	Discharge to Regular Nursing Floor (RNF) or extended recovery/ICU
Airway management	Airway assessment Ventilator settings as ordered/O_2 as ordered Monitor O_2 saturation Vital signs per protocol	Assess for readiness to wean	Wean ventilatory support/O_2 per protocol	Wean to room air Incentive spirometry q2h after extubation
Hemodynamic management	Hemodynamic monitoring Hemodynamic support as necessary	Monitor need for hemodynamic support	Wean from hemodynamic support as tolerated	
Nursing and medical interventions	Identify patient by name and arm band Identify allergies Level of consciousness assessment Dressing assessment Systems assessment Dermatome assessment Report from anesthesia Initiate surgical-specific protocols Pain management—provide pharmacologic therapies Rewarming initiated IV and arterial line management Initiate stir-up regimen (wake up) Place necessary consults Admission documentation	Review chart for patient information Pain management—provide pharmacologic and non-pharmacologic therapies Review orders Implement physician orders Continue stir-up regimen Emotional support Treat nausea/vomiting if necessary Monitor for potential surgical complications	Labs, x-rays complete Consults complete Wean from rewarming devices Patient repositioned Mouth care given Monitor for potential surgical complications Assess need for extended observation	Monitor for potential surgical complications Assess need for extended observation or ICU care
Patient education	Family notified patient in PACU Orient to person, place, and time Explain activities of care while providing care	Answer patient questions Reinforce pain scale	Family called for update on patient's condition Orient to expectations of PACU discharge	Family visit for 15 minutes Instruct on postop pain management Instruct on importance of coughing, deep breathing, and exercising limbs
Outcome criteria	Vital signs within normal parameters Oxygenation within normal range Dressing and drains intact	Vital signs within normal parameters Dressing and drains intact No excessive bleeding Pain minimized	Oriented to person and place/returned to baseline mentation Hemodynamically stable	Postanesthesia score >8 Temp 35.5°-38.4° C Coughing and deep breathing Pain < 4 Minimal nausea/vomiting No evidence of surgical complications All appropriate physician orders initiated

Courtesy Cleveland Clinic Foundation, Department of Advanced Practice Nursing, Cleveland, Ohio.

FIGURE 15-1 Clinical pathway: postanesthesia care unit coordinated care track for pediatric patient.

The IOM defines patient-centered care as "providing care that is respectful of and responsive to individual patient preferences, needs, and values and ensuring that patient values guide all clinical decisions" (Mitchell, 2008). The health care team partners with patients and families to plan care that reflects the patient's needs and preferences and ensures that the patient has the information needed to make health care decisions. All nursing care delivery systems must include these elements of patient-centered care (see Chapter 10).

THE HIDDEN NURSING SHORTAGE

Hospitals and health care, as well as nursing, have always been considered to be "recession-proof." Nursing jobs in acute care were widely available until the recession of 2008. As people lost jobs nationwide, they also lost health insurance benefits. Many postponed needed and elective health care. Nurses began having difficulty finding jobs in acute care facilities. This situation began to ease in some parts of the country in 2010. Reasons for the sudden downturn in acute care jobs include the following:

- A stock market drop in 2008 caused older RNs to delay retiring in order to allow their retirement funds to recover.
- Some nurses retained their jobs because a spouse was laid off.
- Nurses working part-time switched to full-time employment.

- Hospital services and programs cut during the recession were not restored.

Since World War II, nursing shortages have been common. With the beginning of retirement for baby boomers in 2011, a nursing shortage currently exists, but it is hidden in the current, more sluggish growth in jobs (Box 15-3). The number of elderly in society and their potential need for increased health care, including long-term care, has resulted in varying projections of the need for nurses in the future. It is difficult to find exact numbers depicting the need for LPNs/LVNs, but numbers are projected for RNs from over 580,000 by 2018 to 260,000 by 2025. Because of the long-term care needs of an aging society and a future general increase in demand for health care services, employment of LPNs/LVNs is expected to grow by 21% between 2008 and 2018 (Bureau of Labor Statistics, 2008).

Box 15-3	Some Causes of the Hidden Nursing Shortage

The need for nurses will increase in the future.
- Ten percent of nurses are younger than age 30.
- Forty percent of nurses are over the age of 50.
- We can expect a large number of LPNs/LVNs to retire in the next 20 years.
- Nursing schools cannot admit all qualified applicants because of a shortage of faculty and clinical facilities.
- The average age of nursing faculty is 55. They face retirement in about 10 years or less.

Get Ready for the NCLEX-PN® Examination

Key Points

- Health care organizations include a large number of specialized services and health care workers to provide these services. Patients in the United States have some of the best and most expensive health care services in the world.
- Each member of the health care team provides a valuable service to the patient. All members of the health care team are equal in importance to each other.
- Members of the nursing team are registered nurses (including nursing management), practical/vocational nurses, student nurses, cross-trained staff, unlicensed assistive personnel, and clerk receptionists.
- To understand where the practical/vocational nurse fits into the health care team, it is important to be aware of the educational background, role, responsibilities, and possible licensing requirements of all levels of personnel on the health care team.

- To understand your position on the health care team, it is necessary to keep up-to-date about new levels of health care workers and the method of delivering nursing care in your health care agency.
- Functional, team, and primary nursing are examples of methods used to deliver nursing care in acute care facilities.
- Nursing case management focuses on achieving patient outcomes within a specified time frame using clinical pathways.
- The IOM defines patient-centered care as "providing care that is respectful of and responsive to individual patient preferences, needs, and values and ensuring that patient values guide all clinical decisions."
- The increasing number of elderly in society increases demand for health care workers.
- In the twenty-first century, practical/vocational nurses are recognized as important members of the health care team in acute care facilities and the community

Additional Learning Resources

evolve Go to your Evolve website (http://evolve.elsevier.com/Hill/Success) for the following FREE learning resources:

- Answers to Critical Thinking Scenarios
- Additional learning activities
- Additional Review Questions for the NCLEX-PN® exam
- Helpful phrases for communicating in Spanish and more!

Review Questions for the NCLEX-PN® Examination

1. Which of the following nurses on the health care team, with the following initials after their name, has the most education?
   1. RN
   2. BSN
   3. ADN
   4. MSN

2. Select the statement that indicates an understanding of a major difference between the RN and LPN/LVN.
   1. The LPN/LVN initiates all health teaching for patients.
   2. The registered nurse formulates nursing diagnoses.
   3. By law, the LPN/LVN functions in an independent role.
   4. The LPN/LVN interprets the results of research studies.

3. Which of the following statements best describes team nursing as a method of delivering nursing care?
   1. The method based on the level of staff skill and patient need.
   2. Task-oriented efficiency is divided among staff of all shifts.
   3. The RN plans and is accountable for total patient care 24 hours a day.
   4. This method utilizes scarce nursing resources in a cost-effective way.

4. Which of the following practical/vocational nurses is working in a typical LPN/LVN position?
   1. A visiting nurse on the day shift of a public health agency in the community.
   2. A charge nurse on the evening shift of an acute care agency in her community.
   3. A staff nurse assuming nurse manager responsibilities on a surgical unit.
   4. An office nurse preparing a child for a physical examination in a pediatrician's office.

Alternate Format Item

1. Which of the following statements differentiates the role of the practical/vocational nurse from the professional nurse? *(Select all that apply.)*
   1. The LPN/LVN is responsible for formulating all nursing diagnoses.
   2. The LPN/LVN has a more limited role in health teaching for patients.
   3. The LPN/LVN is not employed in any management positions.
   4. The LPN/LVN joins and is actively involved in NFLPN and NAPNES.
   5. The LPN/LVN interprets many research findings in the clinical area.

2. Which of the following are methods of delivering nursing care in acute care agencies? *(Select all that apply.)*
   1. Primary care
   2. Case method
   3. Team method
   4. Functional method
   5. Client-centered care
   6. Case management method

Critical Thinking Scenarios

Scenario 1
From the beginning of her PN student year, Amy set her sights on working as an LPN on the medical-surgical unit of an acute care facility. As she neared graduation, Amy kept hearing of nursing graduates of all nursing programs having trouble finding a job. Give Amy suggestions for finding a job.

Scenario 2
During Paul's medical-surgical clinical rotation, an assigned patient, Mr. R., is preparing to go home after a 2-day hospitalization. The patient shows Paul a list of health care workers he has come in contact with during his hospitalization and marvels at the number of people involved in his care in only 2 days of hospitalization. Mr. R. asks Paul to explain why there are all types of nurses, RNs, LPNs, and SPNs. What is Paul's explanation?

Objectives

On completing this chapter, you will be able to do the following:

1. Define in your own words the following terms:
   a. Culture
   b. Cultural competence
   c. Cultural diversity
   d. Cultural uniqueness
   e. Ethnocentrism
   f. Cultural bias
   g. Cultural sensitivity
   h. Stereotype
2. Explain in your own words nine basic daily needs of all persons.
3. Describe your culture in the areas of:
   a. Family
   b. Religion
   c. Communication
   d. Educational background
   e. Economic level
   f. Wellness, illness, birth, and death beliefs and practices

4. Identify how all persons are unique and similar.
5. Explain in your own words the philosophy of individual worth as it applies to health care.
6. Describe general differences among cultural groups frequently served in your geographic area that may have importance in patient care situations.
7. Explain the importance of the following in developing an ability to provide culturally competent care:
   a. Increasing awareness of your own cultural self
   b. Obtaining general knowledge about culturally diverse groups
   c. Gathering data about specific beliefs and health practices of individual patients to be used in care plan development
   d. Negotiating plans of care for culturally diverse patients

Key Terms

assimilation (ă-SĬM-ă-LĀ-shŭn, p. 194)
biomedicine (BĪ-ō-MĔD-ĭ-sĭn, p. 201)
complementary and alternative medicine (CAM) (KŎM-plĕ-MĔN-tĕ-rē, ăl-TŬR-nă-tĭv, p. 201)
cultural bias (BĪ-ăs, p. 193)
cultural competence (KŎM-pĭ-tĕns, p. 193)
cultural diversity (dĭ-VŬR-sĭ-tē, p. 197)
cultural sensitivity (SĔN-sĭ-TĬV-ĭ-tē, p. 193)
culture (p. 193)
customs (p. 193)
discrimination (dĭ-SKRĬM-ĭ-NĀ-shŭn, p. 193)
enculturation (ĕn-KŬL-chŭr-Ā-shŭn, p. 193)

ethnic groups (ĔTH-nĭk, p. 197)
ethnocentrism (ĔTH-nō-SĔN-TRĬZ-ĕm, p. 193)
melting pot (p. 197)
naturalistic system (NĂCH-ŭr-ăl-LĬS-tĭk, p. 203)
nonjudgmental (NŎN-jŭj-MĔN-tăl, p. 198)
personalistic system (PŬR-sŏ-năl-LĬS-tĭk, p. 203)
prejudice (PRĔJ-ŭ-dĭs, p. 193)
repatterning (p. 209)
stereotype (STĔR-ē-ō-TĪP, p. 193)
wellness and illness (p. 201)
worldview (p. 193)

 Keep in Mind

With knowledge comes responsibility. With knowledge of cultures, that responsibility entails a respect for differences.

You have chosen a career that will give you an opportunity to meet people who are different from you.
- Some of these people will be your patients.
- Some will be your peers at school.
- Some will be your coworkers.
- Some will be a different age than you.
- Some will belong to a different social class.
- Some will have disabilities.
- Some will have different health care beliefs about what causes them to get sick.
- Some will have different values.
- Because of ethnic group status, some of your patients and coworkers will have different cultural backgrounds.

- Regardless of cultural background, some differences will be the result of a growing diversity in individual and family lifestyles.

You will discover that people think, feel, believe, act, and see the world differently from you and your family and friends. Log on to www.minoritynurse.com/about/index.html, sign up for the free quarterly email newsletter, check out featured articles about issues facing minority nurses, and find out if your school subscribes to *Minority Nurse Magazine*.

Review the standards of the National Association for Practical Nurse Education and Service, Inc. (see Appendix A) and the National Federation of Licensed Practical Nurses (see Appendix B). You will note that both organizations have embraced statements that describe the need of the practical/vocational nurse to provide health care to all patients regardless of race, creed, cultural background, disease, or lifestyle. This is an ethical expectation. Review your state's Nurse Practice Act. You might find that failing or refusing to render nursing services to a patient because of the patient's race, color, sex, age, beliefs, national origin, or handicap is listed as unprofessional conduct. The ethical expectation now becomes a legal mandate. Nurses could risk legal suits because of their ignorance of the culture of the patient and resulting poor nursing judgment.

Not only do practical/vocational nurses need to provide care for all persons, but they also need to provide culturally competent care. Cultural competence is the *continuous* attempt of practical/vocational nurses to gain the knowledge and skills that will allow them to effectively provide care for patients of different cultures. Cultural competence is not gained by reading a chapter in a textbook or by looking up a culture in a reference book. It is developing an awareness of different cultures (cultural sensitivity) and continually learning about people who are different from you.

When differences are identified in a health care situation, the practical/vocational nurse needs to suggest adaptations to the plan of care so the plan recognizes these differences. In doing so, the patient will be encouraged to follow suggestions, avoid treatment failures, and return to health as quickly as possible. Practical/vocational nurses will then be able to say that they have truly met the patient's needs.

DEFINITION OF CULTURE

Culture is a way of life. It is the total of the *ever-changing* knowledge, ideas, thoughts, beliefs, values, communication, actions, attitudes, traditions, customs, and objects that a group of people possess and the ways they have of doing things. Culture also includes standards of behavior and sets of rules to live by. Customs are the generally accepted ways of doing things that are common to people who share the same

culture. Basic concepts about culture can be accessed at http://www.culturediversity.org.

CHARACTERISTICS OF CULTURE

An important point about culture is that it is *learned behavior*. The culture of a group is passed on from generation to generation. From the moment you were born, you began to learn about the culture of the group into which you were born. The process of learning your culture (the way your group does things) is called enculturation. A result of enculturation is a worldview that is generally shared by persons with the same cultural background. The worldview, or similar ways of seeing and understanding the world, becomes the reality of the group. This reality fills every aspect of life. It is a cultural bias (a mental leaning) that is never proved or questioned by the individual. The worth of everything, either within or outside the group, depends on whether it fits the worldview of the cultural group. One's worldview can lead to ethnocentrism, prejudice, and discrimination, unless modified by knowledge and experience.

Socialization is the process by which a person of one culture learns how to function in a larger culture. Right now you are being socialized into the career of practical/vocational nursing. You are learning how to think and act like a practical/vocational nurse.

DANGER: ETHNOCENTRISM, PREJUDICE, AND DISCRIMINATION

People who belong to the same cultural group may develop the attitude, through their worldview, that their way of doing things is superior, right, or better than that of groups with different cultures (ethnocentrism). The group uses its culture as the norm against which to measure and evaluate the customs and ways of others. The group is uncomfortable with people who display customs and behaviors that differ from their cultural group. Ethnocentrism is common to all cultural groups. When intolerance of another cultural group occurs, prejudice results. When rights and privileges are withheld from those of another cultural group, discrimination is the result.

AVOIDING FALSE ASSUMPTIONS

Nursing students sometimes think that somewhere there is a manual that will tell them how to care for people who are different from themselves. This type of approach can lead to false assumptions, which are called stereotypes. A stereotype is an assumption used to describe all members of a specific group without exception. It is an expectation that all individuals in a group will act exactly the same in a situation just because they are members of that group. Stereotypes ignore the individual differences that occur within every cultural group. Members of any culture may have modified the degree to which they observe the values and practices of the culture.

Critical Thinking

Example of a False Assumption

While speaking about a particular function at a seminar on business practices, the presenter singled out an engineer in the group who was of Japanese descent. He used the engineer as an example of someone who thinks differently from "Americans" because he is Asian. The engineer was a third-generation American and had no clue what the presenter was talking about.

How did the presenter in this situation go wrong in his assumption?

THINK LIKE AN ANTHROPOLOGIST!

Anthropologists are scientists who study physical, social, and cultural characteristics of human groups. It is helpful to understand how these scientists conduct their studies:

- Anthropologists start the study of cultural groups by identifying common trends in a cultural group.
- These common trends found in the group are called "generalizations."
- Then anthropologists gather data to determine if the common trends (generalizations) apply to all individuals within that cultural group.

Automatically generalizing cultural information about a group's health practices to one person in that group might be drawing a wrong conclusion. Does the individual follow the traditional practice of the group? Has the individual rejected the practice? Does the individual use the practice only in certain situations? If so, what situations? Is the person an immigrant? How recently? When people immigrate to a new country, culturally different groups do adopt some of the culture of the new country. The process of giving up parts of their own culture and adopting parts of the culture of the dominant group is called assimilation. Complete assimilation, however, rarely occurs. Members of the generations that follow the original immigrants may retain some elements of their original culture in addition to assimilating parts of the new culture. For these reasons, generalizations help explain observed behavior, but they do not *predict* behavior.

KNOWING YOURSELF

WHAT MAKES YOU UNIQUE?

To become aware of different cultures, you need to be aware of yourself as a person. Several activities are included in this chapter to help you with cultural self-awareness. The exercises also help you develop an awareness of cultural differences with peers.

Try This

What Makes You Unique?

Let your uniqueness show! Divide the class into small but equal-sized groups. Find one item that makes you unique from other members of the group. Share with your class the item that makes you unique.

HOW MANY HATS DO YOU WEAR?

Most people have several roles in life. People speak of "wearing many hats" or "having a full plate." Some of these roles are played out individually, one at a time, and others are performed simultaneously. The exercise in the Try This: Identifying the Roles You Play in Your Life box gives you the opportunity to identify your roles.

Try This

Identifying the Roles You Play in Your Life

The following categories describe the roles you play in several areas in your everyday life.

CATEGORY 1: ECONOMIC STATUS ROLE

Although standards are available to assign persons to each of the following economic classes, people generally place themselves in one of the following categories by how they perceive their economic status.

Place a check mark next to the economic class that best describes you.

I am in the

_____ Lower economic class
_____ Middle economic class
_____ Upper economic class

CATEGORY 2: POLITICAL ROLE

Put a check mark next to the word(s) that best describe(s) the political role you play in society.

I am

_____ Republican
_____ Democrat
_____ Independent
_____ Liberal
_____ Conservative
_____ Moderate
_____ Indifferent
_____ To the left of liberal
_____ To the right of conservative
Other _____

CATEGORY 3: RACIAL OR ETHNIC ROLE

Place a check mark beside the racial or ethnic terms that best describe you.

I am a (an)

_____ African American	_____ Ethnic
_____ American	_____ Gypsy
_____ American Indian	_____ Hispanic
_____ Amerindian	_____ Indian
_____ Anglo	_____ Latin American
_____ Anglo-Saxon	_____ Latvian American
_____ Arab American	_____ Native American
_____ Asian American	_____ Spanish-speaking
_____ Asian	_____ White
_____ Black	Other _____
_____ Chicano	

Try This

Identifying the Roles You Play in Your Life—cont'd

CATEGORY 4: SOCIAL ROLE

Circle the social roles that describe you.

I am (a)

female, male	stepsister, stepbrother
married, single	half-sister, half-brother
separated, divorced	godmother, godfather
blended family	godchild
wife, husband	grandmother
significant other	granddaughter
mother, father	aunt
daughter, son	niece, nephew
sister, brother	cousin
stepmother,	Other_____
stepfather	
stepdaughter,	
stepson	

CATEGORY 5: WORK ROLE

Place a check mark beside each work role you play in your life.

I am (a)

_____ Blue-collar worker	_____ Student
_____ Businessperson	_____ Technician
_____ Laborer	_____ Unemployed
_____ Professional	_____ White-collar worker
_____ Service provider	Other _____
_____ Skilled worker	

Summarize the hats you wear by listing the items you have checked and circled in the five categories.

Category 1: Economic status role _____
Category 2: Political role _____
Category 3: Racial or ethnic role _____
Category 4: Social role _____
Category 5: Work role _____

_____
_____

Try This

Who Am I Based on My Roles?

Make up a sentence using all the words you listed in the five role categories. This sentence describes you by the roles you play in your life. Have each student write the sentence on a piece of paper (do not put the name of the writer!) and put it in a paper bag. Have someone take a piece of paper out of the bag, read the sentence, and then give the class the opportunity to guess the identity of the person described (adapted from Randall-David, 1992).

WHAT WE SHARE IN COMMON

Because of our genes, each of us is different from every other person in the world. (The only exception is identical twins.) Before you start to think about the differences among people, it is a good idea to think about what people have in common.

Try This

What We Have in Common

When you are among a group of your peers (e.g., eating lunch in the cafeteria or walking to the parking lot), take a few minutes to play the "What We Have in Common" culture game. Excluding sex, age, marital status, and culture group, try to find five items you share in common with each member of the group. This activity is especially helpful when the group includes classmates you perceive as "different" from you.

1. _____
2. _____
3. _____
4. _____
5. _____

- In a class situation, discuss the items you have in common. Did any items you share in common with other members of the group surprise you?
- Did you discover any stereotyping in *your* thinking regarding your peers?

BASIC DAILY NEEDS: ANOTHER COMMONALITY

All people share the same basic daily needs regardless of age, sex, economic status, lifestyle, religion, country of origin, or culture. Chapters 10 and 20 discuss human needs as understood by the psychologist Abraham Maslow. Registered nurse Vivian Culver (1974) compiled a list of people's nine essential daily needs. This list has stood the test of time. These essential needs are a simple yet helpful place to start in learning to understand that all people, regardless of background, share the following things in common:

1. Personal care and hygiene
2. Sleep and rest
3. Nutrition and fluids
4. Elimination
5. Body alignment and activity
6. Environment
7. Emotional and spiritual support
8. Diversion and recreation
9. Mental hygiene

These nine basic daily needs can form the basis for planning patient care. However, you need to understand the meaning of these basic needs for well persons, including yourself, before you can apply them to individuals in the clinical area. Once you gain understanding of these needs and the variety of ways people meet them, applying these needs to patients will be easier. As you read about the nine basic needs of all people, think about how you specifically meet each need in your own daily life. Do some of your peers meet their daily basic needs in different ways than you meet your needs? You will find that this is the case with patients as well.

Personal Care and Hygiene

Clean hair, skin, nails, teeth, and clothing serve two general purposes: protection from illness and promotion of well-being. Skin constantly secretes sebum, the cold cream–like substance of the body, to keep the skin supple. Daily, epidermal skin cells (the outer layer of the skin) are shed as new cells push toward the outer layer. Skin eliminates fluid in the form of perspiration to help keep body temperature stable. Sebum and perspiration are odorless substances. Ever-present bacteria on the skin are responsible for the body odor we associate with the body's oils and perspiration. We meet personal care and hygiene needs by bathing, shampooing, hand washing, maintaining oral hygiene, and grooming.

- Do you prefer a shower, a bath, or another method of cleansing your body?
- How often do you cleanse your body?
- During what part of the day do you cleanse your body?
- How often do you shampoo?
- What products do you use to style your hair?
- How often do you visit the dentist?

 Professional Pointer

Appearance is (almost) everything (Pagana, 2008).

Sleep and Rest

Sleep is needed to refresh us. The actual number of hours of sleep required varies with the individual. Rest and periodic relaxation are just as important because they also help the body restore itself.

- How many hours of sleep do you get each night or day?
- Where do you rest or relax?
- What do you do to rest or relax?
- Do you take naps during the day?

Nutrition and Fluids

Preparing meals from the suggested food selections, as you studied in nutrition, is necessary to stay healthy. We all need a variety of food daily. Fluids help our body to complete its many chemical reactions, transport nutrients, regulate temperature, and lubricate body parts. Fluids include the water content in food, as well as the beverages we drink.

- How many calories do you consume each day?
- How many meals do you eat each day?
- When do you eat your meals?
- How many glasses of fluid do you drink each day?
- What fluids do you prefer to drink?

Elimination

Elimination of wastes from the body is primarily accomplished by the kidneys (in the form of urine) and the large intestine (in the form of feces). The skin is not as good at elimination as these organs, but it does eliminate some body wastes through perspiration.

- What do you consider to be "normal" time intervals for urinary and intestinal elimination?

Body Alignment and Activity

Body alignment, or the relationship of the body parts to one another, is better known as posture. When posture is "good," the body can be used in a comfortable manner without danger of injury. Good posture also enhances the functioning of the respiratory, gastrointestinal, and circulatory systems. You will not tire as quickly if good posture is maintained. Daily exercise may also enhance the function of these body systems. Exercise also helps maintain muscle tone.

- Have a peer evaluate your posture while you are sitting and walking
- How much exercise do you get each day?
- How do you get your exercise?

Environment

Environment refers to the space that surrounds us. Our environment changes many times during a day. Regardless of our specific environment, the most essential component of our surroundings is oxygen. After that environmental need has been met, the next most important need is safety. When oxygen and safety needs have been met, the individual can focus on changing his or her environment to accommodate comfort and personal taste.

- Describe your home environment.
- Do you feel safe in your environment?

Emotional and Spiritual Support

Our emotions greatly influence our health because the body and the mind are linked. This link enables the body to influence the mind and the mind to influence the body. All emotions, including excitement, fear, anger, worry, grief, joy, surprise, and love, can influence our bodies positively or negatively. Spiritual and emotional needs are closely related, yet different. People meet their spiritual needs in a variety of ways that are unique to their personal beliefs (see Chapter 17). Do you acknowledge spiritual needs? If so, how do you meet them?

- How do you express anger, worry, joy, grief?

Diversion and Recreation

We all need to turn aside (diversion) from our usual activities and refresh our bodies and minds with activities other than work (recreation). What is work to one person can be play to another.

- How much time do you spend studying each week?
- How many hours do you work outside of school?
- What type of recreation do you engage in each week?
- How many hours do you devote to recreation each week?

Mental Hygiene

Mental hygiene involves the care and hygiene of the brain. Just as there are good health habits for the body, there are also good daily health habits for the mind.

You need to strive to understand and accept yourself, be optimistic, work well with others, accept criticism, know your abilities and limitations, trust and respect others, and accept responsibility for yourself.

- Who is responsible for your success in the practical/vocational nursing program?
- What is your attitude toward constructive evaluation?
- What kind of a team member are you in the clinical area?
- How do you control your stress level?

 Try This

Basic Daily Needs

Choose one basic daily need and discuss with classmates how you meet that need.

KNOWING OTHERS: CULTURAL DIVERSITY

In the nineteenth century, waves of immigrants from all over the world came to the United States. The United States was eventually called a melting pot, meaning that these immigrants had given up their native cultures and adopted the culture of the American people.

The 2010 U.S. Census included the categories of Hispanic/Latino/Spanish origin (if so, indicate if Mexican, Mexican American, Chicano, Puerto Rican, Cuban, or Argentinean, Colombian, Dominican, Nicaraguan, Salvadoran, Spaniard, and so on), White, Black, African American or Negro, American Indian or Alaska Native, Asian Indian, Chinese, Filipino, Japanese, Korean, Vietnamese, other Asian (Hmong, Laotian, Thai, Pakistani, Cambodian, and so on), Native Hawaiian, Guamanian or Chamorro, Samoan, other Pacific Islander, or other race United States. Today, the melting pot is more like a "casserole," with each ingredient (i.e., different culture) adding to the quality of the whole. The concept of the melting pot has been replaced by the concept of cultural diversity, which refers to the many differences in the elements of culture in groups of people in American and Canadian society. Examples of groups that have been identified as culturally diverse in the United States are Hispanics, African Americans, American Muslims, Asians, American Indians, and Caucasians. American Muslims are discussed in Chapter 17.

Cultural diversity goes beyond racial and ethnic groups. As a practical/vocational nurse, you need to define this concept more broadly so culturally diverse groups can also mean single parents, people who live in poverty, homosexuals, bisexuals, the wealthy, the poor, the homeless, the elderly, and people with disabilities.

The concept of race as a means of categorizing people by biologic traits has come under attack by social scientists. These scientists suggest using ethnicity as a more accurate means of capturing the great diversity found in over 7 billion people in the world (http://www.census.gov/main/www/popclock.html). Members of ethnic groups are a special type of cultural group, composed of people who are members of the same race, religion, or nation, or who speak the same language. They derive part of their identity through membership in the ethnic group. Examples of ethnic groups in the United States include Irish Americans, African Americans, American Indians, Asian Americans, German Americans, Mexican Americans, Jews, Arab Americans, Greek Americans, Finnish Americans, and many more.

IMPORTANCE OF CULTURAL DIVERSITY

Health care today and into the future needs to be able to accommodate patients of many different cultural backgrounds. Failure to develop sensitivity to and competence in handling this diversity could lead to misunderstandings between you and the patient, resulting in stress for both. The plan of treatment for the patient could fail. You could make false assumptions based on generalizations. You might label patients as difficult or uncooperative when their lack of cooperation with the plan of care could be related to a conflict with their personal health belief system. Patients may experience less-than-adequate care when cultural diversity and the differences it represents are overlooked or misinterpreted.

Philosophy of Individual Worth

The philosophy of individual worth is a belief shared by all members of the health care team. The philosophy includes the uniqueness and value of each human being who comes for care, regardless of differences that may be observed or perceived in that individual. Practical/vocational nurses need to realize that each individual has the right to live according to their personal beliefs and values, *as long as they do not interfere with the rights of others.* Each individual deserves respect as a human being.

 Professional Pointer

Respect cultural differences.

Many factors are responsible for differences in patients. They may think and behave differently because of social class, personal income, religion, ethnic background, or personal choice. Regardless of these differences, all patients have the right to receive high-quality nursing care. As a practical/vocational nurse you cannot decrease the quality of the care you give because of differences you observe or perceive.

Practical/vocational nurses need to guard against making judgments about people who are culturally different. This does not mean you must adopt differences as part of your behavior. It means being open-minded and non-judgmental. It means taking the difference at face value, accepting people as they are, and giving high-quality care. Be aware of your own attitudes, beliefs, and values as they affect your ability to give care. If you do identify biases, see them for what they are. Become sensitive to cultural differences, and acknowledge that they exist. Gather knowledge about them so you can work on trying to modify your biases and provide more culturally competent care.

LEARNING ABOUT CULTURAL DIVERSITY
How to Begin
You have been given exercises that help you to discover your own uniqueness and that of others, as well as similarities. Unless you understand your own culture, it will be difficult to understand the culture of others. You need to look inside yourself to learn about your own cultural beliefs, values, and worldview and the influence they have on how you think and act. Some elements of your culture are obvious, such as your language, celebrated holidays, and how and what you eat. However, other aspects of your culture are hidden. Elements such as aspects of communication, beliefs, attitudes, values, sex roles, use of space, concept of time, structure of the family, and family dynamics may be more difficult to recognize and discuss. Some areas of cultural diversity may be taken for granted in patient situations. Examples include food preferences, religion, educational background, economic level, wellness and illness beliefs and practices, the birth experience, and terminal illness and death beliefs and practices.

The first step to developing knowledge about patient differences in these areas is to become aware of and explore *your* cultural patterns in these areas. Read the general information about each area. Develop an awareness of your own cultural patterns in these areas by answering the group of statements or questions included with each area. Sharing this information with peers will highlight the cultural diversity that exists in your nursing class, regardless of cultural background. The questions also provide examples of areas to be discussed with patients when collecting data about their personal beliefs and health practices.

AREAS OF CULTURAL DIVERSITY
Family Structure
No matter what culture is being discussed, the family is the basic unit of society. The role of the family is to have children, if desired or as they come, and to raise them to be contributing members of the group. Actual child-rearing practices vary from culture to culture. Families generally socialize the young to the culture of the group. They meet the physical and psychological needs of the young in culturally specific ways. Some cultures expect only the nuclear family (mother, father, and children) to live in the same house. Others

may expect the extended family (the nuclear family plus the grandparents and other relatives) to do so. Some Vietnamese families are examples of extended families, with three or more generations living in the same house. In many of these families, ties are strong. Behaviors that enhance the family name are encouraged, such as obedience to parents and those in authority.

The single-parent family continues to challenge the traditional nuclear family as the typical family structure. A parent may become a single parent on the death of a spouse, by electing not to marry at the time of pregnancy, or by divorce. Health care workers who have not been in the same situation may be unaware of, and insensitive to, the special way of life of this type of family.

 Try This

Cultural Patterns: Family

Respond to the following statements. Your responses will help you discover your own cultural patterns in regard to the family.
1. Describe your family structure (nuclear, extended, or alternative lifestyle).
2. Describe the role of children, if any, in your family.
3. Discuss who gives permission for hospitalization in your family.
4. List factors that influence the decision of your family members to visit or not visit the hospital when a member is ill. If visiting is acceptable, how long does your family think it is appropriate to visit?
5. Describe the effect that your hospitalization today at 4 PM for emergency surgery would have on you and your family.

Food Preferences
All cultures use food to provide needed nutrients. However, what they eat, when they eat, and how they eat differ vastly by cultural group. Knowledge of nutrition as a science differs by culture. It is interesting that the soil of some cultures (e.g., Mexico) encouraged the growth of two complementary foods that together make up a complete protein source (corn and beans) and became a staple of that culture's diet. Specific foods in different cultures have different meanings. All cultures use food during celebrations. Through generations of experience, different cultures have learned to use different foods to promote health and cure disease.

 Try This

Cultural Patterns: Food

To assist you in identifying your own cultural patterns in regard to food preferences, respond to the following statements or questions.
1. What is your favorite food?
2. Identify one special occasion in which your cultural group participates. What foods, if any, are part of this celebration?
3. Describe your favorite recipe or meal from your mother and from your grandmother. What special ingredients or techniques are used to make the recipe? Is there a written recipe?

Religious Beliefs

Religious beliefs are personal to the individual. Religion is an important aspect of culture. Religion can have different meanings in people's lives. For some, religion is a brief, momentary, and sporadic part of daily life. For another person, it may influence every aspect of life and have a profound effect on personal outlook and on how one lives his or her life. For others, religion may not play a part in their lives at all. Chapter 17 deals with spirituality and religious differences, but it is important to discuss it in this chapter as well. There is a close relationship between religious beliefs and the concept of wellness and illness in some groups. Practical/vocational nurses need to be aware of their own religious beliefs, obligations, and attitudes. They need to know whether these beliefs and attitudes influence the care that is given to patients.

 Try This

Cultural Patterns: Religion

Answering the following questions will help you discover your own cultural patterns in regard to religion.
1. Do you have a religious affiliation? If so, indicate your affiliation.
2. What role does religion play in your life?
3. Is prayer helpful to you?
4. What is your source of strength and hope?
5. What rituals or religious practices are important to you?
6. What symbols or religious books are helpful to you?
7. What dietary inclusions or restrictions are part of your religious beliefs?
8. How does your religion view the source and meaning of pain and suffering?
9. When ill, does your religion prohibit people from the opposite sex from giving care?
10. Does your religion have special days when certain behaviors/activities are mandatory or prohibited?

Concept of Time

Some people follow clock time. An hour has a beginning and an end (after 60 minutes). People who follow clock time eat, sleep, work, and engage in recreational activities at definite times each day. Other people live on linear time. For them, time is a straight line with no beginning and no end. People who follow linear time eat when they are hungry and sleep when they are tired.

 Try This

Cultural Patterns: Time

The questions that follow give you an opportunity to discover your own cultural patterns in regard to time.
1. What determines when it is time for you to eat or sleep?
2. When you are not in the clinical area, do you keep track of time?
3. Are you on time for appointments?

Communication

Chapter 13 introduced you to the types of communication and potential barriers to the communication process. A major barrier to communication in health care is when the patient or nurse speaks a different language. A person's language gives a view of reality that may differ from yours. For example, in English, the clock "runs," but in Spanish, it "walks." This illustrates the different concept of time between the two cultures. For a person who speaks English as a first language, time could move quickly, and there may be a rush to get things done. For some who speak Spanish as a first language, time may move more slowly. Following is a list of areas of communication that may vary for people who are culturally different.

Forms of Hellos and Good-byes
- You may greet your patient and want to get right down to business.
- The patient might expect some light conversation before getting to the matter at hand.
- In some cultural groups, people take an hour to say good-bye, whereas people from other cultures may get up and leave without saying anything.

Appropriateness of the Situation
- Some groups prefer people to sit, not stand, while they converse.
- In some groups the sharing of food is a good way to relate to others and get them to verbalize.

Confidentiality
- All information the patient gives the nurse is considered confidential.
- Some patients do not want their spouse questioned or informed about their problems of the reproductive organs. They fear the spouse may think they are less desirable sexually.

Emotions and Feelings and Their Expression
- Emotions are universal, but the cues to those emotions vary considerably. A lack of awareness of this fact can cause unnecessary stress between the patient and the nurse.
- In some cultural groups, people cannot display affection in public, show disapproval or frustration, or vent anger.
- Some members of cultural groups cannot take criticism.
- You may show dissatisfaction with other members of the health care team by approaching them directly, whereas some team members may show dissatisfaction with you by being polite to your face but then complaining about you to the rest of the staff. The same applies to your classmates.

Pain Expression
- Pain has two parts: sensation and response. All individuals experience the same sensation of pain.
- One's culture influences the definition of pain and the response to the sensation.

- Pain is whatever the person says it is. It exists whenever the person says it does.
- One's culture provides guidelines for approved ways of expressing one's response to the pain sensation and ways to relieve the pain.
- Some cultures teach individuals that it is acceptable to cry, moan, and exhibit other behavior that calls attention to the pain. These behaviors may be considered a cure for pain in their culture.
- Other cultures encourage uncomplaining acceptance of pain and passive behavior when pain is experienced (stoic behavior).

Tempo of Conversation

- You may tend to speak quickly and expect a quick response.
- The patient may be accustomed to pausing and reflecting before giving a response.

Meaning of Silence

- Silence can mean anything from disapproval to warmth, but generally it does not indicate tension or lack of rapport.
- Silence can be difficult for some nurses to tolerate. Resist the temptation to jump in at a pause in the conversation by forcing yourself to concentrate on listening.

Box 16-1 provides some hints to keep in mind when using interpreters or other language resources.

 Critical Thinking

Stoic Behavior in Patients

Discuss some nursing situations in which a stoic (seemingly unaffected by pain) reaction to pain could have negative consequences if a practical/vocational nurse lacked knowledge of cultural differences in pain expression (e.g., a woman in labor or a patient having a heart attack).

 Try This

Cultural Patterns: Communication

Develop an awareness of your own cultural patterns in communication by answering the following questions:
1. What is your first (native) language?
2. Do you speak additional languages?
3. What facial or body habits are you aware of in yourself while you are talking?
4. How do you greet people, and how do you say good-bye?
5. How do you express the following emotions?
   a. Love
   b. Hate
   c. Fear
   d. Excitement
   e. Disappointment
   f. Dissatisfaction
   g. Humor
   h. Anger
   i. Sadness
   j. Happiness

6. Do you make eye contact when talking to people?
7. Do you touch people while talking?
   a. If so, how do they react?
   b. How do you react when people touch you while they are talking to you?
8. How do you express pain? How do you react to pain?

| Box 16-1 | Hints for Using Interpreters and Other Language Resources |

Interpreters provide an invaluable service when patients do not speak English or do not have sufficient experience with the English language to understand complex medical information. Another communication skill for the nurse is learning to work with an interpreter. To decrease the possibility of difficulties in an interpreter situation, follow these suggestions:

- The ideal interpreter should be trained in the health care field, proficient in the language of the patient and the nurse, and understand and respect the culture of the patient.
- If the ideal interpreter is not available, make sure that the individual chosen has training in medical terminology, understands the health matter that needs to be translated, and understands the requirements for confidentiality, neutrality, and accuracy.
- Use family members as interpreters cautiously. Patients of specific cultures may be embarrassed to discuss intimate matters with family members who are younger or older or of the opposite sex. Family members may censor information to protect the patient or the family.
- Make sure the interpreter is acceptable to the patient.
- Look at and speak directly to the patient, not the interpreter.
- Speak clearly and slowly in a normal voice. Use short units of speech.
- Avoid slang and professional jargon.
- Observe the nonverbal communication of the patient.
- Be patient. Remember that interpretation is difficult work.
- Other resources to assist with patients with language other than English include foreign language classes offered to staff in the language of patients commonly served.
- Language Line is a telephone-based interpreting service. Information about Language Line is available at http://www.languageline.com. You can sign up for their health care e-newsletter at http://www.languageline.com/page/newsletter.
- *Say It in Spanish* by Joyce and Villanueva de Gonzalez (2004) is a reference book for health care workers that contains commonly used Spanish phrases.
- Hablamos Juntos is a program whose mission is to improve communication between health care providers and their patients with limited proficiency. Information about this program can be accessed at http://www.hablamosjuntos.org/mission/default.mission.asp.
- Google "translation" lets you enter a phrase and instantly translates it into over 50 languages.

Adapted from Reinhardt E: *Through the eyes of others—intercultural resource directory for health care professionals.* Minneapolis: University of Minnesota School of Public Health, 1995.

Educational Background

The 2003 National Assessment of Adult Literacy assessed the English health literacy of adults in the United States and found that 14% do not have basic health literacy skills (able to understand a simple health pamphlet), while 22% have these skills (able to understand a more complex health pamphlet). Adults assessed got most of their information about health issues from radio and television (Kutner, 2006). Differences in educational background and literacy need to be taken into consideration when teaching patients. When in the clinical area, try to adapt your explanations to the patient's level of understanding.

 Try This

Cultural Patterns: Education

Your responses to the following statements will help you identify your own beliefs and practices in regard to education.
1. Calculate the number of years of education you have.
2. State your ultimate educational goal.
3. Discuss the role education plays in your life.
4. Describe your feelings toward a person who has less education than you.
5. Describe your feelings toward a person who has more education than you.
6. Describe your feelings if you were referred to your school's skills center.
7. Discuss the effect of your cultural background on your values and practices with regard to education.
8. Who in your family has graduated from high school, technical school, junior college, or a college or university?

Economic Level

Economic level is often related to educational background. Sociologists use these two factors to determine the social class of individuals. You will meet patients who are very wealthy and patients who are at or near the poverty level. Others have midlevel incomes. Patients' annual incomes determine the type of house they live in, the neighborhood where they live, the availability of food, and the ability to participate in certain types of preventive health care. Practical/vocational nurses need to take economic level into consideration while reinforcing patient teaching and should adapt their approach accordingly.

 Try This

Cultural Patterns: Economic Level

Identify your personal patterns in regard to economic level by responding to the following statements or questions.
1. Describe how your economic background affects your daily life in the following areas:
   a. Availability of food
   b. Availability of shelter
   c. Availability of clothing
   d. Amount and type of recreation
2. Discuss your feelings toward a person who has less money than you.

3. Discuss your feelings toward a person who has more money than you.
4. Describe how these feelings fit with those of your cultural group.
5. Discuss your ability to afford to go to a physician when you get sick.
6. If you work, do you have health insurance benefits?

Wellness and Illness Beliefs and Practices

Wellness and illness can have different meanings for persons who are culturally different. *Wellness* and *illness* are relative terms. What is good health to one person can be sickness to another. Wellness may not be a high-priority matter to some patients.

Preventing Illness. Some patients believe that illness can be prevented; they practice elaborate rituals and engage special persons to carry out those rituals in an attempt to prevent disease. Other patients look at prevention as an attempt to control the future. They may consider this an impossible feat in the way they view their lives. They may wonder about the necessity of making a trip to a health care provider for preventive care, such as immunizations. Others may think prevention is tempting fate and following through with prevention is risky.

Curing Illness. When disease does strike, some people blame pathogens (germs), some blame spirits, and others blame an imbalance in the body. Some cultural groups have folk medicine practices, such as rituals, special procedures (e.g., rubbing the skin with the edge of a coin to release the toxins causing illness), and special persons in the group to cure disease (e.g., physician, herbalist, shaman). Some groups believe that special foods or food combinations (e.g., "cold" foods for "hot" illness) and herbs (e.g., echinacea and feverfew) can prevent or cure illnesses. Others see no relationship between diet and health.

Complementary and Alternative Medicine. The dominant health system in the United States is biomedicine (Western medicine). Biomedicine focuses on symptoms, with the goal of finding the cause of a disease and then eliminating or relieving the problem. Over 50% of Americans are seeking methods that avoid side effects from medications and treatments and/or that focus on the whole body and not just symptoms when treating disease. They are spending billions of dollars a year, mostly out of pocket, on complementary (used in conjunction with biomedical treatments) and alternative (substitute for conventional medicine) medicine. Complementary and alternative medicine (CAM) focuses on assisting the body's own healing powers and restoring body balance. The diversity of non-Western health care practices among the many cultural groups in the United

States has helped increase the interest and use of CAM. The National Center for Complementary and Alternative Medicine (NCCAM) of the National Institutes of Health conducts research and evaluates the effectiveness and safety of CAM. NCCAM's website (http://www.nccam.nih.gov) provides information about CAM.

Modesty. Individuals in some cultures are embarrassed when they have to discuss bodily functions or allow certain body parts to be examined. Hygiene practices vary according to beliefs, living conditions, personal resources, and physical characteristics.

Mental Illness. Some cultural groups attach a stigma to mental illness and psychiatrists but are accepting of impairments to physical health. Other groups believe that the mental symptoms manifested are a healthy reaction to an emotional crisis. Yet others believe that the mind and body are united and are not separate entities. These cultures may have traditional healers who are experts at healing both the mind and the body. Some people may seek out traditional healers to heal the mind, while at the same time consult Western medicine to heal the body.

 Try This

Cultural Patterns: Wellness Beliefs and Practices

To assist you in identifying your own cultural patterns in regard to wellness beliefs and practices, respond to the following statements and questions.
1. Describe what it means to you to be in good health.
2. What are some of your own practices or beliefs about staying well?
3. Describe what it means to you to be sick.
4. List some foods in your diet that you believe help prevent illness.
   a. How does eating these foods prevent illness?
   b. What are some foods you must avoid to prevent illness?
5. List some foods in your diet that help you recover when you are sick.
   a. What illnesses do they cure?
   b. How do they cure illness?
6. Discuss complementary and alternative medicine (CAM) used by your family.
7. If you use CAM and biomedicine, do you inform the physician of CAM use, including herbs, during a clinic visit?
8. Describe your attitude toward mental illness.
   a. Describe what you think causes mental illness.
   b. Who do you think should treat mental illness?
   c. How do you believe mental illness is best treated?

Pregnancy and Birth Beliefs and Practices
Different cultures welcome a new member into the world in different ways. The Try This: Cultural Patterns: Pregnancy and Birth Beliefs and Practices box helps you to identify your own beliefs about pregnancy and birth.

 Try This

Cultural Patterns: Pregnancy and Birth Beliefs and Practices

To assist you in identifying your own cultural patterns in regard to birth beliefs and practices, respond to the following statements and questions about your family's customs regarding pregnancy and birth.
1. Do the women in your family receive prenatal care?
2. How is "discomfort" expressed during labor?
3. Who attends the birth?
4. Where does birth take place?
5. Who delivers the baby?
6. Is bonding encouraged?
7. What special practices take place after birth and during the postpartum period?
8. Are there special practices regarding the placenta and umbilical cord?
9. Is breastfeeding encouraged?
10. Are there precautions regarding breastfeeding?
11. Is birth control encouraged? Is it permitted?

Terminal Illness and Death Beliefs and Practices
Generally, death and terminal illness bring out strong emotions in most people. Be aware that some cultures have special taboos and prohibitions when a death occurs. Roles that family and friends carry out at the time of death may vary. There are many differences in the way different cultures handle terminal illness for a member. When death does occur, the rituals practiced are numerous and varied.

 Try This

Cultural Patterns: Terminal Illness and Death Beliefs and Practices

To assist you in identifying your own cultural patterns in regard to terminal illness and death beliefs and practices, respond to the following statements and questions pertaining to a death in your family.
1. Is it acceptable to tell a terminally ill family member the diagnosis? If yes, who tells the family member?
2. Where does an anticipated death usually occur (at home, in a hospital)?
3. Who should be present when the death occurs?
4. Does your family require specific treatment of the body after death?
5. Does your family permit/encourage autopsy or organ donation?
6. Who makes the burial arrangements?
7. Describe what you believe happens to you after death.
8. Does your family permit cremation?
9. Does your family have a funeral or memorial service?
10. Do you have a get-together after the burial? If so, for whom? What occurs during the get-together?
11. How does your family remember the dead?
12. Is autopsy and/or organ donation allowed?

Try This

Areas of Cultural Diversity

With your classmates, discuss your answers to statements and questions about various areas of cultural diversity, especially wellness and illness, birth, and death practices.

Regardless of which cultural group you belong to, these exercises about cultural diversity have given you the opportunity to think about the many ways you and your peers differ. You will observe some of these differences in patients in the clinical area. Along with that awareness of and sensitivity to differences, a tolerance may develop for ways of doing things that may be different from yours.

INCREASING YOUR KNOWLEDGE OF CULTURALLY DIVERSE GROUPS

No one can be an expert on every culture in the world. Even those who are experts on a particular culture do not like being labeled as such. These people are aware of the ever-changing nature of cultures and of the important individual variations that occur within any cultural group. Experts are always cautious about stereotyping persons in any particular cultural group.

CATEGORIES OF MAJOR HEALTH BELIEF SYSTEMS

Anthropologists have developed a helpful framework for generally discovering and understanding health belief systems of groups. They divide health beliefs into three major systems: biomedicine, personalistic, and naturalistic.

- Biomedicine is the primary belief system of the United States and is also called "Western medicine." There is an effort to transform nursing curriculums so they reflect multicultural concepts in nursing. However, it is possible that the curriculum of your school of practical/vocational nursing is set up to reflect biomedicine (Box 16-2).
- The personalistic system is found among groups native to the Americas, as well as those south of the

Sahara (e.g., Chad and Niger) and among the tribal peoples of Asia (Jackson, 1993) (Box 16-3).
- The naturalistic system of beliefs developed from the traditional medical practices of the ancient civilizations of China, India, and Greece. Variants of this belief system are found today in the Philippines and among low-income African Americans and indigent white southerners (Jackson, 1993) (Box 16-4).

Box 16-2 Biomedical Health Belief

CAUSE OF DISEASE
- Abnormalities in structure and function of body organs, bacteria, viruses, biochemical alterations, immune system disturbance, environmental factors

HOW DISEASE IS DIAGNOSED
- Physical exam, x-ray, CT scan, MRI, identification of pathogens by lab studies

HOW DISEASE IS TREATED
- Drugs, surgery, diet

WHO CURES THE DISEASE
- Physician

HOW DISEASE IS PREVENTED
- Hand washing, covering mouth when sneezing, lifestyle (diet, exercise, etc.), immunizations

Adapted with permission from Jackson L: Understanding, eliciting, and negotiating patients' multicultural health beliefs. *Nurse Practitioner* 18 (4):30-32, 37-38.

Box 16-3 Personalistic Health Belief

CAUSE OF DISEASE
- Punishment by a ghost, god, evil spirit, sorcerer, ancestor spirit, witch
- Breach of taboo, sin, evil eye, curse
- Above results in soul loss or theft, possession of spirit, poisoning, curse

HOW DISEASE IS DIAGNOSED
- By a person with magic or supernatural powers

WHO CURES THE DISEASE
- Shaman, diviner, herbalist, magic/religious specialist

HOW DISEASE IS TREATED
- Counteract cause with herbs, prayer, rituals, laying on of hands

HOW DISEASE IS PREVENTED
- Faithful observance of rituals (for example, honor ceremonies for ancestors), protective spells, wearing objects that have magic properties against evil eye or injury (amulets)

Adapted with permission from Jackson L: Understanding, eliciting, and negotiating patients' multicultural health beliefs. *Nurse Practitioner* 18 (4):30-32, 37-38.

Box 16-4 Naturalistic Health Belief

CAUSE OF DISEASE
- Imbalance of body elements
- Yin (cold)/yang (heat)
- Wet/dry
- Emotions
- Bad luck

HOW DISEASE IS DIAGNOSED
- Cause of excess heat or cold identified

HOW DISEASE IS TREATED
- Regain body balance, foods, acupuncture, coining, cupping

WHO CURES THE DISEASE
- Physician or herbalist—no supernatural or magical powers

HOW DISEASE IS PREVENTED
- Maintain balance of hot and cold in body, mind, spirit, and environment

Adapted with permission from Jackson L: Understanding, eliciting, and negotiating patients' multicultural health beliefs. *Nurse Practitioner* 18 (4):30-32, 37-38.

- Rarely does a group ascribe to all the beliefs in one system. You might see elements of each of the three systems at work in one individual. For example, a Hispanic patient with a strep throat might take an antibiotic as prescribed by the medical doctor, drink herbal teas as suggested by the curandero, and say prayers as suggested by the religious authority.

DIVERSITY PROFILES OF PREDOMINANT CULTURAL GROUPS IN THE UNITED STATES

At the beginning of the twentieth century, the majority of immigrants to the United States were of European ancestry. According to preliminary reports of the 2010 Census, the total population of the United States can be broken down as white: 65%; Hispanic: 16%; Asian: 5%; African American: 12%; and American Indian/Alaskan Native: 1.4% (Yen, 2011). If current immigration and birth trends continue, it is projected that by the year 2050, non-Hispanic whites will become a minority (Yen, 2011). Box 16-5 provides profiles of these culturally diverse groups.

DEVELOPING CULTURAL COMPETENCE IN HEALTH CARE SITUATIONS

You have started the long road to becoming a practical/vocational nurse who gives culturally competent care. Up to this point, participating in this chapter has given you the opportunity to do the following:

- Identify your culture and its strengths and limitations.
- Recognize how your culture affects your thinking and behavior.
- Discover how persons are similar despite their cultural group.
- Discover how persons are unique despite their cultural group.

Box 16-5 Diversity Profiles of Predominant Cultural Groups in the United States

These profiles are intended to be a general sketch of the culture of the group.

AFRICAN AMERICANS
- **Origin:** From Africa as slaves
- **Family structure:** Matriarchal, nuclear and extended family, fictive kin (not really relation—for example, "Aunt" Bessie)
- **Religion:** Protestant denominations, Catholicism, and Islam
- **Food preferences:** Chicken, fish, leafy greens, yams, grits, and cornbread
- **Illness beliefs:** Illness results from bad spirits, a hex, a spell, as punishment from God. May treat illnesses with home remedies, teas, herbs, compresses. May wait until illness becomes serious before seeking medical care. May visit a spiritualist or folk healer.

HMONG
- **Origin:** Vietnam, Laos, Thailand, Burma
- **Family structure:** Patriarchal. Nuclear family plus extended family (father, mother, brothers, sisters, uncles, aunts, nieces, and nephews) considered one family.
- **Religion:** Animism (worship of deceased ancestors). This may be replaced by or combined with Catholicism and Buddhism.
- **Food:** Rice the main food and served at each meal. Noodles, rarely eat fruit, adults rarely consume dairy products.
- **Illness beliefs:** Imbalance between spirit and the body. Natural and supernatural causes of illness. Natural plants, roots, and herbs used to cure a sick person. Shaman may be called to visit sick person in hospital. Healing rituals performed at home. May use cupping, coining, and pinching of skin as cure.

HISPANICS
- **Origin:** Mexico, Puerto Rico, Cuba, Spain, Central America (El Salvador, Guatemala, Honduras, Nicaragua, Panama, Costa Rica, Belize), South America (Colombia, Ecuador, Peru, Argentina, Venezuela, Chile, Bolivia, Uruguay, Paraguay).
  The following information may vary by country.
- **Family structure:** Nuclear, extended, patriarchal. Family not always defined by blood or marriage.
- **Religion:** Catholic but changing to various Protestant Evangelical religions, Pentecostal and other sects/groups, African spirit religion, voodoo, or a combination of these.
- **Food:** Rice, beans, spices; food choices vary due to socioeconomic status, country of origin, and location within country. Many have "hot" and "cold" foods. Some think American food is bland.
- **Illness beliefs:** A punishment from God for bad behavior or God's will, evil eye (*mal de ojo*), evil spells, fright (*susto*) magic, "hot" and "cold" imbalance, lack of cleanliness, humoral (body fluids) imbalance.

AMERICAN INDIANS/ALASKAN NATIVES
- **Origin:** North America. The U.S. federal government recognizes 550 tribes, bands, and nations, with an additional 200 tribes not federally recognized. This population is very diverse, and retention of traditional customs and the level of acculturation are vastly different. Tribes in different geographic areas differ, as do people in tribes (Lipson and Dibble, 2006).
- **Family structure:** Matriarchal, patriarchal, kinship roles extensive and fictive at times.
- **Religion:** Traditional beliefs, Christian, combine different religious practices.
- **Food:** Diet high in fat, salty, and sugary.
- **Illness beliefs:** Violation of taboos, body, mind, spirit out of harmony with God, nature. May use native healers and ceremonies to restore harmony in conjunction with Western medicine. Sacred objects should not be touched or moved by staff.

Box 16-5	Diversity Profiles of Predominant Cultural Groups in the United States—cont'd

ARAB AMERICANS

- **Origin:** The Arab world consists of 22 countries and territories, and, as with other cultural groups, there is great variation based on country of origin, social class, education, urban or rural origin, and time in the United States. Most of the people in these countries are Muslim (Lipson and Dibble, 2006). Approximately 128 countries have people of the Muslim religion. Not all of these people are Arab, but the culture of the Islam religion links people from these various countries. Islam and how it affects your patient care are discussed in Chapter 17.

Notes

Information about "yin" and "yang" can be accessed at http://www.taopage.org/yinyang.html.

Information about cupping can be accessed at www.medscape.com/viewarticle/487333.8.

Information about "evil eye" can be accessed at http://www.culturediversity.org/hisp.htm.

Information about humoral pathology can be accessed at http://anthro.palomar.edu/medical/humoral_pathology.htm.

Information about curanderos can be accessed at http://www.brighthub.com/health/alternative-medicine/articles/21775.aspx.

Adapted from Reinhardt E: *Through the eyes of others—intercultural resource directory for health care professionals.* Minneapolis: University of Minnesota School of Public Health, 1995, pp. 5-6, 8-14; Lipson J, Dibble S: *Culture and clinical care.* The Regents, University of California School of Nursing, 2006, UCSF Nursing Press.

- Gain knowledge of the three major health belief systems to increase your awareness of different worldviews about the cause, treatment, and prevention of disease.
- Gain awareness of ethnocentrism that can help you respect the health beliefs and practices of others when they are different from your own.
- Learn to respond flexibly when your values and assumptions differ from those of your patients.

Your next step to cultural competence is to develop a knowledge base for a few cultures that are different from yours.

IDENTIFY YOUR AGENCY'S CULTURAL GROUPS

Identify the cultural groups in your community that are served by local health care agencies. Use the following blank lines to list the groups. It is necessary to be knowledgeable about the cultural groups that you frequently come across in your community.

_____

_____

_____

_____

Try This

Your Area's Cultural Groups

1. A helpful learning activity is to hear reports from peers about various cultural groups.
2. Remember to think beyond the more traditional cultural groups, based on ethnicity. Include the disabled, elderly, single parents, alternative lifestyles, and so on.
3. Read about the different cultures that are served in your area. Use the References and Suggested Readings listed at the back of this book for this chapter, Internet sources in the text, and the resources of your learning resource center (LRC), as suggested in Chapter 5, to find texts and articles about specific cultural groups. Google a specific group to obtain information (http://www.google.com), and remember to check your sources.

4. View documentaries on television about cultural groups.
5. Attend community events sponsored by cultural groups.
6. Attend graduations, weddings, birth celebrations, and funerals of different cultures when the opportunities present themselves.
7. Attend a religious service of a cultural group.
8. Read novels involving different cultures.
9. Attend seminars about cultural groups.
10. Invite a member of a cultural group to class to talk about the health/illness beliefs of the group of whom he or she is a member.

MODIFY YOUR WORK SETTING

The health care environment can be made more "welcoming" to culturally diverse patients. Many of these changes require little cost or time to implement, but the results can promote better health and compliance among culturally diverse patients. Box 16-6 presents suggestions for modifying the workplace environment for the practical/vocational nurse working in health care agencies with culturally diverse patients.

CARE PLANNING FOR CULTURALLY DIVERSE PATIENTS IN YOUR SERVICE AREA

Imagine this scenario: Because of short staffing and heavy workloads, your 55-year-old Hmong patient's cultural assessment on admission was not done. This patient speaks limited English. For the past 2 days, this patient has not eaten his breakfast, which arrives on the floor at 7:30 AM. You refer to the topic "Hmong in Culture and Nursing Care" in Lipson and Dibble's (2006) book *Culture and Clinical Care.* According to the book, Hmong usually eat two to three meals a day, but if only two meals are eaten, the first meal is usually eaten at 9 AM or 10 AM. The licensed practical/vocational nurse sends a note to the Dietary Department to schedule two meals a day for this patient (breakfast at 9:30 AM

Box 16-6	**Modifying the Environment to Accommodate Culturally Diverse Patients**

- Identify the various cultural groups that use the health care facility.
- Post welcome signs in the languages of the groups you serve.
- Arrange for messages on answering machines to include the languages of the patients you serve. Place magazines in waiting rooms that reflect the diversity of the patients you serve.
- Include background music that reflects the diversity of the patients you serve.
- Provide handouts, appointment cards, and patient education materials in the languages of the patients you serve.
- Decorate the environment (pictures, posters, objects, etc.) to reflect the diversity of the patients you serve.
- Stock adhesive bandages that do not match any specific skin tone—for example, Walt Disney characters for children and fluorescent or varied colors for adults.
- In waiting areas, provide books, toys, and multicultural videos for children that promote acceptance of diversity. Sesame Street and SpongeBob SquarePants themes are especially effective and accepted.

Adapted from Reinhardt E: *Through the eyes of others—intercultural resource directory for health care professionals.* Minneapolis: University of Minnesota School of Public Health, 1995, pp. 19-20.

and the evening meal at the regular time that trays are delivered).

Each patient of a different culture needs to have data gathered regarding activities of daily living (ADLs) and personal health beliefs and practices. Develop a fact sheet for collecting data for each patient (Box 16-7). Use your culture resources and select topics and questions from the exercises found in this chapter. Clarify ADLs and health beliefs and practices for your patient.

Use reference guides that present general information about different cultural groups. These guides are helpful when you are dealing with a patient from a culture with which you are not familiar because they offer general information about, for example, wellness and illness beliefs and practices, nutritional preferences, and communication issues. These quick sources of generalities of various cultural groups are a starting point for learning which topics to include when collecting data (assessing) that must be clarified and validated with the individual patient. Examples of reference guides include the following:

- Lipson and Dibble, *Culture and Clinical Care.* This book lists information for the same topics used for learning activities, plus more topics for 24 ethnic groups found in the United States.
- D'Avanzo and Geissler, *Pocket Guide to Cultural Assessment.* This *truly* pocket-sized reference book contains information on many of the topics you have been using for learning activities, plus more general information for 180 different cultures throughout the world, listed by country.
- Dibble and Robertson, *Lesbian Health 101: A Clinician's Guide* provides information about health

Box 16-7	**Sample Data-Gathering Sheet Using a Traditional Hmong Patient as an Example**

The following 12 questions are assessment items for all patients. In parentheses are generalizations from the text about traditional Hmong culture that explain the data collected for this patient. The explanations are applicable to the culture of the traditional Hmong group only.

PATIENT: CULTURE: TRADITIONAL HMONG

1. What language do you use to speak/read? (The Hmong written language developed in the 1950s. Most elderly Hmongs are illiterate in their own language.)
2. Observe eye contact during questions. (Consider prolonged, direct eye contact rude.)
3. Observe reaction to handshake when introducing self. (Handshakes are appropriate.)
4. How long have you lived in the United States? (Assimilation may occur the longer a person is in the dominant culture.)
5. What is your religion? What is its importance in your daily life? (May have animistic beliefs in which spirits inhabit objects and natural settings. Worship ancestors with ceremonies so ancestors will bring good fortune and protect the family from harm. Buddhism.)
6. What caused your present illness? (Traditional causes of illness might be soul loss or illness caused by an ancestral spirit.)
7. How can your illness be best treated? (In traditional religious/spiritual beliefs, a shaman is necessary to communicate with the spirit world to learn why the person is ill and what sacrifice is required to make the person well.)
8. Do you use home remedies to cure illness? (Cupping, coining, and pinching are used to release evil spirits or illness-causing toxins from the body.)
9. What is your usual meal pattern at home? (Hmong usually eat two to three meals a day. If two meals are eaten, the first meal is usually eaten at 9 AM or 10 AM.)
10. What foods are in your usual diet? (Rice with small amounts of meat, fish, and green vegetables. Fruit is rarely eaten.)
11. Will you accept visitors while in the hospital? (Visitors are welcomed and helpful in recovery.)
12. Who in your family has decision-making authority? (Women allowed opinions; father/husband makes final decisions.)

Topics and explanations for data-gathering sheet were taken from Lipson and Dibble: *Culture and nursing care: a pocket guide.* San Francisco: UCSF Nursing Press, 2006, pp. 250-263.

issues in lesbians, an underserved minority, that are different from those of heterosexual women.

- The Transcultural Nursing website (http:// www.culturediversity.org) provides information pertaining to people from diverse cultural backgrounds with a range of cultural behaviors in health and illness.

These books explain the limitations of their use in introductory chapters. *Be sure to read the preface and introductory material!* The website presents generalizations about cultural groups. When using this information, it is important to avoid stereotyping your patient. Use Box 16-8 as a guide to help you avoid falling into the stereotype trap.

Suspect cultural differences when a patient is not following the plan of care, refuses treatment, is a "problem" patient, and so on. Question the patient about his or her ADLs and wellness and illness beliefs. When cultural differences are identified, follow Jackson's (1993) suggestions for negotiating patient care with culturally diverse patients. Doing so will result in fewer dissatisfied patients and more compliance with the plan of care.

Box 16-8	How to Avoid Stereotyping Culturally Diverse Patients

- Avoid automatically applying the information you gain to all individuals in a cultural group. Doing so is called the "cookbook method" of learning about different cultures.
- Applying information with the cookbook method makes you guilty of stereotyping individuals—that is, assuming that everyone in that cultural group is the same.
- You have learned that classifying people as being the same just because they share the same religion, lifestyle, or ethnic background is stereotyping.
- Expect personal variations in each cultural group about which you gather information.
- Behaviors found in articles, reference books, and on the Internet containing culture and nursing care for various cultural groups can be applied generally to cultural groups as a whole but cannot automatically be applied to every individual in that group.
- Variable, individual differences exist because of the changing nature of the culture, the patient's personal life experiences (including hospitalization), age, religion, and adaptation to a new culture.
- No individual is a stereotype of one's culture of origin. Individuals are a unique blend of the diversity found within each culture.
- Gather cultural data for each patient. Discover the behaviors in your culture guide that apply to your patient.
- Look at information about cultural groups as explaining behavior in patients, not predicting behavior.

Adapted from D'Avanzo and Geissler: *Pocket guide to cultural assessment.* St Louis: Mosby, 2008.

If the Hmong patient in the scenario had a cultural assessment on admission, or if his nurse had asked him why he refused to eat breakfast, the staff would have found out that he did not like oatmeal and bacon and eggs! The staff chose these foods for him because they were uncertain if he could read the hospital menus. Because, according to Lipson and Dibble (2006), "Hmong people are very polite and reticent," he did not bring this matter to the attention of the staff. He merely did not eat. When questioned about his continued refusal of breakfast, he admitted that he liked Rice Krispies and frequently eats this cold cereal for breakfast at home. The principle governing this situation is that general group behavior *sometimes explains* observed behavior (he did not complain out of respect), but it is *not predictive* of individual behavior (he did not eat because the meals were served at inappropriate times; he did not eat breakfast because he did not like the foods that were served).

ADAPTING PLANS OF CARE FOR CULTURALLY DIVERSE PATIENTS

Jackson (1993) offers suggestions for finding out about patients' health beliefs, along with guidelines for developing plans of care that incorporate those beliefs through a process of negotiation with the patient. Jackson points out that discovering specific health beliefs is easier if the nurse is familiar with a specific culture, but this is not absolutely necessary. Jackson suggests ways of negotiating a treatment plan with culturally diverse patients. The practical/vocational nurse can collaborate with the professional nurse to incorporate these beliefs into the patient's plan of care:

1. *Discover the health beliefs of the individual.* Be respectful and open-minded when you question the patient about the cause of the health problem, when it started, its severity, its course, the problems it has caused in the patient's life, and the treatment the patient thinks will cure the disease. *Avoid assuming anything.* When you are unsure of anything, ask! In situations of cultural diversity, our patients are the teachers and we are the students.

2. *Negotiate treatment plans with the patient.* Avoid trying to change patients' beliefs. Cultural health practices are deeply ingrained. Tradition means more than your word does, even though you are a representative of a health profession. Instead, involve the patient in making decisions about his or her own care. Do so in a way that does not threaten the patient's beliefs and practices or conflict with them. Explain from the biomedical point of view the cause of the disease, how the disease alters the body, the role of treatment, and the

expected outcome. Then compare the patient's belief system with that of biomedicine. All patients need to have this information to help ensure their cooperation with the plan of care. See Box 16-9 for an example of negotiating treatment plans with the patient.

3. *Preserve the beliefs and practices that are helpful to the patient.* Starting in 1993, the Office of Alternative Medicine of the National Institutes of Health began to identify, study, and bring together the best healing practices of other cultures with those of Western medicine. Many of the beliefs and practices of non-Western systems of health beliefs have proved beneficial. Two examples are acupuncture and acupressure, and more are about to be approved. Collaborate with your professional nurse about patients' practices that have not yet been researched or found effective. If the practices seem to help the patient and do no harm, include them in the plan of care, regardless of your ability to see the benefit of the practice. These practices have special significance and meaning to some individuals, despite the fact that you may be unable to see how or whether they help. Box 16-10 provides an example of preserving the beliefs and practices that are helpful to the patient.

Box 16-9   Negotiating Treatment Plans with the Patient

SITUATION

Nancy Thai, a Cambodian refugee, resides in Chicago with her husband and three children. She delivered an 8-pound boy early this morning at St. Mary's Hospital. The practical/vocational nurse who was assigned to Mrs. Thai on the day shift reported to the evening staff that the patient was "uncooperative." Specifically, Mrs. Thai refused to eat and take her pills. In frustration the nurse said, "I just don't know what to do with her."

CULTURAL HEALTH BELIEFS IN THIS SITUATION

Mrs. Thai's health beliefs include the belief that pregnancy and birth weaken the body. Also, blood loss during delivery is considered a yin (cold) condition. Mrs. Thai believes that for 1 month after delivery, a mother must have a yang (hot) diet to restore strength, keep the stomach warm, counteract heat loss, prevent incontinence, and prevent itching at the site of the episiotomy. "Cold" refers to foods that are cold in their physical form as well as considered cold in nature. "Cold" foods (e.g., salt, crab, salad, bananas, sour foods [e.g., tomato, tangerine, plum, lemon, grape, vinegar, grapefruit, olives]), as well as cold water, are viewed as bad for the stomach and the teeth. "Warm" refers to foods that are warm in their physical form as well as considered warm in nature. Among preferred "warm" foods are rice, fish, and chicken.

NEGOTIATING TREATMENT PLANS

The nurse assigned to Mrs. Thai on the evening shift informed her that the doctor had ordered pills to help prevent bleeding after delivery. After discussing this, Mrs. Thai agreed to take her pills with warm water. In a respectful manner, the evening nurse asked Mrs. Thai if she did not like the hospital food. Mrs. Thai smiled and explained her need for a yang diet. The evening nurse said that she could arrange to have the dietary department send rice, chicken, or any other food Mrs. Thai would find helpful after childbirth. Mrs. Thai said her husband would bring rice and chicken from home. The nurse canceled Mrs. Thai's food order but requested a pot of hot water, silverware, and napkins for her use.

Box 16-10   Preserving the Beliefs and Practices That Are Helpful to the Patient

SITUATION

Ted Washington, a 72-year-old African American, lives in a rural area of South Carolina. He was admitted to Brent Hospital with pneumonia and advanced osteoarthritis. John, an LPN, is his nurse. John cannot understand how anyone can get to such a state of ill health without seeing a doctor. John is especially upset because Mr. Washington could have prevented much of his disability from arthritis if he had followed a preventive program when he first developed symptoms of this disease.

CULTURAL HEALTH BELIEFS IN THIS SITUATION

Mr. Washington has lived in poverty for his entire life. As with any person in this situation, his main concern in life has been the present and getting through his problems on a day-to-day basis. Mr. Washington's time orientation is the moment (present), not the future; therefore, preventive regimens have not been central to his way of thinking. Persons with similar backgrounds and situations delay care until the disease interferes with their ability to work or results in a disability.

It cannot be said that Mr. Washington ignored his condition. He participated in self-treatment by using cultural health practices in the form of topical application of oils and ointments to his aching joints. These self-treatments helped Mr. Washington deal physically and psychologically with his condition. Mr. Washington looks at his disability as a punishment from God, who let something get into his joints. His belief stems from the wellness and illness beliefs brought to this country from Africa. These beliefs center on wellness as a state experienced when one is in harmony with nature. Illness is experienced as a state of disharmony with nature.

PRESERVING THE BELIEFS AND PRACTICES THAT ARE HELPFUL TO THE PATIENT

John supported Mr. Washington's application of oils and ointments. He applied massage lotion to Mr. Washington's joints at bedtime. John arranged for Mr. Washington's friend to bring his ointment from home. After clarifying self-treatment with the patient, John realized that such applications could give psychological comfort to the patient, as well as relieve pain. In the future John will make it a point to ask all newly admitted patients about self-treatment for their diseases.

4. *Repattern harmful practices.* Harmful practices that are prevalent in Western society include smoking, diets high in fat, refined grains and refined sugar, and lack of exercise. In Burma, when a woman is pregnant, extreme dietary restrictions are imposed. In Cambodia, mud is placed on the umbilicus of newborns. These practices are dangerous and if followed could lead to high blood pressure, heart disease, maternal toxemia, poor fetal development, and tetanus in the newborn. Explain your reasons for opposing a harmful practice, and offer alternatives. Box 16-11 provides an example of repatterning harmful practices.

When practical/vocational nurses demonstrate awareness of and respect for the many cultural groups in their service area, knowledge about these cultural groups, and skill in applying their knowledge in a caring manner, they are on the road to delivering culturally competent care.

| Box 16-11 | Repatterning Harmful Practices |

SITUATION
Over a 2-month period during the summer, a Chinese infant was seen in a New York clinic for diarrhea that did not respond to treatment. Stool cultures showed no unusual organisms. A change in formula did nothing to stop the diarrhea. During a home visit, the visiting nurse found a hot apartment with several bottles of home-prepared formula on the windowsill. Several other full bottles were in the refrigerator.

CULTURAL HEALTH BELIEFS IN THIS SITUATION
The child's mother explained that she had recently given birth. Because of this, she had to avoid cold. To avoid her exposure to the cold of the refrigerator, her husband would remove the bottles from the refrigerator that she needed during the day before he left for work and line them up on the windowsill.

REPATTERNING THE PATIENT'S HARMFUL PRACTICES
The visiting nurse explained that by being exposed to the heat of the day, the formula would grow germs that could cause diarrhea. She asked if there was a way that the bottles could be kept cold until needed. After some thought, the mother said she could put on a hat, coat, and gloves before removing the bottles from the refrigerator. The nurse agreed with this plan. The baby had no further episodes of diarrhea.

Reproduced with permission from Jackson L: Understanding, eliciting and negotiating patients' multicultural health beliefs. *Nurse Practitioner* 18:30-32, 37-38, 42, 1993.

Get Ready for the NCLEX-PN® Examination

Key Points

- A good place to start learning about how people are different is to remind yourself that all persons are unique but have similarities as well.
- Everyone shares the nine basic daily needs. How individuals meet these needs varies with their culture, the learned ways they have of doing things.
- One guideline in health care is the philosophy of individual worth, the confidence that all persons are unique and have value regardless of the way they view their world, and they deserve the best nursing care you can give.
- Awareness of cultural diversity is important for practical/vocational nurses so they can avoid false assumptions and misunderstandings about the patients in their care.
- The first step in understanding other people's culture is to understand your own culture. It is important to be aware of your personal beliefs and practices in the areas of family, religion, communication, educational background, economic level, pregnancy, wellness and illness beliefs and practices, and death and dying.
- Some ways to learn about cultural diversity include reading about different cultures, especially those found in your geographic area, and actively listening to reports from your peers who are culturally different.
- Cultural characteristics of groups are not predictive of behavior of individuals in a group. They are generalizations. *Always allow for individual variations within specific groups.*
- Understanding your own culture, attaining sensitivity to cultural diversity, gaining knowledge about other people's cultures, and adapting the plan of care to reflect the patient's health and illness beliefs put you well on the road to providing culturally competent nursing care.

Additional Learning Resources

evolve Go to your Evolve website (http://evolve.elsevier.com/Hill/Success) for the following FREE learning resources:
- Answers to Critical Thinking Scenarios
- Additional learning activities
- Additional Review Questions for the NCLEX-PN® exam
- Helpful phrases for communicating in Spanish and more!

Review Questions for the NCLEX-PN® Examination

1. Select the term practical/vocational nurses need to avoid when studying different cultures.
   1. Stereotyping
   2. Socialization
   3. Enculturation
   4. Assimilation

2. Select the statement that best illustrates the philosophy of individual worth.
   1. All individuals are unique and have value regardless of their differences in how they meet daily needs.
   2. People who belong to ethnic and minority groups have different daily needs in most needs categories.
   3. People of different cultures need to be approached as if their culture is the best of all culture groups in the area.
   4. People of color are sensitive about their differences and need to have them downplayed in patient situations.

3. An Asian-American resident in a nursing home does not want to follow the nursing care plan regarding diet. The best course of action for the nursing staff would be to:
   1. Insist the resident accept the diet as ordered.
   2. Document the stubbornness of this resident.
   3. Avoid making an issue of his noncompliance.
   4. Consider the possibility of cultural differences.

4. Mr. Metoxen, a member of the Oneida Tribe of Indians, was admitted to the medical floor with a diagnosis of angina. He is to receive nitroglycerin PRN for chest pain. Select the priority cultural concern of the practical/vocational nurse for administering pain medication to a patient whose culture values stoic behavior.
   1. That the drug be kept in a dark container to protect it from light.
   2. That the drug is always kept with the patient when he is walking.
   3. That nonverbal signs of pain not be overlooked in this situation.
   4. That the patient's pain level be assessed at the beginning of the shift.

Alternate Format Item

1. Practical/vocational nurses use culture and nursing care guides to gather information about different cultures. Which of the following suggestions apply to the use of culture reference guides? *(Select all that apply.)*
   1. Avoid applying information automatically to all members of a culture.
   2. Variation in any member of the same cultural group does not occur.
   3. Assume that all members of a cultural group are the same in all aspects.
   4. Information obtained explains behavior but does not predict behavior.
   5. Once you gather data for one patient, this information can be applied to others.

Critical Thinking Scenario

Hector Santiago, a legal Mexican immigrant, has been in the United States for only a short time. He was admitted to the hospital after experiencing 3 days of intermittent chest pain. He is not taking well to bed rest and has attempted to walk down the hall several times when he should stay in bed. Using gestures only, Mr. Santiago has been indicating that he is in pain, but he consistently refuses drugs. During visiting hours, Mr. Santiago's wife, children, sisters, brothers, and parents visit. Dr. Jones plans to order a diagnostic study to evaluate Mr. Santiago's coronary arteries. He asks Mr. Santiago's wife for permission, and she refuses. Mr. Santiago has a stroke, and after a few days, the doctor tells Mrs. Santiago that he must go to a nursing home. Mrs. Santiago is horrified to hear this news. Why did Mr. Santiago wait three days to get care? Why did he attempt to walk down the hall when he knew he was on bed rest? Why did he refuse drugs for pain? Why did he have so many visitors? Why did Mrs. Santiago refuse coronary artery studies for her husband? Why did she become upset when nursing home placement was suggested for her husband?

Spiritual Needs, Spiritual Caring, and Religious Differences

Objectives

On completing this chapter, you will be able to do the following:

1. Differentiate between spirituality and religion.
2. Identify the difference between the spiritual and emotional dimensions of individuals.
3. Discuss the practical/vocational nurse's role in providing spiritual care to the patient and the family.
4. Discuss nursing interventions that can be used to meet the spiritual needs of patients.
5. List members of the health care team who can help provide spiritual care for patients.

6. Discuss personal religious and/or spiritual beliefs, or the absence of them, and how these beliefs will influence nursing practice.
7. Discuss the general beliefs and practices that account for the differences among various Western, Middle Eastern, and Eastern religions, philosophies, and groups in the United States and Canada.
8. Describe nursing interventions/considerations of patients of various religions, philosophies, and groups.

Key Terms

agnostic (ăg-NŎS-tĭk, p. 214)
Allah (ĂL-ă, p. 220)
atheist (Ā-thē-ĭst, p. 214)
Buddha (BŪ-dă, p. 225)
emotional needs (ē-MO-shŭn-ăl nēds, p. 212)
Jesus Christ (krīst, p. 216)
parish nurse (PĀR-ĭsh, p. 212)
pastoral care team (PĂS-tě-RĂL, p. 213)
reincarnation (RĒ-ĭn-kăr-NĀ-shŭn, p. 223)

religion (rē-LĬ-jŭn, p. 211)
religious denomination (dě-NŎM-ĭ-NĀ-shŭn, p. 214)
rituals (RĬ-choo-ăls, p. 214)
spirit (SPĬ-rĭt, p. 211)
spiritual caring (SPĬR-ĭ-chūăl CĀR-ĭng, p. 212)
spiritual dimension (SPĬR-ĭ-chūăl dĭ-MĔN-shŭn, p. 212)
spiritual distress (SPĬR-ĭ-chūăl dis-TRĔS, p. 214)
spiritual needs (SPĬR-ĭ-chūăl nēds, p. 212)
spirituality (SPĬR-ĭ-chū-ĂL-ĭ-tē, p. 211)

 Keep in Mind

If you were hospitalized, is it important to you that the staff be informed of your spiritual practices?

Jan, the evening nurse, found Thomas Bernes, age 32, sitting up in bed, crying and moaning with what she interpreted as pain after a testicular biopsy that was positive for cancer. After assessment, she volunteered to get Thomas some pain medication, but he refused. Thomas shouts, "Why did I have to get cancer? Why me?" Then he says, "Oh, I'll be fine. Just leave me alone and I will get rid of the pain myself." Jan quickly and quietly leaves the room so Thomas can be alone.

In its *Nursing Diagnoses: 2009–2011* edition, the North American Nursing Diagnosis Association (NANDA) includes "spiritual distress" as a nursing diagnosis. In the foregoing patient situation, Thomas was in spiritual distress. A minister or priest might have been able to address Thomas's problem, but Thomas needed immediate spiritual care. It would have been helpful to Thomas if his

nurse had offered to spend time with him and encouraged him to talk about what he was thinking and feeling at that time. Nursing has always embraced a holistic approach to patient care: care of the body, mind, and spirit. Despite the NANDA-I diagnosis, some nurses are uncomfortable with matters of the spirit. Some have not had adequate education in how to deal with patients in this aspect of care.

SPIRITUALITY AND RELIGION

Spirituality is an essential part of being human. The word comes from the Latin word *spiritus*, which means "breath" or "air." The spirit is the very essence of a person, the innermost part of a person that provides animation. The spirit is a life force that penetrates a person's entire being. It includes the beliefs and value systems that give people strength and hope. The spirit gives meaning to life. It is hoped that the spiritual self grows and matures throughout one's life.

The terms *spirituality* and *religion* are related, but they have different meanings. Religion may be a spiritual experience that contains specific beliefs and rituals. It can include spirituality, but spirituality, one's life force, does not necessarily include religion. Participation in a religion may include spirituality, but spirituality does not necessarily include participation in a religion. According to LeGere (Carson, 1989), spirituality is not a religion. Spirituality is related to experience, but religion has to do with giving form to that experience. Spirituality focuses on what happens in the heart, and religion tries to make rules and capture that experience in a system.

SPIRITUAL VERSUS EMOTIONAL DIMENSION

Meeting the spiritual needs of patients through spiritual caring differs from providing emotional support. The spiritual dimension of a person gives insight into the meaning of life, suffering, and death. This dimension refers to the relationship of an individual to a higher power. Emotional needs include how people respond and deal with feelings of joy, anger, sorrow, guilt, remorse, and love. The spiritual dimension of a patient's life requires the same emphasis that other daily needs receive. When spiritual needs of patients exist and are met, practical/vocational nurses can say they have directed care to the total person.

IMPORTANCE OF SPIRITUAL CARE

Spiritual care involves helping patients to develop an awareness of and maintain the following:

- Inner strength
- Self-awareness
- Life's meaning and purpose
- Relationship to others
- Relationship to a higher power

Florence Nightingale encouraged nurses to be instruments of spiritual caring in all situations. Nurses should avoid waiting for crisis situations to occur before they become concerned about spiritual care. The Joint Commission requires spiritual assessments and interventions to support the spiritual needs of patients and families. As a practical/vocational nurse, you have the responsibility to provide spiritual care to patients and families.

WHO NEEDS SPIRITUAL CARE?

An individual's spiritual dimension is a very private and personal area. Although all people have a spiritual dimension, needs that arise in this area depend on a variety of situations and the individual's ability to cope with them. An example of nurses who routinely recognize spiritual needs are nurses who work with patients in various church settings in a health ministry. The goal of these parish nurses is to keep their groups happy and healthy by treating the whole

person—body, mind, and spirit. Parish nurses recognize the relationship between spirituality and health and encourage spiritual growth in their patients.

Crisis situations occur in all health care situations, but they especially arise in acute health care. Patients' beliefs and values can profoundly affect their response to these crises, their attitude toward treatment, and their rate of recovery. Be alert for the following patient situations that may intensify the need for spiritual care for patients and families:

- Hospitalization
- Patients who are in pain
- Patients who have a chronic or incurable disease
- Patients who are dying
- Families who have experienced the death of a loved one
- Patients who are facing an undesirable outcome of illness, such as an amputation
- Patients who have emotionally lost control of themselves

In her article "Called to Care: Addressing the Spiritual Needs of Patients," Schoenbeck (1994) said, "When the body and mind are battered by time and use, the spirit, the very essence of the patient, remains."

GATHERING DATA FOR SPIRITUAL ISSUES

The first step to providing spiritual care for patients is to strive to become comfortable dealing with spiritual matters. The second step is to become aware of your own spirituality and the spirit that is the essence of *you*. Gather data about your spiritual self. The exercise in the Try This: Your Personal Spirituality box can help you increase awareness of your personal spirituality.

 Try This

Your Personal Spirituality

1. How do you cope?
2. Who is your source of support?
3. Who are the significant people in your life?
4. With whom do you laugh?
5. Do you feel loved?
6. Do you have someone with whom to cry?
7. What gives your life meaning?
8. What brings joy to your life?
9. Do you believe in the power of prayer?
10. What are your beliefs about a higher power?
11. Do you have a relationship to a higher power?
12. Do you have a religious affiliation? If so, how do your religious beliefs affect your spirit?
13. What is your philosophy about life and death?

 Critical Thinking

My Spiritual Sensitivity

Have you ever said or heard others say, "My spirit is broken"? What does this remark mean to you?

MEETING THE SPIRITUAL NEEDS OF PATIENTS AND THEIR FAMILIES

Once you know your spiritual self, you will be better able to help others meet their spiritual needs. When you acknowledge that your beliefs are effective for you but not necessarily for others, you will be able to set your beliefs aside when helping patients and families meet their spiritual needs. The questions in the Your Personal Spirituality box can also be used to gather data for patients' spiritual condition. Respect for the belief system of patients and families can give strength, hope, and meaning to their lives. When working with patients and families, try to do the following:

- Ask questions to help patients and families verbalize beliefs, fears, and concerns, such as "What do you think is going to happen to you (your father/mother)?" and "Who is your source of support?"
- Show interest through supportive statements (see Chapter 13).
- Listen with an understanding attitude. Be sure your body language and affective response reflect what you are saying.
- Respond as naturally to spiritual concerns as you do to physical needs.
- Help patients face the reality of a terminal illness without abandoning hope.
- Encourage the patient's active involvement in self-care, which can help uphold hope.
- Allow families to participate in caregiving (e.g., offering fluids/ice chips, when allowed; wiping the patient's brow).
- Avoid false assurances such as "Everything will be okay."
- When a patient faces death, you can help to make the remaining days meaningful by attending to needs, respecting their beliefs and death practices, and approaching the patient in a supportive and empathetic manner. Feeling loved helps bring peace to the dying.

Box 17-1 lists spiritual care interventions that can be used by practical/vocational nurses.

PASTORAL CARE TEAM

The pastoral care team is made up of ministers, priests, rabbis, consecrated religious women (i.e., nuns/sisters), representatives of other religious organizations, and laypersons. All are educated to meet spiritual needs, in addition to religious needs, in a health care setting. The members of this team are allies with nurses in providing spiritual care. You can notify this team if a patient requests a visit. When members of the pastoral care team come to the unit to fill the request, inform them of the patient's background and condition. Describe the interventions you have incorporated into the patient's care to provide spiritual care. Remember

---

Box 17-1   Spiritual Care Interventions
• Ask open-ended questions. • Actively listen to the patient. Sit beside the patient. Make eye contact. • Be nonjudgmental of patients and their responses. • Avoid giving advice or a lecture to the patient. • Avoid being a proselytizer (i.e., a person who tries to convert another person to one's religion). • Be aware of nonverbal messages from the patient. • Understand the feelings of the patient, but avoid adopting those feelings for yourself. (See Chapter 13 for a discussion of sympathy versus empathy.) • Expect to learn from patients. • Stay with the patient after the person has received an unfavorable diagnosis. • When patients request help with prayer, offer to pray with them. • When a patient requests help with specific readings, offer to read to him or her. • Assist the patient to participate in desired religious/spiritual rituals. • Protect the patient's religious/spiritual articles.

that the pastoral care team does not relieve you of your responsibility to provide spiritual care.

By visiting, talking, and listening, the pastoral care team explores the patients' fears, hopes, and sources of strength. Because of federal privacy standards (see the Health Insurance Portability and Accountability Act [HIPAA] in Chapter 12), the health care facility may not make a patient's name available to church representatives without the patient's permission. Before being hospitalized/admitted, patients can personally notify their clergy regarding a planned hospitalization and desire for a visit. If an admitted patient requests a visit of personal clergy, follow the facility directive for arranging this request. Agency policies vary and are being tested nationwide.

HOW PATIENTS MEET SPIRITUAL NEEDS

PATIENTS' SPIRITUAL PRACTICES

Regardless of religious beliefs, or lack of them, *all* patients have a spiritual self. They also have spiritual needs and personal spiritual practices to meet those needs. Spiritual practices help individuals to develop an awareness of self, an understanding of the meaning and purpose of life, and an appreciation of their relationship to a higher power. Examples of personal spiritual practices may include gardening, reading inspirational books, listening to music, meditating, watching select TV shows and movies, communing with nature, walking a labyrinth, practicing breathing techniques, enjoying art, enjoying fresh flowers, volunteering, expressing gratitude, counting blessings, walking, talking with friends and relatives, and participating in crafts and hobbies.

Try This

My Spiritual Practices

Identify the spiritual practices that you use to meet spiritual needs.

RELIGION AND THE PATIENT

The religious self refers to the specific beliefs an individual holds in regard to a higher power. Some patients help to meet their spiritual needs by belonging to a specific religious denomination. A **religious denomination** is an organized group of people who share a philosophy that supports their particular concept of God or a higher power, as well as worship experiences.

Agnostics hold the belief that the existence of God can be neither proved nor disproved. **Atheists** do not believe that the supernatural exists, so they do not believe in God. Christians may find comfort and solace in their refuge in God, including passing into another life after death. The atheist does not have this belief. It may be difficult for the nurse who believes in the supernatural to relate to a person with atheistic beliefs. The nurse may feel unsuccessful in meeting the total needs of the patient who is an atheist because atheists do not believe in the supernatural. The spiritual aspect, however, is present in all individuals. Spiritual assessment and interventions are appropriate for agnostic and atheist patients. Encourage these patients to express personal feelings about life, death, separation, and loss.

Professional Pointer

Avoid imposing your personal beliefs and values on the patient.

VALUE OF RITUALS AND PRACTICES

The different rituals and practices of a religion are stabilizing forces for the patient. **Rituals** are a series of actions that have religious meaning. They can bring the security of the past into a crisis situation. Concrete symbols such as pictures, icons, herb packets, rosaries, statues, jewelry, and other objects can affirm the patient's connection with a higher power.

The value of patients' rituals and religious practices is determined by their faith. Value is not determined by scientific proof of their benefit. Studies have shown that people who have faith recover more quickly from illness, surgery, and addiction and are less likely to die prematurely from any cause. When patients are not allowed to practice their religious rituals, practices, and responsibilities, they may feel guilty and uneasy. This can also affect their recovery. As a practical/vocational nurse, you need to develop an awareness of the general religious philosophy of the patient's belief system. If membership is claimed in a specific denomination, question the patient about the rituals and exercises that the patient believes in and practices. **Spiritual distress** can be observed in patients who are unable to practice their religious rituals. It also can be observed in patients who experience a conflict between their religious and spiritual beliefs and the prescribed health regimen (e.g., a Catholic patient with continuous, severe psychiatric problems who is advised to avoid pregnancy).

THE PATIENT AND PRAYER

Prayer is a spiritual practice of some individuals whether or not they are members of an organized religion. Prayer can put a patient in touch with a personal higher power. Sometimes prayer can decrease anxiety as effectively as a drug. Prayer helps some patients cope with their illness or situation. Honor the request of the patient who wants to pray privately. If the patient requests prayer, the nurse needs to assist the patient or seek assistance in this matter. When patients express an interest in praying, ask what prayer they would like to say. Try to accommodate the request.

In her book *Spiritual Dimensions of Nursing Practice* (1989), Carson comments on conversational prayer, one of the many forms that prayer can take. In this type of prayer, the specific concerns and needs of the patient are included in the prayer. Carson provides the following interaction between a patient awaiting a cesarean section and a nurse who noticed the patient had been crying. It is an excellent example of the simplicity and effectiveness of conversational prayer.

Nurse: You have been crying. What's wrong?
Patient: I wanted to see my minister this morning, but he will not be able to get here before my surgery. I wanted him to pray for me and my baby.
Nurse: Well, I'd be happy to pray for you and the baby. Would that be okay?
Patient: Oh, yes, would you please? This surgery really scares me.
Nurse: Dear God, please comfort this mother as she enters surgery. Lift her fear, and in its place give her peace and strength. Let her know that you are with her and the baby.
Patient: Thanks so much. That really means a lot to me.

THE RELIGIOUS AMERICAN

Examples of the religious American include Hindu, Jew, Buddhist, Muslim, Lutheran (Evangelical Lutheran Church in America, Wisconsin Synod, Missouri Synod, and English Synod), Catholic (Roman Rite, Eastern Rite as Ukrainian Catholic, and Greek Catholic), Eastern Orthodox (Russian Orthodox and Greek Orthodox), Quaker, Presbyterian, Methodist, Church of Christ, Mennonite, Seventh-Day Adventist, Assembly of God, Mormon, Baptist (Independent and Southern Baptist Convention), Wiccan, Jehovah's Witness, Episcopalian, African Methodist Episcopalian, Christian Science, United Church of Christ, Moravian, Evangelical, Salvation Army, and nondenominational.

The First Amendment of the U.S. Constitution allows the free exercise of religious choice. Starting with the Pilgrims, America has a long history of religious freedom and tolerance. As the preceding list shows, the United States is religiously diverse.

RELIGION IN THE UNITED STATES

The U.S. Census Bureau does not ask about religion on the census questionnaire. The number of persons belonging to specific religious denominations and groups in the United States can be found at www.adherents.com. The approximate sizes of Protestant, Catholic, Jewish, and Islamic denominations in the United States follow:

- There are approximately 66 million members of Protestant denominations. The number of mainline Protestants continues to decline, and it is predicted that in the future Protestantism will not be a majority religion (Lindner, 2010).
- The *2011 Yearbook of American and Canadian Churches* identified the Catholic Church as the largest single denomination in the United States with over 68 million members and 1.18 billion worldwide (Lindner, 2010).
- According to *The American Jewish Yearbook 2006*, over 6 million Jews comprise the largest non-Christian, organized religion in the United States (Sheskin and Dashefsky, 2006).
- There are approximately 6-7 million Muslims in the U.S. and 2.1 billion Muslims worldwide.

AVOIDING FALSE ASSUMPTIONS AND STEREOTYPES

The suggestions presented in Chapter 16 regarding the avoidance of false assumptions and stereotyping when caring for culturally diverse patients also apply when caring for patients of different religions. Some nursing students may think there is also a guidebook that supplies nursing interventions when caring for patients who belong to different religions. As with different cultures, this type of approach can lead to false assumptions and stereotyping. Not only is there diversity among religious groups, but there is also diversity among members of a specific religion or group. It is a false assumption to expect that all individuals of a specific religion or belief system will believe exactly the same just because they are members of that religion or belief system. Avoid assuming that all Protestants, Catholics, Jews, Muslims, Buddhists, and Hindus, for example, believe in and follow all the aspects of their formal religion/belief system. *Individual differences occur in every religious or belief systems group.* Members may have modified the degree to which they observe the practices of their religion or belief system based on age, experience, education, social group, and so on. Avoid judging patients if their religious beliefs do not conform to the traditional ones for that religion.

Box 17-2	Gathering Data for Religious Beliefs and Practices of Patients

- Do you have a religious affiliation? If so, state it.
- What role does religion play in your life?
- Is prayer helpful to you?
- What is your source of strength and hope?
- What brings you comfort and joy?
- What religious rituals or practices are important to you?
- What symbols or religious books are helpful to you?
- What dietary inclusions or restrictions are a part of your religious beliefs?
- How does your religion view the source and meaning of pain and suffering?
- When ill, does your religion prohibit people of the opposite sex from giving care?
- Does your religion have special days when certain behaviors are mandatory or prohibited?
- If a death is imminent, does your family have any special practices at the time of death?

Data must be gathered about each patient's specific beliefs and religious practices (Box 17-2).

The nursing interventions provided in Boxes 17-3 to 17-8 and Tables 17-1 and 17-2 will serve as a reference to be used in meeting the religious needs of specific patients during your time as a student practical/vocational nurse. This information can also be used in your nursing career after you graduate. Each religion has specific beliefs and practices. Sometimes an individual will adapt them to fit his or her own circumstances. Clarify with the patient the specific beliefs and practices that offer comfort to them and that they prefer. Develop an awareness of health issues and decisions that may involve religious or philosophical beliefs. The references at the end of this book can be used to learn more about a specific religion when such information is needed. Also, check www.beliefnet.com.

WESTERN AND MIDDLE EASTERN RELIGIONS IN THE UNITED STATES AND CANADA

Judaism, Christianity, and Islam are examples of monotheistic (belief in one Supreme Being) Western and Middle Eastern religions found in the United States.

JUDAISM

Judaism is the oldest of faiths that have a belief in one deity. In 2010, there were 14 million Jews worldwide. The prophet Abraham founded Judaism in approximately 2000 BC. The holy books of the Jews are the Torah and the Talmud. The Torah contains the written teachings, laws, and stories of Judaism. The Talmud contains the oral teachings and explanations. Followers of Judaism are called Jews, and Jewish clergy are called rabbis. Jews worship in buildings called temples or synagogues, and a

FIGURE 17-1 Star of David. This is a generally recognized symbol of Judaism.

common symbol of the Jewish faith is the Star of David (Figure 17-1). The following are the major divisions of Judaism:

- **Orthodox Judaism:** Orthodox Jews follow the traditional faith and strictly adhere to rituals, including a kosher diet (see Box 17-3) and keeping of the Sabbath. They consider the Torah and the Talmud as revealed by God and do not believe in completely integrating into modern society. Hasidism is an ultraorthodox form of Judaism.
- **Conservative Judaism:** Conservative Jews follow most traditional practices but adapt traditions to the modern world.
- **Reform Judaism:** Reform Jews stress the ethical and moral teachings of the prophets and autonomy of the individual. Rituals are performed that will promote a Jewish, God-filled life. Reformed Jews regard Judaism as evolving and subject to change. Reform Judaism does not accept the binding nature of Jewish law and believes that the Torah was written by human sources rather than by God. Traditionally, Jewish identity is considered to be passed on through the mother. Reform Jews accept Jewish identity passed on through the father. Reform Judaism is the largest, fastest-growing division of Judaism.

Box 17-3 lists the beliefs and practices that need to be clarified for each patient and nursing interventions that have importance for health care workers in contact with patients who are Jewish.

CHRISTIANITY

Christianity is a 2000-year-old religion based on the belief that **Jesus Christ** was the son of God. Followers of Christianity are called Christians, and a common symbol of this faith is the cross (Figure 17-2).

General Beliefs of Christians

The Bible. The Bible is the sacred book of Christians. It contains writings divided into two sections: the Old Testament, which was written before Jesus's birth,

---

Box 17-3	Beliefs, Practices, and Nursing Interventions for Jewish Patients

GENERAL
Beliefs and Practices
Jews believe in God but do not have a belief in Jesus Christ.
Nursing Interventions
Avoid references to heaven or Jesus.

OBSERVATION OF SABBATH
Nursing Interventions
If observed, provide time for rest, prayer, and/or study from sunset on Friday until after sunset on Saturday.
If observed, provide yarmulke (skullcap) or prayer shawl. Ask family to provide these items.

OBSERVANCE OF DIETARY RULES (KOSHER DIET)
Beliefs and Practices
If following a kosher diet, meat may be consumed a few minutes after drinking milk, but 6 hours must pass after eating meat before drinking milk.
Some Jews do not eat pork, ham, Canadian bacon, eel, oysters, crab, lobster, shrimp, or eggs with blood spots.
Nursing Interventions
Clarify if patient follows these dietary rules.
If desired by patient, make arrangements for separate utensils for preparing and serving meat and milk dishes. If separate dishes are not available, these foods can be served in the original containers or on paper plates.

DYING JEWISH PATIENT
Beliefs and Practices
Family and friends may want to be with the patient at all times.
Some Jews do not believe in autopsies, embalming, or cremation.
Some Jews may not want the nurse to touch the body of a deceased Jew.
Nursing Interventions
Some Jews may request that the nurse notify the Burial Society for preparation of the body for burial.

FIGURE 17-2 The cross represents the instrument of the crucifixion of Jesus Christ.

and the New Testament, which was written after his birth. Different Christian groups use different versions of these writings. The numbers and names of the books in the Bible differ in the Catholic and Protestant versions.

Many Christian patients will find comfort in reading or having someone read to them selected passages from the Bible. Treat the patient's Bible with respect. In addition to believing it contains the inspired word of God, some people received their Bibles as gifts commemorating special occasions, such as a wedding, a graduation, Confirmation, an anniversary, or a jubilee. Some Bibles list passages that can be used in specific patient situations, such as pain, sorrow, sleeplessness, and so on.

Baptism. Baptism is the rite of admission to the Christian community. Christian groups give different meanings to baptism. Some consider this rite a means of salvation, a way of washing away sin, a means of receiving the Holy Spirit (the third person of the Holy Trinity, the belief of some Christians of three persons in one God), an imprinting of character on the soul, or a promise of divine grace. Christian groups differ as to the age (infant, adult) at which a person may be baptized. Although water is used for baptizing, the method differs among groups (pouring, sprinkling, immersion).

If an infant is in danger of death, baptism may be given if the religious beliefs of the parents include infant baptism. If the patient is Protestant and baptism is desired, it is preferable to have a witness. If death is imminent and the patient is Catholic, a witness is not necessary, and anyone with the right intention may baptize. The procedure for baptism can be found in Box 17-4. Baptism beliefs and practices of Catholics and some Protestant denominations are included in Boxes 17-5 and 17-6.

Box 17-4   **Procedure for Baptism**

If baptism is desired/allowed:
Nursing Interventions
Allow water to flow over and contact the patient's skin while saying the words "Name (if known), I baptize you in the name of the Father, and of the Son, and of the Holy Spirit."
If the patient desires to be Catholic, death is imminent, and it is uncertain whether baptism was received in the past, baptism is administered conditionally. In this situation, the following words are used: "If you are not baptized, I baptize you in the name of the Father, and of the Son, and of the Holy Spirit."
Report the baptism to the chaplain or pastoral care team and the family.
Document the baptism in the patient's record.

Box 17-5   **Beliefs, Practices, and Nursing Interventions for Catholic Patients**

ROMAN CATHOLIC (WESTERN)
Baptism Beliefs
Necessary for salvation and initiation into the community. This sacrament removes all sin. Person receives the Holy Spirit. Infant or adult may be baptized, usually by pouring of or immersion in water.
Nursing Interventions
If the patient is a gravely ill infant, a stillbirth, or a fetus, the nurse may baptize without a witness.
If a patient or family member requests baptism and death is imminent, the nurse may baptize before the priest arrives.
Communion Beliefs
Believe that the bread and wine become the body and blood of Jesus Christ.
Nursing Interventions
If sacrament is desired, follow agency privacy policy, developed to carry out HIPAA guidelines, to receive communion.
Medicine and water may be taken before Communion.
If the patient's mouth is dry, water may be given after Communion.

SACRAMENTS
Nursing Interventions
If requested, follow agency privacy policy to arrange for the sacrament of Reconciliation and provide privacy when the priest hears the patient's confession.

If desired by patient, follow agency privacy policy for arranging the sacrament of the Anointing of the Sick. (Some Roman Catholics may refer to this as the Sacrament of the Sick. Older Catholics may refer to this as the Last Rites or the sacrament of Extreme Unction.) This sacrament is for anyone seriously ill or weakened by old age. This sacrament is believed to offer hope, consolation, and peace; assist in physical, mental, and spiritual healing; and provide strength to endure suffering.
If requested, follow agency's privacy policy to make arrangements for the priest to administer this sacrament.
Dietary Restrictions
If there are no health restrictions, Roman Catholics 14 years of age and older are to abstain from meat on Ash Wednesday and all Fridays during Lent. Catholics ages 14 to 59 must fast (eat only one full meal, although food that does not add up to a full meal can also be eaten) on Ash Wednesday and Good Friday. Fasting and abstaining are excused during hospitalization. Eastern Rite Catholics may be stricter about fasting.
Nursing Interventions
Clarify practices with patient.
Sexuality
Abortion is not allowed. Natural methods of family planning are strongly promoted.
Dying Catholic Patient
Catholic patients facing death may want to receive the last sacrament of the Christian. In addition to the anointing of the sick, the sacraments of Reconciliation and Viaticum (the

Continued

| Box 17-5 | Beliefs, Practices, and Nursing Interventions for Catholic Patients—cont'd |

last Communion that provides food for the journey from this life to the next) are administered.

Nursing Interventions

Follow agency privacy rules to make arrangements for the priest to administer this sacrament. Cremation and organ donation are allowed.

EASTERN ORTHODOX CHURCHES

Baptism Beliefs

Necessary for salvation. Infants are baptized by sprinkling or immersion.

Communion Beliefs

Believe the bread and wine are the body and blood of Jesus Christ.

Follow procedure for Communion as with Catholic patient.

Sacraments

Celebrate seven sacraments.

Nursing Interventions

Follow procedure for Anointing of the Sick as with Catholic patient.

Dietary Restrictions

Abstain from meat and dairy products on Wednesdays and Fridays during Lent.

Ill patients are excused from this requirement.

Sexuality

Birth control and abortion are not allowed.

Dying Eastern Orthodox Patient

The Last Rites are obligatory.

Beliefs and Practices

Autopsy and organ donation are not encouraged. Euthanasia and cremation are discouraged.

Nursing Interventions

Follow agency privacy policy to arrange for priest to administer the Last Rites, preferably while the patient is conscious.

| Box 17-6 | Beliefs, Practices, and Nursing Interventions for Protestant Patients of 10 Denominations |

NURSING CONSIDERATIONS THAT PERTAIN TO ALL PROTESTANT PATIENTS

Nursing Interventions

Because of federal privacy laws, inform patient that if a visit by a personal minister or pastor is desired for Communion, Anointing, and other sacraments, the patient must follow agency policy.

Provide privacy if patient reads the Bible.

Include on data-gathering list:

If patient is an infant and condition is serious, do parents desire baptism if child is not baptized?

If patient is dying, what are family's beliefs about death and dying?

OLD ORDER AMISH (HOUSE AMISH)

Amish are a conservative division of the Mennonites. Old Order Amish worship in private homes. The Amish do not believe in health insurance and Social Security, and they rely on mutual aid in time of need. Patients may believe that sudden fright or blood loss may cause loss of the soul. Female patients may object to cutting their hair because of their belief that Holy Scripture forbids it.

Baptism: Adult baptism.

ASSEMBLY OF GOD

One of several American Pentecostal denominations. May believe in the power of prayer for healing.

Baptism: Receive Jesus Christ as Lord and Savior. Administered by immersion when person understands the meaning of baptism.

Communion: Yes.

BAPTIST

Started in the seventeenth century in the United States. Baptists regard the Bible as a complete, sufficient, and final authority in matters of faith. Interpret the Bible literally. Stress personal relationship with Jesus Christ. Discourage alcohol consumption.

Baptism: No infant baptism. Person needs to understand the meaning of baptism. Adults are baptized by immersion. Baptism not considered a means of salvation.

Communion: Considered a symbol and a remembrance of Jesus Christ's death.

EPISCOPALIAN

Began in the sixteenth century in England. Also called the Anglican Church in England. Service book is Book of Common Prayer. Clergy include bishops, priests, and deacons. Priests may marry. Women may be ordained.

Baptism: Believe baptism is necessary for salvation. Infant baptism is performed by sprinkling.

Communion: Believe that Jesus Christ is present in the bread and wine.

LUTHERAN

There are several Lutheran bodies in the United States. Ministers may marry. Believe in anointing and blessing when ill.

Baptism: Conveys grace. Infants are baptized at 6 to 8 weeks of age by pouring, sprinkling, or immersion. In case of illness, invasive procedures, and emergent situations, infants may be baptized by their pastor, if possible. Baptism by a layperson is acceptable.

Communion: Believe the presence of Jesus Christ is real. Conveys grace.

METHODIST

Methodism started in the eighteenth century. There are several branches of the Methodist Church.

Baptism: An outward and visible sign of an inward and spiritual grace. Infant and adult by sprinkling or immersion.

Communion: Conveys grace. Open to everyone.

PRESBYTERIAN

Began in Scotland and evolved from John Calvin in the sixteenth century. May avoid alcohol.

Continued

| Box 17-6 | Beliefs, Practices, and Nursing Interventions for Protestant Patients of 10 Denominations—cont'd |

Baptism: Infant, usually by sprinkling. Signifies the beginning of life in Jesus Christ and not its completion.

Communion: Believe Jesus Christ is present in spirit.

QUAKERS (RELIGIOUS SOCIETY OF FRIENDS)
Beliefs and Practices

Believe they receive Divine Truth from "inner" light supplied by the Holy Spirit. Services called "meetings." Generally regard sacraments as nonessential to Christian life.

Nursing Interventions

Clarify baptism beliefs with patient. At birth, infant's name recorded in official church book.

SEVENTH-DAY ADVENTIST

Adventists observe the Sabbath from sunset on Friday to sunset on Saturday. Do not pursue their jobs or worldly pleasures during this time. Many Adventists are vegetarians and use soybean products as a protein source. These dietary practices are not mandatory. Adventists generally do not smoke or drink alcoholic beverages. Some Adventist patients may avoid beverages with caffeine. They believe that at death the body rests in the grave until the second coming of Jesus Christ. Organ donation is acceptable.

Nursing Interventions

Clarify diet restrictions.

Baptism: Makes one a church member. Adult by immersion. Opposed to infant baptism.

Communion: May practice washing of the feet in preparation.

UNITED CHURCH OF CHRIST

Formed in 1957 by merger of Congregational and Evangelical and Reformed Churches.

Baptism: Infant by pouring, sprinkling, or immersion. When baptized, become church members.

Communion: Celebrated and open to all.

Holy Communion. Holy Communion (or Holy Eucharist) is partaking of consecrated (blessed) elements of bread and wine. Depending on the group, the bread is leavened (with yeast) or unleavened. Some groups use grape juice instead of wine. Holy Communion has different meanings for different denominations. Examples of these differences include a remembrance of the Last Supper and a remembrance of Jesus Christ's death. Some groups consider the bread and wine to be only symbols of Jesus Christ, whereas others believe they are the body and blood of Jesus Christ. When caring for a patient of a specific affiliation, question the patient and family regarding specific beliefs and practices regarding Communion. Boxes 17-5 and 17-6 include Communion beliefs and practices of Catholics and some Protestant denominations.

Major Divisions of Christianity

The major divisions of Christianity are Catholicism, Protestantism, and Eastern Orthodoxy.

Catholicism. Catholicism consists of the Western or Roman Catholic Church, including Catholics of the Eastern Rite. Sometimes there is confusion between the Eastern Churches and Roman Catholicism. The Eastern Churches are either Catholics of the Eastern Rite or Eastern Orthodox

Catholics of the Roman Rite. There are 1.18 million Catholics worldwide (Rocca, 2011). Catholics trace their faith from Jesus Christ through an unbroken line to the pope. The pope is considered to be the representative of Jesus Christ on earth and is considered infallible—that is, incapable of being in error when speaking of matters of faith and morals. Beliefs are found in the Bible and tradition. Catholic clergy, called priests, are not allowed to marry because of tradition (custom), not dogma (law). Women cannot be ordained. The administrative hierarchy of the Catholic Church consists of cardinals, archbishops, bishops, priests, and deacons. Buildings of worship for Catholics are called churches and cathedrals. A cathedral is the headquarters of a bishop, archbishop, or cardinal. Celebration of the Mass is the center of worship. The seven sacraments of the Catholic Church are Baptism, Confirmation, Holy Eucharist, Penance, Anointing of the Sick, Holy Orders, and Matrimony. The Society of St. Pius X is an example of an ultraconservative branch of the Roman Catholic Church that is in schism (separated from Rome).

Catholics of Eastern Rites. Catholics of Eastern Rites have the same beliefs as the Western or Roman Catholic Church. They recognize the Vatican and the pope. They keep their own canon law, customs, and liturgy. Clergy are priests and bishops, and priests of this Eastern Rite (with the exception of monks) may marry. Bishops are selected from among monks. Examples of Catholics of Eastern Rites include Armenian Catholic, Chaldean Catholic, Maronites, and the Catholics of the Byzantine Rite (e.g., Greek Catholics, Bulgarian Catholics, and Russian Catholics).

Eastern Orthodox Churches. There are over 250 million members of Eastern Orthodox churches worldwide. The Eastern Orthodox Church considers itself catholic (that is, universal) but does not recognize the pope. The Roman Catholic Church considers these churches to be in schism because they refuse to submit to the authority of the pope. Beliefs come from the Bible and tradition. Clergy are bishops, priests, and deacons. Priests may marry before ordination. *Matuska*, meaning "Little Mother," is a title given to wives of Orthodox priests. Monks may not marry, and bishops are selected from among monks. These Eastern churches have no central authority. They are self-governed by a board consisting of a bishop and laypersons. Some of these churches are headed by a patriarch. Seven sacraments are celebrated. The Virgin Mary is respected. Liturgies differ among nationalities but have similarities to the Roman Catholic Church, although the services are more elaborate than Roman Catholic liturgies. Examples of Eastern Orthodox Churches are Orthodox of the Byzantine Rite (e.g., Greek Orthodox and Russian Orthodox), Armenian Orthodox, and Jacobite churches. Box 17-5 lists beliefs and practices that need to be clarified for each patient and nursing implications for patients who are Catholic (Roman and Eastern). Eastern Orthodox beliefs and practices are also listed.

Protestantism. In the sixteenth century, Germany was part of the Holy Roman Empire and almost entirely Roman Catholic. Protestantism began in 1517 when Martin Luther separated from the Catholic Church in protest because of the many scandals that were taking place in the church. This was the beginning of the Reformation and Lutheranism. As Lutheranism spread throughout Germany, Catholic clergy tried to limit changes affecting the Catholic Church and to retain its authority in all church matters. John of Saxony led a group to a Catholic Church assembly, where they objected to the Catholic Church's plans to limit innovations in doctrine and practices in the Catholic Church. The group then signed a *protestation* and became known as *Protestants* from then on (Gritsch, 2002). Protestants believe that their convictions are closer to New Testament Christianity. The chief characteristic of Protestantism is the acceptance of the Bible as the sole authority in matters of faith. It is believed that Christians are justified in their relationship to God *by faith alone and not by good works.* Examples of denominations and sects that came from the Reformation include Lutheran, Reformed, and Presbyterian. Depending on the denomination, Protestant clergy are called ministers or pastors. Protestant places of worship are called churches or temples. During the second half of the nineteenth century, opposition to changes in Protestantism resulted in a conservative type of Protestantism called Fundamentalism. Southern Baptists are an ultraconservative form of Protestants. Box 17-6 lists beliefs and practices that need to be clarified for each patient and nursing interventions for patients of 10 Protestant denominations.

ISLAM

The word *Islam* implies "peace." In the sixth century AD, the prophet Muhammad founded Islam in Arabia. Followers of Islam are called Muslims. There are 2.1 billion Muslims worldwide. Muslims believe in one God: Allah. Salvation depends on one's commitment to Allah and his teachings in the Qur'an (Koran). This holy book contains the words of Allah as he spoke to Muhammad. Muslims pray in Arabic and worship in mosques. The imam is the leader of the Muslim congregation (Figure 17-3).

Muslims have many beliefs that are similar to Judeo-Christian doctrine—for example, angels and

FIGURE 17-3 Crescent moon and star is an internationally recognized symbol of Islam.

prophets such as Abraham, Moses, and Jesus. Muslims believe in heaven, hell, the last judgment, prayer, fasting, and giving to the poor.

Islam is not one entity but has many interpretations, resulting in diversity in its practice. The two main divisions in Islam are the Sunni and Shi'ite sects. The majority of Muslims worldwide are Sunnis. Because Muhammad did not designate a successor when he died, the Sunni sect chose a successor, who became the political leader of the community. Sunnis believe they must follow the Sunnah, the ethical and religious code from the sayings of Muhammad and vest religious and political authority with the community as guided by Islamic law and consensus of the Qur'an and the leaders. The Shi'ite sect believes that Muhammad designated his cousin and son-in-law, Ali, to be the leader of Islam after his death and vest all authority with the imam (the leader of a Muslim congregation) and ultimately the ayatollah (a high-ranking religious and political leader), and these leaders guide the teachings of Islam (Gellman and Hartman, 2002). Wahhabism is an ultraconservative form of Islam. Information about this reform movement can be obtained at www.pbs.org/wgbh/pages/frontline/shows/saudi/analyses/wahhabism.html.

Despite different sects and divisions, the Five Pillars are the essential and obligatory practices all Muslims accept and follow:

1. **The Profession of Faith:** This is a verbal pledge that there is only one God, Allah, and that Muhammad is the messenger of God. (Muslim mothers may whisper this pledge into a newborn's ear.)
2. **Prayer:** Muslims are called to prayer five times a day.
3. **Almsgiving:** This involves an annual payment of a certain percentage of a Muslim's wealth and assets. This money is distributed among the poor.
4. **Fasting:** During Ramadan, the ninth month of the Islamic calendar, adult Muslims abstain from dawn to sunset from food, drink, and sexual activity.
5. **Pilgrimage:** Adult Muslims who are physically and financially able are expected to perform the pilgrimage to Mecca (Islam's holiest shrine) at least once in their lifetime.

Jihad, meaning "to strive or struggle" in the way of God, is sometimes referred to as the Sixth Pillar of Islam, although it has no such official status. In his book *Islam: The Straight Path*, Esposito (1998) explains as follows:

> In its most general meaning, [jihad] refers to the obligation incumbent on all Muslims, as individuals and as a community, to exert themselves to realize God's will, to lead virtuous lives, and to extend the Islamic community through preaching, education, and so on. A related meaning is the struggle for or defense of Islam, a holy war. Despite the fact that jihad is not supposed to include aggressive warfare, this has occurred, as exemplified by early extremists like the Kharijites and contemporary groups like . . . jihad organizations in Lebanon, the Gulf States, and Indonesia.

Male infants are circumcised. Islamic law does not prohibit contraception for married couples. No permanent damage to reproductive organs is allowed. Abortion is permitted if the mother's life is at stake and the fetus is not older than 4 months' gestation. Saving a life is one of the greatest merits and imperatives in Islam. Box 17-7 lists beliefs and practices that need to be clarified and nursing considerations for Muslim patients.

 Critical Thinking

Avoid Stereotyping Your Patients

How would you avoid stereotyping and making false assumptions about a Muslim patient who is dying. Do the same for a patient of a religious group that is frequently seen in your community.

ADDITIONAL CHRISTIAN AND NON-CHRISTIAN RELIGIOUS GROUPS

Box 17-8 lists beliefs and practices that need to be clarified for each patient and nursing interventions for patients of various religious groups.

EASTERN RELIGIONS AND PHILOSOPHIES IN THE UNITED STATES AND CANADA

Because the Western and the Eastern worlds contain different value systems, the two worlds represent different ways of thinking that have molded the culture, including the worldview, of two different parts of the world. In the twenty-first century, cultures and religious practices of other countries have become more known to us because of travel, the mass media, and immigration of people from all over the world to the United States and Canada.

The Eastern world (e.g., India, China, Japan, and Korea) emphasizes the following virtues:

- Self-discipline and control
- The inner nature of self
- Moderation in all things
- Nonattachment to worldly things
- Awareness that selfish desire is the cause of much suffering
- Tolerance of other religions and points of view
- Respect for family, elders, and authority
- The principle of not harming any living creature

Box 17-7 Beliefs, Practices, and Nursing Interventions for Muslim Patients

GENERAL BELIEFS

Members of Islam may desire to pray to Allah five times a day (after dawn, at noon, in midafternoon, after sunset, and at night). Friday is a day for communal prayer.

Beliefs and Practices

Rules of cleanliness may include eating with the right hand and cleansing self with the left hand after urinating and defecating.

Nursing Interventions

If patient requests to face Mecca, the holy city of Islam, a bed or chair may be positioned in a southeast direction from the United States.

If a Muslim brings the Koran, the holy book of Islam, to the health care facility, do not touch it or place anything on top of it.

If a Muslim wears writings from the Koran on a black string around the neck, arm, or waist, these writings need to be kept dry and remain on the patient because they are passages from the Koran.

OBSERVATION OF DIETARY RULES

Beliefs and Practices

Some Muslims might not eat *haram* (prohibited food)—for example, pork and pork products (ham, bacon), meats from animals that have not been bled to death by a Muslim, and gelatin.

Foods that are permitted are called *halal* (legal).

Some Muslims might not drink alcoholic beverages.

Nursing Interventions

Clarify dietary restrictions.

OBSERVATION OF FEMALE MODESTY

Beliefs and Practices

Some Muslim women prefer to be clothed from head to ankle.

Nursing Interventions

During a physical examination, female Muslims may prefer to undress one body part at a time.

DEATH PRACTICES

Beliefs and Practices

Women may be barred from the room of a dying family member.

The family may pray for the dying family member. The imam usually reads from the Koran for the patient after death.

After death, the body is turned toward Mecca.

After death, the family washes the body, including all orifices, and seals them with cotton.

The body is wrapped in a white cloth for burial.

The family may not permit organ donation, autopsies, or cremation in order to keep the body intact so the person may meet God with integrity. These decisions may vary by country of origin.

No embalming of bodies after death. No cremation.

Muslims try to bury the dead within 24 hours.

Nursing Interventions

The nurse may touch the body only after donning gloves.

Box 17-8	Beliefs, Practices, and Nursing Interventions for Additional Christian and Non-Christian Religious/Spiritual Groups

CHRISTIAN SCIENTIST (CHURCH OF CHRIST, SCIENTIST)

Founded in nineteenth century by Mary Baker Eddy, who wrote *Science and Health with a Key to the Scriptures*.

Beliefs and Practices

Believe sin causes sickness and studying Eddy's book and the Bible will heal them.

Patient may believe that sickness can be overcome through prayer and spiritual understanding that God is good and the only reality.

Healing considered an awakening to this belief.

There are no clergy, but patient may want a Christian Science practitioner to give treatment through prayer.

No baptism.

Consider the Lord's Supper a spiritual communion with God and may sit quietly during this time.

No smoking or drinking alcohol. They do not accept blood transfusions or surgery.

Nursing Interventions

Clarify baptism beliefs with patient.

JEHOVAH'S WITNESSES

Originated at the end of the nineteenth century in the United States. Witnesses base their beliefs on the Bible.

Beliefs and Practices

Believe the Second Coming has begun, Armageddon is imminent, and the millennium will soon follow. At that time, repentant sinners will have a second chance for salvation.

They do not believe in the Trinity. Consider Jesus inferior to God, the Father, Jehovah.

No ordained ministers.

No churches but worship in Kingdom Halls. Publications include *Awake* and *Watch Tower*.

Witnesses will refuse to receive whole blood products, including plasma. Receiving such products is viewed as a violation of the law of Jehovah (Genesis 9:3-4; Leviticus 17:14; Acts 15:28-29). They will accept blood transfusion alternatives.

Alcohol and tobacco are discouraged.

Believe the soul dies at death. Autopsy decided by family.

Cremation is acceptable.

Organ transplants are a private decision. Before transplant, organs must be cleansed with a nonblood solution.

Baptism: Necessary for salvation. Considered a symbol of dedication to Jehovah. Adult by immersion. No infant baptism.

Communion: Occurs one time a year.

MORMONS (CHURCH OF JESUS CHRIST OF LATTER DAY SAINTS)

In the nineteenth century, Joseph Smith founded the Mormon Church. The headquarters are in Salt Lake City, Utah.

Beliefs and Practices

Revelation is emphasized to establish doctrine and rituals.

The Book of Mormon contains accounts of ancient peoples in America. This book is considered complementary scripture to the Bible.

Mormons emphasize tithing and community welfare.

Mormons worship in temples and tabernacles.

Mormon adults wear undergarments at all times as a symbolic gesture of the promises made to God.

There is no ordained clergy. High priests are members of the church and form the Council of Twelve and exert spiritual leadership. Three high priests vested with supreme authority form the first presidency of the church.

A Mormon may be anointed and blessed before planned hospitalization.

Abortion is not allowed unless the mother's life is in danger.

Natural methods of birth control are allowed. Artificial means may be used when the physical or emotional health of the woman is in question.

May avoid tobacco, alcohol, coffee, and tea.

Baptism: Considered necessary for salvation. Causes remission of sins. Allows the person to receive the gifts of the Holy Spirit. Baptism is given at age 8 or older by immersion. Baptism may be given after death by proxy.

Communion: The Lord's Supper with bread and water. Considered a symbol and renewing of covenant with Jesus Christ.

BAHA'I

Founded in the nineteenth century in Persia (now southern Iran).

Beliefs and Practices

Believe in world peace, the unity of all religions and humanity, and the equality of men and women.

There is no clergy.

Members meet in homes. The house of worship in the United States is in Wilmette, Illinois. There is an annual 19-day fast from sunrise to sundown during the last month of the Baha'i calendar. You can find more information at www.bahai.us/welcome/principles-and-practices/bahai-calendar/.

May avoid alcohol.

At death, the soul, the real self, journeys through the spiritual world, which is the timeless, placeless extension of the universe.

No embalming, unless required by state law. Cremation discouraged.

Burial to take place within 1 hour's travel time of death.

There is no baptism or Communion.

Their special book is *The Book of Certitude*.

The Western world (e.g., Europe, Canada, and the United States) emphasizes the following virtues:

- The value of individual worth
- The need to be responsible for one another, which gives rise to many social programs
- A personal relationship with one God that translates into love of neighbor and environment

Because of immigration and acculturation of Eastern peoples and interest in and adoption of Eastern philosophies by Western society, both traditions can be seen in the other. For example, there are a large number of Christians among Eastern peoples. Westerners have adopted meditation, yoga, complementary therapies (including use of herbs and oils), and a focus on inner development.

HINDUISM

Hinduism dates back to prehistoric times. This oldest religion is the third largest religion in the world and is comprised of a diverse system of thoughts and beliefs (Figure 17-4). The essence of Hinduism is based on a vast body of scriptures, including the Vedas and the Bhagavad-Gita. These texts teach the path to

FIGURE 17-4 Om (Aum). This represents Brahman, the impersonal Absolute of Hinduism, the source of all manifest existence.

the proper way of living through *dharma* (ethics, duties), *karma* (action, deeds), and *bhakti* (devotion and knowledge that God is the ultimate power and exists in many forms). With these in mind, Hinduism is more a way of life than a religion. Hindus believe in **reincarnation**: One is reborn to a higher or lower level of existence based on one's moral behavior in the prior phase of existence. The cycle of birth and death continues until the soul achieves *moksha* (or Nirvana), the self-realization and unification of the soul with the ultimate being.

There is no common creed or doctrine in Hinduism; it is based on the accumulated treasury of spiritual laws discovered by different people in different times. Most Hindus venerate many gods and goddesses, including the Trinity: *Vishnu*, the Protector; *Shiva*, the destroyer; and *Brahma*, the Creator. These gods, along with their equally powerful consorts, are worshipped in their various incarnations and forms. One good site of information about Hinduism can be accessed at www.religionfacts. com/hinduism/fastfacts.htm. Tables 17-1 and 17-2 present general beliefs and practices of Buddhist

Table 17-1	General Religious Beliefs/Practices and Nursing Interventions for Buddhist and Hindu Patients	
BELIEFS/PRACTICES	**NURSING INTERVENTIONS**
Not having a central authority or dictated doctrine, the approximately 550,000 **Buddhists** and 1.3 million **Hindus** in North America exhibit a variety of traditions, beliefs, and practices.	Clarify with the patient his or her preference of practices to be observed.
Buddhists believe pain and suffering result from actions in this or a past life.	Accept the patient's right to this belief; neither agree nor disagree.
Buddhist and **Hindu** patients accept traditional medical treatment. However, to maintain a clear state of mind, **Buddhists** may refuse drugs that alter the state of the mind.	Inform physician of patient's concern. Explain to patient/family the action of all medications before administering them. Report to physician and chart any medications refused and reason for refusal.
Generally, **Buddhists** do not believe in healing through faith. Healing for **Buddhist** patients may be promoted by awakening to the laws of Buddha. After many years of searching, Siddhartha Gautama, the founder of Buddhism, finally found the truth of existence and became the Buddha—the Enlightened One. Many persons since then have become Buddhas by becoming enlightened.	Avoid references to "God" (e.g., "God will help you get through this").
Hindu patients may prefer a light diet in the morning and evening and a heavy meal at noon. Some **Hindu** patients may fast on a specific day of the week or month.	Allow patient/family to select diet for each meal. Encourage patient/family to write in food preferences when not listed. Arrange for visit by dietitian.
Hindus may practice Ayurveda, the traditional Indian science of health that uses herbs to treat disease. Some **Hindus** also practice folk medicine.	As with patients of all cultures and in all settings: Question use of herbs in daily life so possible drug interactions can be avoided. Question use of folk medicine. If practice is not harmful, include practice in plan of care. If practice is harmful, repattern practice. (See examples of adapting care plans for culturally diverse patients, pp. 207-208.)

Continued

Table 17-1   General Religious Beliefs/Practices and Nursing Interventions for Buddhist and Hindu Patients—cont'd

BELIEFS/PRACTICES	NURSING INTERVENTIONS
Buddhist patients may use incense, images of Buddha, and/or prayer beads in worship.	Respect these objects if used by patient. Provide these personal objects if patient asks for them.
Hindu patients may have a thread on their torso or around their wrist to signify a blessing.	Avoid removing the thread.
Buddhist patients may have a visit from a Buddhist priest, monk, or nun to conduct a religious ceremony. **Hindu** priests generally are not involved with illness care.	Provide privacy for visit of priest, monk, or nun.
Buddhist families may perform traditions with patient.	Arrange the environment to accommodate the family.
Significant others of **Hindu** patients may do the same.	Provide quiet and privacy.
Buddhist patients may chant or meditate to help calm and clear their minds.	Avoid interrupting the patient during meditation or chanting.
Puja, the worship of **Hindu** deities, is preceded by outer purification. **Hindu** patients may request a daily bath.	Provide necessary equipment for bathing for ambulatory patients. If patient requires assistance, assist with bath before meal. If bathing required in bed, add hot water to cold water (Lipson and Dibble, 2006).

Table 17-2   Death Beliefs, Practices, and Nursing Interventions for Buddhist and Hindu Patients

Buddhists believe in many reincarnations until they achieve Enlightenment and are freed from worldly illusion, passions, and suffering. Until this is achieved, death provides the opportunity to improve in the next life. Understanding the Four Noble Truths and the Noble Eightfold Path will allow one to achieve Enlightenment and enter Nirvana (a state, the absence of self, extinguishing of desire and suffering), at which time the cycle of rebirths and deaths ends. Resources within the person to achieve Enlightenment are stressed rather than reliance on ancient gods.

Hindus believe in the wheel of birth, life, and death (reincarnations) until they break through the illusions of the world and participate in the manifestation of the true self (Atman, the deathless self, the soul). Meditation and grace will help the Hindu believer to realize the Supreme self, which is hidden in the heart. When this occurs, eternal peace or Brahman (the universal soul and source, the Absolute Truth) is the reward.

BELIEFS/PRACTICES	NURSING INTERVENTIONS
Buddhists and **Hindus** believe in rebirth and death (reincarnation). They do not believe in the concept of an immortal soul.	Accept the patient's right to this belief; avoid agreeing or disagreeing.
Buddhists and **Hindus** believe in karma, the law of cause and effect by which thoughts, words, and deeds of each person create his or her own destiny. One reaps what one sows. Karma is carried over to the next life and determines the form of each new existence. **Buddhists** believe it is the state of one's consciousness at the time of death that usually determines one's rebirth.	For dying patients, make provision for rites and ceremonies by the family and/or spiritual leaders. Avoid interfering with praying, singing, and chanting. **Buddhist Patients** Provide an environment for the dying patient that will allow a clear, calm state of mind and a peaceful death. **Hindu Patients** Allow the family/spiritual leader to place water in the mouth of Hindu patients.
Buddhists and **Hindus** treat the body with respect. Cremation is common for **Buddhists** and **Hindus**. The **Hindu** patient's ashes are saved, to be disposed of in a holy river (e.g., the Ganges). Family may want to wash the body in preparation for cremation.	Inform funeral director of patient's religion. **Hindu Patient** When requested, provide family with equipment to wash the body. Present possibility of organ donation to family in a private environment.
Organ Donations	
Buddhists may allow organ donation if it will help someone pursue enlightenment. **Hindus** allow organ donation.	Follow agency policy for obtaining permission for organ donation.
Autopsies	
Buddhists and **Hindus** permit autopsies	Follow agency policy for obtaining permission for autopsy.

FIGURE 17-5 Buddhist Wheel of Life. The eight spokes symbolize the Noble Eightfold Path. The three swirling segments in the center represent the Buddha, the teachings, and the spiritual community.

and Hindu patients, nursing interventions, and items that need to be clarified.

BUDDHISM

Siddhartha Gautama (Buddha) founded Buddhism in the sixth century BC in India. Buddhism can be considered a religion, a philosophy, and a way of life (Figure 17-5). Much of Eastern beliefs have evolved from Buddhism. Well before Christianity, Buddhism originated in India, as did Hinduism. It shares much with Hindu philosophy but also radically departs from it (see Table 17-1). Buddhism spread to China, Japan, Korea, Tibet, Burma, Sri Lanka, Laos, Cambodia, and Vietnam. As Buddhism spread, the core beliefs were adapted to the culture of the host country. The beliefs were shaped and influenced by rituals and the belief system of each country. Two core beliefs of Buddhism that remained constant, however, are the Four Noble Truths and the Noble Eightfold Path leading to Nirvana:

1. Life is suffering.
2. Suffering is caused by desire. Desire is described as the craving or longing for the pleasures of the senses and life itself. Suffering is also caused by ignorance, which is interpreted as not being able to see things as they are.
3. Suffering can be eliminated by eliminating desire (craving or longing for the pleasures of the senses and life itself).

4. To eliminate desire, follow the Noble Eightfold Path:
   a. Right views
   b. Right intention
   c. Right speech
   d. Right action
   e. Right livelihood
   f. Right effort
   g. Right concentration
   h. Right ecstasy

Because of the variation in beliefs and history of Eastern groups, the time interval since immigration, and the degree of socialization, it is difficult to provide clear-cut examples of what a Japanese American or East Indian Hindu American believes and practices. As much diversity exists among Eastern religions and philosophies as exists among Christians.

NURSING INTERVENTIONS FOR EASTERN RELIGIONS

In patient care, the practical/vocational nurse can come in contact with a Japanese Buddhist, a Korean Buddhist, and a Tibetan Buddhist, among others, as well as American/Canadian patients who have blended Buddhism with their chosen religion. Apply the principles from Chapter 16. Develop an awareness that not everyone sees the world as you do. Avoid stereotyping individuals and considering them all the same just because they are Buddhist or Hindu. Table 17-1 presents a comparison of general religious beliefs and practices that *may* be found in Buddhist and Hindu patients, along with appropriate nursing interventions. Table 17-2 presents general death beliefs and practices of Buddhist and Hindu patients and appropriate nursing interventions.

 Try This

Learning About Different Belief Systems

Gather information about a religion, philosophy, or group (not discussed in this chapter) other than your own that interests you. Focus on nursing interventions appropriate for the topic you chose to research. Use Chapter 5 as a resource to gather information.

Get Ready for the NCLEX-PN® Examination

Key Points

- The practical/vocational nurse has a responsibility to care for the total person, including physical, emotional, and spiritual needs.
- Spiritual needs of patients arise from their desire to find meaning in life, suffering, and death.
- Gathering data about spiritual needs and providing spiritual care are routine parts of all patients' care, not only in times of crisis.
- To meet the spiritual needs of patients, you need to be aware of the patient's personal spiritual beliefs or the absence of them.
- Members of the health care team who assist the practical/vocational nurse in providing spiritual care to patients are the minister, priest, rabbi, chaplain, and other representatives of religions, groups, and philosophies and the pastoral care team.
- Many patients help to meet their personal spiritual needs by their participation in an organized religion.
- Spirituality can be part of religion, but religion is not necessarily part of spirituality.
- Spiritual distress can occur when patients cannot fulfill the rituals and practices of their religion or when they experience conflict between their spiritual beliefs and their health regimen.
- For these reasons, you need to develop an awareness of religious differences and an understanding of the basic beliefs, rituals, and practices of the many religious denominations, groups, and philosophies that exist today.
- Avoid assuming that patients who belong to a specific religion or belief system adopt all of the beliefs and practices of that religion or belief system.
- Clarify personal religious beliefs and practices for all patients.
- Although many patients in the United States are Protestant, Catholic, and Jewish, you will encounter other denominations and groups, such as Muslims and members of Eastern religions and philosophies, as well as persons who have no religious affiliation. By learning more about these groups, you will be able to accommodate their beliefs and practices and will be able to say you have met the needs of the total person.

Additional Learning Resources

evolve Go to your Evolve website (http://evolve.elsevier.com/Hill/Success) for the following FREE learning resources:
- Answers to Critical Thinking Review Scenarios
- Additional learning activities
- Additional Review Questions for the NCLEX-PN® exam
- Helpful phrases for communicating in Spanish and more!

Review Questions for the NCLEX-PN® Examination

1. The deity to whom a Muslim patient prays is:
    1. Jesus Christ
    2. Zeus
    3. Allah
    4. Yahweh

2. Select the statement that **best** describes the role of the pastoral care team.
    1. The pastoral care team is the social services department in acute care facilities and extended care.
    2. The pastoral care team works with the nursing staff to help meet the spiritual and religious needs of patients.
    3. Religious care and spiritual support are offered to seriously ill and dying patients by the pastoral care department.
    4. Because of pastoral care, the nursing staff does not have to worry about meeting the spiritual needs of patients.

3. If a Catholic patient requests Last Rites before surgery, the practical/vocational nurse responds by:
    1. Reassuring the patient that he is not going to die during surgery.
    2. Notifying the patient's family that his condition has changed.
    3. Calling the patient's physician to report the patient's mental state.
    4. Notifying the pastoral care team of the patient's preoperative request.

4. If a patient with a bleeding peptic ulcer is a Jehovah's Witness and refuses to receive an ordered blood transfusion preoperatively, select the priority action of the licensed practical/vocational nurse.
    1. Notify the nursing supervisor STAT and report the patient's refusal.
    2. Encourage the patient to accept the transfusion as a life-saving measure.
    3. Explain that the transfusion is needed because of severe blood loss.
    4. Alert family members of the crucial need to notify church authorities.

Alternate Format Item

1. A Jewish patient is admitted to the extended care unit on your shift. Which of the following nursing interventions apply to this situation? *(Select all that apply.)*
    1. Provide quiet time for prayer on the Sabbath.
    2. Ask the family to bring in the patient's yarmulke.
    3. Order all meals to be served using kosher preparation.

4. Arrange for milk to be delivered at least a half hour before meals.
5. Clarify personal beliefs and practices with the patient.

2. Najid, age 76 and a devout Muslim, has died on your shift after an illness with pancreatic cancer. Family wishes and his traditional belief system have been documented. Select the interventions the LPN/LVN would include in Najid's care. *(Select all that apply.)*

1. Turn Najid's bed in a southeast direction.
2. Provide the family with bathing supplies.
3. Obtain permission for an autopsy.
4. Arrange for Najid's body to be wrapped in a white cloth.
5. Only touch Najid's body with gloved hands.

Critical Thinking Scenario

Amy has an assigned patient who is Muslim. His wife visits daily and always wears a scarf over her head. Amy sees this manner of dress occasionally in her town. She is puzzled about this practice. Help Amy understand the reason for wearing a scarf in this manner if one is a Muslim female.

Health Care Settings: Potential Job Sites

Objectives

On completing this chapter, you will be able to do the following:

1. Compare public and private health care agencies according to the following criteria:
   a. Source of funding
   b. Services provided
   c. Examples of agencies in your geographic area
   d. Possible places of employment for practical/vocational nurses
2. Differentiate between official and voluntary agencies.
3. Explain what is meant by private health care agencies as the usual entry into the health care delivery system in the United States.
4. Give an example of an:
   a. Official government public health care agency in your area
   b. Official government public health care agency in your state
   c. Official government public health care agency at the federal level
5. Identify the federal health care agency in the United States that is headed by an appointee of the president and advises the president in health matters.
6. List eight agencies that make up the U.S. Public Health Service (USPHS).
7. Describe the responsibility of the World Health Organization (WHO).
8. Provide examples of two voluntary health care agencies in your area that are not listed in this chapter.
9. Explain the difference between proprietary and nonprofit health care agencies.
10. Discuss how primary care relates to family practice physicians.
11. Differentiate between general and specialized hospitals.
12. Explain the purpose of teaching and research hospitals.
13. Discuss the difference between ambulatory and acute care settings.
14. Describe free clinics as a source of primary care.
15. Differentiate among the following types of long-term care:
    a. Home care
       —Home health nursing
       —Community health nursing
    b. Adult day care
    c. Residential care settings
       —Assisted living
       —Continuous care retirement communities
    d. Institutional settings
       —Subacute care
       —Long-term care facilities
       —Intermediate care facility (ICF)
       —Skilled care facility
    e. Green House homes
    f. Hospice care

Key Terms

acute care (ă-KŪT, p. 232)

adult day care center (ă-DŬLT, p. 234)

ambulatory care facilities (ĂM-bū-lă-tŏr-ē kar fă-sil-i-tēs, p. 233)

ambulatory surgery centers (ĂM-bū-lă-tŏr-ē SŬR-jĕr-ē SĔN-tĕrs, p. 233)

assisted care (ă-SĬS-tĕd kăr, p. 234)

board and care homes (bŏrd kăr hōms, p. 234)

community health nursing (kŏm-Ū-nĭ-tē, p. 234)

continuous care retirement community (CCRC) (kŏn-TĬN-ū-ŭs, p. 234)

Department of Health and Human Services (DHHS) (p. 230)

free clinic (frē KLĬ-nĭc, p. 233)

freestanding (frē STĂN-dĭng, p. 233)

general hospitals (JĔN-ĕr-ăl HŌS-pĭ-tăls, p. 232)

Green House (grēn hŏws, p. 235)

home health nursing (hōm hĕlth, p. 233)

hospice care (HŎS-pĭs, p. 237)

long-term care (LTC) (lŏng tĕrm kăr, p. 236)

official (government) health care agencies (ō-FĬSH-ŭl, p. 230)

outpatient clinic (ŎWT-pā-shĕnt KLĬ-nĭc, p. 233)

post–acute care (PAC) (pōst ă-KŪT kăr, p. 236)

primary care (PRĪ-măr-ē kăr, p. 232)

private health care agencies (PRĪ-vĭt, p. 229)

proprietary hospitals (for profit) (prŏ-PRĪ-ĭ-tĕr-ē, p. 232)

Keep in Mind

What is your passion? Choose carefully, and make that first job worthy of you.

All health care agencies are not the same. They differ in size, focus, quality of service, and how they are financed. Do some research before making an application for a job so you can make an informed choice about employment after you graduate. Compose questions to ask during an employment interview. Refer to Chapter 22 for ideas.

 Critical Thinking

Personal Vision of Working as a Nurse

What is your vision for working as a nurse after you complete nursing school?

PUBLIC VERSUS PRIVATE HEALTH CARE AGENCIES

The various health care services in the United States can be grouped into two general categories: services delivered by the public sector and services delivered by the private sector. Table 18-1 outlines the major differences between public and private health care agencies. As you read about public and private health care agencies, think of them as potential sources of employment for the LPN/LVN.

PUBLIC HEALTH CARE AGENCIES

There are two types of public health care agencies—official and voluntary. Official (government) health care agencies have the following characteristics:

- Government agencies supported by tax money
- Are accountable to the taxpayers and the government
- Government agencies put primary emphasis on the delivery of disease prevention and wellness promotion programs
- Provide direct health care services

Voluntary health care agencies have these characteristics:

- Are supported by voluntary contributions
- Sometimes charge a fee for services
- Are tuned in to public opinion but are accountable to their supporters
- Activities determined by supporter interest, not legal mandate
- Primary emphasis is on research and education
- May offer direct health services to the patient

Some official and voluntary health care agencies operate at the local, state, federal, and international levels.

EXAMPLES OF PUBLIC HEALTH CARE AGENCIES

Official Government Agencies

Local. The official health agency at the local level is the city or county health department. These agencies have the following characteristics:

Table 18-1   Comparison of Health Care Agencies in the Public and Private Sectors

	PUBLIC		PRIVATE
	OFFICIAL (GOVERNMENT)	**NONOFFICIAL (VOLUNTARY)**	**PRIVATE**
Support	Tax money	Voluntary contributions and fees for service	Fees for service
Primary service	Programs of disease prevention and wellness promotion	Research and education	Curing disease and illness
Additional services	Sometimes direct service of health care	Offer direct health services	Disease prevention and wellness promotion
Accountability	Taxpayers and government	Supporters, boards, and so forth	Owners
How programs determined	Mandated and nonmandated	Supporter interest	Defined goals of the organization

- They are funded by local tax money, as well as by subsidies from the state and federal levels of government.
- They carry out state laws (mandated) concerning community health.
- They carry out nonmandated programs, such as health promotion programs.

State. Each state has a state health department. This official health agency has the following characteristics:
- It is funded by state tax money.
- It sometimes receives money from the federal government.

Federal (National). The official health agency at the federal level in the United States is the Department of Health and Human Services (DHHS). DHHS has the following characteristics:
- It is funded by federal taxes.
- A person appointed by the president of the United States is head of the agency. This person advises the president in health matters.

The DHHS division that is concerned primarily with health is the U.S. Public Health Service (USPHS), which is made up of the following eight agencies:
- *Food and Drug Administration (FDA).* Administers Federal Food, Drug, and Cosmetics Act and several related public health laws.
- *Centers for Disease Control and Prevention (CDC).* Lead agency related to surveillance and identification of disease through epidemiologic and laboratory investigations. It is also the primary agency for administering grants to support public health programs such as HIV/AIDS, sexually transmitted diseases, injury protection, immunization, and cancer screening.
- *National Institutes of Health (NIH).* Funds biomedical research in its own laboratories and in universities, hospitals, private research institutions, and private industry. New knowledge can potentially improve health, quality of medical care, and understanding of disease process.
- *Health Resources and Services Administration (HRA).* Improves access to medical care for indigent, uninsured, rural residents, and special-needs populations.
- *Substance Abuse, and Mental Health Services Administration (SAMHSA).* Improves the quality and availability of prevention, treatment, and rehabilitation services for persons suffering from alcoholism, substance abuse, and mental illness.
- *Agency for Healthcare Research and Quality (AHRQ).* Focuses on quality of care and medical care outcomes.
- *Agency for Toxic Substance and Disease Registry (ATSDR).* Works to prevent exposure and to minimize adverse health effects associated with waste management emergencies and pollution by hazardous substances.
- *Indian Health Services (IHS).* Constitution is the legal basis for the federal government's responsibility to provide health services to American Indians and Alaskan Natives. Goal is to provide comprehensive, culturally acceptable personal and public services.

The preceding definitions are based on the *Gale Encyclopedia of Public Health.*

International. Health activities take place at the international level through the World Health Organization (WHO), an agency of the United Nations (UN). It acts as a coordinating authority on international public health.
- WHO is located in Geneva, Switzerland.
- The major objective of WHO is the highest possible level of health for people all over the world.
- WHO defines *health* as a state of complete physical, mental, and social well-being and not merely as the absence of disease or infirmity.
- WHO is funded through fees paid by member nations of the UN.
- Coordinates international efforts to control outbreaks of infections, such as SARS, malaria, tuberculosis, influenza, and HIV/AIDS. Also sponsors programs to prevent and treat such diseases.

 Try This

Local Health Care Agency

Identify an official and voluntary health care agency in your geographic area. What services does each agency provide locally?

VOLUNTARY HEALTH CARE AGENCIES

Voluntary or nonofficial health care agencies (Table 18-2) are so named because they are nonprofit. The health services they provide are complementary to official (government) health care agencies. They often meet the needs of persons with specific diseases (e.g., heart disease) and certain segments of the population (e.g., those with disabilities). Although paid personnel work in voluntary health agencies, volunteers form a major part of their support system. Voluntary organizations are sites for volunteer service for practical/vocational nursing students and LPN/LVNs. Some examples follow. Refer to your local telephone directory for additional names and numbers of voluntary health care agencies.

Visiting Nurse Association

The Visiting Nurse Association (VNA) is a public voluntary agency that has the following characteristics:
- Provides home nursing care for persons with acute and chronic diseases. Care includes health supervision, education, counseling, bedside care, and carrying out physicians' orders.
- Visits mothers with newborn infants.

Table 18-2 Examples of Voluntary Agencies

AGENCY	PURPOSE	CONTACT
American Cancer Society (ACS)	Cancer research, public information resource to patients, families, professionals	(800) ACS-2345, *www.cancer.org*
American Lung Association (ALA)	Research, professional education, resource for professionals and public	(800) LUNGUSA, *www.lungusa.org*
American Heart Association (AHA)	Research and education on heart disease and stroke	(800) 242-8721, *www.americanheart.org*
American Stroke Association	Research and education on stroke	(888) 4STROKE, *www.strokeassociation.org*
Alcoholics Anonymous	Rehabilitation help and support to patients and families	Check telephone book's local listing. Also (800) 511-9225, *www.alcoholics-anonymous.org*
ALS Society of America	Collects data on persons with amyotrophic lateral sclerosis (Lou Gehrig's disease) for research purposes; resource for public and professionals	(800) 782-4747, *www.alsa.org*
Easter Seals National Headquarters	Research and rehabilitative services for disabled children and adults	(800) 221-6827, *www.easterseals.org*
La Leche League	Information and support for breastfeeding mothers; breast milk for infants because of health reasons but lack a source	(800) LALECHE, *www.lalecheleague.org*
United Ostomy Association of America (UOA)	Education, information, and advocacy for patients undergoing intestinal or urinary diversion procedures	(800) 826-0826, *www.ostomy.org*
American Diabetes Association (ADA)	Resource for type 1 and type 2 diabetes, nutrition information, referrals to doctors, and educational programs	(800) 342-2383, *www.diabetes.org*

- Engaged in health teaching.
- Frequently involves the family in the care of its own members.
- Assists with referrals for patients to other community services.
- Staffed primarily by BSN nurses and home health aides trained for specific tasks of personal bedside care.

⊙ Try This

Voluntary Health Care Agencies

Discover if there is a VNA or equivalent agency in your area. If so, do they employ LPNs/LVNs? What are the skills that LPNs/LVNs are able to perform with registered nurse (RN) supervision?

PRIVATE HEALTH CARE AGENCIES

You may be most familiar with private health care agencies:

- Entrance to the health care delivery system in the United States is generally gained through private health care agencies.

- Although some voluntary or nonprofit agencies are found in the private sector, private health care agencies are generally proprietary (i.e., for profit).
- Charge a fee for their services.
- Primary emphasis has been on curing disease and illness, but a change in emphasis to include disease prevention and wellness promotion has occurred.

EXAMPLES OF PRIVATE HEALTH CARE AGENCIES

Private health care agencies have the following characteristics:

- Complement and supplement government agencies.
- In general, are proprietary (for profit).
- Corporations that own a chain of health care facilities often operate them.
- Occasionally owned by an individual or by doctors who practice in the agency.
- Compared with public health services, the greatest changes in health care services have been noted in the area of private health care agencies.

Family Practice Physicians

Primary care is the term used to describe the point at which an individual enters the health care system. Family practice physicians are a source of primary care. They provide diagnosis and treatment. The patient is billed a fee for these services. If further diagnostic evaluation is needed, the patient is referred to a specialist. Medical doctors function within the Medical Practice Acts of their respective states.

Private Practice Nurses

Specializing in primary health care, advanced practice registered nurses (APRN) provide consulting and counseling services to groups or individuals. These nurses practice in all areas of health care. APNs fill an especially acute need in rural areas where physician services are sometimes difficult to obtain. The nurses function within the Nurse Practice Act of their respective states. See Chapter 12.

TYPES OF HOSPITALS

PROPRIETARY HOSPITALS

Proprietary hospitals are for-profit hospitals operated for the financial benefit of the owner of the hospital. The owner may be an individual, a partnership, or a corporation. With good management techniques, the hospital can be run efficiently, and a profit can be realized. Today, when patients are admitted to the hospital, they are more acutely ill and require more skilled nursing care. This setting for health care is called acute care. There are more than 6500 general and specialized hospitals in the United States. Most are general hospitals, which are set up to deal with a full range of medical conditions experienced by patients. More than 1000 hospitals are set up to deal with a particular disease or condition (e.g., rehabilitation, cancer, orthopedics, mental illness). Specialized hospitals are limited to one type of patient, such as children, women, cardiac patients, and so on.

For most conditions, a general hospital is able to accommodate a patient's needs. However, a general hospital may not have specialists with expertise for treating serious or unusual medical problems. The patient may need to be treated in a hospital center that has highly skilled specialists with advanced knowledge of the condition.

TEACHING AND RESEARCH HOSPITALS

Teaching and research hospitals can be private or public. They have a variety of goals, including the following:

- Treating patients, especially those with serious or unusual conditions
- Training sites for physicians, nurses, and other health professionals

- Researching and developing treatments for disease conditions

These hospitals are almost always affiliated with medical schools and have access to highly skilled practitioners.

PUBLIC HOSPITALS

Public hospitals include Veteran's Administration, state, county, and municipally owned and operated nonprofit hospitals. Hospitals for people with serious mental illness continue to be funded by federal, state, or county funds.

VOLUNTARY COMMUNITY HOSPITALS

Community associations and religious organizations operate voluntary community hospitals. These non-profit hospitals provide short-term inpatient care for people with acute illnesses and injuries. Voluntary community hospitals are heavily dependent on gifts and donations to supplement sources of revenue. Ultimate responsibility for the hospital rests with the board of trustees, usually chosen from the community's business, and professional people, who serve without pay. The board of trustees appoints a paid administrator to manage the hospital.

Try This

Hospitals

What kind of hospitals do you have in your area? Do they currently employ LPNs/LVNs? If so, which nursing units employ LPNs/LVNs?

AMBULATORY SERVICES

The continual rise in cost of inpatient care has resulted in the rapid development of a variety of ambulatory services. As a consequence, the number of inpatient days and the length of stay in acute care facilities have decreased. Ambulatory services offer less expensive care because admission to an acute care facility is avoided. People come to these facilities for assessment, advice, monitoring, teaching, treatment, evaluation, and care coordination.

Private sector ambulatory settings are located in the following places:
- University hospital outpatient departments
- Community hospital outpatient departments
- Physician group practices
- Health maintenance organizations (HMOs)
- Physicians' offices
- Freestanding ambulatory centers
- Nursing care centers

Public sector ambulatory settings include the following:
- Community health clinics
- Indian Health Service
- Community and migrant worker health centers

OUTPATIENT CLINICS

Outpatient clinics provide follow-up care to patients after hospitalization and have the following characteristics:

- Manage disease on an ambulatory basis for those who do not need to be hospitalized.
- Are a part of health care facilities or are freestanding (i.e., not attached to a hospital).
- Function by appointment only.
- Include specialty areas, such as diabetes, neurology, allergy, and oncology.
- Number of specialized clinics depends on the population of the area.
- Employ full-time staff.

URGENT CARE CENTERS

Services are available in ambulatory care facilities for walk-in patients who do not have an appointment. For some individuals, they replace doctor's offices. These facilities have the following characteristics:

- Make primary health care available as an alternative to care by a family physician or care offered in a more expensive emergency room.
- People who do not have a family physician use them.
- Patients who desire faster service outside of regular office hours use them.
- Names given to ambulatory care services reflect the type of care provided (e.g., convenience clinics, express care, quick care, urgent care).

ONE-DAY SURGICAL CARE CENTERS

One-day surgical care centers (ambulatory surgery centers) perform surgery at a scheduled date and time. Patients are discharged when they have recovered from anesthesia and are considered to be in stable condition. These surgery centers have the following characteristics:

- Eliminate the need and monetary charge for being hospitalized overnight.
- Services are also known as outpatient surgery within an established hospital.
- Freestanding outpatient surgery centers provide outpatient surgery as their only service.
- Approximately 80% of surgical procedures are performed in this type of setting.

◎ Try This

Ambulatory Care Providers

What are ambulatory health services in your area called? Do any of them employ LPNs/LVNs? If so, what skills will the LPN/LVN perform under RN supervision?

FREE CLINICS

Some communities have established free clinics as an alternative means of providing primary health care. These free clinics have the following characteristics:

- Persons who cannot afford traditional health services or are reluctant to use more traditional services use the clinics. Cost is based on income.
- Generally have an age and/or income limit.
- Environment is as free of red tape as possible.
- Generally staffed by one salaried administrator and volunteer physicians and nurses.
- A volunteer board makes policy decisions for the clinic.

ALTERNATIVES TO NURSING HOMES

IN-HOME CARE

Most older adults live at home, but a small percentage reside in institutional settings.

Home Health Nursing

Home health agencies are public or private agencies that provide home health services, supervised by a licensed health professional in the patient's home, either directly or through arrangements with other agencies. Some examples of home health agencies include the following:

- Public, nonprofit (e.g., visiting nurse association)
- Public, nonprofit, freestanding (e.g., city, county, including county visiting nurse associations, and state health departments)
- Private or nonprofit hospital-based (e.g., hospital home health agency)
- Private, for-profit, freestanding (e.g., home health care owned by person or corporation)

Home health nursing differs from hospital and nursing home care by increased focus on family and the patient's environment. The purpose is to promote, maintain, or restore health or minimize the effects of illness or disability. An important role is to teach the patient and family self-care. Skilled services in home health care include the following:

- Skilled nursing
- Physical therapy
- Speech-language therapy
- Occupational therapy
- Medical-social services
- Homemaker–health aide services
- Other therapy services may be offered (e.g., respiratory, nutritional, podiatry)

Skilled nursing services are provided and directed by RNs. Basic nursing services are provided by LPNs/LVNs under the supervision of an RN. *Depending on state regulations and agency policy,* LPNs/LVNs are able to provide many home health services. The plan of care for all disciplines requires a treatment plan signed off by a physician and recertified every 60 days. Examples include, but are not limited to, the following:

- Teaching, supervising, or setting up medications
- Injections
- Ostomy care

- Wound care and dressings
- Finger sticks for blood glucose testing
- Catheter care

 Try This

Community Health Services

Are there community health nursing services or home care agencies available where you live? What services do they offer? Which of them employ LPNs/LVNs? What skills are the LPNs/LVNs expected to perform under RN supervision?

Community Health Nursing Services

Nurses have always been at the forefront of community health nursing activity. The major focus of community health nursing is to improve the health status of communities or groups of people through public education, screen for early detection of disease, and provide services for people who need care outside the acute care setting.

Community health nurses work with many different people and groups on prevention and modification of health issues. Among the many possible roles are advocate, caregiver, case finder, health planner, occupational health nurse, school nurse, teacher, and so on. Community health nursing services may exist as a part of an outpatient clinic service, a service attached to an HMO, or a freestanding private service.

Adult Day Care Centers

Hospital-based and freestanding adult day care centers provide services for individuals who need supervision because of physical or safety needs but are not candidates for nursing home placement. Patients with families who are able to assist the person during evening hours and on weekends may prefer adult day care centers instead of nursing home placement.

The purpose of adult day care is to provide mental stimulation, socialization, assistance with some ADLs, and basic observation skills. Some typical services include transportation, meals, therapeutic activities, nursing interventions, and rehabilitation activities. The supervisor is often a social worker or RN. Certified nursing assistants (CNAs) and personal care assistants who meet state requirements assist with ADLs. Volunteers play a major role in some of the adult day care centers.

 Try This

Adult Day Care Services

Is adult day care available in your area? Where are the centers located, what services are offered, and who staffs them? Do they employ LPNs/LVNs? If so, what are the LPNs/LVNs' responsibilities?

RESIDENTIAL CARE

Independent Living Apartments

Independent living apartments are not licensed or regulated. People living in these facilities are not there for personal or medical care, but they like to live with seniors who share their interests. Generally, planned activities and trips and bus service for shopping are offered.

Assisted Living Programs

Assisted living programs (ALPs) provide "a home with services" (assisted care) that emphasizes a resident's privacy and choice. Living quarters are used by older adults who want to remain as independent as possible but cannot manage all of their ADLs. Residents typically have private, locking rooms and bathrooms (or apartments), shared only by choice. Living quarters are handicap accessible and are planned to accommodate the changing needs of residents as they age. Help with daily routine is available but not 24-hour care. These services include bathing, dressing, daily activities, and health maintenance. Care management and skilled nursing services, when needed, come from an outside agency. ALPs accept private pay, Medicaid, and Social Security Supplemental Income (SSI) recipients. The facilities are family oriented, provide activities, and assist the resident with travel to outside appointments. The fee for one- or two-bedroom apartments includes utilities, weekly housecleaning, linen changes, and so on. An additional fee is charged for meals. The assisted-living facilities are often connected to a skilled nursing facility, and the resident can be moved into the skilled nursing facility if that level of care becomes necessary.

Continuous Care Retirement Community

A continuous care retirement community (CCRC) provides a continuum of living options from independent living, enriched living, assisted living, and skilled nursing home, all on one campus. Residents can move from one level of care to another as their needs change. A complete range of housing and health care are offered. Residents generally enter when relatively healthy and transition to care according to need.

Board and Care Homes

Board and care homes are also known as adult care homes, group homes, or family-type homes. The facilities offer temporary or long-term residential care, housekeeping, and custodial care (personal care services) for a small number of adults unrelated to the operator. Assistance with activities of daily living (ADLs), self-administration of medication, preparation of meals, special diets, and transportation are usually supervised and provided by the owner or manager.

The residence may be a single-family home. The residence is licensed as an adult family home or adult group home. The Department of Social Services oversees the operation.

INSTITUTIONAL SETTINGS

Nursing Facilities

Nursing facilities specialize in skilled nursing care (SNF), intermediate nursing care (INF), and long-term care (LTC). The care is paid for by:

- Private pay
- Health insurance
- Medicaid
- Medicare. Health care plans will pay for skilled services but not for custodial services unless they are a part of a skilled care service plan of care. See www.longtermcarelink.net/eldercare/long_term_care.htm for more information.

HOW THE OMNIBUS BUDGET RECONCILIATION ACT RELATES TO SKILLED NURSING AND INTERMEDIATE NURSING FACILITIES

The Omnibus Budget Reconciliation Act (OBRA) of 1987 was in large measure a response to evidence of mistreatment, abuse, and neglect of nursing home residents during the 1970s and 1980s. The Institute of Medicine set out detailed recommendations for improving care, and these recommendations became the basis of OBRA 1987. The Centers for Medicare and Medicaid Services (CMS) implemented the law over a period of years. Rules were not strongly enforced, and by 1998, changes were made in the law. The change omitted language regarding nursing coverage for skilled nursing facilities (SNFs) and intermediate nursing facilities (ICFs). In 1999, the language for nursing care was reinstated. It mandates that all SNFs and ICFs would be required to have 24-hour licensed nursing services 7 days a week and at least one RN employed 8 hours a day, 7 days a week. Requests for waivers for LPN and RN coverage are reviewed and approved by the CMS.

According to *www.healthaffairs.org/,* the following evidence exists of improvement in care:

- Declining use of physical and chemical restraints
- Lower rates of urinary infections and use of catheters
- Fewer hospitalizations

Areas that have shown no change include the following:

- Pressure sore rates
- Malnutrition
- Dehydration
- Other feeding problems
- Increase in bowel incontinence cases

TYPES OF CARE

WHAT IS SKILLED NURSING CARE?

Skilled Nursing Facility

In a skilled nursing facility, services and supplies can be provided by or under the supervision of skilled or licensed nursing personnel. Skilled care is considered care that is medically necessary to improve the quality of the patient's health or to maintain or slow decompensation of a patient's condition, including palliative treatment. See www.longtermcarelink.net/eldercare/long_term_care.htm for more information.

- Registered nurses do wound care and change dressings after major surgery, or they administer and monitor IV antibiotics for a severe infection.
- Physical therapists help to correct strength and balance problems that have made it difficult for a patient to walk or get on and off the bed, toilet, or furniture.
- A speech therapist helps to regain the ability to communicate after a stroke.
- An occupational therapist may also be needed on a long-term basis if the patient requires adaptive assistance using the upper body.

Monitoring vital signs, giving medications, dressing wounds, and so forth are normally associated with skilled care. Delivery of skilled care is based on a written care plan. Residents who meet Medicare requirements and are classified as skilled care receive payment from Medicare and private sources.

Alternative Elder Living: Eden Alternative and Green House Homes. In the early 1990s, Dr. William Thomas and his wife Judy (Jude) Meyers-Thomas developed the Eden Alternative, a philosophy to alleviate the "three plagues" of boredom, helplessness, and loneliness. They offered a creative way to change the culture of nursing homes by bringing growth and laughter into the lives of elders. It was a fundamental change in the relationship between the staff and management, introducing pets, gardens, and children to the nursing home. This concept led to the Green House model of care.

The Green House model is a radical departure from traditional skilled nursing homes and assisted living facilities. The Green House model alters facility size, interior design, staffing patterns, and methods of delivering skilled professional services. It was designed to deinstitutionalize long-term care by eliminating large nursing facilities and creating habilitative, social settings where assistance and support with activities of daily living and clinical care are not the focus of existence.

The Green House residence is a home with 6 to 12 elders in a residential setting. The home includes vibrant outdoor space as well as aesthetically appealing interiors. Each elder has a private room and bathroom. Rooms have a high level of sunlight and are situated around the hearth, an open kitchen and dining area. While adhering to all codes required by regulations, Green House homes look and feel like a typical home and have very few indications of the medical care being provided.

The small size of the Green House home promotes less need for wheelchairs. There is easy access to all areas of the house, including the kitchen and laundry, an outdoor garden, and a patio. Safety feature are built into the house. The elder is free from the limitations of an institutional schedule and lives a comfortable daily life, sleeping, eating, and engaging in any activities he or she chooses. Meals are prepared in the open kitchen and served at the large dining room table, where staff, elders, and visitors enjoy pleasant dining (called convivium). Fresh food and good conversation with people who mingle with one another stimulates the appetite and make for an unhurried mealtime. (This portion was written by Peggy Callantine RN, Board Member of Sheridan Green House Alternative for Living Project.)

Short-Term or Acute Care. Short-term care, also called post–acute care (PAC) or transitional care, is for individuals who have been hospitalized recently and typically have more complicated medical needs. It is provided by many long-term care facilities or hospitals. Included are rehabilitation services, specialized care for certain conditions such as stroke and diabetes, postsurgical care, and other services associated with the transition from hospital to home. The goal is to discharge residents to their home or to a lower level of care.

Intermediate Care Facility. Intermediate care facilities (ICFs) provide 24 hours of licensed nursing services, based on changes in the OBRA law (1999). The difference between skilled and ICF care is more a matter of who delivers the care, rather than the actual care. Not all states license ICFs that provide less than 24-hour RN coverage. It has been suggested that because residents receive lesser services, these homes should more accurately be called "small nursing homes" (see www.longtermcarelink.net/eldercare/long_term_care.htm).

LONG-TERM CARE FACILITIES

Long-term care (LTC) includes a range of medical services designed to help people who have disabilities or chronic care needs. Common reasons for long-term care include cardiovascular disease, mental and cognitive disorders, and endocrine disease (Christensen and Kockrow, 2011). All long-term facilities focus on promoting independence, maintaining function, and supporting autonomy. Medicare, Medicaid, and the Veterans Administration will cover the cost of long-term care under certain conditions. If a veteran is at least 70% service-connected disabled, the VA will cover the cost of nursing home care indefinitely (see www.longtermcarelink.net/eldercare/long_term_care.htm).

Long-Term Skilled Nursing Facility

Long-term care (LTC) facilities provide a range of services for people with severe disabilities or chronic care needs. One such facility is known as a skilled nursing facility for the severely disabled (SNFSD). It provides 24-hour-a-day care for persons with severe mental disabilities. Many of these facilities are locked or secure areas where residents reside for their own protection and the protection of others.

 Try This

Long-Term Care Facilities

What long-term care facilities are located in your area? What level of care do they offer? Do they hire LPNs/LVNs? If so, what skills will the LPN/LVN be expected to perform?

CUSTODIAL OR PERSONAL CARE

Custodial care is when individuals who are neither trained nor licensed can safely and reasonably provide services and supplies. It includes assistance with activities of daily living such as the following:

- Bathing
- Dressing
- Eating
- Grooming
- Getting in and out of bed
- Walking around
- Toileting (incontinence care)

OTHER TYPES OF FACILITIES

REHABILITATION SERVICES

After a patient has been stabilized following an acute illness or injury, a rehabilitation phase, lasting from days to years, may follow. Rehabilitation may take place in the following facilities:

- Rehabilitation centers
- Long-term care facilities
- Outpatient facilities
- Group residential homes
- Patient's home

The focus, regardless of the setting, is the return of function and prevention of further disability. Nurses play an important role on the rehabilitation team.

Try This

Rehabilitation Services

Where are the rehabilitation health services available in your area? What kind of rehabilitation is available? Do they hire LPNs/LVNs? If so, what skills will the LPN/LVN perform with RN supervision?

Wellness Centers

An emphasis on promoting wellness continues to result in a multitude of services being offered in this area of health care. Not only have hospitals developed programs to detect disease in early stages, but they also have developed programs to promote wellness. Wellness center programs include nutritional counseling, exercise programs, stress reduction, and weight control. The private sector continues to be active in the wellness area. People have developed an interest in exercise and fitness clubs, weight-reduction programs such as Weight Watchers, smoking cessation classes, stress control, and parenting classes.

 Try This

Wellness Programs

Choose one wellness program in your area. Find out what services it offers and the qualifications of the staff who provide the information. Which programs employ LPNs/LVNs?

HOSPICE CARE

Hospice, or end-of-life, services are available in many areas to persons who have been certified as terminally ill. The philosophy of hospice care is to maintain comfort as death approaches. The hospice may be in an institutional setting, such as a hospital or a freestanding agency. Hospice care is offered in the institution, especially if pain and symptom management is necessary, the family caring for the person needs respite, or for terminal care. Hospice home care is also available to those who wish to die in their own home. Because RNs, LPNs/LVNs, home health aides, CNAs, and volunteers all staff a hospice, home care can be tailored to the person's needs.

 Try This

Develop Your Own Style

Using clustering (concept mapping) as shown in Chapter 3 as your guide, develop your own style/form to summarize the health care settings described in this chapter.

 Critical Thinking

Has My Vision Changed?

Throughout your course of study, you will find that your interest in a particular area of nursing may change or be modified. Based on what you have learned from reading this chapter, what kind of health care setting is most appealing to you at this time?

Get Ready for the NCLEX-PN® Examination

Key Points

- Health care services are delivered in public and private sectors.
- Public health care agencies are classified as official and voluntary.
- Official public health care agencies are supported by taxes.
- Official public health agencies are local, state, and federal agencies.
- FDA, CDC, NIH, HRSA, AHRQ, ATSDR, IHS, and SAMHSA make up the USPHS.
- The public health care agency of the United Nations is WHO.
- Voluntary health care agencies are supported by contributions and provide complementary services to official health care agencies.
- Private health care agencies are generally proprietary (for profit).
- VNA provides home nursing care for persons with acute and chronic conditions.
- Primary care describes the point at which people usually enter the health care system.

- General hospitals deal with a full range of medical and surgical conditions.
- Specialized hospitals are limited to patients with specific diseases.
- Teaching and research hospitals offer treatment for serious or unusual conditions and usually are a training site for health professionals.
- Ambulatory health care services are available in both private and public sectors.
- Free clinics provide primary care for persons who cannot afford traditional health care services.
- Short-term care, also known as post–acute care or transitional care, provides rehabilitation services and specialized care as a transition between hospital and home.
- Long-term care facilities provide a range of services for people with severe disabilities and chronic care needs.
- Green House homes are a radical departure from traditional skilled care and assisted living facilities.
- Board and care homes, also known as adult care homes, group homes, or family-type homes, offer housing and custodial care.

- Assisted care residences are a "home with services."
- Continuous care retirement communities provide a continuum of living options as needs change.
- Community health, public health, and home health share many responsibilities. A major difference in home health is providing direct patient care.
- Adult day care centers provide socialization, mental stimulation, and assistance with ADLs, basic observation, and health referrals.
- Wellness centers provide nutritional counseling, exercise programs, stress reduction, weight control, and other services.
- Hospice staff maintain comfort of the person as death approaches.
- Responsibilities of care agencies continue to be modified because of changes in the health care system.

Additional Learning Resources

evolve Go to your Evolve website (http://evolve.elsevier.com/Hill/Success) for the following FREE learning resources:
- Answers to Critical Thinking Review Scenarios
- Additional learning activities
- Additional Review Questions for the NCLEX-PN® exam
- Helpful phrases for communicating in Spanish and more!

Review Questions for the NCLEX-PN® Examination

1. Which of the following is an official health agency funded by the UN?
   1. WHO
   2. CDC
   3. NIH
   4. FDA

2. How do official and voluntary agencies differ?
   1. Official agencies are proprietary.
   2. Voluntary agencies are tax supported.
   3. Official agencies provide primary care.
   4. Voluntary agencies emphasize research.

3. How will you explain the different levels of long-term health care to someone planning to seek placement for an elderly relative?
   1. Board and care homes provide "a home with services" added on, as needed.
   2. Intermediate care is suitable for persons who do not need acute or skilled care.
   3. Residential care provides 24-hour transitional care after hospitalization.
   4. Assisted care facilities offer 24-hour supervision and housing for 3 to 16 residents.

4. What quality would not be helpful when working with hospice?
   1. Knowledge of the physiologic process occurring as death approaches.
   2. Ability to sit without the need for dialogue, if desired by the individual.
   3. Feeling the need to tell the individual your beliefs about life after death.
   4. Willingness to honor the person's request for food, conversation, visitors, and so on.

Alternate Format Item

1. What is the difference between community health nursing services and home health agencies? *(Select all that apply.)*
   1. Home health agencies provide direct nursing services to people in their home.
   2. Community health nursing services work on prevention and case finding.
   3. The VNA and the County Health Department are examples of home health agencies.
   4. Home health agencies have an increased focus on family and the patient's environment.

2. How do Green House homes differ from traditional nursing homes? *(Select all that apply.)*
   1. Traditional homes provide personal care by assigning an LPN/LVN to give total care to the resident.
   2. Green House homes follow strict schedules for eating, bathing, and so on to provide a sense of security.
   3. Green House elders have flexibility in when they get up, eat, bathe, go outdoors, and receive visitors.
   4. Sharing a room helps the traditional nursing home residents become friends who can rely on one another.

Critical Thinking Scenarios

Scenario 1
Joni is graduating soon and is thinking about where she would like to work. While working in a nursing home, she developed an interest in working with elders. How might Joni go about finding information about what is available in her area and what her responsibilities will be in each facility?

Scenario 2
Carman, a soon to graduate SPN, is interested in learning more about Green House homes as a potential place of employment. It turns out that a neighboring community is in the process of building four Green House homes. How can Carman find out more details about Green Houses?

The Health Care System: Financing, Issues, and Trends

Objectives

On completing this chapter, you will be able to do the following:

1. Discuss the provisions of the Affordable Care Act.
2. Describe two general methods of financing health care costs, as follows:
   a. Fee-for-service
   b. Capitation
3. Explain the following methods of payment options for patients:
   a. Personal payment (private pay)
   b. Private health insurance (nongovernment)
   c. Public health insurance (government-sponsored)
      1) Medicare
      2) Medicaid
4. Identify sources of funding for public (government) health programs and private health insurance.
5. Discuss the following issues and trends that affect the direction of health care:
   a. Quality
   b. Safety
   c. Cost
6. Explain how the practical/vocational nurse participates in increasing the quality and safety of health care and decreasing the cost of care.
7. Discuss the effect of the restructuring of the health care system on health care and employment opportunities for licensed practical/vocational nurses (LPNs/LVNs).
8. Identify your reaction to change involving your nursing career and personal life.
9. Develop a personal plan to help you adapt to change in your nursing career and personal life.

Key Terms

alliances (ă-LĪ-ăns-ĕs, p. 247)
capitation (kăp-ĭ-TĀ-sŭn, p. 240)
coinsurance (KŌ-ĭn-sur-ăns, p. 240)
continuous quality improvement (CQI) (kŏn-TĬN-ū-ŭs KWĂL-ĭ-tē ĭm-PROOV-mĕnt, p. 246)
copayment (KŌ-pā-mĕnt, p. 240)
cost containment (KŎST kŏn-TĀN-mĕnt, p. 247)
deductibles (dĭ-DŬK-tĭ-bŭlz, p. 240)
diagnosis-related group (DRG) (p. 244)
entitlement program (ĭn-TĪ-tĕl-mĕnt PRŌ-grăm, p. 242)
fee-for-service (SĔR-vĭs, p. 240)
health care provider (hĕlth kār pră-VĪ-dĕr, p. 240)
health maintenance organization (HMO) (p. 240)
Institute of Medicine (IOM) (p. 246)

managed care (MĂN-ăgd kār, p. 240)
marketplace (MĂR-kĕt-PLĀS, p. 247)
Medicaid (mĕd-ĭ-KĀD, p. 244)
Medicare (mĕd-ĭ-KĀR, p. 242)
National Patient Safety Foundation (NPSF) (p. 246)
out-of-pocket (p. 243)
preferred provider organizations (PPOs) (prĕ-FĔRD, p. 240)
premium (PRĒ-mē-ŭm, p. 242)
private pay (PRĪ-vĭt, p. 240)
prospective payment system (PPS) (pră-SPĔK-tĭv pā-mĕnt, p. 244)
restructuring (rē-STRŬK-chŭr-ĭng, p. 247)
"seamless" systems (SĒM-lĕs SĬS-tĕm, p. 248)
third-party coverage (thĭrd PĂR-tē KŌV-răj, p. 241)

 Keep in Mind

Do you pay federal or state taxes? If you do, then you help pay for health care for others. (See Evolve: Payroll Deductions.) Do you have health insurance? If you do not, who pays for your health care?

THE AMERICAN HEALTH CARE SYSTEM

The U.S. health care system has been described as a poorly organized and complicated maze of services that lacks preventive care, wastes resources, is low quality, and is unsafe. Over 50 million people in the

United States do not have health insurance. When people do have access to health care through some type of health insurance plan, problems of quality, service, and cost can arise.

 Critical Thinking

Who Deserves Health Care?

1. Should all individuals in our society have access to health care?
2. Do you think health care is a right or a privilege?

HEALTH CARE REFORM: THE AFFORDABLE CARE ACT

In 2009, the Affordable Care Act was signed into law. It is the first wide-sweeping piece of legislation to address health care reform in the United States since 1965, when Medicare was added to the Social Security Act.

◎ **Try This**

Health Care Reform: The Affordable Care Act

How well do you understand how this law affects you and your patients? Answer True or False to the following questions about the law.
1. The law requires all Americans to have health insurance, or they must pay a fine.
2. The law allows a government panel to make decisions about end-of-life care for people on Medicare.
3. The law cuts benefits that were previously provided to all people on Medicare.
4. The law expands the existing Medicaid program and will cover low-income, uninsured adults regardless of whether they have children.
5. The law will result in the rationing of health care.
6. The law prohibits insurance companies from denying coverage if you have a preexisting condition.
7. The law requires all businesses to provide health insurance for employees.
8. The government will run an insurance program to compete with private plans.
9. The law will provide health insurance to illegal immigrants (Health Reform Quiz, 2011).
   Explanations for the answers in the quiz and additional information that applies to the Affordable Care Act will be included *in italics* as the chapter evolves. More information about the Affordable Care Act can be found at healthreform.kff.org. A timeline for implication of the A.C.A. can be found at www. healthcare.gov.

Answers: 1 = T and F; 2 = F; 3 = F; 4 = T; 5 = F; 6 = T; 7 = F; 8 = F; 9 = F

FINANCING HEALTH CARE COSTS

The two most common ways to finance health care services are **fee-for-service** and **capitation.**

FEE-FOR-SERVICE

The traditional method of paying health care bills is the system called fee-for-service. In this method, physicians are paid a fee for each service they provide.

- Physicians are directly reimbursed for most ordered diagnostic tests and treatments for illness.
- Some insurance companies do not reimburse the tests and treatments that could keep patients healthy or could identify illnesses in their early stages when they are less expensive to treat.
- To improve their margins of profit, insurance companies charge deductibles, copayments, and coinsurance.

CAPITATION

- Capitation is an alternative to the traditional fee-for-service method of payment.
- Capitation involves a set monthly fee charged by the provider of health care services for each member of the insurance group for a specific set of services.
- Managed care plans that use the capitation method of payment include health maintenance organizations (HMOs), preferred provider organizations (PPOs), and open access plans.
- If health care services cost more than the monthly fee, the provider absorbs the cost of those services.
- At the end of the year, if any money is left over, the health care provider keeps it as a profit.
- Suddenly, if a provider of health care services can keep a member of the insurance group healthy, that provider will make a profit!

Before continuing, review Table 19-1 for a comparison of the fee-for-service and capitation methods of payment for health care services and Box 19-1 for health insurance terms. See Box 19-2 for different types of managed care plans.

HOW PATIENTS PAY FOR HEALTH CARE SERVICES

PERSONAL PAYMENT

Payment directly by the patient (i.e., private pay) was the primary method of payment of health care costs before the 1940s. Although some patients may use this method of payment today, the cost of health care services discourages the millions of people in the United States who do not have health care insurance from using this method.

PRIVATE HEALTH INSURANCE

Health insurance, like any insurance, spreads risk. The risk that is spread in health insurance is that the young and the healthy generally subsidize (support financially) the sick and older individuals in the health insurance group. Those who are likely to have high medical bills are denied coverage. *The Affordable Care Act prohibits discriminating against children with preexisting conditions—for example, cystic fibrosis. By 2014, insurance companies will be prohibited from refusing coverage to anyone based on their medical history or health status. The Affordable Care Act also prohibits individual and group health plans from placing lifetime limits on the dollar value*

Table 19-1   **Comparison of Methods of Payment for Health Care Services**

	FEE-FOR-SERVICE	CAPITATION
Services covered	Each health care service claimed by the physician (e.g., diagnostic tests, treatments)	Health care services in group contract
Are preventive tests or treatments covered?	Depends on the plan	Wellness practices covered
Cost	Set fee per member of group	Set fee per member of group
How revenue is increased	Increase health care services Increase patient visits	Decrease health care services Increase number of persons served
Advantages	All tests and treatments for illness covered	Wellness encouraged No deductibles and copayments
Disadvantages	Emphasis on illness Deductibles and copayments keep patient from reporting illness in early stages	To realize a profit, needed tests may not be ordered

Box 19-1   **Health Insurance Terms**

Premium: The monthly fee a person must pay for health care insurance coverage.

Deductible: The yearly amount an insured person must spend out-of-pocket for health care services before a health insurance policy will begin to pay its share.

Copayment: The amount an insured person must pay at the time of an office visit, when picking up a prescription, or before a hospital service.

Coinsurance: Once a deductible is met, the percentage of the total bill the insured person must pay. The remainder is paid by the insurance company.

Health care provider: A licensed health care person, such as a physician, dentist, or nurse practitioner, whose health care services are covered by a health insurance plan.

of coverage and prohibits insurance companies from rescinding coverage—for example, for a patient on chemotherapy.

Administrative costs of private health insurance can run to 31% of premiums. These costs involve screening of applicants for denial of coverage, reviewing claims for reimbursement, profits to investors, and marketing.

Private Group Health Insurance

Group health insurance is a method of pooling individual contributions for a common group goal: protection from financial disaster as a result of health care bills. When insured, an individual is said to have third-party coverage (a fiscal middleman). This financial middleman pays the individual's health care bills. Employers offer most of the private group insurance in the United States. *The Affordable Care Act does not require all employers*

Box 19-2   **Managed Care Plans**

HEALTH MAINTENANCE ORGANIZATIONS

- Are generally located in buildings that are used solely for HMO business, and all physicians working in the HMO are hired specifically for the HMO.
- Receive a prepaid fee to provide comprehensive care to members of the enrolled group.
- Encourage prevention of disease by the practice of preventive medicine.
- Discourage physicians from ordering excessive diagnostic tests and treatments.
- Patients may not have the option of choosing their physician each time treatment is needed. If a physician is chosen outside the HMO network, the cost has to be paid by the patient.
- Depending on the HMO, a member may go outside the HMO to see a desired physician with a point-of-service (POS) option. With the POS option, the member pays an extra fee.

OPEN ACCESS PLANS

- Allow members to see specialist physicians in the network for treatment without need of a referral, as in traditional

HMOs. This option may affect the subscriber's coinsurance.

PREFERRED PROVIDER ORGANIZATIONS

- PPOs are an alternative to the strict utilization review system of some managed care plans.
- Fees are paid by fee-for-service, and health insurance companies contract with physicians and hospitals and negotiate discount fees. These members of the network are "preferred" providers.
- Patients may choose to see any general physician or specialist in the network. If a patient chooses a preferred provider, a larger amount of the cost will be covered by the health care plan.
- Family practice physicians may be hired as members of a PPO. These physicians remain in the same office in which their family practice is located and continue to belong to the same physician group. Part of their day is spent treating patients in their own family practice, and part of the day is spent treating patients who are enrolled in the PPO under the rules of the PPO.

to provide health benefits. However, it imposes penalties on larger employers (those with 50 or more workers) that do not provide insurance to their workers or that provide coverage that is unaffordable. Beginning in 2010, small businesses that offered health insurance received a tax credit. No member of the group insurance plan is denied coverage based on past medical history.

Blue Cross and Blue Shield is an example of private group health insurance. Blue Cross covers hospital inpatient costs and Blue Shield covers inpatient physician costs. A major medical plan is available to include the cost of outpatient services.

Private Individual Health Insurance

Many major insurance companies offer health insurance to individuals who are not part of a group. Premiums are based on a person's health risk (if not denied coverage for a preexisting condition) and age.

PUBLIC HEALTH INSURANCE

Medicare: A Program of Social Security

People of retirement age find themselves ineligible for group insurance plans because they are not employed. This inability to get insurance occurs at the very time when individuals are more likely to encounter medical costs because of chronic disease.

- In 1965, Medicare was added to the Social Security Act.
- This federally sponsored entitlement program and public health insurance plan helps finance health care for all persons older than age 65 (and their spouses) who have at least a 10-year record in Medicare-covered employment and are a citizen or permanent resident of the United States.
- Coverage is also given to persons younger than age 65 who are permanently and totally disabled, persons with end-stage renal disease, and persons with Lou Gehrig's disease.
- No person is denied coverage based on past medical history. Approximately 48 million elderly and disabled U.S. citizens are on Medicare.
- Approximately 10,000 baby boomers each day become eligible for retirement benefits, placing huge demands on Social Security, including Medicare.
- A current Medicare handbook can be accessed by typing "Medicare Handbook" into Google.

Medicare Health Care Plans

- The Original Medicare Plan (Traditional Plan/Parts A and B). This fee-for-service plan allows the beneficiary to go to health care providers or hospitals that accept Medicare patients. The health care provider gets paid for each Medicare-covered service provided. Medicare pays its share and patients pay their share (Boxes 19-3 and 19-4).
- Administrative costs to run the Medicare fee-for-service program are approximately 2%. Money is saved by not having to work at screening out high-risk patients.

Part C (Medicare Advantage Plan)

- Medicare Advantage Plans are government-approved health plan options that are offered by private insurance companies. These plans are alternatives to original (traditional) Medicare plans.
- Coverage includes parts A and B, and in some plans, Part D of the traditional plan.
- Generally, lower copayments and additional benefits (vision care, hearing aids) are offered in these plans, but there may be a limit on where care can be obtained, which physician can be seen, and how often the beneficiary can see the physician. Benefits can change from year to year.
- Different types of Advantage Plans are described in Box 19-5.
- The Congressional Budget Office paid Medical Advantage Plans (i.e., private insurance companies) 12% to 19% more than it would have cost for the same care in traditional Medicare.
- *The Affordable Care Act reduces payments to the privately administered Medicare Advantage Plans to be more in line with traditional Medicare.*
- *Medicare Advantage Plans will still be required to provide all benefits that are covered by traditional Medicare. See "What Will Happen to Medicare Advantage Plans" at healthreform.kff.org.*

Box 19-3   Medicare Part A Provisions

Medicare Part A helps pay for inpatient hospital care. Part A is available without cost and is funded by a payroll tax; it includes a deductible and a coinsurance fee that starts on day 61 of hospitalization. In 2011, Medicare Part A helped pay for the following types of situations:

- Inpatient hospital care (e.g., a semiprivate room, meals, drugs, supplies, lab tests, radiology, and intensive care units) and care in certified Christian Science sanatoriums.
- Twenty days' posthospitalization skilled nursing facility care (full cost) for rehabilitation services. The next 80 days are paid after a daily coinsurance.

- Under certain conditions, home health care services with coinsurance charges for medical equipment and hospice care for terminally ill beneficiaries.
- Part A does *not* pay for long-term care custodial services (e.g., patients who need help only with activities of daily living [including feeding]), private rooms, telephones, or televisions provided by hospitals, skilled nursing facilities, or Christian Science practitioners. You can find Medicare premiums and coinsurance rates at http://questions.medicare.gov.

Box 19-4   Medicare Part B Provisions

Medicare Part B is similar to a major medical insurance plan. Part B is funded by monthly premiums that are income related. The premium is deducted from the monthly Social Security, Railroad Retirement, or Civil Service Retirement payment. Part B requires a deductible and pays 80% of covered charges. The remaining 20% of charges are the patient's responsibility. In 2012, Medicare Part B helped to pay for medically necessary (needed for diagnosis and treatment of a medical condition) services, which included the following:

- Physician visits and other medical services
- Outpatient hospital services (including emergency room visits) and outpatient mental health
- Clinical laboratory services and diagnostic tests (x-rays, MRIs, CT scans, EKGs)
- Ambulance transportation
- Durable medical equipment (wheelchairs, walkers, oxygen, hospital beds)
- Kidney supplies and services
- Some diabetic supplies

- Physical, occupational, and speech therapy in a hospital outpatient department or a patient who resides in a Medicare-certified bed in a rehabilitation agency
- Limited chiropractic services
- Preventive services: "Welcome to Medicare" physical exam in the first 6 months after enrolling in Plan B; cholesterol, lipid, and triglyceride blood levels once every 5 years; mammography every 12 months; Pap test and pelvic exam every 2 years; fecal occult blood test every year; screening colonoscopy every 10 years; PSA test and rectal digital exam every year; flu shot once a year; pneumococcal vaccine once a lifetime; bone mass measurements every 24 months, if at risk for osteoporosis; and diabetic screening
- Part B does *not* pay for most prescription drugs, routine physicals, services not related to treatment of illness or injury, dental care, dentures, cosmetic surgery, routine foot care, hearing aids, routine eye examinations, or routine glasses.

Source: *Medicare and You 2012* (CMS Publication Product Number 10050). Baltimore, MD: U.S. Department of Health and Human Services.

Box 19-5   Medicare Advantage Insurance Plans

Shopping for Advantage Health Plans involves comparison of plans to find the right plan, at the right price, to meet personal needs. An online visit to www.medicare.gov can connect individuals to sites that present health plan options in a specific area of any state.

- **Medicare HMO:** The Medicare patient can go to only doctors, specialists, and hospitals that are in this plan's network. A point-of-service (POS) option offered by some Medicare HMO plans allows the patient to go to doctors and hospitals outside the network for an additional fee.
- **Medicare PPO:** This plan has a network like HMOs but allows patients to go outside the network for an additional fee.
- **Medicare private fee-for-service plans (PFFS):** Any physician or hospital that accepts the plan's payment can be chosen. The insurance company pays its share of doctor and hospital bills, and the patient pays his or her share. The private insurance company, not Medicare as in the original plan, decides how much the patient will pay.

Source: *Medicare and You 2012* (CMS Publication Product Number 10050-24). Baltimore, MD: U.S. Department of Health and Human Services.

Part D

- Medicare drug legislation, passed in 2003, provided prescription drug coverage that helps to pay for brand-name drugs at participating pharmacies. See Box 19-6 for Medicare reform prescription drug benefits.
- HMOs and other private health plans use their buying power to negotiate fairer prices through discounts for the drugs they purchase. The Medicare drug legislation of 2003 bars the federal government from using its power to negotiate lower prices from drug companies for the drug bill. However, the

Veteran's Administration negotiates lower drug prices for the VA system.

- *The Affordable Care Act gradually reduces the amount that Medicare Part D enrollees are required to pay for their prescriptions when they reach the coverage gap. The coverage gap will be eliminated by 2020.*

See Evolve for sources of revenue for government health insurance.

Medigap Coverage. Because of the items Medicare does not cover, beneficiaries are encouraged to purchase private supplemental insurance, called Medigap, in addition to Medicare to cover copayments, deductibles, coinsurance, and limited-coverage situations that exist in the federal program. These policies are sold by private insurance companies. Enrollment in a Medicare prescription drug plan is also encouraged if it is not included in the selected health care plan. See Evolve: What the Patient Pays When on Traditional Medicare for an example of **out-of-pocket** expenses a patient would pay when having surgery.

Diagnosis-related groups. Payment for Medicare is a major item in the federal budget. In 2010, Medicare spending totaled approximately $528 billion. Before 1983, hospitals submitted a bill to the government for the total charges they incurred for Medicare patients and were reimbursed for this amount. This was called a "retrospective payment" system because payment was based on actual costs.

- In 1983, the federal government attempted to stop the skyrocketing cost of health care.
- The former Health Care Financing Administration (now the Centers for Medicare and Medicaid Services [CMS]) adopted a system of paying hospitals a set fee or flat rate for Medicare services.

Box 19-6 The Medicare Prescription Drug, Improvement, and Modernization Act of 2003: Prescription Drug Benefit

Participation is voluntary in the traditional Medicare plan and premiums depend on the private plan chosen.

COVERAGE FOR 2012

- Most plans have a coverage gap (the donut hole). After the patient's drug plan and the patient spend a total of $2840 for drugs, the patient is in the "donut hole" and receives a 50% discount on brand name formulary drugs and a 7% discount on generic formulary drugs.
- After the patient spends $4550 out-of-pocket for drugs, he or she is out of the donut hole. For the remainder of the year, catastrophic coverage "kicks in," requiring $2.50 for generic drugs or $6.30 for brand-name drugs or 5% of retail drug costs—whichever is highest.
- *The A.C.A. gradually reduces the amount that Medicare Part D enrollees are required to pay for their prescriptions when they reach the coverage gap. The coverage gap will be eliminated by 2020.*
- Information about the coverage gap can be found at http://healthreform.kff.org/faq/how-does-law-change-the-medicare-part-d-donut-hole.aspx.

Source: *Medicare and You 2012* (CMS Publication Product Number 10050-24). Baltimore, MD: U.S. Department of Health and Human Services.

- Hospitals were told in advance how much they would be reimbursed.
- Because the federal government announces to a hospital in advance what it will pay for health care costs, this system is called the prospective payment system (PPS).
- Under the diagnosis-related group (DRG) system, a math formula is used to arrive at the fee the government will pay for hospitalization. This fee depends on the DRG category (illness) causing the patient's hospitalization.
- Hospitals receive a flat fee for each patient's DRG category regardless of length of stay in the hospital. Hospitals have an incentive to treat patients and discharge them as quickly as possible. If the hospital keeps the patient longer than the government's fee will cover and the patient cannot be reclassified in the DRG system, the hospital has to make up the difference in costs.
- If the acute care facility can treat the Medicare patient for less than the guaranteed reimbursement, the facility can keep the difference as profit.

Because Medicare patients, like all patients, are discharged sooner from hospitals than they were in the past (as a result of the PPS), extended care units are often used to continue convalescence.

Medicaid

The Medicaid program (Title XIX) was added to the Social Security Act in 1965. This program provides medical assistance for eligible families and individuals with low incomes and resources.

- Medicaid is a cooperative venture jointly funded by the federal and state governments. Table 19-2 provides a comparison of Medicare and Medicaid.
- The federal government establishes broad, national guidelines for Medicaid.
- Each state establishes its own program services and requirements, including eligibility. For this reason, when eligible for Medicaid in one state, an individual is not automatically eligible in another state.
- *Under the Affordable Care Act, Medicaid will be expanded to cover nearly all individuals under age 65 with incomes up to 133% of the federal poverty level. The*

Table 19-2 Comparison of Medicare and Medicaid

	MEDICARE	MEDICAID
Purpose of program	Health care for persons 65 years and older who are eligible for Social Security, the disabled, and persons with end-stage renal disease and Lou Gehrig's disease	Medical and health-related services for persons with decreased income and resources that meet eligibility requirements
Source of funding	Federal government (i.e., your tax money) An entitlement health care program. Congress must fund Medicare each year, as opposed to a discretionary program, in which funding must be approved yearly.	An entitlement program jointly financed by the federal and state governments (your tax money). Medicaid is a major expenditure in federal and state budgets.
Who administers the program?	The federal government	Individual states. *There is wide state variation in levels of eligibility and services provided that will be removed by the Affordable Care Act in 2014.*
Cost to individual to enroll	Part A: Hospital insurance for inpatient care. No cost for persons who meet eligibility requirements for Social Security. Part B: Medical insurance covering doctors' fees and so on. A premium or monthly fee is taken out of the monthly Social Security check when person registers for program.	No fee Must meet income eligibility requirements

Affordable Care Act creates a uniform Medicaid eligibility level and income definition across all states and eliminates a prohibition that prevented states from providing Medicaid coverage to adults without dependent children. Undocumented immigrants and legal immigrants who have resided in the United States for less than five years are not eligible for Medicaid.

 Try This

How Have Medicare and Medicaid Provisions Changed/ Evolved?

What changes in legislation at the federal level and at your state level have affected the Affordable Care Act and Medicare and Medicaid since the seventh edition of *Success in Practical/ Vocational Nursing* was published?

COST OF HEALTH INSURANCE

The continual rise in health care costs has resulted in annual increases in health insurance premiums for employers. *The Affordable Care Act requires the federal government to create a process in conjunction with states where insurers have to justify unreasonable premium increases.*

 Critical Thinking

What Services Should Medicare Offer?

1. Should Medicare pay for new technological procedures that are developed to treat common medical problems of the elderly?
2. Should cost-effectiveness enter the picture for treating Medicare patients?

THE UNINSURED

Over 50 million Americans do not have health insurance. These include:

- **Low-wage employees.** This class of people is employed in low-wage jobs that are less likely to offer insurance benefits.
- **The middle class.** Some of these workers are unemployed. Those employed may be priced out of the health care insurance market by rapidly rising health insurance premiums.
- *Starting in 2014, citizens and legal residents must obtain health insurance or pay a penalty.*
- *Groups exempt from this requirement include those who would have to pay more than 8% of their income for health insurance, those with incomes below the threshold required for filing taxes, those who qualify for religious exemptions, undocumented immigrants, those who are incarcerated, and members of American Indian tribes.*
- *Some alternatives to paying for health care include Medicaid (if they qualify), private pay (if they can afford it), and charity care (if they can find it); some may become*

victims of medical bankruptcy. Thirty-five states have high-risk, preexisting condition insurance plans for persons with medical conditions that make them uninsurable. In July 2011, the federal government reduced premiums of high-risk insurance plans that are running in 17 states by up to 40%.

- Unemployment and a downturned economy increase the number of uninsured who seek treatment in emergency rooms.
- Lack of access to health care prevents individuals from receiving preventive care and seeking treatment when a health problem develops.
- These individuals may seek treatment during the later stages of illness, usually at greater expense. Cancer is an example of a disease that is best treated and possibly cured when diagnosed in its early stage.
- Consider the case of a sinus infection. The most cost-effective means of diagnosing and treating a sinus infection is an assessment by a family physician or nurse practitioner. However, this solution is not realistic if you do not have health insurance, your insurance company does not cover this type of visit, or you do not have the money to pay for deductibles, copayments, coinsurance, or a retail clinic visit such as at Walmart. When the sinus infection reaches an acute stage, the individual might seek treatment at the local emergency department. Many people rely on emergency departments for all levels of health care due to lack of insurance.
- Emergency room treatment is expensive and is intended for seriously ill or injured persons and not for less serious illnesses.

 Critical Thinking

Who Pays the Health Care Bill?

If a patient does not have health insurance or the ability to pay the emergency room fee, who pays the bill?

QUALITY, SAFETY, AND COST OF HEALTH CARE

Each year, the United States spends over $2.3 trillion on health care. (See Evolve: What Is a Trillion Dollars?) Some reasons for the high cost of health care are the costs of prescription drugs, medical malpractice lawsuits, and continual development and use of medical technology. The United States has the highest health care spending of industrialized countries but has lower life expectancy and higher infant and maternal mortality than most of the industrialized countries of the world. The 2010 National Healthcare Quality and Disparities report states that Americans too often do not receive care that they need or receive care that causes harm. For all the money spent on health care, patients are not experiencing quality and safety in their health care.

The **Institute of Medicine (IOM)** is an independent, nonprofit organization that serves as an advisor to improve the nation's health. The IOM has released the following two reports that address the issue of quality, safety, and cost in health care. These reports have influenced the direction of health care and education of nurses in the twenty-first century.

- *To Err Is Human: Building a Safer Health Care System* (1999): This report found that up to 98,000 people die each year from preventable medical errors and presents a comprehensive strategy to prevent such errors.
- *Crossing the Quality Chasm: A New Health System for the 21st Century* (2009): This report provided six aims for improving the quality and safety of health care in the United States that should be adopted by all personnel providing health care.

IMPROVING QUALITY IN HEALTH CARE

1. *Continuous quality improvement (CQI)*: Quality by inspecting patient incidences of harm or mistakes *after* they had occurred during care. CQI focuses on *preventing* problems or adverse events.
   - Checklists are an example of a method used to ensure quality and safety when giving care. Checklists are a list of items or actions for a task where each item is checked off when completed. This helps the nurse remember parts of a procedure or intervention.
2. *Aims of the IOM for improving quality in health care:* The six aims of the IOM (2001) to increase quality in health care are referred to as STEEEP:
   - *Safe:* Avoid injuries to patients from the care that is intended to help them.
   - *Timely:* Reduce waits and sometimes harmful delays for both those who receive and those who give care.
   - *Effective:* Provide services based on scientific knowledge to all who could benefit and refrain from providing services to those not likely to benefit.
   - *Efficient:* Avoid waste of equipment, supplies, ideas, and energy.
   - *Equitable:* Provide care that does not vary in quality because of personal characteristics such as gender, ethnicity, geographic location, and socioeconomic status.
   - *Patient-centered:* Provide care that is respectful of and responsive to individual patient preferences, needs, and values, and ensure that patient values guide all clinical decisions.

? Critical Thinking

Increasing Quality in Providing Care

Provide examples of content from your practical/vocational nursing program and this text that help you meet the IOM aims to increase quality in health care.

3. *Continued competency:* An important component of quality health care is that the providers of that care be able to demonstrate competency throughout their careers. Current nursing licensure considers nurses from all levels of educational preparation minimally competent upon receiving the initial license, and continued competence is assumed throughout a career. Patients, lawmakers, employers, and professional organizations question this assumption. As this matter is debated and a method is devised to assure patients that their health care providers are competent and qualified, practical/vocational nurses need to update themselves continually in their area of practice.

 Try this

Identify How You Will Stay Current in Your Career

Identify ways that practical/vocational nurses can remain current in their areas of employment.

IMPROVING SAFETY IN HEALTH CARE

1. *The Joint Commission (TJC) National Patient Safety Goals:* Nursing has always promoted safety first with patients: First, do no harm. TJC reviews adverse incidents studies on causes of serious harm and death to patients. The results are startling. For example, the Institute of Medicine's 1999 study estimated that 44,000 to 98,000 Americans die each year as a result of medical errors. High on the errors list is medication error. Improper patient identification is often a problem in giving medication and also in doing wrong-site surgery. Nurses are often involved in patient preparation for surgery and marking the site so no confusion exists during the surgical process. Additional information is available at http://www.jointcommission.org/PatientSafety Goals. Box 19-7 provides a list of TJC 2011 Patient Safety Goals for hospitals.
2. *National Patient Safety Foundation (NPSF):* Since 1997, the mission of the NPSF (2011) has been to improve the safety of care provided to patients and to eliminate health care errors. As a central voice for patient safety, NPSF is committed to a team approach to prevent health care mistakes by avoiding errors of commission (doing the wrong thing), omission (not doing the right thing), or execution (doing the right thing incorrectly). The NPSF is planning a professional credentialing process for 2012 and has formed the American Society of Professionals in Patient Safety (ASPPS) as the first and only individual membership program for the patient safety field. ASPPS was established to advance patient safety as a unique and vital health care discipline.
3. *Transition to Practice:* The Transition to Practice initiative is being tested in pilot studies by the National

Box 19-7 TJC 2011 National Patient Safety Goals

TJC National Patient Safety Goals have been revised yearly since their conception. There are gaps in numbering of the 2007 goals. Some original goals have been retired, usually because the requirements were integrated into the standards. The number of the old goal is dropped, and the numbering for new goals is continued. This is done so there will be no confusion about the content of a goal that is current. See National Patient Safety Goals (http://www.jointcommission.org/PatientSafetyGoals).

- **Goal 1:** Improve the accuracy of patient identification. For example, before giving medication, have at least two ways to identify the patient (neither one can be the room number). The patient's wristband, with identifying data, and the patient's chart, with matching name and patient number, are acceptable.
- **Goal 2:** Improve effectiveness of communication among caregivers. For example, use standard abbreviations and the 2005 TJC "do-not-use" abbreviation list. Check with your instructor if you are unable to read a doctor's order or other notes on the chart. Review the patient care plan you developed with your instructor before giving care.

- **Goal 3:** Improve safety in using high-alert medications. For example, prepare a medication such as insulin or a narcotic under instructor observation.
- **Goal 7:** Reduce the risk of health care–associated infections. Comply with current Centers for Disease Control and Prevention hand-washing guidelines and other recommendations for preventing and transferring infection to the patient or your family.
- **Goal 8:** Accurately and completely reconcile medications across the continuum of care. Patient's current medication is compared with what was ordered while cared for in a health facility. If the patient is transferred, a complete list of medications accompanies the patient. A complete list of medications is provided to the patient upon discharge from the health facility.
- **Goal 15:** The hospital identifies safety risks inherent in its patient population. This goal applies to psychiatric hospitals and patients being treated for emotional or behavioral disorders. Be aware of the patient's verbal, nonverbal, and affective communication. Avoid discounting what you hear and what you suspect. Report your concerns to the instructor or nurse in charge.

Council of State Boards of Nursing as an effort to improve the quality and safety of health care. Beyond orientation to a facility, the pilot studies will determine the best way to transition from a student role to a newly licensed role in a health care setting (see Chapter 24).

 Critical Thinking

Patient Safety Goals

Discuss how you implemented TJC Patient Safety Goals in your last clinical experience.

IMPROVING THE COST OF HEALTH CARE

A driving force today in health care agencies is cost containment (the need to hold costs to within fixed limits) while remaining competitive in the health care marketplace. Practical/vocational nurses need to remember that health care agencies are interested in improving their agency's "bottom line" by reducing waste and inefficiency. Practical/vocational nurses who identify wasteful practices and inefficient routines in their work settings while maintaining quality may in fact be saving their own jobs. The following are the LPNs/LVNs' roles in containing health care costs in the work setting:

- Follow facility policy for charging patients for all supplies used in their care.
- Follow facility policy for documenting patient care for reimbursement.
- Organize patient care for effective and efficient use of your time.

- Be efficient and effective in delivering patient care. If some aspect of care needs to be "redone," it means you could have done it right the first time.
- Ensure reimbursement, and decrease the patient's length of stay by implementing nursing care to help prevent complications.
- Meet the patients' needs, not yours.

Nurses are an essential factor when it comes to addressing quality, safety, and cost in health care. These attributes of health care need to be understood and brought to all clinical situations by all nurses, regardless of educational preparation (Kovner and Spetz, 2011).

 Professional Pointer

Remember to consider quality, safety, and cost in your practice.

RESTRUCTURING THE HEALTH CARE SYSTEM

The changes in health care to improve the delivery of health care (*service*), increase the *quality* and *safety* of that care, and decrease the *cost* of care are continual. A major change that continues to take place in health care services today is the restructuring of the health care system. This is a response to escalating health care costs.

Changes in the delivery of health care in the community involve new organization and structure of health care organizations:

- Alliances (partnerships) are formed among hospitals, clinics, laboratories, health care systems, and physicians. By joining together, or *networking*, these alliances can coordinate the delivery of care and contain costs among providers of health care services; for example, supplies can be purchased in bulk, and the staff can share a computer. Patient records can be more readily available on referral to another health care provider in the network. For this reason, alliances are called "seamless" systems.

- Consolidated systems of health care include hospital systems found nationwide. An example is the Aurora Health Care system that is a for-profit system of hospitals. Any profits realized go to the investors in a for-profit system.

Try This

Identify Restructuring of Health Care in Your Area

1. Identify health care alliances, networks, or consolidated systems that have formed in your area of the country.
2. Do these systems employ practical/vocational nurses?

DEALING WITH CHANGE

If you had no prior experience in health care before entering the student practical/vocational nursing program, you may not be aware of the changes taking place in the workplace. If you had prior experience in the health care field, some of the changes you now observe in health care services may be obvious, whereas others may be subtler. Even new workers in a health career will see changes as their program of study progresses. How do you react to changes in your life? Whether changes occur in your personal life or career, it is important for you to remember that you have choices. You can be a victim, a survivor, or a navigator of change. When change is in the wind, are you a victim, a survivor, or a navigator?

- **Victims** look at change in a negative way. They fear the worst will happen because of the proposed change and feel helpless in the situation. They do not willingly participate in the change process, allowing change to control them.
- **Survivors** resist change but go along for the ride. They claim the change will never work, and if their prediction comes true, they say, "I told you so!"
- **Navigators** of change feel in control of the situation. They feel confident and excited about the possibility of being part of the solution to a problem. Navigators believe they have some control over change rather than being controlled by the change.

 Professional Pointer

Be a self-directed, motivated, problem-solving employee.

In the twenty-first century, practical/vocational nurses need to define their role as more than the list of nursing tasks and duties they perform. Less trained, unlicensed persons on the health care team are also performing these nursing tasks and duties. *Practical/vocational nurses need to define their role in light of their assisting role in the nursing process.* Practical/vocational nurses are effective in noting new patient problems and collaborating with RNs in setting patient goals, performing nursing interventions, and evaluating the results of planning. It is these problem-solving and critical thinking aspects of nursing that make practical/vocational nurses valuable members of the health care team.

Practical/vocational nurses need to present themselves in clinical situations as invaluable to the health care agency. Be self-directed, motivated, positive, and a problem solver in your daily work. Avoid being known as the person who always asks what needs to be done next. Identify what needs to be done, prioritize, and do it. Respond flexibly to changes that are presented. Identify tasks or protocols that could be done more efficiently. Use the critical thinking skills that were encouraged in your nursing program to devise innovative suggestions to make these areas more efficient, effective, and safe. Be a role model for practical/vocational nurses.

Get Ready for the NCLEX-PN® Examination

Key Points

- The quality, safety, and cost of health care are major concerns in today's health care system.
- Reports of the Institute of Medicine highlight concern for the quality, safety, and cost of health care.
- Traditional fee-for-service and capitation are the main ways of financing health care.
- Insurance plans, both private and government-sponsored, are the major third-party payment systems in existence today.

- The number of uninsured is a major concern in health care.
- Continuous quality improvement, aims of the Institute of Medicine, continued competency, the Joint Commission National Patient Safety Goals, the National Council of State Boards of Nursing's Transition to Practice Model, and the licensed/practical nurse's role in containing health care costs address the issues of quality, service, and cost of health care.
- Changes in health care delivery include patient-centered care, HMOs, PPOs, open access plans, and health care

alliances. Practical/vocational nurses need to be self-directed, motivated, and positive problem solvers in their areas of employment.

- Changes in health care need to be approached with flexibility and viewed as an opportunity to improve the quality and safety of patient care.
- Practical/vocational nurses need to ensure quality and safety of patient care by keeping updated and current in their areas of employment.

Additional Learning Resources

evolve Go to your Evolve website (http://evolve.elsevier.com/Hill/Success) for the following FREE learning resources:
- Answers to Critical Thinking Review Scenarios
- Additional learning activities
- Additional Review Questions for the NCLEX-PN® exam
- Helpful phrases for communicating in Spanish and more!

Review Questions for the NCLEX-PN® Examination

1. A driving force in health care today is:
   1. Safety concerns
   2. Patient demands
   3. Technological explosion
   4. Labor negotiations

2. Select the statement that best explains Medicare as a prospective payment system.
   1. Hospitals like the prospect of being paid by the federal government for health care services for elderly people.
   2. When the patient is discharged, the hospital calculates the bill and sends it to the federal government.
   3. Because of DRGs, the federal government tells the hospital in advance how much will be paid for an illness.
   4. The benefits covered by Medicare are changing rapidly because of new legislation by the federal government.

3. A patient tells the LVN about the new HMO that his employer has chosen to cover employees with health care benefits. Select the statement that indicates the patient understands the coverage of an HMO.
   1. "Each time I go to the doctor, I pay the charges as I leave the office, and I send the bills to the HMO for reimbursement."
   2. "My annual physical is covered by the HMO, and I do not have to pay deductibles or copayments when I use the HMO."
   3. "The doctors hired by the HMO submit their bills to the HMO and receive reimbursement for the services they provided."

   4. "I must call the HMO each time I need to go to the doctor and obtain permission to be seen by a physician, or they will not pay."

4. You have been elected by your state as the first practical/vocational nurse to be a member of the U.S. Senate. When you arrive in Washington, D.C., you find that the Senate's focus during your first year in office will be health care reform. Each of the following projects would reform health care. Select which project would have the greatest effect on reforming health care.
   1. Reform Medicare and Medicaid to reduce fraud, waste, and inefficiency.
   2. Develop a plan for complete health care coverage for all the uninsured.
   3. Expand the Children's Health Insurance Plan to include their parents.
   4. Provide prescription drug coverage for all people on Medicare and Medicaid.

Alternate Format Item

1. Which of the following source(s) of revenue help finance state and federal government health care programs? *(Select all that apply.)*
   1. FICA
   2. FICA-Medical
   3. Group health insurance
   4. State withholding tax
   5. Federal withholding tax

2. Select the statements that describe provisions of the Affordable Care Act. *(Select all that apply.)*
   1. The health reform law will give all Americans health insurance.
   2. Insurance companies will not be able to exclude me because of medical history.
   3. Undocumented immigrants are covered under the Health Reform Act of 2010.
   4. Persons with Medicare will retain all the benefits they had before the new law was passed.
   5. The federal government will have death panels to evaluate persons on Medicare.

Critical Thinking Scenario

During break, a group of LVN students are discussing new health reform legislation. Jason is upset because the Affordable Care Act is socialized medicine. Mike tells the group his grandfather told him the new law will make it necessary to have death panels evaluate care for Medicare patients. Mike said he heard that the new law rations care. How would you address these statements?

Objectives

On completing this chapter, you will be able to do the following:

1. Describe the expanded role of the practical/vocational nurse (LPN/LVN), as written in your state's Nurse Practice Act.
2. Identify the location of the practical/vocational charge nurse on the organizational chart of a long-term care facility.
3. Explain the difference between leadership and management.
4. Identify your personal leadership style.
5. Explain the following leadership styles in your own words:
   a. Autocratic
   b. Democratic
   c. Laissez-faire
   d. Situational
6. Identify ways to attain competency in the following five core areas, in which knowledge and skills are needed to be an effective first-line leader:
   a. Motivate team members to accomplish goals.
   b. Communicate assertively.
   c. Problem solve effectively.
   d. Build a team of cooperative workers.
   e. Manage stress effectively.
7. Identify ways to obtain competency in the following three specific areas, in which knowledge and skills are needed to be an effective first-line leader:
   a. Occupational skills
      1) Nursing (clinical) skills, including the nursing process
      2) Documentation
      3) Legal aspects
      4) Federal, state, and private organization regulations
   b. Organizational skills
      a) Time management
      b) Continuous quality improvement
      c) Conflict resolution

   c. Human relationship skills
      a) Anger management
      b) Performance evaluations for nursing assistants
      c) Empowering team members
8. Describe how the Howlett Hierarchy of work motivators can help the practical/vocational nurse leader influence nursing assistants to motivate themselves.
9. Identify the importance of documenting objective, not subjective, charting entries in long-term care.
10. Use the problem-solving approach to set up a plan to solve a clinical problem.
11. Read the mission statement for your current area of clinical assignment.
12. Using suggestions in this chapter, write a plan that could be used to build a team to work on a long-term care unit.
13. Develop a plan to decrease stress in the clinical area.
14. Using the ABCD method of Ellis, identify an irrational thought you have had on the clinical area, and convert it to a rational thought.
15. In your own words, explain specific skills required of the practical/vocational charge nurse in long-term care because of Omnibus Reconciliation Act of 1987 (OBRA) regulations.
16. Prioritize tasks that need to be completed for your next clinical assignment.
17. Identify areas to improve efficiency in your current area of clinical assignment.
18. Practice giving positive and negative feedback, in measurable terms, to peers in a mock clinical situation.
19. Develop a plan for personal growth as a practical/vocational charge nurse.

Key Terms

autocratic style (ĂW-tō-kră-tĭk, p. 254)
Centers for Medicare and Medicaid Services (CMS) (p. 262)
conflict resolution (KŎN-flĭkt, p. 264)
continuum (kŏn-TĬN-ū-ŭm, p. 254)
Howlett Hierarchy (HĪ-ĕ-RĂR-kē, p. 256)
irrational thinking (ĭ-RĂ-shŭn-ăl, p. 264)

leadership (LĒD-ĕr-shĭp, p. 253)
management (MĂN-ĭj-mĕnt, p. 253)
mission statement (MĬ-shŭn, p. 259)
Nursing Home Reform Act (p. 262)
Omnibus Budget Reconciliation Act of 1987 (OBRA) (RĔ-kŏn-SĬL-Ē-Ā-shŭn, p. 262)
patient outcomes (PĀ-shŭnt ŎWT-kŭms, p. 264)

Keep in Mind

"The manager does things right. The leader does the right things."

—Warren Bennis, *On Becoming a Leader* (2003)

Grace and Emily, nursing assistants at Quality Care Home, collapsed in their chairs in the lunchroom. "I had forgotten how hectic mornings can be," said Grace. "I am exhausted." This was the first day back on the day shift on the Evergreen Wing for both nursing assistants. Both women had substituted for a week for vacationing nursing assistants—Grace on nights and Emily on the evening shift.

"I don't care how tired I am, I sure am glad to be back with our charge nurse," said Grace. "I missed Sal Sytchuashun's way of running things," she continued. "On nights, being with that LVN Gina Ivanapleze was like working with mass confusion. Anything you wanted to do was fine with her. It seemed the most important thing to her was the happiness of the nursing assistants, not the residents' care. Anything we wanted to do was hunky-dory. Sal listens to my suggestions but also offers input when I need it."

"That sure is different from my experience," said Emily. "Being with RN Priscilla Pittbul taught me the real meaning of her initials—"real nasty." She commanded us to do everything; she never suggested. Never a 'thank you' or 'good job.' We had a task list and a time sequence to follow, and, no matter what cropped up, heaven help us if we didn't stick to it precisely. We couldn't even ask questions about her assignment sheet. The only time I appreciated Priscilla barking her orders was the evening we had a code. I was shaking in my boots, but she knew exactly what to do. And the resident pulled through."

"I'm glad we didn't have a code with Gina in charge," said Grace. "We have so few codes around here. That is a situation in which I would appreciate having some direction."

"I liked the way Sal handled the situation this morning in the lounge when a resident complained of chest pain," Grace added. "Sal gave us each something to do STAT. After the situation was over, we all discussed the emergency as a team. Sal listened to our suggestions on how to make things go more smoothly in the next emergency situation. Sal makes me feel like a real team member and not a slave!"

Grace and Emily finished their lunches. As they went back to Evergreen Wing, they both agreed that LVN Sal had a way about him that gets the job done, makes you feel comfortable about going to him with a concern or question, and makes you want to come back to work for the next shift. Both agreed he is a good role model for the vocational nurses and nursing assistants.

PRACTICAL/VOCATIONAL NURSE AS FIRST-LINE LEADER

Have you ever experienced employment situations similar to the ones just described by Gina and Priscilla? Perhaps you received directions as a nursing assistant or in another job capacity and did not like the way you were approached by your supervisor.

Nurses at all levels need to manage patient care. Some nurses will also be leaders. Licensed practical/vocational nurses have proved themselves effective as first-line leaders. First-line leaders are responsible for supervising nursing assistants who deliver care in long-term care units. Such positions are referred to as charge nurse positions. If you are a manager of patient care and a leader, you will be more effective in this expanded role in practical/vocational nursing.

Practical/vocational nurses need to develop leadership and management skills so they can direct and supervise others in a manner that will effectively meet the goals of the employing agency. In your practical/vocational nursing program, you started to build a strong, solid base in these skills. This chapter and Chapter 21 will help you to continue to develop skills to lead and manage. This chapter focuses on the leadership role and provides 20 Leadership Hints, 5 Leadership Activities, and 1 Critical Thinking exercise to get you started thinking in a leadership mode. Chapter 21 provides 11 Management Hints, 12 Management Tools, and 7 Critical Thinking exercises to help you apply the knowledge and skills needed to be a charge nurse. The interactive format of both chapters, especially Chapter 21, will have you thinking as a new charge nurse and solving some of the problems new charge nurses face. This chapter and Chapter 21 can both be used as reference tools of skills while orienting to a practical/vocational charge nurse position.

ORGANIZATIONAL CHART

The organizational chart is a picture of responsibility in an employment situation. In the traditional organizational chart, individuals who are lower on the

FIGURE 20-1 Sample traditional organizational chart for the practical/vocational nurse in the charge nurse role.

FIGURE 20-2 Sample contemporary organizational chart for the practical/vocational nurse in the charge nurse role.

organizational chart report to the person directly above them on the chart. Figure 20-1 shows where the practical/vocational nurse fits into the traditional organizational chart as a first-line leader. In Figure 20-1, the practical/vocational nurse reports to the nurse manager, who is a registered nurse. Nursing assistants report to the practical/vocational nurse. To whom does the nurse manager report?

Because of changes in the structure of organizations, organizational charts have become more horizontal than vertical in appearance. Figure 20-2 provides an example of a contemporary organizational chart. This "flattening out" has eliminated some of the middle manager positions in organizations. As a result, the remaining middle managers have taken on more responsibilities and are spread thin. Middle managers in this system have more persons reporting to them than in the past. Middle managers depend on the people who report to them, such as the practical/vocational charge nurse, to think critically and problem solve. Middle managers expect to be contacted when you have tried and are unable to solve your own problems. See the Coordinated Care, Leadership Activity: Examining Organizational Charts box.

Coordinated Care
Leadership Activity

Examining Organizational Charts

Resources needed:
- Organizational charts from clinical sites used by students in your practical/vocational nursing program

Organizational charts may differ by region of the United States. Obtain organizational charts of long-term care facilities in your area. Clarify specific levels of responsibility as they apply to the practical/vocational nurse. Identify whether these charts reflect a traditional or contemporary style of organization.

EXPANDED ROLE OF PRACTICAL/VOCATIONAL NURSING

It is important for you to review the current Nurse Practice Act of your state. This law legally defines the exact role and boundaries for practical/vocational nurses. Also review the following for more guidelines related to the expanded role of the practical/vocational nurse:

1. Appendix A: NAPNES Standards of Practice and Educational Competencies of Graduates of Practical/Vocational Nursing Programs
2. Appendix B: NFLPN Nursing Practice Standards for the Licensed Practical/Vocational Nurse

See the Coordinated Care, Leadership Activity: Determining Your State's Requirements to Assume the Position of Practical/Vocational Charge Nurse box.

 Coordinated Care

Leadership Activity

Determining Your State's Requirements to Assume the Position of Practical/Vocational Charge Nurse

Resources needed:
- Your state's Nurse Practice Act

Obtain a current copy of your state's Nurse Practice Act. Identify the part of the act that addresses your state's position on the practical/vocational nurse who is assuming the charge nurse position in the following areas:

1. Requirements before assuming the practical/vocational charge nurse position
2. Site of employment
3. Scope of practice

If your state's Nurse Practice Act does not address the issue of charge nurse, how can this information be obtained?

An example of the expanded role of the practical/vocational nurse is the first-line manager position, also called charge nurse, in a nursing home or long-term care facility. In these situations the practical/vocational nurse has the responsibility of supervising the care given by nursing assistants and other personnel. The practical/vocational nurse will direct, guide, and supervise these health care workers as they attempt to meet the goals of the resident's plan of care.

The most recent practice analysis of entry-level practical/vocational nurses by the National Council of State Boards of Nursing (NCSBN, 2010) for which data are available occurred in 2009. This survey identified that 45.2% of practical/vocational nurses responding to the survey reported they had administrative responsibilities, with 65.8% of these respondents working in long-term care. Fifty-two percent of respondents in long-term care reported the charge nurse position as their administrative responsibility. To carry out the first-line manager/charge nurse role effectively, you will need the abilities found in both a leader *and* a manager. The 2009 practice analysis can be obtained at www.ncsbn.org.

PREPARING FOR A LEADERSHIP AND MANAGEMENT ROLE

The topic of leadership and management for the practical/vocational nurse is a vast one. All practical/vocational nurses are already managers in the sense that they consistently need to direct, handle, and organize care for assigned patients. It is worthwhile for you to review the ways in which your practical/vocational nursing program helps prepare you for a management position. The practical/vocational nursing program encourages

development of the following skills, which are necessary for functioning successfully as a first-line manager:

1. Basic nursing skills, including the nursing process
2. Time-management techniques for home and clinical time
3. How to learn new information, including using resources for learning
4. The power of positive self-talk and thinking
5. Rules for assertiveness
6. Communication skills
7. Ethical aspects of health care
8. Legal aspects of health care
9. Problem solving and critical thinking
10. Stress management
11. Participation in clinical evaluation

Learning leadership and management involves much more than taking one course or reading one chapter about becoming a leader. Learning leadership is a process (continual development) that includes many skills and is something that evolves over time. This chapter encourages you to think specifically of a leadership role, and it provides leadership hints that practical/vocational nurses need.

DIFFERENCE BETWEEN MANAGEMENT AND LEADERSHIP

Management is the organization of all care required of patients in a health care setting for a specific period.
- The focus of management is planning and directing to meet patient goals.
- Management is a formal role given to a person by the employer.
- Managers are appointed by their employers.
- The tools needed for management could be written in a step-by-step manner and given to you to follow.
- Following the directions for using the management skills would possibly get the job done in an efficient manner.

Leadership is the manner in which the leader gets along with coworkers and accomplishes the job.
- The focus of leadership is to produce changes in the workplace that will meet the goals of the employing agency.
- Leadership is an informal role that is given to a person by a group of workers. You become a leader when your team members decide to follow you.
- Leaders cannot be appointed.
- The leader needs to influence others in the work setting to want to implement desired change.
- Directions for leadership skills can also be written, but it is through experience that leadership skills are truly developed.

The practical/vocational nurse who has the skills of both management and leadership will get the job done in the most efficient and effective manner, and the practical/vocational nurse manager and coworkers will enjoy the experience that much more! A manager is not automatically an effective leader, and a leader is not automatically an effective manager. Your goal will be to develop skills of leadership *and* management.

WHAT KIND OF LEADER ARE YOU?

You can lead in several different ways. What is your predominant leadership style? Each of the statements given in the Coordinated Care, Leadership Activity: Discovering Your Personal Leadership Style box is an extreme. The responses are not positive or negative. One answer does not have value over another answer. They just are.

 Coordinated Care
Leadership Activity

Discovering Your Personal Leadership Style

Put a check mark next to the statement that *best* describes the way you *might* be at work, not how you *want* to be.

A SHORT TEST OF LEADERSHIP STYLE

1. My primary goal at work is to:
   a. Get the job done.
   b. Get along with the people with whom I work.
   c. Do the job correctly.
   d. Hope the work I do is noticed.
2. My clinical coworkers would say I am:
   a. Domineering in my relationships.
   b. Friendly and personable in my relationships.
   c. Likely to attend to details of the resident care plan.
   d. Creative and energetic in giving care.
3. At work, I feel like I have to be:
   a. In control of the resident situation.
   b. Liked by my coworkers.
   c. Correct in giving care.
   d. Recognized and praised for my care.
4. When I communicate on the nursing unit:
   a. I am usually direct and to the point.
   b. I am more considerate of the person to whom I am talking rather than strongly getting my point across.
   c. I usually give detailed information.
   d. I usually elaborate on the point at hand.
5. My coworkers would say I am a person who:
   a. Gets the job done regardless of what shift I work.
   b. Is very likable and patient.
   c. Is precise and accurate in giving nursing care.
   d. Is optimistic and has good verbal skills.

6. My charge nurse might describe my behavior while on my shift by saying that:
   a. Sometimes I alienate people.
   b. Sometimes I waste time and fall for excuses others may give.
   c. Sometimes I can be stubborn with coworkers.
   d. Sometimes I appear flaky to my coworkers.
7. I react to a stressful incident on the nursing unit:
   a. By being rude, blaming other departments, and yelling at coworkers.
   b. By being accommodating to the person in charge and by passive behavior.
   c. By becoming silent and withdrawing from the situation.
   d. By talking faster and louder.
8. When I deal with my coworkers on the nursing unit regarding patient matters, I like them to:
   a. Get to the point and be businesslike in their behavior.
   b. Be casual and sincere in their behavior.
   c. Use the facts of the matter and go step by step when explaining a resident-care situation.
   d. Be enthusiastic about the situation and use demonstrations to explain their points.

Add up your "a" and "c" answers. These answers are more characteristic of a task-oriented person. In leadership terms, this person is called an *autocratic* leader. Add up your "b" and "d" responses. These are more characteristic of a people-oriented person. In leadership terms, this person is called a *laissez-faire* leader.* Your score can give you a rough estimate of the tendency of your leadership style.

*French for not interfering in the affairs of others.

LEADERSHIP STYLES

The literature abounds with examples of leadership styles. Figure 20-3 illustrates a continuum (a line with extreme opposites at each end) of leadership styles. Box 20-1 compares and contrasts the leadership styles found on this continuum.

BENEFITS AND DISADVANTAGES OF LEADERSHIP STYLES

A purely task-centered leadership style (called autocratic style) thrives on power. It involves telling someone what to do, with little regard for the employee as a person who may have ideas about how to improve resident care or reach the goals of the employer. Adopting the autocratic or laissez-faire style in Box 20-1 to use consistently as a leadership style is unrealistic. Its consistent use could be disastrous. However, there is room for an autocratic leadership style—for example, in

AUTOCRATIC STYLE	DEMOCRATIC STYLE	LAISSEZ-FAIRE STYLE
Concerned with the task	Balances concern with task and employee	Concerned with the employee
Extreme	Midpoint	Extreme

FIGURE 20-3 Extremes of leadership styles on a continuum.

| Box 20-1 | Comparing Autocratic, Democratic, and Laissez-Faire Styles of Leadership |

GENERAL DESCRIPTION
Autocratic: Does not share responsibility and authority with employees
Democratic: Shares responsibility and authority with employees
Laissez-faire: Gives away responsibility and authority to employees

IMPORTANCE OF AGENCY'S POLICIES
Autocratic: Emphasis is on policies
Democratic: Enforces policies but with concern for employees
Laissez-faire: Puts employees before policies

HOW LEADER GETS THE JOB DONE
Autocratic: Tells employees what tasks to do; does not seek input from employees

Democratic: Seeks input from employees and encourages problem solving
Laissez-faire: Tries to please everyone

WHAT GETS DONE
Autocratic: May reach goals
Democratic: Because of involvement of employees, goals may be achieved with positive staff feelings
Laissez-faire: Maybe nothing, but at least staff feels good

WHEN STYLE CAN BE USED
Autocratic: Crisis situations, code situations, emergencies
Democratic: Daily nursing care situations, meetings, committees, review of care plans
Laissez-faire: When agency goals/policies are not a consideration

times of emergency. On the following lines, list two additional examples of situations that might require the autocratic style of leadership.

1. _____
2. _____

A purely people-oriented style (laissez-faire) focuses on people's feelings but ignores the task at hand. It allows employees to act without any direction. The goals of the employer will be compromised when the laissez-faire leadership style is used. At times, persons in leadership roles may feel the need to be liked by all team members and use this leadership style, but the task of accomplishing goals will be compromised.

Focusing on both the task and the employee is characteristic of the democratic style of leadership. In this style the practical/vocational charge nurse displays concern for the work that needs to be done, as well as for the team performing the work. When using this leadership style, the practical/vocational charge nurse encourages supervised nursing assistants to discuss resident care, make decisions, and problem solve improvements in care. It may take longer than the autocratic style for work to be accomplished, but patient goals (outcomes) will be achieved, with staff having positive feelings about their supervisor and the experience. Examples of situations in which the democratic style of leadership is useful include daily nursing care situations, unit meetings, and reviews of patient care plans.

Situational Leadership
A popular system of leadership for the twenty-first century is called situational leadership. **Situational leadership** involves varying your leadership style to meet the demands of the situation in the work environment. According to this system, the practical/vocational nurse needs to pick a leadership style that fits the work situation at hand.

USING THE LEADERSHIP CONTINUUM AS A GUIDE

The value of a continuum, as shown in Figure 20-3, is that as you move along the continuum from each extreme toward the center or midpoint, the two extremes begin to blend together. You have some of each style, depending on where you are on the continuum. A blend, to some degree, of the two extremes in the appropriate work situation would be the leadership style needed at the moment.

 Coordinated Care
Leadership Activity

Plotting My Leadership Style Score

Using your leadership style score from the Discovering Your Personal Leadership Style box, place an "X" on the continuum in Figure 20-3 to indicate where you are at this point in general leadership style tendencies.

Do the exercise in the Coordinated Care, Leadership Activity: Plotting My Leadership Style Score box. Remember, this score is your tendency. If your "X" is far to the left or right, it will benefit you to be aware of this tendency and to avoid using this style consistently. Remember the continuum and the need to be flexible in your style. Balance task and people orientation as needed. Knowing what your predominant style of leadership is will be helpful in your evaluation of work situations and the style needed at that time. Some situations require a supportive style, whereas others require a more directive approach.

CORE KNOWLEDGE AND SKILLS NEEDED FOR LEADERSHIP

To function well in your expanded role as practical/vocational charge nurse, you will strive to be a good leader. The scenario at the beginning of this chapter provides examples of what not to do as a nurse leader.

Much research in learning about the business of leading others and the theories that go with leading is available in the literature. *Core knowledge and skills lay the foundation for leadership.* They will help you develop other necessary knowledge and skills for your leadership role. We identify five core areas of knowledge and skills that are necessary for the practical/vocational charge nurse to be an effective leader. These core areas include the ability to do the following:

1. Motivate team members to accomplish team goals.
2. Communicate assertively.
3. Problem solve effectively.
4. Build a team of cooperative workers.
5. Manage stress effectively.

UNDERSTANDING MOTIVATION AND HUMAN NEEDS

As a leader, you will have the task of getting your team members to meet goals set by your employer. Getting people to do what needs to be done is a complex task. What motivates one person does not necessarily motivate another. Understanding motivation and human needs will help you get started.

Motivation

Motivation is a drive that causes individuals to set personal goals and behave in a way that will allow them to reach those goals. The motivation drive comes from within an individual and is intrinsic. Recognition for accomplishing something, a sense of achievement, praise, and opportunity for growth and development are examples of intrinsic factors that help motivate a person (Murray, 2009). Research has shown that paychecks and benefits that are initiated by an employer are extrinsic factors. These factors do not act as motivators once basic needs are met (Murray, 2009). Research has also shown that rewarding desired behavior of employees is instrumental in having that behavior repeated (Pink, 2009).

Human Needs

All individuals have needs that must be filled to meet goals. Individuals are internally motivated to engage in various activities to meet these needs. The activity they engage in is called behavior and can be observed. Here are some facts about needs:

- Abraham Maslow, a psychologist, presented a pyramid of human needs that ranks those needs and can assist the learner in understanding self and others (see Figure 10-1A).
- Meeting needs on one level of the pyramid acts as a motivator for meeting the needs on the next level.
- Progression through these levels is not clear-cut. In reality, as most of your needs are met on one level, you are already beginning to check out the next level.
- When faced with overwhelming difficulties, physical or emotional, some regression takes place—for example:

- Physiologic needs become a priority if you have lost your job or housing.
- Safety and security needs become a major issue if you are facing a serious illness, move into an unsafe neighborhood, or are facing a divorce.
- Once these issues have been dealt with or resolved, higher needs will reemerge.

Motivating Nursing Assistants

Maslow's Hierarchy of Needs can be adapted to help the first-line LPN/LVN leader understand motivation of team members in a health care setting, based on needs (Figure 20-4). Remember, all behavior is internally motivated. As an LPN/LVN manager, you can influence what nursing assistants might be motivated to do. If nursing assistants see that doing a good job helps them meet personal needs, they will also be meeting the goals of their employer.

All levels of the pyramid in Figure 20-4 are considered to be needs of employees in an employment situation. As you go up the Howlett Hierarchy, strategies could be used to encourage meeting needs of nursing assistants at each level. The opportunity to meet these needs can be encouraged or discouraged by the employer and/or the work environment, including the charge nurse (extrinsic motivators). If these needs are met, the person can proceed to the next highest level of the pyramid. If these needs are not met, a person may become dissatisfied with the work situation. Strategies for levels 3 and 4 can play an important role in motivation for team members at any level of the Howlett Hierarchy. Praise, recognition, and rewards are extremely important tools for leaders.

 Try This

What Motivates You as an Employee?

List what motivates you specifically in clinical situations to get your assignment completed.

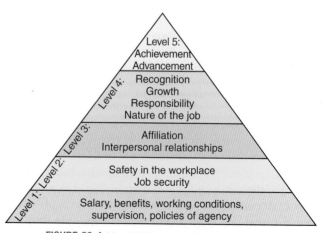

FIGURE 20-4 Howlett Hierarchy of work motivators.

Critical Thinking

Motivating Nursing Assistants

Resources needed:

- Readings on motivation, the Howlett Hierarchy, and your creativity to find ways to meet the needs of nursing assistants.

This exercise encourages the charge nurse to be creative in finding ways to encourage motivation in nursing assistants. Examples of behaviors that encourage meeting needs at each level of the hierarchy are given; the person responsible for the behavior is listed in parentheses. Space is provided for you to fill in additional suggested behaviors at each level to encourage motivation of nursing assistants. Identify whether the employer needs to initiate the strategy or whether the strategy could be initiated by the first-line practical/vocational nursing leader.

LEVEL 1. SALARY, BENEFITS, WORKING CONDITIONS, SUPERVISION, AND POLICIES OF AGENCY

Examples

- Explanation of policies that affect employees (employer)
- Cafeteria-style benefits—pick and choose benefits (employer)

LEVEL 2. SAFETY IN THE WORKPLACE AND JOB SECURITY

Examples

- Provision of adequate equipment to carry out standard precautions (employer and first-line LPN/LVN leader)
- Establish policy for hostile patients (employer and first-line LPN/LVN leader)

LEVEL 3. AFFILIATION AND INTERPERSONAL RELATIONSHIPS

Examples

- Plan monthly potluck dinners, pizza lunches, get-togethers (first-line LPN/LVN leader)

LEVEL 4. RECOGNITION, GROWTH, RESPONSIBILITY, AND NATURE OF THE JOB

Examples

- Encourage attendance at continuing education seminars, in-service training, and so on (employer and first-line LPN/LVN leader)
- Recognize employees when working short-staffed (employer and first-line LPN/LVN leader)

LEVEL 5. ACHIEVEMENT AND ADVANCEMENT

Examples

- Recognition of successful completion of class or seminar (employer and first-line LPN/LVN leader)
- Provide objective examples of how you can implement each of your suggested behaviors. For example, level 5 could be implemented by the following examples:
  - A written account in the facility's newsletter
  - Posting an announcement on a special section of the bulletin board
  - A personal note of congratulations from the charge nurse

APPLYING COMMUNICATION SKILLS AS AN LPN/LVN LEADER

One of the LPN/LVN leader's most productive tools is the effective use of verbal and nonverbal communication. The principles of communication in Chapters 13 and 14 are building blocks for the communication skills you will need as a practical/vocational charge nurse. See the Coordinated Care, Leadership Hint: Communication of the Practical/Vocational Charge Nurse box and the Coordinated Care, Leadership Hint: Encouraging Verbal Communication from Nursing Assistants box.

 Coordinated Care

Leadership Hint

Communication of the Practical/Vocational Charge Nurse

VERBAL

1. When talking to nursing assistants, deliver your message with clear, specific language. Spell out objectively what has to be done for residents. If you work with nursing assistants who do not speak English as a first language, determine their proficiency with English. Verify that intended messages were received.
2. As a practical/vocational charge nurse, you are a role model for nursing assistants. Discourage profanity, personal criticisms, gossip, and rumors.
3. Use "I" instead of "you" messages. "I" messages indicate you take the responsibility for the message—for example, "I saw you tie the patient's wrist restraint to the side rail. This could cause injury to the patient when the side rail is lowered. I suggest you review the videotape on application of restraints. Also review the policy this home has about the danger of restraint application." You messages imply that you are blaming the person to whom you are speaking—for example, "You did a poor job applying that wrist restraint." Take responsibility for your messages.
4. When talking with your supervisor, be valued for your input. Avoid being known as someone who just brings up problems. After objectively stating the problem, offer solutions.

NONVERBAL

1. Be sure your body language and message are consistent and professional. For example, avoid smiling when you are delivering a needed reprimand. Face the person to whom you are speaking.
2. When delivering your message, appear sure of yourself. Have an attentive posture.

WRITTEN

1. Use language that all staff will understand.
2. Review your written messages before posting them to be sure the intent of the message is clear.
3. Provide written work assignments that do not require the nursing assistant to make judgments.
4. Provide written reports of all meetings. If information is not restricted, a report from a meeting with management can dispel/prevent rumors about what "they" are planning now. The reports can be placed in a loose-leaf binder in an area that is accessible for nursing assistants.

TELEPHONE

1. Gather your thoughts before you make a call. This includes the purpose for the call.
2. With a smile in your voice, greet the person by name, identify yourself, and offer a brief inquiry as to his or her well-being, if you know the person you called. For example, say, "Hello, Mrs. Kylie, this is Tricia Zak from The Home. How are things going?"
3. State the reason for the call: "I need to order a video and wanted to know if you had any specific needs."

4. You initiated the conversation. Terminate it when your business is completed. The exception is when the person you called brings up a work-related question.
5. Avoid long conversations about non–work-related topics. This is what is considered allowing the telephone to extend into your time.
6. Arrange to have incoming calls answered quickly, by the second or third ring.
7. When you answer, identify the facility and give your name and title: "The Home, Tricia Zak, charge nurse."
8. Speak clearly in a moderate tone of voice. Most people talk too loudly on the phone.
9. Callers are "customers." Treat the caller respectfully and cordially.
10. If it is necessary to put the person on hold, ask permission to do so.
11. If it is necessary to put the person on hold, try to get back to her or him within 30 seconds. If you are still delayed, ask for a number so you can call back.
12. Provide the information requested.

Coordinated Care

Leadership Hint

Encouraging Verbal Communication from Nursing Assistants

1. Actively listen to nursing assistants. Avoid distraction and inattention.
2. Stay focused on what the nursing assistant is saying.
3. Avoid forming a response while the nursing assistant is speaking.
4. Avoid judging the message or the nursing assistant.
5. Rephrase the message when the nursing assistant is done to verify that you understand the message.
6. Encourage comments. Your goal is to have the nursing assistant go back to the team and say, "That charge nurse really listened to me!"
7. Encourage constructive evaluation. Create an environment in which nursing assistants are encouraged to give their input, whether positive or negative.
8. Respect all opinions. Nursing assistants need to feel safe to speak up, ask questions, identify problems, and suggest solutions to those problems.

APPLYING PROBLEM SOLVING AS AN LPN/LVN LEADER

The basic hint for successful problem solving is *identify the real issue and solve it.* What is the problem? Avoid spending precious time on finding solutions for what is not really the problem. Chapter 9 introduced you to the nursing process, an excellent problem-solving process. You have been using this problem-solving method throughout your student practical/vocational nursing program. For problem solving, the nursing process can be used to solve resident problems as well as staff problems. The nursing process also works at home, as well as in the clinical area (Figure 20-5).

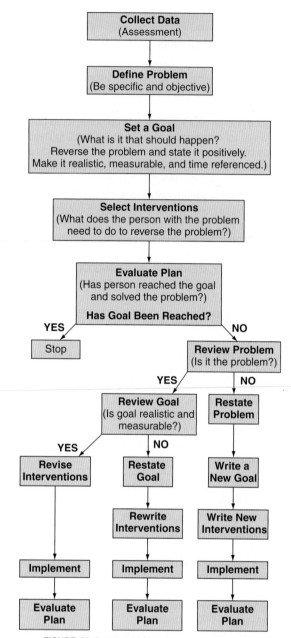

FIGURE 20-5 Decision tree for problem solving.

Scenario: Late for Assigned Shift

Penny, a nursing assistant, is assigned to the day shift in a long-term care facility. Her shift begins at 6:45 AM with a verbal report from the day practical/vocational charge nurse for her wing. All nursing assistants are expected to attend this report and receive their assignments at this time.

Data Collection. On May 8, 10, 15, 16, 23, and 24, Penny came to work either during the charge nurse report or after the charge nurse had finished. When questioned about this behavior, she states she has problems getting her teenagers up and ready for school.

Problem. A record of Penny's tardiness indicates this is a recurring problem and not an isolated incident. A pattern has been established in being late for report.

Goal. Starting immediately, Penny will be on time for the day charge nurse's report and will hear the entire report.

Intervention. As the charge nurse, it is your responsibility to talk to Penny about this tardiness. This includes the times and days of her tardiness. Select a private location for your discussion. Encourage Penny to think through why this behavior is inconvenient for the staff and residents. Review the long-term care unit's policy on punctuality. Encourage Penny to come up with ideas that will allow her to be on time. Set limits with Penny. Identify that she needs to be on time for her assigned shifts. Plan to meet with her in 1 week to discuss her performance. At that time, if she has not improved her performance, a written reprimand will be given and included in her personal file. At the end of the meeting, compliment Penny on an area of her work that has been going well.

Evaluation. During the next week, continue to document Penny's arrival for her assigned shifts. If she complies, note and praise her change in performance.* If she continues to be late for her shift, issue a written reprimand. Place a copy in her file, give a copy to your supervisor, and keep a copy in your file. Be sure the warning contains objective information, such as the following:

1. Days and times late for shift
2. Date of oral warning
3. Seriousness of situation
4. Consequences

TEAM BUILDING

Mission Statements
Mission Statement of The Home

- The Home is a private, nonprofit, long-term care facility. The Home provides 24-hour nursing care in a manner and setting that maintain or improve each resident's quality of life, health, and safety.

The practical/vocational charge nurse needs to be aware of the mission statement of the long-term care facility. A mission statement defines the purpose and goals of the organization. The foregoing mission statement contains what staff must do to meet the goals of The Home.

Each unit in the long-term care facility can write a specific statement of goals that spins off the facility mission statement. This will get the nursing assistants on your team thinking about what they believe and value in regard to resident care. One example of a unit mission statement that is a spin-off of The Home's mission statement follows.

The Home—Team A Goals

- Nursing assistants of Team A of The Home are committed to providing competent, caring, safe, and personalized service to residents and their families.

The team you supervise has the goal to carry out the mission statement of the long-term care facility. As charge nurse, you are in charge of creating the climate of the work environment that will motivate staff to meet this goal. In this situation the goal is maintaining or improving quality of life, health, and safety of residents at The Home. You are a role model for attitudes and behavior. Your team will model the attitudes and behavior you expect of them. Suggested practical/vocational charge nurse attitudes to convey while attempting team building include the following beliefs:

1. Most employees want to do a good job at work.
2. Most employees want to reach their full potential.

See the Coordinated Care, Leadership Hint: Using Unit Mission Statements box and the Coordinated Care, Leadership Hint: Practical/Vocational Charge Nurse Behaviors That Encourage Team Building box.

 Coordinated Care
Leadership Hint

Using Unit Mission Statements

1. Using input from nursing assistants, develop a unit mission statement for your unit.
2. Unit mission statements can be printed on small cards and carried in the pockets of nursing assistants.
3. Unit mission statements can be handed to residents and families on admission. The nursing assistant's first name and title can be included on the card.
4. Unit mission statements need to be reviewed on a regular basis to refresh nursing assistants about their goals. These cards are a written reminder of common values in resident care.

 Coordinated Care
Leadership Hint

Practical/Vocational Charge Nurse Behaviors That Encourage Team Building

1. Review the mission statement of the facility with nursing assistants.
2. Review the unit mission statement with nursing assistants.
3. Use teamwork language, such as "we" and "us." Convey the attitude "We have common goals, and together we will meet them."
4. Encourage politeness, cooperation, trust, and respect among nursing assistants.
5. Encourage honest feedback among nursing assistants.
6. Provide an opportunity for sharing of ideas among nursing assistants.
7. Ask nursing assistants for ideas on how to do unit tasks more effectively.
8. Provide occasions for nursing assistants to spend time together.

---

*In the next week Penny actually arrived a few minutes before the other nursing assistants. The practical/vocational charge nurse allowed her to choose her break and lunch times. Penny had never experienced this before and was very pleased.

9. Create a positive environment in the clinical area that nursing assistants will want to be a part of.
10. Use rewards to provide positive reinforcement of behaviors that contribute to team goals.
11. Reward group accomplishments.
12. Treat nursing assistants on your team as you would like to be treated.

STRESS MANAGEMENT

Stress is a part of all work environments. The long-term care area has its fair share because of increased workloads (especially when a nursing assistant calls in sick) and conflicts with nursing assistants, physicians, families, and residents. Stress and anxiety in the clinical area can result in dysfunctional behavior on the job. Examples of dysfunctional job behaviors include the following:

1. Decreased performance of nursing assistants
2. Negative interactions with nursing assistants
3. Ineffective communication
4. Inappropriate body cues, such as sharp tone of voice
5. High staff turnover
6. Unhappy residents, families, physicians, and nursing assistants

As a practical/vocational charge nurse, you have the responsibility to be a stress manager and role model for the team. Your goal will be to do the following:

1. Display the ability to cope with stress as it affects you.
2. Create a work environment with decreased stress levels.
3. Guide and support nursing assistants when they experience stress.

The practical/vocational charge nurse needs to learn how to detect stress in the clinical environment. A good place to start is to be aware of your own stress level. See the Coordinated Care, Leadership Hint: Life Skills That Help Control Stress box and the Coordinated Care, Leadership Hint: Creating a Less Stressful Work Environment box.

Coordinated Care
Leadership Hint

Life Skills That Help Control Stress

1. The actual stress reduction/relaxation technique you choose is personal. Whatever works for you is the skill to choose.
2. Review Chapter 6 regarding meditation, relaxation techniques, imagery, and so on.
3. Massage.
4. Daily exercise: Walking is the easiest and least expensive form of exercise. No special equipment is required, except good walking shoes.
5. Apply the principles you learned in nutrition and let the MyPlate be your guide for getting the fuel your body needs. Review Chapter 6 for nutrition updates.

6. Get the amount of rest you need to function at your best.
7. Take your breaks when at work. You will be reenergized and increase your productivity.
8. Develop leisure activities you enjoy (or rediscover activities you put on the back burner during nursing school).

Coordinated Care
Leadership Hint

Creating a Less Stressful Work Environment

1. Your ability to organize your shift will help prevent some stressful situations.
2. Have available the equipment that nursing assistants need to get their job done.
3. Encourage nursing assistants to take breaks.
4. Create a calm environment.
5. Treat nursing assistants with respect. Remember your communication skills, especially "please," "thank you," and "I sure appreciate _____."

Coordinated Care
Leadership Activity

Identifying Signs of Stress

Resources needed:
• Any textbook identifying physical and emotional signs of stress

The next time you feel yourself getting stressed, identify how you are feeling and what you are thinking. List the physical and emotional symptoms you experience.

Stress Control Skills for the Practical/Vocational Charge Nurse

Controlling Stress by Altering How You Think. Stress is the body's reaction to the mind's analysis of a situation. It is not the situation, but your reaction to the situation, that creates stress. You have the only stress management tool you will ever need right inside your head. If you learn to manage how you think about the many interactions you have daily with nursing assistants, residents, and family members, you can control your reaction and therefore your stress level. See Chapter 6 for additional stress-reduction techniques.

Thinking Before "Irrational Thinking" Class

Nursing assistant (on telephone): "I cannot come in today. I have a headache."

Practical/vocational charge nurse (*thinking*): "*I'll just bet she has a headache. She probably spent half the night partying.*"

The LPN/LVN becomes abrupt with the nursing assistant and hangs up. She feels angry and allows the incident to ruin her entire day. Nursing assistants can sense that the charge nurse is upset and will try to avoid any contact with her.

Ellis (1994) discusses rational versus **irrational thinking**. When we are in a situation, we engage in self-talk about what is happening. This self-talk is often irrational because it is based on judgments we make about the situation. Judgments are subjective and have no bearing on facts. The irrational thinking then causes negative emotions, and stress often results. Ellis offers the ABCD way of increasing awareness of irrational thinking and changing how we think to a more rational way. In learning to do so, we control our emotions and thus the stress that results. The following are examples of how Ellis's ABCD method of controlling irrational thinking applies to the practical/vocational charge nurse.

A—Activating event: The nursing assistant called in sick with a headache.

B—Belief (self-talk) about the situation: The charge nurse thinks the nursing assistant must have been out partying.

C—Consequences: The LPN/LVN manager was abrupt with the nursing assistant on the telephone. She allowed herself to feel angry about the absence. She allowed it to ruin her whole day. Nursing assistants avoided her like the plague.

D—Dispute irrational thoughts: Choose a more rational, assertive response to the situation. Focus on the objective facts (nursing assistant has a headache). Avoid the subjective judgments that your beliefs (self-talk) call up (the nursing assistant was partying). You will avoid the anger over this incident and its effect on nursing assistants. Stress is avoided for all.

Thinking After "Irrational Thinking" Class

Nursing Assistant (on telephone): "I cannot come in today. I have a headache."

Practical/vocational charge nurse (tempted to use irrational thinking but remembers Ellis's ABCD instead): "I'm sorry to hear that. I hope you feel better after you get some rest."

See the Coordinated Care, Leadership Hint: Avoiding Irrational Thinking box.

 Coordinated Care

Leadership Hint

Avoiding Irrational Thinking

1. Be aware that beliefs about the situation are self-talk. Self-talk sometimes makes judgments. These judgments, if negative, can cause an emotional reaction. The emotional reaction leads to stress.
2. See situations objectively. Rational thinking is based on facts. Objective facts do not cause emotion. The situation "just is."
3. Avoid thinking that nursing assistants *should*, *must*, or *always* do something. This is another example of irrational thinking and can lead to anger. When you use these words for yourself, they can lead to anxiety and guilt.

4. We do not have the power to make nursing assistants do anything. We can encourage or prefer that nursing assistants do something.
5. For yourself and team members, use the words *want*, *choose*, and *prefer* in your thinking.

SPECIFIC KNOWLEDGE AND SKILLS NEEDED FOR LEADERSHIP

To be a leader in long-term care, it is necessary to use the aforementioned core areas of knowledge as a base and to develop the following skills in three specific areas:

1. *Occupational (clinical) skills:* The knowledge and skills of nursing.
2. *Organizational skills:* Skills necessary to function in the organization that delivers health care.
3. *Human relationship skills:* The ability to get along with and relate to people.

OCCUPATIONAL SKILLS FOR FIRST-LINE LPN/LVN LEADERS

Nursing (Clinical) Skills, Including the Nursing Process

Solid clinical skills are a must to be a good nursing leader. Visible expertise in clinical skills is a plus with the nursing assistants and also gives you an informal power base. See the resident situation for yourself, assist in providing care, and demonstrate nursing skills to nursing assistants as needed. This conveys the attitude that resident care comes first. This action demonstrates that the facility mission statement and unit goals are not just a written exercise. It communicates that practical/vocational charge nurses are there to support their staff.

Knowledge of your role in the nursing process is an important part of organizational skills. Your practical/vocational nursing program has started your skill development in this area. You will need to keep this area current and fresh. Refer to Chapter 9 for more about your role in the nursing process.

Documentation

Use the guidelines in nursing fundamentals for your charting. Practical/vocational charge nurses need to be aware of the documentation requirements of federal and state laws and accrediting agencies. Specific, objective documentation demonstrates whether or not the standard of care has been met. Effective nursing documentation is the basis for payment of resident fees or denial of payment by Medicare, insurance, and/or the state. This is especially important when these agencies mandate patient outcomes. Incomplete or questionable documentation could also result in a citation for the facility. It cannot be emphasized often enough that you must make sure all your charting is specific, objective, and complete. Avoid subjective comments and personal judgments in your charting. Students sometimes find this area of charting difficult, especially if they see examples of general and subjective entries on charts by licensed staff in the clinical area.

Legal Aspects

The nursing assistants and you, the practical/vocational charge nurse, are the people who have direct contact with residents and their families on a daily basis. You have the ability to ensure resident and family satisfaction with care. You are also a vehicle to voice concerns. This in turn will decrease the need for legal action to resolve disputes. Chapter 12 provides you with information for being legally sound in your nursing career.

Be aware of your state's Nurse Practice Act, health care facility policies and procedures, state and federal regulations, and published standards of your nursing organizations and codes of conduct (see NAPNES and NFLPN in Appendixes A and B). The standards and codes are guidelines to evaluate safe practice. Keep current and informed.

Federal Regulations. Your facility must be in compliance with federal, state, and local laws. The impact of federal regulations in your facility is most strongly felt in the Omnibus Budget Reconciliation Act of 1987 (OBRA) and the Centers for Medicare and Medicaid Services (CMS).

The Omnibus Budget Reconciliation Act of 1987. OBRA contains the Nursing Home Reform Act. The basic objective of the Nursing Home Reform Act is to ensure that residents of nursing homes receive quality care that will result in their achieving or maintaining their "highest practicable" (reasonable) physical, mental, and psychosocial well-being. The act also established a Resident's Bill of Rights. A copy of one state's Resident's Bill of Rights can be found at www.forltc.org/nhrbillrights.html. OBRA regulations will be reviewed with you at the time of your orientation. See the Coordinated Care, Leadership Hint: OBRA Provisions That Deal Specifically with Nursing Assistants box.

Coordinated Care
Leadership Hint

OBRA Provisions That Deal Specifically with Nursing Assistants

1. Nursing assistants require 75 hours of instruction before taking a state-approved written and skills competency evaluation. This establishes a baseline proficiency and competence of nursing assistants.
2. Each state must have a nursing assistant registry. This registry is an official list of individuals who have successfully completed nursing assistant training and competency evaluation. To be listed in a state directory, the history of the nursing assistant must be free of incidents of abuse, neglect, or dishonest use of property.
3. Your state's registry must be notified by the employer before employment of nursing assistants. The registry of some states is available online.
4. Nursing assistants' work must be evaluated "regularly."
5. Nursing assistants must have 12 hours of in-service training per year.
6. If two consecutive years have passed without a person being employed as a nursing assistant, training and competency evaluation must be repeated.

Centers for Medicare and Medicaid Services. This agency was formerly called the Health Care Financing Administration (HCFA). The Centers for Medicare and Medicaid Services (CMS), a federal agency of the Department of Health and Human Services (HHS), certifies nursing homes for Medicare and Medicaid reimbursement. To receive payment, facilities are required to meet conditions of participation. The long-term care unit will have the conditions of participation in its policies. Current CMS regulations will be presented during your orientation.

Your State's Regulations. Long-term care units and nursing homes are licensed by the state in which they are located. Each state sets regulations that must be met to be licensed. Periodically, inspectors will visit the facility to determine whether the facility has any deficiencies. Being cited for deficiencies can affect licensing. Your state's regulations will be reviewed at orientation.

The Joint Commission (TJC) is an independent, not-for-profit organization. The purpose of this organization is to improve quality of care by creating a safe environment for patients through the accreditation process. The Joint Commission reviews organizations such as hospitals, long-term care facilities, and home health agencies. Accreditation is a voluntary activity. If your facility participates in The Joint Commission accreditation, its requirements will be explained to you at your orientation. Detailed information about The Joint Commission and long-term care can be obtained at www.jointcommission.org.

ORGANIZATIONAL SKILLS FOR FIRST-LINE LPN/LVN LEADERS

Organizational skills are an essential ingredient for leaders as well as team members. The emphasis on the personal and vocational issues/concepts course in your student practical/vocational nursing program has given you the opportunity to learn and apply the principles of time management (see Chapter 2). Continuous quality improvement (see Chapter 19) and conflict management (see Chapter 13) are also necessary skills for the development of any nursing leader in today's health care organizations, including long-term care.

Time Management

Whether your dominance is on the left or right side of the brain, you have been given the opportunity this year to develop time management skills by applying the content of Chapter 2. Your school year has certainly provided the need to use your time effectively (doing the right thing) and efficiently (doing it right the first time, and in the appropriate amount of time) for class, clinical, and home. The step-by-step procedures learned in the nursing skills lab helped you prioritize your care for efficiency and the safety and comfort of the patient. You have experience organizing work for one or two patients in the clinical area. As a practical/vocational charge nurse, you will direct the care of approximately 30 residents and supervise a team of possibly 3 to 4 nursing assistants.

Time management is more about management and less about time. Your ability to manage time will help you organize tasks and allow you to be successful as a charge nurse. Once again, the nursing process will be the tool to help you get organized. See the Coordinated Care, Leadership Hint: Applying the Nursing Process to Organize Your Shift box.

Coordinated Care
Leadership Hint

Applying the Nursing Process to Organize Your Shift

ASSESSMENT (DATA COLLECTION) OF TASKS

1. Make a "to-do" list that reflects unit routines and schedules. When new to the job, listing unit routines and schedules is helpful until you experience the actual routine. This list includes break times, staff meal times, resident meals and nourishments, scheduled physician rounds, and routine times for vital signs, capillary blood testing, medicine administration, treatments, and so on.
2. Develop a worksheet to use during report. Use a style you are comfortable with. Some charge nurses develop a list according to a sequence of room numbers. Others list residents that need special assessments. Others list treatments, vital signs, and so on by time.
3. Prioritize the list. Use Maslow's Hierarchy of Needs to set priorities for residents. Remember, physiologic needs must be met before other needs are considered. "A's" are most important needs and must be done. They could be life-threatening or urgent resident needs. "B's" must be done, but there is more leeway in the exact time they are accomplished. Some "C's" are necessary but not of urgent status. Some of the "B's" and "C's" can be assigned to unlicensed assistive personnel (UAPs) or postponed. Some "C's" might not need to be listed at all.

Here are some examples:

Tasks	Examples	Comments
"A" tasks	STAT med, PRN med, q2h neuro check after resident's fall on prior shift	New "A" tasks always surface during the shift, requiring modification of the "to-do" list. These needs are unpredictable and cannot be planned in advance.
"B" tasks	Routine medicine administration, dressing changes, routine resident personal care, ambulation, activities, routine treatments, nourishments, meals	These needs are recurring and predictable.
"C" tasks	Mail and flower delivery, chitchat with family	Important but can be delayed.

PLANNING USE OF TIME (GOAL SETTING)

1. Plan tasks within a time frame of 2 to 3 hours. Arrange blocks of time according to unit routine. Planning allows you to have the feeling you are in control of the situation. Take resident preferences into consideration when you are planning. For example, one resident prefers to eat breakfast at 6 AM, but breakfast is served at 8 AM. Arrangements could be made for coffee and crackers at 6 AM, if diet allows.
2. Use the same guidelines for setting goals for planning time as with care plans or personal goals. Focus on goals as outcomes (the results expected after a given period). Using action verbs, make sure goals are realistic and measurable. A measurable goal states specifically and objectively what results are expected after a specified period. Set minigoals for timed tasks to keep you on task.
3. Planning involves having the equipment and supplies that the team needs for the shift and the shift that follows. As you collect data about residents when first starting your shift, check rooms and treatment closets for needed supplies. This includes linen, a well-stocked floor refrigerator, supplies for treatments, supplies for medicine administration kept on a med cart, and so on.
4. Make sure you have your personal tools for the shift: your watch (working), a pen that writes, bandage scissors, a stethoscope, and a small notebook. Use the notebook to quickly jot down the equipment that is needed and the results of data collection.

IMPLEMENTING YOUR PLAN

1. Remember, your plan is written in soft, non–trans fat margarine, not marble. Be flexible.
2. As you carry out your plan for the shift, expect interruptions of your planned activities. You know they will occur but not when. These include telephone calls, changes in residents' conditions, transfer of a resident, and staff injury.
3. When unexpected events occur, planning assists you to rearrange tasks. If you have a plan, you can return to the plan after interruptions. You can continue or revise the plan as needed.

EVALUATING YOUR USE OF TIME

1. As nursing assistants give you reports for their assigned residents, seek input from them about the effectiveness and efficiency of the shift.
2. Ask for suggestions to improve staff and your use of time at the next shift you work.
3. Keep a log of your shift activities. Look for a pattern of inefficient use of time. Examples of time wasters are putting things off, allowing unnecessary interruptions, socializing with staff, inability to say "no," and allowing telephone calls to exceed needed time for business.
4. At the end of your shift, take a few minutes to plan for the next day. This will allow you to leave work-related activities at work, and it will allow you to enjoy your much-needed leisure time.

Continuous Quality Improvement

Continuous quality improvement (CQI) is a program found in all health care facilities. The principles of CQI found in health care are borrowed from those of the business world. The focus of CQI is quality of care. Quality is indicated by patient outcomes. Patient outcomes are observable, measurable results of nursing activities. The CQI program involves all departments of health care facilities, including long-term care. You will receive information about the CQI program during orientation at your facility. See the Coordinated Care, Leadership Hint: CQI Components That the Practical/Vocational Charge Nurse Needs to Incorporate into the Leadership Role box.

The Centers for Medicare and Medicaid Services (CMS) is involved with quality improvement in nursing homes and long-term care facilities. The Quality Improvement Organization (QIO) program consists of a national network of 53 QIOs that are under the direction of CMS. The requirements of QIO include the following:

- Improve quality of care for beneficiaries.
- Ensure that Medicare pays only for services that are reasonable and medically necessary and that are provided in the most appropriate setting.
- Protect beneficiaries by expeditiously addressing individual complaints, notices, and appeals, such as noncoverage (HHS, 2006).

Coordinated Care
Leadership Hint

CQI Components That the Practical/Vocational Charge Nurse Needs to Incorporate into the Leadership Role

1. Review job descriptions with your nursing assistants. Emphasize the role they have in achieving quality and safety in care and resident service for a reasonable price (do it right the first time).
2. Remember that CQI is a continuous, daily part of your unit.
3. Encourage nursing assistants to report safety issues in resident care and the work environment.
4. Encourage nursing assistants to offer suggestions to solve safety issues in number 3 of this list.

5. When safety issues are noted, initiate a plan for improvement.
6. Consider volunteering for a CQI committee. Policies and nursing procedures are revised based on the input you and your nursing assistants provide regarding resident care and the functioning of the unit. It is personally rewarding to be included in policy and procedure revision because revisions improve resident care.
7. Document resident information in an objective and specific manner. Your documentation will be used to measure the effectiveness of CQI efforts.

Conflict Resolution

Conflict can occur whenever two or more persons interact. In long-term care, conflicts can arise with nursing assistants, staff, residents, families, and physicians. Conflict is not always a bad thing; sometimes it is an opportunity for growth and learning. Other times the presence of conflict can point out the need for change in an organization. When conflicts are out in the open, the opportunity exists to settle issues. This is preferable to leaving conflicts unsettled. Unsettled conflicts can act like cancer, slowly growing into something much larger that may be more difficult or impossible to resolve. Tools to reduce conflicts include clear communication and the ability to work well as a team. Conflict resolution involves people settling their differences. Resolution of the conflict is an exercise in problem solving. See the Coordinated Care, Leadership Hint: Applying the Nursing Process for Conflict Resolution box.

Coordinated Care
Leadership Hint

Applying the Nursing Process for Conflict Resolution

DATA COLLECTION: OBTAIN ALL THE FACTS

1. When a conflict arises, avoid pursuing it on the spot. Arrange for the involved parties to meet in an area that will provide privacy.
2. Separate the person from the problem. Attack the problem, not one another.
3. Each party has its own perception and strong emotions about what happened. Unclear communication may result. Clarify subjective statements and generalizations. You need to obtain objective and specific facts. For example, clarify what is meant by "she always does that" and "they."
4. Actively listen to the person presenting "the facts."
5. Avoid formulating your response while the other party is giving "the facts."

STATE THE PROBLEM: IDENTIFY THE SPECIFIC ISSUE

1. After hearing all sides, state in your own words what you understand to be the conflict. Use "I" messages when presenting your perspective. For example, say, "Emma, I heard you say that Hannah always leaves the utility room in disarray and does not offer to help the other nursing assistants when she has completed her work and they are swamped."

2. Ask parties for feedback as to the accuracy of your understanding of the conflict: "Emma, am I clear about the nature of your complaint? Is there anything you would like to add or correct?" and "Hannah, is there anything you would like to add or correct about the situation?"

INTERVENTIONS (PLANNING)

1. Convey the attitude of working side by side to settle the conflict. For example, sit side by side to work on the problem.
2. Involve all parties in identifying and discussing possible solutions to the conflict. The more alternatives, the better. The goal is a solution that will be agreeable to everyone's interests.
3. *Avoid* bargaining over *positions* (*what you want*). Egos are identified with positions. The parties involved will focus on defending their positions. In the end, all parties need to save face.
4. *Focus* on *interests* (*why something is wanted*). Behind a *position* is a *motivating interest*. Behind opposite *positions* lie shared and compatible *interests*. *Compromise* involves giving up aspects of an issue that are important to one of the parties involved. This is not a good intervention. *Collaborate* for a win-win solution that focuses on shared or compatible interests.

IMPLEMENTATION: IMPLEMENT THE SELECTED SOLUTION

On a sunny, cool day in the fall, two residents are sitting in the sunroom of a long-term care facility. Resident A's *position* is that he wants a window open, and Resident B's *position* is that he wants the windows shut. The practical/vocational charge nurse asks Resident A why he wants a window open. He replies, "So I can get some fresh air." The charge nurse asks Resident B why he wants the windows closed. He replies, "So it won't be drafty."

A solution built on *collaboration* would involve the charge nurse wrapping Resident B in a blanket and moving his wheelchair to the north end of the sunroom. She would move Resident A to the south end of the sunroom and open a window near him. This is a "win-win" solution. A solution built on *compromise* would involve the practical/vocational charge nurse returning one of the residents to his room and accommodating the other in the sunroom. This is an "I win-/you lose" solution.

EVALUATION: EVALUATE THE EFFECTIVENESS OF INTERVENTIONS IN MEETING THE GOAL

In the preceding situation, the practical/vocational charge nurse returns 30 minutes later and finds both residents peacefully asleep in their wheelchairs.

HUMAN RELATIONSHIP SKILLS FOR FIRST-LINE LPN/LVN LEADERS

Practical/vocational charge nurses can have excellent clinical skills, use the nursing process expertly, and document to the letter of the law. The practical/vocational charge nurse can have a good understanding of federal and state laws and requirements of accrediting agencies. Charge nurses can get the job done efficiently, but perhaps human relationship skills are the most important skills for an LPN/LVN leader to have. Gina Ivanapleze and Priscilla Pittbul *might* get the job done. Leaders with human relationship skills will get the job done with style and tact, without sacrificing quality. Nursing assistants will value their leader's

style a whole lot more and be more effective in reaching the goals of the unit. Because success depends on what is accomplished through others, the ability to relate well to others is crucial.

 Professional Pointer

Human relationship skills are important skills for an LPN/LVN to have in any clinical setting.

Practical/vocational nurses are well versed in clinical skills. They risk bringing *clinical* problem-solving skills to the practical/vocational charge nurse role when leadership/management skills, in the area of human relationship skills, are needed in this position.

Anger Management

Besides providing money on which to live, work provides people with the opportunity to be recognized for what they do, to belong to a group, and to display their competence. (Review the Howlett Hierarchy of work motivators.) When any of these needs is threatened in the course of the workday, or when you feel like a victim in a workplace with lack of control, you may get angry. Anger is not automatically bad; it gives you a cue that something is wrong. If your anger is justified, it can help you get your needs met by stimulating you to action. Harassment and discrimination are examples of situations in which anger is justified. If your anger is unjustified, or displayed inappropriately, it can get you and others in trouble. See the Coordinated Care, Leadership Hint: Preventing Anger in Nursing Assistants box, the Coordinated Care, Leadership Hint: Personal Anger Management Techniques for the Practical/Vocational Charge Nurse box, and the Coordinated Care, Leadership Hint: Prevention of Workplace Violence box.

 Coordinated Care
Leadership Hint

Preventing Anger in Nursing Assistants

1. Meet the needs above level 2 (e.g., belonging, affiliation, and recognition) on the Maslow and Howlett hierarchies.
2. Use assertive communication, especially "I" messages. This will prevent the practical/vocational charge nurse from being perceived as a threat. In your "I" messages, remember to include what you observed, the possible result of that observation, and your recommendations.
3. Actively listen, using direct eye contact and alert body posture, to convey to nursing assistants that you are interested in understanding their point of view.
4. Successful team building helps nursing assistants feel like part of the group.
5. Seek input of nursing assistants to find solutions for unit problems. This provides a sense of control over one's work environment.

6. Use win/win strategies in conflict resolution to provide a feeling of having control over situations and being treated with respect.
7. Encourage nursing assistants to participate in objective evaluation of their clinical performance to maintain self-esteem, and give nursing assistants some control over what happens to them.
8. Encouraging self-evaluation also helps tone down an important but potentially volatile area, especially when areas for improvement are noted.
9. Attempt to help nursing assistants become self-confident, reach their full potential, and achieve the higher levels of the Maslow and Howlett hierarchies. When needs are met at these higher levels, nursing assistants are more satisfied in their work environment.

Coordinated Care
Leadership Hint

Personal Anger Management Techniques for the Practical/Vocational Charge Nurse

1. Learn your personal signs that communicate you are becoming angry. Pay attention to what you are thinking and feeling.
2. How you appraise events causes the anger response. Change irrational thoughts to rational thoughts.
3. If your heart is pounding, take deep breaths.
4. If you feel tension in a body area, rub the area for a few seconds.
5. When angry, speak slowly and in a lower tone of voice, acknowledge how you feel, and take a time-out.
6. View a stimulus to anger as a problem. Use the problem-solving process to arrive at a solution.

Coordinated Care
Leadership Hint

Prevention of Workplace Violence

1. Suggest in-service education in anger management for all employees.
2. Create a work environment that is respectful and fun.
3. As a practical/vocational charge nurse, be a positive role model for anger management.
4. Take conflicts in the work environment seriously.
5. Refer to/use your facility's employee assistance program (EAP).
6. If your facility does not have an EAP program, suggest that such a program be developed.

Performance Evaluation of Nursing Assistants

The thought of performance evaluation can send shivers up the spine of the person doing the evaluating, as well as of the person being evaluated. Perhaps this goes back to bad evaluation experiences in prior situations. Perhaps it even goes as far back as grade school. Perhaps you and the nursing assistants have learned to associate evaluation with constructive criticism and weaknesses. Keep sight of the main purpose of evaluation, which is to encourage personal and career growth. Constructive evaluation gives you and your team members a profile of strong behaviors and behaviors for improvement, along with a plan to improve. Evaluation encourages the development of employees who will meet the facility's objectives and fulfill the mission statement. See the Coordinated Care, Leadership Hint: Providing Feedback to Nursing Assistants box.

Coordinated Care
Leadership Hint

Providing Feedback to Nursing Assistants

POSITIVE FEEDBACK IDENTIFIES STRONG BEHAVIORS TO BE ENCOURAGED
1. Most nursing assistants know what it is like to be caught doing something "wrong." Catch them doing something "right." This encourages them to repeat the behavior.
2. Let nursing assistants know you notice their efforts, believe in them, and feel good about their contributions to the long-term care facility.
3. Praise people in measurable terms (specific and objective) so that the behavior can be repeated. For example, say, "When you disinfected the shower, I noticed that you paid special attention to the corners and the shower chair. Great job!"

NEGATIVE FEEDBACK IDENTIFIES BEHAVIORS THAT NEED IMPROVEMENT
1. Provide verbal feedback as close to the event as possible. The purpose of negative feedback is to point out behaviors that need to be modified. Focus on the behavior as one needing improvement. Avoid addressing the behavior as a criticism.
2. Without emotion, objectively point out what is wrong with the behavior and its consequences. You want the nursing assistant to remember the message, not the manner in which it was delivered. You also want the team member to know it is performance that is being evaluated.
3. Negative feedback needs to be accompanied by suggestions to correct the behavior. These suggestions need to be so specific that the nursing assistant will be able to correct the behavior by following them. For example, you might say, "I noticed that the ties of your isolation gown were untied while you were in the room with the patient who has TB. Once you remove the gown, you risk spreading the bacteria to other patients, staff, and your family because the back of your uniform was not protected. When getting into an isolation gown, be sure to cover the back of your uniform and tie the gown at the waist."
4. Mention behaviors that need improvement first. Offer praise at the end of a reprimand. The message will be heard more clearly. The impact of the praising will not be ruined.

As a practical/vocational charge nurse, your responsibilities in evaluating nursing assistants include the following:
1. Observing skill performance and attitudes of nursing assistants
2. Providing daily oral/written feedback, including suggestions for improvement

3. Documenting observations
4. Presenting a final evaluation form

Review the evaluation process and form for your facility. What you are evaluating is not subject to your personal judgment. You will be objectively evaluating the skills and attitudes of nursing assistants. These work-related activities are expected of nursing assistants and are found in their job description and the facility's policy manual. If a checklist format is used for daily observations, be sure you understand the scale used by the long-term care facility. In observing nursing skills, you will be evaluating the application of nursing assistant knowledge of a skill to actual skill performance. Attitudes are more difficult to evaluate. They are stated as observable behaviors and usually involve areas such as dress and grooming, attendance, functioning as a team member, and interpersonal skills.

The performance evaluation is written documentation of what you have been discussing and documenting throughout the period before the formal process of evaluation. Documentation is a time-consuming task. When you are used to the system for the long-term care facility, you will find it can be completed more quickly.

OBRA mandates regular evaluations for nursing assistants. In addition to scheduled performance evaluations, you will be giving spontaneous feedback to nursing assistants. Evaluation is the responsibility of the practical/vocational charge nurse and the nursing assistant. No one needs to "give" another person an evaluation. Evaluation needs to be a joint process. Evaluation is not a secret that you surprise team members with at the end of the evaluation period. It is a tool for personal and career growth. A team member has the right to be able to correct areas for improvement as time goes by. It is unfair to have your discrepancies unloaded (i.e., dumped) on you during the final evaluation interview. See the Coordinated Care, Leadership Hint: Encouraging Nursing Assistants to Participate in the Evaluation Process box and the Coordinated Care, Leadership Hint: Meeting for the Final Evaluation Interview box.

Coordinated Care
Leadership Hint

Encouraging Nursing Assistants to Participate in the Evaluation Process

1. Provide nursing assistants with their own copy of the evaluation form at the beginning of the evaluation experience. Tell them it contains the elements you will be evaluating. Encourage them to read it.
2. Encourage nursing assistants to evaluate themselves daily and record their evaluation on their copy of the form. This also gives them the opportunity to become familiar with the form.
3. Remind them to include their strong areas. People are good at identifying areas for improvement but sometimes need

reminders to acknowledge their strong points. Dispel the myth that doing so is egotistical or boastful. It is merely stating what is.
4. Encourage nursing assistants to include a plan on the evaluation form for improving areas that need improvement.

Coordinated Care
Leadership Hint

Meeting for the Final Evaluation Interview

1. Remember that the goal of evaluation is to encourage personal and professional growth. In preparation for the evaluation, summarize strong behaviors of the nursing assistant and behaviors that need improvement on your copy of the evaluation form. Develop a suggested plan for improvement. Attach this summary to the front of the evaluation. Remind nursing assistants to do the same and to bring their copy of the completed evaluation form to the meeting.
2. Schedule the interview for a private location.
3. Allow 10 to 20 minutes for the interview.
4. Conduct the interview in a neutral manner. Check your verbal and nonverbal messages.
5. Use "I" messages when discussing the summary sheet. For example, say, "The following are the behaviors that I observed when you were working with residents and staff...."
6. Start with strong behaviors and compare them with the nursing assistant's list. This creates a good mood.
7. Compare behaviors for improvement.
   a. Similar behaviors appearing on both evaluation forms can indicate insight into the problem. Both the nursing assistant and the practical/vocational charge nurse have noted similar behaviors in the clinical area.
   b. When the nursing assistant includes behaviors not noted by the practical/vocational charge nurse, this can indicate the value of self-evaluation. The charge nurse cannot observe everything.
   c. If the practical/vocational charge nurse includes behaviors not included by the nursing assistant, this can indicate lack of self-evaluation by the nursing assistant.
8. Finish the evaluation interview with the plan for improvement for any behaviors that need to be modified. The nursing assistant's plan is especially valuable because it indicates personal thinking through of interventions needed for improvement.
9. Check feedback throughout the interview to ensure clear communication. Have the nursing assistant rephrase feedback to see whether your intended message was heard. Some people may distort the message. Clarify messages given by the nursing assistant for information not understood. Encourage questions about any areas on the evaluation that are not understood. For example, say, "What did you understand me to say regarding your areas of strength that I have identified?"
10. Have the nursing assistant sign and date both evaluations. You do the same. The signature indicates that the forms were discussed and all questions were answered.

Your nonthreatening, objective approach to constructive evaluation will result in positive evaluation experiences for you and the nursing assistants on your team. Occasionally you may experience a situation in which a nursing assistant feels threatened and becomes defensive during evaluation. If the defensiveness begins to escalate or the person displays anger, terminate the meeting. Set a new time for another meeting. Have your supervisor present at this time. Such experiences are the exception, not the rule.

Empowering Team Members and Encouraging Personal Growth and Development of Confidence

It is rewarding to see the nursing assistants on your team increase their self-confidence and display career and personal growth. You can encourage personal growth in nursing assistants by demonstrating the leadership skills you have developed in your position as practical/vocational charge nurse. The nursing assistant must do the actual work to achieve confidence and grow. See the Coordinated Care, Leadership Hint: Strategies to Increase Self-Confidence in Nursing Assistants box and the Coordinated Care, Leadership Hint: Strategies to Encourage Personal Growth in Nursing Assistants box.

Coordinated Care
Leadership Hint

Strategies to Increase Self-Confidence in Nursing Assistants

1. Provide opportunities to be successful in new situations.
2. Praise beginning successes in new situations.
3. On clinical evaluation forms, include positive statements as well as negative statements.
4. With administration's support, plan educational opportunities for nursing assistants (e.g., seminars and in-service programs).
5. Include nursing assistants in planning meetings, in-service ideas, and so on.
6. Stand up for and support nursing assistants.
7. Actively listen to problems involving the clinical area.
8. Coach/mentor nursing assistants on a new skill and/or how to improve an old one.
9. Provide challenging assignments.

Coordinated Care
Leadership Hint

Strategies to Encourage Personal Growth in Nursing Assistants

1. Display a balanced interest in the personal problems of nursing assistants.

2. Encourage nursing assistants to solve their own problems.
3. Suggest referral when nursing assistants are unable to solve personal problems. Follow facility policies.
4. Think of nursing assistants as individuals. Clip and give pertinent cartoons, articles, and so on.
5. Be a mentor/coach.
6. Be a role model. Display a positive work ethic; demonstrate good clinical skills; get out from behind the desk and see what is going on with residents; display good grooming; give objective, specific feedback; address the problem, not people; and actively listen.

ADDITIONAL RESOURCES FOR THE LPN/LVN TO DEVELOP ORGANIZATIONAL, OCCUPATIONAL, AND HUMAN RELATIONSHIP SKILLS

There are many ways to add occupational, organizational, and human relationship skills for survival in the workplace. Some of the following suggestions for additional learning for the practical/vocational charge nurse offer continuing education credits. See the Coordinated Care, Leadership Hint: Sources of Learning Skills for the Practical/Vocational Charge Nurse Position box.

Coordinated Care
Leadership Hint

Sources of Learning Skills for the Practical/Vocational Charge Nurse Position

1. Check with your local vocational/technical school for a practical/vocational nursing leadership course.
2. Ask your boss to consider in-service programs on leadership techniques, as well as updates on nursing skills. Suggest cosponsoring such in-services with the local technical college and making them available to a wide geographical area.
3. Form a network with other persons who fill first-line leadership positions. Be sure to go outside your institution, as well as the discipline of nursing. You will find that the leaders have similar problems regardless of the discipline.
4. Attend seminars relating to leadership topics as well as nursing topics.
5. Read books and articles that offer hints for leaders. Be sure your personal nursing library is up to date.
6. Enroll for certification courses to enhance your knowledge and skills. See Chapter 24 for tips on making your career grow.

Get Ready for the NCLEX-PN® Examination

Key Points

- When the state's Nurse Practice Act allows, practical/vocational nurses are used as first-line leaders as charge nurse in the nursing home/long-term care unit.
- The basic student practical/vocational nursing program offers students the opportunity to develop skills in nursing procedures, the nursing process, critical thinking, communication, time management, assertiveness, and stress control. These are skills needed for everyday practice, as well as leadership positions.
- Development of a leadership style is important in guiding nursing assistants to meet the goals of the long-term care facility.
- Established leadership styles range from the extreme of autocratic, with a pure emphasis on the task, to laissez-faire, which solely emphasizes concern with the employee.
- Situational leadership adapts a leadership style to the environment and situation at hand. It is the suggested way of leading in the twenty-first century.
- The five core skills of leadership involve the ability to (1) motivate team members, (2) communicate assertively, (3) problem solve effectively, (4) build a team of cooperative workers, and (5) manage stress effectively. These core skills lay the foundation for the development of other specific skills for leadership.
- Specific skill areas for nursing leadership include occupational skills, organizational skills, and human relationship skills.
- No one chapter or course can teach you how to become a leader. The development of leadership skills is a process and evolves over time.
- In addition to training given by the institution, first-line practical/vocational nursing leaders need to educate and update themselves continually in the five core and three specific skill areas noted.

Additional Learning Resources

evolve Go to your Evolve website (http://evolve.elsevier.com/Hill/Success) for the following FREE learning resources:
- Answers to Critical Thinking Review Scenario
- Additional learning activities
- Additional Review Questions for the NCLEX-PN® exam
- Helpful phrases for communicating in Spanish and more!

Review Questions for the NCLEX-PN® Examination

1. Select the highest level of work motivator from the following list.
   1. Recognition and praise
   2. Job safety and security
   3. Social activities at work
   4. Policies, salary, and benefits

2. An LPN/LVN is interviewing for a charge nurse position in a long-term care facility. The employer questions the nurse about knowledge of situational leadership. Which of the following responses describes this leadership style?

   1. After report, tell nursing assistants the exact care to be given that shift and not to deviate from the care plan.
   2. In all situations, put nursing assistants before the policies of the nursing home and strive to be friendly and personal.
   3. To decrease workplace stress, seek suggestions from nursing assistants during a code for how to handle the situation.
   4. Evaluate the circumstances in the work environment and vary your leadership style to meet the needs of the situation.

3. Select the charting entry that is considered to be an objective entry describing the resident's response to the nursing intervention "force fluids."

   1. Nursing assistant spent much time forcing fluids from 8 AM to 11 AM.
   2. Resident drank a lot of fruit juice and cola soft drinks from 3 PM to 9 PM.
   3. Resident drank a total of 310 cc of liquids from 3 PM to 11 PM.
   4. Resident loves 7-UP, Coca-Cola, and orange juice without pulp.

4. Laura, a nursing assistant, has been absent four times this month, each absence occurring on the weekend. Which of the following practical/vocational charge nurses is using problem solving to handle this situation?

   1. Focuses feedback on Laura's frequent absences for assigned shift.
   2. Downplays the importance of absences to make Laura feel better.
   3. Provides Laura with all the suggestions needed to correct the problem.
   4. Assumes being present for assigned shift is something Laura cannot do.

Alternate Format Item

1. A work-related conflict has surfaced between two nursing assistants on their shift at the long-term care facility, where a licensed practical/vocational nurse is charge nurse. Which of the following crisis intervention strategies does the charge nurse use to resolve the conflict? (Select all that apply.)

   1. Develop a collaborative solution to solve the conflict so the two parties are satisfied with the solution.
   2. To save time for resident care, limit the number of possible solutions offered to solve the conflict.
   3. Instead of focusing on what solution each assistant wants, focus on why they want that specific solution.
   4. Actively listen while each nursing assistant presents his or her side of the conflict and solutions.
   5. Arrange to meet with the nursing assistants away from the site of the conflict to discuss the situation.

2. Select the internal motivation factors in this list. *(Select all that apply.)*

   1. Cheyenne gets a "good job" from the charge nurse during report.
   2. Matt's paycheck includes a bonus this week for a job well done.
   3. Tera posts a sign on the bulletin board about Kim's perfect attendance.
   4. Nursing assistants receive notice that The Home now will extend sick days.
   5. The CNAs will now have weekly pizza parties paid for by the nursing home.

Critical Thinking Scenario

Jill, an LPN, is the new charge nurse on the evening shift at the local nursing home. The nursing assistants on the evening shift are complaining to the nursing assistants on the day shift about the way Jill gives them directions about their assignments. What suggestions would you provide?

LPN/LVN Charge Nurse Skills: Management, Including Assignment and Delegation

Objectives

On completing this chapter, you will be able to do the following:

1. Using your state's Nurse Practice Act, identify the following as they apply to the charge nurse position for practical/vocational nurses:
   a. Requirements before assuming the licensed practical/vocational nurse (LPN/LVN) charge nurse position
   b. Site of employment
   c. Scope of practice
2. Review charge nurse job descriptions.
3. Identify specific institutional policies, regulations, and routines that the practical/vocational nurse needs to clarify when assuming a charge nurse position.
4. Collect a list of data that are needed before reporting a change of condition of a resident to a physician.
5. Discuss strategies for handling the following common LPN/LVN charge nurse problems:
   a. When nursing assistants bring problems from home
   b. Encouraging nursing assistants to be accountable for learning skills
   c. Dealing with the demanding/complaining family
6. Describe elements that need to be focused on when receiving and giving a change-of-shift report as charge nurse in the long-term care facility.
7. Discuss the assignment of tasks versus the delegation of duties with regard to the following factors:

   a. Your state's laws regarding the role of the practical/vocational nurse and the delegation of duties in the charge nurse position
   b. Differences between assigning nursing tasks and delegating nursing duties
   c. Legal aspects of assigning nursing tasks and delegating nursing duties
   d. The following criteria that need to be considered when assigning nursing tasks and delegating nursing duties:
      1. Right task
      2. Right person
      3. Right circumstance
      4. Right direction/communication
      5. Right supervision (monitoring), feedback, and evaluation
8. Using nursing process as a guide, discuss the method for assigning and delegating the following:
   a. Collecting data
   b. Planning
   c. Implementing
   d. Evaluating
   e. Putting it all together
   f. Reporting at the end of your shift

Key Terms

accountability (ă-KŎWNT-ă-BĬL-ĭ-tē, p. 281)
assigning (assignment) (ă-sīn-ĭng, p. 280)
change-of-shift report (chānj, p. 284)
delegating (delegation) (DĔL-ĕ-GĀT-ĭng, p. 280)
duties (DOO-tēs, p. 280)

goals (outcomes) (gōlz, p. 283)
Nurse Practice Act (nŭrs PRĂK-tĭs ăkt, p. 273)
scope of practice (skōp, PRĂK-tĭs, p. 281)
tasks (tăsks, p. 280)

 Keep in Mind

"Effective leadership is putting first things first. Effective management is discipline, carrying it out."

-Stephen R. Covey

Tricia was always a "saver," as her several well-constructed scrapbooks and boxes of books and papers from nursing school testified. Tricia looked at the carefully clipped classified ad she had saved from 5 years ago, when she had applied for her current nursing position. Five years ago, her husband was transferred to the neighboring state of Oz. After 3 years' experience as an LVN in a nursing home, postgraduate courses in leadership at the local technical college, seminars, in-service programs, personal reading, and workshops, Tricia thought that she was qualified for a charge nurse position.

Tricia smiled as she pictured herself going in for the interview. That navy blue blazer sure paid off! And all her preparation for the interview served her well. What a sage

Mrs. Kelly had been in Personal/Vocational Issues (PVI) class to recommend that a job applicant obtain a copy of the facility's mission statement before the interview. Although she did not have LPN/LVN charge nurse experience, she was sure her knowledge of the facility's emphasis on and pride in providing quality care was a big plus in landing the job. And this was in addition to the enthusiasm and positive attitude she displayed to the interviewer about her willingness to learn and her confidence that she would be able to do the job. Also, following the textbook suggestion to obtain the state of Oz's Nurse Practice Act before employment gave her the opportunity to learn how an LPN/LVN could delegate in the state of Oz and helped her to think of some delegation-related questions to ask at the interview.

Five years had passed since she had gotten the job as LPN/LVN charge nurse. Tricia loved her job and smiled as she remembered many of the challenges she had faced early in her job as charge nurse. She began to page through that old seventh edition of her PVI textbook....

LPN/LVN

> Full-time position available for an experienced LPN/LVN to join our long-term care facility as a charge nurse on the evening shift. Must have excellent communication and customer service skills, needs to be team-oriented, and must have current state of Oz license. We offer a competitive salary and full benefits package. If you qualify, submit resume and cover letter to: cradant@email.abc or Quality Care Home, 982 Brick Lane, Wayback, OZ 00005. For more information, contact Claudette Radant, DON at 987-123-4516 (cell).

Before continuing with Tricia's story, review the Coordinated Care, Leadership Activity: Determining Your State's Requirements to Assume the Position of Practical/Vocational Charge Nurse box in Chapter 20.

Tricia looked at the job description the director of nurses gave her during her job interview. It all seems such a routine and comfortable part of her job, but Tricia remembers how overwhelming it was to read through the 12 areas of responsibility, along with the 15 duties of the charge nurse.

WHERE TO BEGIN? JOB DESCRIPTION FOR CHARGE NURSE

Read the Coordinated Care, Management Tool: Reviewing LPN/LVN Charge Nurse Job Descriptions box. The charge nurse job description might seem overwhelming at first, but it illustrates the reason state laws require that practical/vocational charge nurses have education, training, or experience beyond the basic practical/vocational nursing curriculum and documentation of such. It is difficult to prepare health care workers in 1 year or less to be able to function in this position immediately after graduation. After additional education, training, and experience, many LPNs/LVNs become charge nurses, also called first-line managers, in long-term care units and nursing homes. They are doing an excellent job in that role. According to the 2009 practice analysis by NCSBN to gather data for content areas for the NCLEX-PN®, 45.2% of LPNs/LVNs stated they regularly had one or more administrative roles; 65.8% of those respondents worked in long-term care; and 52.8% of those with administrative roles in long-term care indicated the charge nurse position as their administrative role (NCSBN Research Brief, 2010).

Quality Care LPN/LVN Charge Nurse—Job Description

QUALIFICATIONS

Licensed practical/vocational nurse with a current license to practice in the state of Oz under Chapter 747. The LPN/LVN should have a certificate of successful completion of an approved course in Medication Administration.

STANDARDS

The job of the LPN/LVN charge nurse is to ensure that residents receive nursing care, treatments, and medications that have been ordered by their physicians. The LPN/LVN charge nurse shall do the following:

- Help coordinate resident care services (e.g., physicians, dietitian, activity director, physical therapist, and social worker).
- Assist the Director of Nurses in the orientation of new employees.
- Evaluate work performance of nursing assistants.

RESPONSIBLE FOR

- Knowledge of residents' conditions at all times.
- Assigning actual nursing care tasks to nursing assistants.
- Providing nursing care according to physicians' orders and in agreement with recognized nursing techniques and procedures, established standards of care as described in Oz state statutes, and administrative policies of this long-term care facility.
- Recognizing symptoms: reporting residents' conditions, including changes, and assisting with remedial measures for adverse developments.
- Assisting physician in diagnostic and therapeutic measures.
- Administering medications and treatments as prescribed.
- Maintaining accurate and complete records of nursing data collection and interventions, including documentation on the electronic medical record (EMR) and Kardex.
- Efficiency of execution of workload, including neatness and orderliness.
- Delegating duties, as appropriate, to nursing assistants.
- Maintaining a safe and hazard-free environment.
- Ensuring the residents' right to privacy.
- Maintaining the dignity of residents.

DUTIES

- Observes and reports symptoms and conditions of residents.
- Administers medications as prescribed by physicians. Gathers data about therapeutic response and side effects of medications.
- Takes and records vital signs when appropriate.

Continued

Quality Care LPN/LVN Charge Nurse—Job Description—cont'd

- Maintains charts and Kardexes, including residents' conditions and medications and treatments received.
- Notifies physician when necessary. Records phone/fax orders.
- Contacts pharmacist for prescription drugs as needed.
- Assists in maintaining a physical, social, and psychological environment for residents that is conducive to their best interests and welfare.
- Receives report at beginning of shift from personnel on previous shift and assigns tasks to nursing assistants under the LPN/LVN charge nurse's supervision.
- Supervises, assists with, and evaluates delegated duties to nursing assistants.
- Evaluates the completion of nursing assistant assignments in a safe and timely manner.
- Provides report to oncoming shift.
- Evaluates nursing assistants in the performance of their job description and reports same to Director of Nursing.
- Attends supervisory staff meetings.
- Interprets state and federal guidelines to employees. Uses authority as LPN/LVN charge nurse to "follow code."
- Participates in orientation of all new employees assigned to LPN/LVN charge nurse.

 Coordinated Care

Management Tool

Reviewing LPN/LVN Charge Nurse Job Descriptions

Resources needed:
- LPN/LVN charge nurse job descriptions of long-term care facilities
  Review LPN/LVN charge nurse job descriptions of long-term care facilities at sites at which you affiliate during your student year.

HOW LONG WILL IT TAKE ME TO PREPARE TO BE A CHARGE NURSE?

You are probably thinking, "How long will it take for me to get to this point in my practical/vocational nursing career?" The answer is individual to the person asking it. The law of some states specifically dictates that the LPN/LVN charge nurse functions in a nursing home and under the direct supervision of a registered nurse. In these states the practical/vocational nurse could not function as a charge nurse in a medical clinic or an acute care facility. Also, the LPN/LVN could not function under general supervision until after passing the NCLEX-PN® examination. *Be sure to check your state's Nurse Practice Act.* Some practical/vocational nursing programs offer a postgraduate course that prepares graduates for an expanded role. The answer to the question "How long will it take for me to get to this point in my practical/vocational nursing career?"

depends on your state's Nurse Practice Act, additional education, your motivation to learn the manager role, your ability to be a risk taker, and how you use your nursing experience.

HOW THIS TEXT CAN HELP YOU TO PREPARE FOR A FUTURE CHARGE NURSE POSITION

This text is unable to provide you with a concise recipe of how to function in the role of charge nurse as an LPN/LVN. This chapter begins with a discussion of areas of responsibilities, problems, and concerns that affect the LPN/LVN charge nurse in a long-term care unit or nursing home. Through active learning and an interactive format, this chapter also presents 12 Management Tools. These tools involve you with the many areas that need to be considered, understood, and investigated when assuming an LPN/LVN charge nurse position. The chapter also includes 10 Management Hints that provide concise information about concepts being presented. Seven critical-thinking exercises present the opportunity to apply learning in the area of assignment and delegation.

Scenarios for three residents are interspersed throughout the nursing process guide for *assigning* and *delegating.* You will be expected to be self-directed, to problem solve, and to think critically as you apply the information in Chapter 20. These are the very attributes employers expect of you as an LPN/LVN charge nurse. References to specific resources that you will need to work through the Management Tools are provided. You are encouraged to use the information from the entire text, your other classes, and your Learning Resource Center to work through the self-directed Management Tools. Your instructor is a valuable resource. Remember, also, the usefulness of peer group discussion.

At times we will flash back to Tricia as she reminisces about her early days in the LPN/LVN charge nurse position. Her initial experiences and adjustment to the charge nurse role will show you the challenges and opportunities the LPN/LVN charge nurse role provides.

Tricia thought back to the orientation phase of her job. It seemed so overwhelming at the time. The thought of going through those thick manuals of policies, regulations, and routines was enough to give her a headache. However, they sure did contain valuable information. Mrs. Kelly gave the class the following sample checklist as a guide when reviewing these manuals.

A CHECKLIST OF POLICIES, REGULATIONS, AND ROUTINES FOR THE LPN/LVN CHARGE NURSE

Not all the areas included in this checklist are the responsibility of the LPN/LVN charge nurse in a nursing home/long-term care facility. However, LPN/LVN charge nurses need to have information for all the areas included so they can carry out their management duties. Because the LPN/LVN charge nurse has the responsibility to supervise nursing assistants, these personnel also need information about policies and routines. Orientation to your facility needs to include these items.

FACILITY ORGANIZATION/LEGAL ASPECTS

—Mission statement
—Organizational chart
—State statutes for all licensed persons on health care team
—Skills checklists for LPNs/LVNs and nursing assistants
—Skills checklists for all cross-trained personnel
—Job descriptions and duties of RNs and LPNs/LVNs
—Job descriptions and duties of unlicensed personnel and cross-trained personnel

FEDERAL, STATE, AND PRIVATE AGENCY REGULATIONS

—Inspection protocols
—Current federal (including HIPAA regulations) and state regulations
—Regulations of the Omnibus Budget Reconciliation Act of 1987 (OBRA)
—Regulations of the Centers for Medicare and Medicaid Services (CMS)
—Regulations of The Joint Commission (if facility seeks TJC accreditation)
—National Patient Safety Standards

PERSONNEL POLICIES

—Employee manual
—Time sheets—location and interpretation
—Vacation, holiday, sick leave policy
—Special request for time off, leave of absence
—Communication—reporting: on and off duty, sickness, absence, memos, bulletin board
—Meal and coffee break
—Smoking regulations
—Use of facility telephones, personal cell phones, and other electronic devices
—Uniform regulations

RECORDS AND UNIT ROUTINES

—General shift routine for days, evenings, and nights
—Duties of each of the three shifts
—Methods of reporting
—Procedure manual
—Facility policy manual
—Procedures specific to each division of the facility
—Nursing care plan system
—Nursing Kardex and Medix systems
—Routine for care planning conferences
—Routine for physicians' visits
—System of transcribing physicians' orders
—Location of reference books

UNIT ADMINISTRATION

—Admission, placement, transfer, and discharge of residents
—Care of clothing and valuables, including personal property list
—Routine for seriously ill residents
—Routine for death of a resident
—Autopsy permit
—Authorization procedure and forms for diagnostic tests and surgery
—Visiting hours
—Notary public

SAFETY POLICIES

—Side rails
—Restraints
—Fire regulations: reporting, evacuation plan, fire exits, location of fire extinguishers, preventive measures, fire drill procedure
—Use of oxygen
—Transportation of residents by cart, wheelchair
—Body mechanics and back safety policy
—Door alarms
—Standard precautions
—Security policies
—Smoking policy

HOUSEKEEPING, MAINTENANCE, AND SUPPLIES

—Linen: how supplied, extra linen
—Care of contaminated linens and dressings
—Unit cleaning procedure and responsibilities
—How to obtain supplies: drugs, sterile supplies, personal care items, kitchen items
—Maintenance and repairs requests
—Conservation of supplies, linen, and equipment

EQUIPMENT: HOW TO USE IT AND WHERE TO OBTAIN IT

—Oxygen
—Suction equipment
—Therapeutic beds
—Respiratory therapy equipment and services

FOOD SERVICE FOR RESIDENTS

—Ordering diets/diet changes
—Tray service
—Unit food stock items
—Special nourishments
—Policy for feeding residents
—Policy for dining room
—Policy for family trays

NURSING CARE PROCEDURES/ASSISTING PHYSICIAN

—Morning and evening cares
—Bathing/showering
—Mouth care
—Bed making
—Temperature (devices used), pulse, and respiration
—Blood pressure
—Catheterization
—Enemas
—Suppositories—rectal
—Recording intake and output
—Systems used for pressure ulcer care
—Collecting, delivering, and labeling specimens
—Assisting podiatrist with foot care
—Policies for sterile technique procedures
—Blood glucose monitoring
—Colostomy care
—Nasogastric and gastrostomy tubes: flushing, feeding, administration of medication
—Standard precautions
—Postmortem procedures

MEDICATIONS

—Medication system
—Policy for reordering
—Unit stock
—Ordering from pharmacy
—Review of metric system, proportions
—Drug errors: reporting, incident reports
—Narcotics count
—Sources of drug administration

DOCUMENTATION

—Method of documenting
—Computer system
—Forms used
—Flow sheets used
—Policy for phone/fax orders
—Incident reports
—Lists for wanderers, hearing aid use, and so on
—Federal and state chart forms and requirements

SPECIAL AREAS

—Emergency supplies
—Central supply area
—Physical therapy
—Occupational therapy
—Laundry
—Maintenance
—Break room
—Dining room
—Kitchen
—Business offices
—Social services
—Director of nurses
—Chaplain services/chapel area
—Staff educator
—Administrator of facility
—Conference rooms
—Activity department

MISCELLANEOUS

—Paging system
—Call light system
—Disaster plan
—Routine for residents who desire cardiopulmonary resuscitation
—Volunteer services
—On-call schedule
—Handling of wanderers
—Procedure for signing resident in and out of facility
—Hair care services
—Podiatrist and dentist list
—Staff break room

See the Coordinated Care, Management Tool: Reviewing Policies and Routines box.

 Coordinated Care

Management Tool

Reviewing Policies and Routines

Resources needed:
- Aforementioned checklist of policies, regulations, and routines for the LPN/LVN
- Your opinion and reasons (rationale)

All policies, regulations, and routines of a health care facility are important. After reading the checklist, complete the following:

1. List the five items from Records and Unit Routines that you think are most necessary for effective running of the resident wings of the long-term care unit. Provide the reason (rationale) for your choices.

Item	Rationale
a.	
b.	
c.	
d.	
e.	

2. List the five items from Unit Administration that you think are most necessary for effective running of the resident wings of the long-term care unit. Provide your reason (rationale) for your choices.

Item	Rationale
a.	
b.	
c.	
d.	
e.	

Tricia came across a data list. Mrs. Kelly had stressed the importance of the LPN/LVN's assisting role in collecting data. Mrs. Kelly always said that what the LPN/LVN did with that data really separated the licensed nurse from unlicensed personnel. Mrs. Kelly had provided a helpful list of signs and symptoms to be aware of in various patient situations. She stressed it would not be a complete list but would be something to get us started. It had been some time since Tricia updated that list.

COLLECTING DATA AS A CHARGE NURSE

As LPN/LVN charge nurse, the *change-of-shift report* when coming on duty provides data for dividing the work of the shift among team members. Baseline data of residents for whom you are in charge also must be obtained. This involves a quick visit of each resident to compare the status of residents to the status reported at change of shift. You will also collect data periodically during your shift. The frequency of data collecting depends on patient condition. Following is a list of signs and symptoms that may indicate illness, exacerbation of a previous disease condition, injury, or decline in prior functioning.

Be observant with each resident interaction. When nursing assistants report that "something does not seem right," visit the resident to collect your own data. After collecting the data, record it on the proper form and report all abnormal observations according to agency policy. The actual data-collecting parameters given here are guidelines. Follow specific parameters given for the resident.

SIGNS AND SYMPTOMS

1. **Weight:** Increase or decrease of 5 to 10 lb in 1 week.
2. **Temperature:** Elevation over 100 °F orally or 100.6 °F rectally; temperature under 96.6 °F orally.
3. **Upper respiratory:** Head congestion, headache, sore throat, ear pain, runny nose, postnasal drip.
4. **Lower respiratory:** Acute onset or worsening of shortness of breath, dyspnea with exertion, orthopnea, cough (productive or nonproductive), wheezing or other abnormal sounds on inhalation or exhalation.
5. **Cardiac:** Blood pressure over 135/85 (new symptom); blood pressure below 80/50; irregular pulse (new symptom); chest, neck, shoulder, or arm pain; fatigue; increased frequency of angina; shortness of breath; orthopnea; peripheral edema; sacral edema or distended neck veins.
6. **Breast:** Lump found on palpation, discharge from nipple.
7. **Abdomen:** Localized or generalized pain, especially of acute onset; epigastric burning or discomfort; constipation; diarrhea; nausea; vomiting; bloody or tarry stools; loss of appetite.
8. **Musculoskeletal:** Swollen and tender joints, loss of strength in limbs, pain, loss of motion, ecchymosis, edema.
9. **Reproductive system:** Vaginal discharge, abnormal vaginal bleeding.
10. **Genitourinary:** Urgency, frequency, dysuria, nocturia, hematuria, incontinence. Male: Dribbling, inability to start or stop stream.
11. **Sleep and rest patterns:** Changes from normal routine, requirement of medication for sleep, nightmares or dreams.
12. **Appearance of skin:** Changes in color, turgor, contusions, abrasions, lacerations, rashes, lesions.
13. **Mobility and exercise:** Need for support in ambulation, changes in posture, weakness of extremities, changes in coordination, vertigo.
14. **Hygiene status:**
    a. *Mouth:* Condition of mucous membranes, gums, teeth, tongue, mouth odor.
    b. *Body:* Cleanliness, odor, especially of body creases and genital area.
    c. *Hair:* Grooming, distribution, scalp scaling, lesions.
    d. *Nails:* Color, texture, and grooming of fingernails and toenails.
15. **Communication:** Verbal, nonverbal, and affective, aphasia, level of understanding.
16. **Sensory-perceptual:** Ability to hear, condition of hearing aid; ability to see, condition of glasses; ability to feel in all extremities; ability to discriminate odors; ability to distinguish tastes.
17. **Cultural/religious:** Food preferences, wellness/illness beliefs, religious practices (e.g., rosary, prayer beads, Bible, Koran, Torah, religious readings, medals, icons, communion, clergy visits, confession, sacrament of the sick).
18. **Psychological status:** Level of consciousness, disorientation, intelligence, attention span, vocabulary level, interests, memory, affect.

Tricia remembered how Mrs. Kelly stressed the importance of getting to a room and personally collecting patient data, especially when there was a change of condition. Tricia found the example Mrs. Kelly gave so that members of the class could avoid the same situation.

THE REPORT THAT WASN'T

A nursing assistant (NA) reported to the LPN/LVN charge nurse (CN) that Mr. Jones "doesn't look too good to me." The charge nurse immediately called the physician.

Doctor Grimm: What seems to be the trouble?
CN to NA: What seems to be the trouble?
NA to CN: I don't know. He just doesn't look right.
CN to doctor: He just doesn't look right.
Doctor: How long has he looked like this?
CN: I don't know. We just noticed.
Doctor: What's his temperature?
CN: Just a minute. I'll find out.

CN to NA: Take Mr. Jones's temperature.

Doctor: What are his other vital signs?

CN: I don't know. The nursing assistant is going to check them.

Doctor: How much fluid has he had?

CN: Just a minute. (She puts the telephone down and goes to check Mr. Jones's IV.)

CN: He's getting an IV now.

Doctor (with sarcasm in his voice): Is he breathing? Never mind, don't send anyone to check. I will be over to check him myself. (The doctor hangs up abruptly.)

CN to NA: I don't know why he gets so upset every time I call him. What am I supposed to do?

See the Coordinated Care, Management Tool: Reporting Change of Condition to the Physician box.

 Coordinated Care

Management Tool

Reporting Change of Condition to the Physician

Resources needed:
- A checklist of signs and symptoms (earlier in this chapter)
- SBAR information from Chapter 13
- A medical-surgical textbook

List the data you would collect and any other pertinent information you would gather before notifying the physician of a "change of condition" in the following residents:
- Resident has history of compensated, left-sided congestive heart failure.
- Resident has cancer of the esophagus and uses a Duragesic patch for pain control.

Tricia began to think of the "people problems" she continually experiences in her job as LVN charge nurse. With each day that passes, handling these problems becomes easier and easier. Mrs. Kelly's basic advice to "treat people as you would like to be treated" has saved the day on many occasions. That was good advice even for reporting change of condition to the doctor: "What information would I need if I was the physician and my patient had a change of condition?" As for dealing with doctors, residents, staff, and families, I sure remember situations that arose as clearly as if they happened yesterday.

 Professional Pointer

Treat others as you would like to be treated

COMMON PROBLEMS OF LPN/LVN CHARGE NURSE

Tricia recalled one morning during the second week of work after orientation to the charge nurse position. The nursing assistants were all tied up in knots. The babysitter for the three young children of Margarita, one of the nursing assistants, had quit the evening before, and when Margarita got up the next morning for work, her car would not start. All the nursing assistants were talking about Margarita's

problems from the time they hung up their coats, straight through lunch and beyond. It was only the week before that Margarita found out she was overdrawn at the bank because she wrote checks before her paycheck was deposited by Quality Care Home and cleared by the bank. It seemed as though "things always happened to Margarita, and she was such a nice person. It just was not right." All the nursing assistants were feeling bad because all these problems happened to Margarita. Everyone was involved with how to get Margarita out of her current mess. Several of the nursing assistants forgot to do some of their tasks/duties, and Margarita needed a lot of assistance to get her assignment completed. As Tricia remembered that particular time, a picture flew through her mind. It was Mrs. Kelly standing in the front of the class with a stuffed toy monkey on her back.

WHEN NURSING ASSISTANTS BRING PROBLEMS FROM HOME

As an LPN/LVN charge nurse, it is important that you do not fall into the "monkey trap," as described by Blanchard, Oncken, and Burrows in *The One-Minute Manager Meets the Monkey* (1991). You fall into the trap each time you take on a responsibility (monkey) that belongs to an employee. Once monkeys are adopted, they take a lot of time in their care and upkeep. LPN/LVN charge nurses can help nursing assistants become aware of this trap and be a role model for avoiding it.

Realize that you do not own any problems that nursing assistants experience. The nursing assistant owns the problem. Avoid feeling bad because you cannot solve the problems of team members. Be supportive and express genuine concern and empathy, but realize that you do not have a license to counsel nursing assistants. Team members need to solve their own problems. Follow facility policies when personal problems interfere with work performance. Report the situation to your supervisor. Professional counseling in the community may be necessary. See the Coordinated Care, Management Tool: When Nursing Assistants Bring Problems from Home box.

 Coordinated Care

Management Tool

When Nursing Assistants Bring Problems from Home

Resources needed:
- Reading: The section in this chapter "When Nursing Assistants Bring Problems from Home"
- Creative thinking

Pretend you are the LPN/LVN charge nurse the morning Margarita comes to work with her problems. Identify a way to handle the situation.

Tricia remembered Betty, a nursing assistant who had been employed at Quality Care Home for 6 months when she told Kay, a nursing assistant on her wing, that she did not know how to use the new patient-lifting device. Kay stated she did not really have time, but Betty coaxed her to take the time to get the resident out of bed for her. Tricia had suggested to Kay a way of handling the situation that she had learned in PV class—a tip that would help Betty be more accountable.

ENCOURAGING PERSONAL RESPONSIBILITY IN NURSING ASSISTANTS

When nursing assistants cannot do something that is in their job description—for example, transferring a resident by a lifting device—it is their problem. Staff persons need to avoid assuming it is a staff problem. Be sure to follow the policy of the facility. For safety reasons, encourage nursing assistants to report to the charge nurse when they are having problems carrying out their assignment. This gives the charge nurse the opportunity to determine what staff member is skilled and available to assist in the situation. Encourage the nursing assistant to offer suggestions for learning to do the part of their job that they do not know how to do. Praise them for coming up with a plan, and add to the plan, if necessary. Write a note to your supervisor explaining the situation objectively and how you proceeded to remedy the situation. If necessary, request additional training for the nursing assistant. Learning who owns problems will help you control a large part of the stress you experience as an LPN/LVN charge nurse and help ensure the safety of resident care. See the Coordinated Care, Management Tool: Encouraging Nursing Assistants to Be Accountable for Learning Skills box.

 Coordinated Care

Management Tool

Encouraging Nursing Assistants to Be Accountable for Learning Skills

Resources needed:
- Reading: The section in this chapter "Encouraging Personal Responsibilities in Nursing Assistants"

  Develop a plan to encourage Betty to approach the lifting-device situation in a more accountable manner.

Tricia remembered instances in her student days and throughout her career when families had complained about care given to their relatives. These complaints troubled Tricia, who had high standards and prided herself on the quality of her nursing care. She would take the complaints seriously and investigate each criticism thoroughly. Sometimes nothing could be found out of order, and sometimes she began doubting her ability to self-evaluate. Once again, Mrs. Kelly offered insight into this common problem, which Tricia still uses today.

DEALING WITH DEMANDING/COMPLAINING FAMILIES

A common problem in the nursing home is dealing with complaints of family members regarding care of their relatives. A common complaint involves physical care. Sometimes the family members become verbally aggressive, express concerns in an angry manner, and are very critical of the charge nurse. Others will be nonassertive and sarcastic. Remember the problem-solving process. First, collect data to determine the real problem. If there is a problem with physical care, identify and correct it. Sometimes when the problem is identified and solved, the complaints continue. Sometimes when no problem with physical care is identified, the family may continue the attack.

It is necessary to consider the situation in which the family finds itself. They are in a position of seeing their loved one progressively aging and decompensating. This is a time of loss for the family. They may feel guilty about placing a relative in a long-term care facility or about not being able to continue caregiving. They may have grieving issues to contend with. Lashing out may be their attempt at relief. To avoid personal issues, family members may unconsciously project blame onto nursing assistants and other members of the nursing staff. It is similar to looking at skeletons in other people's closets so you do not have to look at those in your own closet. This behavior may make a family feel better. It is important for staff to understand these issues to avoid hurt feelings. Avoid personalizing the situation. Suggested interventions to deal with the demanding or complaining family are included in the Coordinated Care, Management Tool: Interventions to Use for the Demanding/Complaining Family box. When family complaints surface, investigate them, but remember to keep broad shoulders. The exercise in the Critical Thinking: Dealing with the Demanding/Complaining Family box can help you to practice dealing with the demanding and complaining family.

 Coordinated Care

Management Tool

Interventions to Use for the Demanding/Complaining Family

See Bauer and Hill's book *Mental Health Nursing* (2000) for interventions for additional specific behaviors.
- Develop a sincere, nonpunitive relationship with the resident's family.
- Encourage the family to ventilate feelings about the resident's placement in a nursing home, aging, and behavior.
- Try to identify the unconscious issue and address it.
- Determine the needs the family is trying to fulfill through their demands, criticism, and complaints.
- Spend time with the family when demands or complaints are not being made.
- Establish rapport with the family to provide emotional support during this difficult time.
- Explain the resident's disease and expected behavior.
- Suggest joining a support group. These groups offer explanations for specific diseases, as well as a place to share feelings and frustrations.
- Encourage the family to stay involved with the resident and continue caregiving and visiting.

Critical Thinking

Dealing with the Demanding/Complaining Family

Resources needed:
- Reading: Chapter 20: Figure 20-5 Decision-Making Tree for Problem Solving on p. 258.

Mrs. Duffy, age 82, was admitted 2 weeks ago to Quality Care Home. You are an LPN/LVN charge nurse on her wing on the evening shift. Mrs. Duffy has osteoarthritis, short-term memory loss, and Parkinson's disease. In the past few days her family has been complaining about her hair care, mouth care, appearance, and missing items in her laundry.
- Develop a plan with specific interventions to investigate and alleviate these complaints.
- Despite modifications in Mrs. Duffy's care plan, the complaints continue. Plan specific interventions to handle the continuing specific complaints.

ASSIGNMENT AND DELEGATION

Tricia stopped at the topic of "Assigning Tasks and Delegating Duties to Nursing Assistants." She remembered well the confusion she experienced in class in trying to understand the difference between "assigning" and "delegating" to nursing assistants. Like most of the students in her class, she thought assigning and delegating meant the same thing. They sure sounded the same. The fact that she went to school in a state that did not allow her to delegate to nursing assistants compounded her confusion in understanding these concepts. Mrs. Kelly, as usual, had the situation well under control. She said that although assigning and delegating had many similarities, there were differences that had legal consequences. The best place to start was to lay down the boundaries of what we were talking about, define and describe the terms, and then go on from there. In case the students thought assigning and delegating were new concepts, Mrs. Kelly read the following quote:

> *To be "in charge" is certainly not only to carry out the proper measures yourself, but to see that everyone else does, too. It is neither to do everything yourself nor to appoint a number of people to each duty, but to ensure that each does that duty to which he is appointed.*

> *Florence Nightingale*
> *Notes on Nursing, 1859*

CHECKING YOUR NURSE PRACTICE ACT

At this time, not every state in the United States allows practical/vocational nurses to delegate in their charge nurse positions. It is crucial that you check your state's Nurse Practice Act (NPA— the state law/statute that regulates your nursing practice) to determine whether you may delegate as an LPN/LVN charge nurse in your state. If you cannot clearly find an answer, contact your state's Board of Nursing (BON). Click on your state at the National Council of the State Boards of Nursing website (https://www.ncsbn.org/contactbon.htm) for contact information. See the Coordinated Care, Management Tool: Reviewing Your Nurse Practice Act for Authority to Delegate box.

 Coordinated Care

Management Tool

Reviewing Your Nurse Practice Act for Authority to Delegate

Resources needed:
- Your state's Nurse Practice Act
  —Locate the section of your state's Nurse Practice Act that discusses your ability to delegate nursing duties as an LPN/LVN charge nurse.
  —In your own words, write that position.

If your state's Nurse Practice Act allows LPN/LVN charge nurses to delegate duties, you will have the authority to delegate duties to nursing assistants (unlicensed assistive personnel). In 1994, the president of the National Council of State Boards of Nursing (NCSBN) stated, "Boards of nursing must clearly define delegation in regulation, promulgate clear rules for its use, and follow through with disciplinary action when there is evidence that the rules are violated" (Rachels, 1994). For this reason, some states may differ in their interpretation of "delegation." This is one reason you need to check with the BON in your state for its interpretation. In addition to your state's Nurse Practice Act, be sure to review the following:

1. Rules and regulations of your state's BON
2. Interpretations, guidelines, and memorandums developed by your state's board of nursing regarding delegation

A state's NPA usually presents information in a general manner. Rules and regulations and interpretations of your BON are more specific statements. They make clearer the intent of the NPA and provide more specific details that describe your nursing practice.

Your state may give you permission to delegate as an LPN/LVN, but to delegate in your place of employment, *your facility must also give permission for that function by including it in its written policies.* For this reason, check facility policy regarding delegation of nursing duties by the LPN/LVN charge nurse.

The standards of nursing organizations are not legal statements, but they provide support to the legal decisions of your state. Be sure to review the standards of your nursing organizations that apply to delegation by the LPN/LVN. See the Coordinated Care, Management Tool: Locating Positions of Nursing Groups and Employer on Delegation Function of LPN/LVN Charge Nurse box.

 Coordinated Care

Management Tool

Locating Positions of Nursing Groups and Employer on Delegation Function of LPN/LVN Charge Nurse

Resources needed:
- Rules, regulations, interpretations, guidelines, and memorandums regarding delegation of your state's board of nursing

- Appendix A: NAPNES Standards of Practice and Educational Competencies of Graduates of Practical/Vocational Nursing Programs
- Appendix B: NFLPN Nursing Practice Standards for the Licensed Practical/Vocational Nurse
- Policies on delegation of employer
  Review the policies/rules and regulations/interpretations/guidelines/standards of the following agencies in regard to delegation:
- Board of Nursing
- National Association for Practical Nurse Education and Service, Inc.
- National Federation of Licensed Practical Nurses
- National League for Nursing
- Health care facility

GENERAL CONSIDERATIONS

Assignment and *delegation* are terms used in reference to allocating patient care activities to team members. Both terms refer to nursing actions or activities, but the terms do not have the same meaning. It is important to think about and use *assignment* and *delegation* in the way they are legally intended. **To help increase your understanding and decrease confusion, the terms *assignment* (assigning) and *delegation* (delegating) are used in this chapter in the following way.**

—When discussing **assignment**, this topic will be used in reference to **"tasks."** Tasks are activities that are carried out by nursing assistants. Nursing assistants learn "how to" perform a task in their nursing assistant training, and these tasks are listed in their job description.

—When discussing **delegation**, this topic will be used in reference to **"duties."** Tasks are functions that are performed by LPN/LVNs because they successfully passed a licensing exam. The duties are included in the state's Nurse Practice Act. The duties are their *scope of practice*. The LPN/LVN learns "why" a duty is performed and "what" could go wrong during performance of a "duty." Resident circumstances can change a "task" for a nursing assistant into a "duty" requiring the LPN/LVN to use the nursing process.

Whenever the title "charge nurse" is used, it will be in the context of the LPN/LVN.

DIFFERENCES BETWEEN ASSIGNING AND DELEGATING

Assigning

Assigning is the way that work is distributed among team members for the shift. Assigning is a skill that every LPN/LVN needs to develop if their state allows them to assume a charge nurse position. Distributing the workload by assignment is a routine part of the LPN/LVN charge nurse's job. Assignment occurs at the beginning of every shift and as the need arises during the shift.

When LPNs/LVNs give assignments to nursing assistants, they are **allotting tasks that are in the job description of these health care workers.** The assigned tasks are tasks that nursing assistants are trained, hired, and paid to perform. The tasks are in *their* job description. These unlicensed personnel have the responsibility to complete the assignment in a safe and timely manner. The LPN/LVN charge nurse shares responsibility with unlicensed personnel for the quality of the care delivered. In assigning situations, the LPN/LVN charge nurse needs to monitor the performance of the task and evaluate the quality and effectiveness of the care that was assigned. See the Coordinated Care, Management Hint: Assigning Tasks box for help in understanding assigning tasks.

Coordinated Care
Management Hint

Assigning Tasks

- The need to assign can occur at any time during the shift but *always* occurs at the beginning of the shift.
- The assigning of tasks is part of the LPN/LVN charge nurse's job.
- The LPN/LVN charge nurse assigns tasks to nursing assistants that are in *their* job description.
- *Nursing tasks* are tasks that nursing assistants are trained, hired, and paid to perform. See p. 284, Specific Tasks for Nursing Assistant Assignment.
- Because assignments involve allocating the tasks that are to be done by nursing assistants in *their* job description, these team members cannot refuse the assignment unless they do not feel qualified to perform the task.
- Nursing assistants assume responsibility for completing assigned tasks safely and in a timely manner.

Delegating

LPNs/LVNs receive the authority to provide nursing care from the nursing license they receive after successfully passing the NCLEX-PN® examination. When allowed by your state's Nurse Practice Act and facility policies, delegating duties in the long-term care unit involves **transferring the authority to perform nursing duties that are in the job description of the LPN/LVN charge nurse (the person doing the delegating)** to competent nursing assistants (unlicensed personnel, known as the delegate) in selected situations. These nursing duties are in *your* job description and "emerge" from your nursing license. These duties are in your scope of practice. **Based on your scope of practice, the most important duty of LPNs/LVNs is the assisting role in the nursing process.** Table 21-1 presents a comparison of assigning tasks and delegating duties.

Delegating is a complex skill requiring sophisticated clinical judgment. Delegation information, including scenarios, might be included in theory classes in your

Table 21-1	Assigning Versus Delegating by the LPN/LVN Charge Nurse	
	ASSIGNING TASKS	**DELEGATING DUTIES**
To whom may tasks or duties be assigned or delegated?	Nursing assistants and other unlicensed personnel	Nursing assistants and other unlicensed personnel
Are tasks or duties in nursing assistant's job description?	Yes	No. The duties delegated are in the job description of the LPN/LVN. Specific duties are not listed. Delegated duties depend on the situation.
May nursing assistant refuse nursing task/duty?	No, unless nursing assistant thinks he or she is unqualified for the assignment.	Yes. In addition, the nursing assistant must voluntarily accept delegation function.
Who has accountability for nursing task/duty?	The nursing assistant is responsible for completing the task and in a safe manner.	The LPN/LVN is accountable for delegating the right duty to the right person.

practical/vocational nursing program, but opportunities to apply the information on clinical may be limited. To be effective, delegation is a skill that needs to be developed with a licensed nurse as a mentor after graduation (Grumet, 2005; NCSBN, 2005).

Delegating duties and assigning tasks are written in the job description of the LPN/LVN charge nurse at Quality Care Home. When allowed by your state's Nurse Practice Act and your facility, **delegating is a voluntary function.** You do not *have* to delegate because the facility allows it. The Coordinated Care, Management Hint: Delegating Duties box contains helpful information for delegating duties.

Coordinated Care
Management Hint

Delegating Duties

- When delegating duties, you are asking nursing assistants (unlicensed personnel) to do part of *your* job.
- Delegation involves the ability to share power with nursing assistants.
- Delegation is *not* asking nursing assistants to do duties that the LPN/LVN dislikes doing.
- As LPN/LVN charge nurse, you are asking nursing assistants to help you perform some of *your* job description so that you may perform other responsibilities, with the ultimate goal of improving resident care and meeting resident goals (outcomes).
- Because you are delegating part of *your* job as charge nurse, nursing assistants must give approval to the assignment. Nursing assistants must voluntarily accept the delegation; they cannot be forced to accept the delegated duty.
- When delegating duties, the LPN/LVN charge nurse needs to provide the nursing assistant with the necessary information, assistance, and equipment to safely carry out the delegated duty.
- Employers may suggest that certain duties be delegated, but the LPN/LVN is ultimately responsible for the following:
  —Deciding *to* delegate a duty
  —Deciding *what* duty to delegate
  —Deciding *to whom* to delegate a duty
  —Deciding *under what circumstances* to delegate a duty

WHY DELEGATING IS IMPORTANT

When allowed by your Nurse Practice Act and facility policies, learning to delegate some of the duties in your job description to nursing assistants can have many advantages. Delegating can do the following:
  —Increase your effectiveness and efficiency as an LPN/LVN charge nurse
  —Be instrumental in realizing patient goals (outcomes) in a cost-effective manner
  —May help nursing assistants increase and improve their job skills

LEGAL ASPECTS OF DELEGATING

In the long-term care facility, the LPN/LVN charge nurse, who is under the *general* supervision of a registered nurse (RN), is managing and directing the activities of nursing assistants. The RN might be in the building on days and evenings. On the night shift the RN might be at the other end of a cell phone. When the RN delegates a duty to the LPN/LVN charge nurse and the charge nurse then delegates to a nursing assistant, the legal principle of *respondeat superior* comes into play. By that principle, the nursing act delegated is the act of the supervising nurse, the RN. The registered nurse is *ultimately* responsible for the supervision of nursing assistants. But the LPN/LVN charge nurse assists in the supervision of these health care workers and shares accountability with the RN for their actions.

Scope of Practice for the LPN/LVN

Never delegate what is in your legal scope of practice. Legal scope of practice is what you are able to do because you are an LPN/LVN. Your scope of practice includes the assisting role in the nursing process. The LPN/LVN charge nurse can delegate to nursing assistants the duty of checking a resident's intravenous (IV) site for intactness and dryness of dressing. However, nursing assistants are not trained in the basics of collecting data. If the resident complained of being cold at the site of the IV, nursing assistants might provide the patient with another blanket, turn up the heat, or turn down the air conditioning. They would not automatically check to see if the infusion device had come out of the resident's vein and was infusing fluid onto the bed sheets.

Although unlicensed assistive personnel obtain data while caring for residents, they do not have the nursing education to make a judgment about or interpret that data. Therefore, nursing judgment cannot be delegated to or expected of nursing assistants. The LPN/LVN charge nurse needs to use his or her knowledge and experience to interpret data gathered by these members of the team.

Your license is at stake in the matter of delegating nursing duties. To be legally sound when delegating duties, see the suggestions in the Coordinated Care, Management Hint: Suggestions for Legal Soundness When Delegating box.

 Coordinated Care

Management Hint

Suggestions for Legal Soundness When Delegating

- Delegate only if allowed by your state's Nurse Practice Act and facility policies.
- Determine stability of the patient's condition.
- Delegate duties for which nursing assistants have demonstrated ability.
- Provide specific, objective, clear-cut directions to nursing assistants for delegated duties.
- Provide assistance and instruction to nursing assistants when you delegate a duty.
- Monitor the activities of nursing assistants when they carry out delegated duties. Depending on the nursing assistant and the situation, this monitoring can mean anything from being "right there" to a periodic check.
- Intervene if correction is needed to maintain safety.
- On completion of the delegated duty, evaluate the safety and effectiveness of duties delegated to nursing assistants.
- If you delegated improperly and a resident was harmed, you are liable. This could result in a disciplinary action against your license and/or a civil suit (see Chapter 12).
- If you delegated properly, including monitoring, and the patient was injured, the nursing assistant is liable.

Tricia continued paging through her PVI text and notes. What memories they brought back! All those shifts of taking report and focusing on important aspects of each patient or resident on the clinical area had a purpose. Tricia remembered the first time she had taken report as an LPN/LVN charge nurse. Her new position of responsibility gave her a heightened sense of awareness of the data being given. Based on the data she received in report, she *had to decide what to assign and what to delegate to nursing assistants for the shift.*

USING THE NURSING PROCESS AS A GUIDE FOR ASSIGNING TASKS AND DELEGATING DUTIES

The nursing process will be used as the device to cover the various aspects that need to be understood and used when assigning or delegating.

- *Collecting data:* Oncoming report, assessment of residents
- *Planning:* Establishing goals (outcomes) for the shift, setting priorities, and assigning/delegating
- *Implementing:* Monitoring, assisting, being available, and intervening
- *Evaluating:* Two-way feedback

COLLECTING DATA

Oncoming Report

National Patient Safety Goals require a standardized approach to communications (for example, change-of-shift report, which is sometimes called "handoff"), including an opportunity to ask and respond to questions during reports. If your facility has TJC accreditation, there may be a standardized form to use when receiving report. The National Patient Safety Goals of TJC are in Chapter 19 and can also be accessed at www.jointcommission.org.

Change-of-shift report allows the LPN/LVN charge nurse to collect data to determine how the work of the shift will be divided. **Always keeping in mind patient goals (outcomes) for shift, report helps guarantee continuity in resident care.**

Report When Starting Your Shift

Reports in long-term care units and nursing homes, as in other health care facilities, are a way to pass pertinent data to the oncoming shift. The report you receive when you are starting your shift will be your basis for collecting data about resident needs. This is legally necessary so you can safely distribute the work of the shift to nursing assistants to provide care for specific residents by keeping in mind patient goals (outcomes). Report may be taped or oral, depending on TJC accreditation or agency policy.

When report is taped, offgoing personnel usually are still on duty. They answer call lights and attend to residents' needs while the oncoming shift listens to report. This enables the charge nurse to question unclear information after report. If facilities do not have a standardized report form, nurses develop personal ways of gathering data when they are taking report, including the use of symbols and abbreviations. See the Coordinated Care, Management Tool: Developing Your Personal Form for Collecting Data During Report box.

Coordinated Care
Management Tool

Developing Your Personal Form for Collecting Data During Report

Resources needed:
- Method of gathering data during report that you have developed during the clinical year
- Sample of forms/method to gather information for report used by clinical sites where you have worked this year
- Your creativity

Develop a form that will help you gather the pertinent information needed to assume responsibility of taking charge of the residents on your wing(s). Include format, symbols, and abbreviations you find helpful and that will allow you to quickly and accurately gather the information. Compare your form with forms of classmates.

Assessment of Patients

Assignment/delegation of patients is usually done after report. Ideally, the LPN/LVN charge nurse makes rounds to personally assess each resident before making assignments. This baseline assessment allows the charge nurse to note any changes in condition of residents or discrepancies that may have occurred since report. If distribution of work for the shift is done before rounds and a change in assignment/delegation is required, the nursing assistant needs to be notified.

PLANNING

"We may be very busy, we may be very efficient, but we will also be truly effective only when we begin with the end in mind."
-Stephen R. Covey

Planning involves deciding goals (outcomes) for the shift, setting priorities of care, and then using specific directions, assigning/delegating the appropriate task/duty to the nursing assistant who can safely and effectively complete the assignment/delegation.

Before Assigning Tasks/Delegating Duties to Nursing Assistants

Distributing the work to be done among nursing assistants follows change-of-shift report. Encourage nursing assistants to take notes and ask questions regarding the directions you give for assigned tasks/delegated duties. Resist the urge to think of work only as tasks to be completed and to just divide the work equally among team members. In other words, just because there are 32 patients and 4 nursing assistants, it does not mean that each assistant automatically gets 8 patients. Take time to plan how work will be distributed. At first this part may seem tedious and time consuming, but planning becomes easier with practice and experience. This part of the nursing process is a good reason why the charge nurse position, by state law, requires experience beyond a new graduate.

Hansten and Jackson (2008) state, "Fail to plan. Plan to fail." When nurses must decide what to assign/delegate, it is important that they identify resident goals (outcomes) and set priorities.

Identifying Resident Goals. To be more effective when assigning/delegating and to make these functions more understandable, think in terms of resident **goals (outcomes)**. Goals are desired results in resident progress after nursing intervention. What should happen after nursing intervention by the nursing assistant? Why is the nursing activity being done? What is the goal (outcome) for each resident for the shift?

Critical Thinking
Formulating Goals/Outcome for Residents

Formulate a goal (outcome) to be met at the end of the shift for each of the following residents:
- **Harold,** an active 90-year-old with osteoarthritis, had a right total hip replacement and is completing his rehabilitation at Quality Care Home, with the goal to go back to his apartment in assisted living. He is to walk x2 with stand-by assist and have one dry clean dressing change daily. His temp went to 100.4 °F last evening, but he is not displaying respiratory symptoms.
- **Goal (outcome) for Harold for day shift:** Harold will maintain hip abduction when turning and getting out of bed to prevent hip dislocation. Harold will have causes of his elevated temp investigated.
- **Adelia,** age 76, and a 2-year resident of Quality Care Home, has type 1 diabetes and receives an intermediate-acting insulin injection each morning and capillary blood glucose monitoring ½ hour before meals with sliding scale short-acting insulin coverage. Adelia can be up ad lib, and today is her shower day, which Adelia is looking forward to. The PM shift had trouble getting a blood sample and had to do *two* fingersticks to obtain a blood sample for testing.
- **Goal (outcome) for Adelia for day shift:** Adelia will have blood glucose monitoring done x2 with only one fingerstick required for each test.
- **Blake,** age 82, has resided at Quality Care Home for 3 years. He has arteriosclerotic heart disease (ASHD). He recently was hospitalized with a cerebral vascular accident (CVA) and is back at Quality Care Home. Blake has weakness on the right side of his body, is allowed up with the assistance of one person, and uses a walker. He has dysphagia (difficulty swallowing).
- **Goal (outcome) for Blake for day shift:** Blake will eat breakfast and lunch without aspirating.

Setting Priorities. Set priorities among the goals (outcomes) for the shift. The priority (most important) care to be done can be evaluated according to the following criteria:
1. *Life-threatening situations—real or potential*
   a. A resident who has unrelieved back pain that started on the last shift. (Goal/outcome: Resident will be pain-free at end of shift.)

b. A resident who is dying. (Goal/outcome: Because of comfort measures provided and presence of family, resident will have a peaceful look on his face and lie still in bed without thrashing and picking at sheets.

c. A resident who is showing untoward effects to a newly ordered drug. (Goal/outcome: Resident will have stable blood pressure and respirations of 22 to 26 per minute. This requires frequent monitoring and reporting PRN to physician.)

d. A resident attempted to flee the building several times on the last shift. (Goal/outcome: Resident will be present in the building at the end of the shift, thanks to constant supervision.)

2. *Essential to safety.* This criterion pertains to residents and the nursing team.

a. Which residents, because of their weight, require two persons to turn and position?

b. Which residents, because of poor balance, need assistance to get out of bed and/or ambulate?

c. Who is going to check special equipment (e.g., the stock of supplies used in emergencies) for shift?

d. Does a resident require standard precautions that infrequently need to be used in the facility? Instruction may need to be given to nursing assistants.

3. *Essential to the medical/nursing plan of care.* Criteria include ordered treatments, facility routines for care, and interventions listed on the nursing plan of care—for example, dressing changes, administration of drugs, measuring vital signs, turning, transferring, ambulating, feeding and encouraging fluids, and monitoring of capillary blood glucose levels.

Criteria for Assigning/Delegating to Nursing Assistants

In 2006, the National Council of State Boards of Nursing (NCSBN) and the American Nurses Association (ANA) issued a joint statement on delegation to assist licensed nurses to delegate safely and effectively in clinical settings. Table 21-2 adapts the NCSBN's decision tree for delegation to nursing assistive personnel. The joint statement and additional materials about delegation can be accessed online at www.ncsbn.org (type "delegation" in the search box).

The joint statement provides a list of five areas to assist LPNs/LVNs in making decisions about delegation. When discussing delegation, the joint statement uses the term "task." Remember, to help differentiate and understand assigning versus delegating, we use "task" to apply to assigning and "duty" to apply to delegating those functions that require the knowledge and judgment of your nursing license and experience.

1. Right task (duty)
2. Right circumstance
3. Right person

4. Right directions and communication
5. Right supervision and evaluation (Some states use the term *monitor* instead of *supervision* when the LPN/LVN performs this function.)

Right Task. A crucial legal consideration in dividing work among nursing assistants is nursing judgment. The LPN/LVN charge nurse needs to avoid real and potential harm to residents when allocating workload to nursing assistants. You are *legally liable* for improper assigning/delegating. Change-of-shift report and rounds for beginning of shift resident data collection gave you the opportunity, as LPN/LVN charge nurse, to collect data about the specific nursing needs of the residents for your shift and the complexity of those needs. Actual tasks/duties allocated depend on the following criteria:

—Laws in your state
—Policies of the long-term care facility
—Needs and condition of the residents on your unit
—Training of nursing assistants

Assigning Tasks. Assigning tasks involves dividing work that is in the job description of nursing assistants. The Coordinated Care, Management Hint: Specific Tasks for Nursing Assistant Assignment box lists specific tasks that could be assigned to nursing assistants.

Coordinated Care
Management Hint

Specific Tasks for Nursing Assistant Assignment

Routine:
- Personal care, including hygiene, dressing, toileting, grooming, and skin care
- Feeding and hydration
- *Basic restorative skills,* including transfer, positioning, ambulation, and maintaining range of motion
- Measuring and recording vital signs, height and weight, and intake and output
- Assistance with elimination, including catheter care and enemas
- Maintaining safety factors, including fall prevention, application of heat and cold, and infection prevention
- Collecting specimens of urine and stool
- Nursing assistants who have displayed an excellent work ethic, job performance, and skills may be offered additional, specialized training to become restorative aides. Additional training occurs for positioning, transferring, performing range of motion, using assistive devices, and preventing pressure ulcers.

Delegating Duties. Remember, delegating involves transferring the authority (the right) to perform a selected nursing duty (a duty your license gives you the right to do after attending a practical/vocational nursing program and passing a licensing exam given nationally). Delegation generally involves selected activities in patient care. A nursing assistant can receive

Table 21-2	Delegation Decision-Making Tree for the Licensed Practical/Vocational Nurse			
Starting with question 1, if you answer "no" to a question, do not delegate. If you answer "yes," proceed to the next question.				
1. Does your Nurse Practice Act give the LPN/LVN permission to delegate?		**No**	**Do not delegate**	**Yes**
2. Does the employing agency give the LPN/LVN permission to delegate?		**No**	**Do not delegate**	**Yes**
3. Is the duty to be delegated within the scope of practice of the LPN/LVN?		**No**	**Do not delegate**	**Yes**
4. Does the LPN/LVN have the education necessary to delegate nursing duties?		**No**	**Do not delegate**	**Yes**
5. Has the LPN/LVN collected data of the patient's needs and condition?		**No**	**Collect data and continue**	**Yes**
6. Is the nursing assistant to whom a duty is being delegated competent to accept the delegation? (See p. 287 for suggestions to determine competency.)		**No**	**Do not delegate**	**Yes**
7. Is the delegated duty performed according to a sequence of steps?		**No**	**Do not delegate**	**Yes**
8. Does the delegated duty occur repeatedly in the daily care of patients?		**No**	**Do not delegate**	**Yes**
9. Does the delegated duty involve little or no modification from one patient situation to another?		**No**	**Do not delegate**	**Yes**
10. Can the delegated duty be performed with a predictable outcome?		**No**	**Do not delegate**	**Yes**
11. Is there danger of affecting the patient's life or well-being if the nursing duty is carried out?		**No**	**Do not delegate**	**Yes**
12. Is the delegated duty in the nursing assistant's job description?		**No**	**Do not delegate**	**Yes**
13. Does the nursing assistant accept the delegated duty?		**No**	**Do not delegate**	**Yes**
14. Does the nursing assistant have the knowledge, skills, and abilities to accept the delegated duty?		**No**	**Do not delegate**	**Yes**
15. Does the nursing assistant's ability match the patient's needs?		**No**	**Do not delegate**	**Yes**
16. Can the delegated nursing duty be performed without requiring nursing judgment?		**No**	**Do not delegate**	**Yes**
17. Are the results of the delegated duty reasonably predictable?		**No**	**Do not delegate**	**Yes**
18. Can the delegated duty be safely performed according to exact, unchanging directions?		**No**	**Do not delegate**	**Yes**
19. Can the delegated duty be safely performed without constant data collection, interpretation of that data, and the need for decisions based on that data?		**No**	**Do not delegate**	**Yes**
20. Does the agency have a written policy, procedure, and/or protocol for the delegated duty?		**No**	**Do not delegate**	**Yes**
21. Is the LPN/LVN who delegated the duty available for monitoring the nursing assistant?		**No**	**Do not delegate**	**Yes → May delegate**

Adapted from National Council of State Boards of Nursing *Decision Tree for Delegation to Nursing Assistive Personnel*, App. B of *2006 Joint Statement on Delegation*, American Nurses Association (ANA) and the National Council of State Boards of Nursing (NCSBN). Available at www.ncsbn.org.

an assignment, and within that assignment might be activities that need to be delegated. *Avoid assuming that simpler duties may be automatically delegated.* The Coordinated Care, Management Tool: Criteria for Delegating Duties box lists criteria for delegating duties to nursing assistants.

Coordinated Care
Management Tool

Criteria for Delegating Duties

The following are criteria for nursing duties that can be delegated for residents whose conditions are stable:
- The delegated duty must apply to an unchanging situation. (If there is a chance for a change in the patient during a procedure, do not delegate.)

- The results of the delegated duty must be predictable.
- The potential for risk during performance of the delegated duty must be minimal (e.g., the patient with difficulty swallowing is a risk).
- The delegated duty should be necessary and routine in daily care.
- The delegated duty should not require nursing judgment (e.g., "I think the blood glucose level is normal").
- The delegated duty should not require frequent, repeated collection of data during performance of the duty.

The following suggestions include information to help decide what duty can be delegated.
- A question that can help the LPN/LVN make a decision as to what to delegate is "What is the intended outcome (goal/desired result) of the nursing care in question?" In their article, "Delegating to

UAPs—Making It Work," Hansten and Washburn (2001) use a bath given for several different reasons (goals/outcomes) as an example.

—If the bath of a patient in long-term care who is recuperating from total hip replacement is being used as a teaching situation for family members to learn how to observe for signs of skin breakdown, then a licensed nurse needs to be part of the procedure.

—If a resident who is recuperating from a stroke has a mobility issue, then a physical therapy assistant may be involved with range-of-motion training for the family during the bath.

—The aforementioned two baths could be given as a team, with the nursing assistant bathing the resident, while the licensed nurse points out pressure points susceptible to skin breakdown or the physical therapy assistant gives range-of-motion training.

—If the desired goal of a bath is to have a long-term care resident bathed before being discharged, then the nursing assistant would be assigned.

- Given *specific* directions, nursing assistants can assist to collect, report, and document simple data, but not interpret that data.
- More complex skills to delegate depend on the following:
  —What is allowed by law in your state
  —Resident needs of your unit
  —Further training of nursing assistants—for example, electronic blood glucose monitoring

A concise, across-the-board list of what nursing duties to delegate and what not to delegate does not exist. The Coordinated Care, Management Hint: Why Lists of Duties to Delegate Do Not Exist box contains the drawbacks of such lists.

 Coordinated Care
Management Hint

Why Lists of Duties to Delegate Do Not Exist

- A duty list for nursing assistants eliminates the need for collecting data of the needs of each patient.
- A duty could be on a list of acceptable duties to delegate to a nursing assistant, but the patient situation might indicate the duty would be dangerous or inappropriate for a nursing assistant—for example, feeding a patient with dysphagia (difficulty swallowing).
- The board of nursing has the responsibility to protect the patient. Licensed nursing personnel carry out this responsibility.
- A duty list for nursing assistants puts the control of nursing care into the hands of unlicensed persons who have had minimal training for patient care.
- The exact duties delegated to nursing assistants are interpreted by each state's board of nursing and by each patient situation.

It is somewhat easier to list what duties of the LPN/LVN should *not* be delegated. The Coordinated Care, Management Hint: Examples of Duties Not to Delegate box contains examples.

 Coordinated Care
Management Hint

Examples of Duties Not to Delegate

- Sterile technique procedures: Nursing assistants do not have training in sterile technique.
- Crisis situations (you must be there): An example of a crisis situation is a resident who develops chest pain.
- Initial patient education by an RN: In most states, LPNs/LVNs may reinforce initial patient teaching given by the RN.
- Although nursing assistants can collect simple data, they have not been trained to make decisions about or interpret that data. For example, nursing assistants cannot evaluate results of capillary blood glucose monitoring or determine when vital signs need to be rechecked.
- Duties that are part of *your* legal scope of practice may *never* be delegated. Your legal scope of practice is your assisting role in the nursing process.

? Critical Thinking

Delegating Duties

You practice in a health care facility that allows the LPN/LVN charge nurse to delegate nursing duties to nursing assistants. List two additional items to consider before actually delegating:
1.
2.

Right Circumstance. NCSBN emphasizes that the setting and patient situation must be considered when delegating. The same criteria must be considered when assigning tasks. Assignment/delegation of duties would not occur if the following is true:

- Resident is unstable. For example, the LPN/LVN would probably work as part of "pair caring" with the nursing assistant when a patient has difficulty swallowing, needs to be fed, and has a history of choking. The LPN/LVN would feed the resident and could use the situation as an opportunity to teach the nursing assistant techniques to use to avoid choking.
- The unit does not have equipment or supplies needed to safely carry out the procedure. The procedure would not be attempted until equipment and supplies were obtained.
- There are safety issues for the nursing assistant, including infection control issues.
- The staffing level is so limited that:
  —Supervision (monitoring) of assigned/delegated duties would not be adequate.

—Assistance from the LPN/LVN might not be available when needed—for example, assistance when the nursing assistant has questions or needs directions.

Right Person. The National Council's guidelines describe delegation as transferring the authority to perform a "selected nursing task" to a *competent* person. These guidelines also apply to assigning tasks to nursing assistants. According to NCSBN interpretation (Working with Others, 2005), a *competent* nursing assistant should be capable of the following in addition to basic care:

- Communicate effectively
- Collect basic subjective and objective data
- Perform noncomplex nursing activities safely, accurately, and according to standard procedures
- Seek guidance and direction when appropriate

The following suggestions will help you determine competence of nursing assistants.

Review Job Descriptions. Legally, you need to know the job descriptions of nursing assistants to whom you assign tasks. Check these job descriptions of the facility in which you are employed or on clinical affiliation as a student. See the Coordinated Care, Management Tool: Reviewing Nursing Assistant Job Descriptions box.

Coordinated Care
Management Tool

Reviewing Nursing Assistant Job Descriptions

Resource needed:
- Job descriptions of nursing assistants

Make a list of the tasks nursing assistants can perform in various health care facilities.

Know Level of Competence. Know the level of clinical competence of nursing assistants you supervise. The following questions can help you determine the competency of nursing assistants on your team:

- Is the nursing assistant certified?
- How much nursing assistant training have they had?
- What skills are taught in their nursing assistant program?
- What is the nursing assistant's job description?
- Does the facility conduct yearly skills list updates? (Some LPNs/LVNs keep a laminated copy of nursing assistant job descriptions and skills lists on their clipboards.)
- What clinical strengths have you observed?
- Have the nursing assistants demonstrated previous competency when performing the activity?
- What clinical weaknesses have you observed?
- Is orientation to your unit completed?
- What activities do nursing assistants say they feel qualified doing?

- What activities do nursing assistants feel unsure doing?
- Ask nursing assistants to describe what they would do in a specific situation—for example, "Tell me how you would get this resident with a total hip replacement out of bed." If the nursing assistant hesitates or looks baffled, suggest that you will assist the nursing assistant when she gets the patient out of bed for the first time and use it as a teaching situation.
- Ask what the nursing assistant would do if a deviation from the normal procedure should develop. For example, you might say, "While getting this resident to stand up, what would you do if he got dizzy when attempting to stand?"
- Ask if the nursing assistant has done the procedure before. If nursing assistants misrepresent themselves by saying they know how to perform a nursing activity when they do not know how to perform the activity, they could be liable in a court of law. For example, if a nursing assistant tells you that he or she can do a fingerstick test and then does it incorrectly, causing injury to the resident, he or she could be liable.

Refusing Assignment. If a nursing assistant does not feel qualified to safely perform an *assigned task* and refuses the assignment, the team member is then reassigned. It is a fine art distinguishing between "I don't want to" and "I don't know how to." If there is a training problem, follow the suggestion in the Coordinated Care, Management Tool: Reviewing Nursing Assistant Job Descriptions box. Make arrangements with the staff educator of your facility for this team member to receive the training necessary to safely perform the task(s). Also see the Coordinated Care, Management Tool: Handling Refusal of Assignment by Nursing Assistants box.

Coordinated Care
Management Tool

Handling Refusal of Assignment by Nursing Assistants

Resource needed:
- Reading: The "Refusing Assignment" section in this chapter.

A nursing assistant on the team has refused your assignment to give a resident a whirlpool bath because he does not feel qualified to do the job safely. Write a brief note to the staff educator of the facility regarding this situation. (In a real situation, also send a copy of the note to your supervisor.)

Once you work consistently with nursing assistants, they will prove their dependability and ability to pursue assigned tasks. Nursing assistants have the right to refuse a delegated duty. The LPN/LVN charge nurse then uses questioning to determine if the team member feels unqualified or simply does not want to do the activity. Feeling unqualified is a training problem; not wanting to do an activity is an attitude problem. Problems in attitude can interfere with a nursing assistant's growth as a member of the health care team.

Tricia chuckled as she thought about the time she asked a nursing assistant to force fluids for a resident with an elevated temperature. When the nursing assistant was approached during the shift, she kept reporting that she was forcing fluids. At the end of the shift, when asked for the volume of fluid taken by the resident during the shift, the nursing assistant replied that although she had forced fluids every hour, the resident took only 80 cc for the entire shift. Tricia thought that response served her right for not explaining the assignment objectively as taught by Mrs. Kelly.

Right Directions and Communication. Using effective communication techniques is an excellent example of the leadership skills that are needed by LPN/LVN charge nurses. The LPN/LVN charge nurse's ability to communicate assignments effectively to nursing assistants for reaching patient goals depends on these skills.

As with all communication, assigning/delegating is a two-way process. The communication skills of LPNs/LVNs and their management styles are crucial for establishing a positive working relationship between charge nurse and nursing assistant. It is not only *what* you say as LPN/LVN charge nurse but also *how* you say it. *Inadequate communication is the most common reason delegated duties are not completed as required.* The communication guidelines for delegating duties also apply to communication for assigning tasks. Communication skills need to be learned by studying and using the techniques. Review Chapter 13 regarding straightforward communication.

Do not just tell a nursing assistant what to do. Be sure to give the rationale for duties assigned or delegated. Explain *why* an assigned or delegated duty must be done first or at a specific time. Explain why you need the results at a specific time. Nursing assistants become frustrated and feel unsafe when expected to complete an activity when too little information is given. See the Coordinated Care, Management Hint: Communication/Direction Responsibilities of the LPN/LVN Charge Nurse When Assigning or Delegating box for communication guidelines that apply to assigning *and* delegating.

Coordinated Care

Management Hint

Communication/Direction Responsibilities of the LPN/LVN Charge Nurse When Assigning or Delegating

When assigning tasks or delegating duties, be sure to provide nursing assistants with the following information:

- Give objective, detailed, clear-cut verbal and written directions. Get to the point!
- Consider writing assignments in a concise, objective manner on a master assignment sheet.
- Clarify if the nursing assistant has performed delegated duty in the past.
- Explain what is expected at the nursing assistant's level of understanding.
- Be specific about the results you are expecting and when to report. Do not ask nursing assistants to "find out how the patient is." Instead, ask a patient who has been itching because of a rash if the rash still itches.
- Provide guidelines for reporting after the delegated duty is completed. Provide the time you expect to be informed and why.
- Make sure your directions are specific and complete. Provide all the necessary information, including time, to get the task or duty done correctly and safely. For example, say, "Please report the numbers immediately after you measure Mr. Smith's blood pressure, pulse, and respirations. I need to know the numbers before his 0900 blood pressure medicine can be given."
- Given specific directions, nursing assistants can collect, report, and document simple data. However, they are unable to make judgments based on that data. For example, say, "Please report the results of Mr. Ettle's fingerstick immediately after you perform it so I can determine if he needs insulin."
- Tell nursing assistants when to consult with the charge nurse during the performance of an assigned/delegated duty. For example, say, "Let me know if you are having trouble getting the specimen."
- Clarify all messages by asking nursing assistants to tell you what it is you expect them to do and when to report.
- A "please" and "thank you" are in order as part of common courtesy.

Inform nursing assistants when you expect a report/rundown on activities. A suggested "routine" for reporting back to the charge nurse is before and after breaks and meals and before going off duty. The exact number of reports depends on your familiarity with how the nursing assistant functions, the condition of the residents, and the nature of the assigned/delegated duty. Examples of delegated duties that need priority or more frequent reporting are blood pressure numbers when the resident is to receive blood pressure medicine and blood glucose monitoring with sliding scale insulin coverage. State *when* you expect to be informed and *why* you need to be informed.

Review Chapter 20 for hints that can be used to motivate team members and the Leadership Activity: Using the Howlett Hierarchy in Leadership Situations.

 Critical Thinking

Identifying Resident Goals/Outcomes

Using the information in the "Identifying Resident Goals/Outcomes" section, the "Signs and Symptoms" list in Chapter 20, and a medical/surgical text, write the following activities/observations to be assigned/delegated to nursing assistants in

specific, objective, clear-cut terms. The directions need to be realistic, measurable, and time referenced.
1. Be sure to clean up Mr. Collar.
2. Make sure Mrs. Thren drinks today.
3. Mrs. Wall must get up today.
4. If Mr. Jones does not pass any urine, let me know.
5. Have Mrs. Neidert ready for her doctor's appointment.

? Critical Thinking Exercise

Communicating Objectively to Nursing Assistants

This is your first month as charge nurse at Quality Care Home. Provide specific, objective, clear-cut data for the nursing assistant to be aware of while giving care in the following resident situations:
1. Resident has compensated right-sided congestive heart failure.
2. Resident is a poorly controlled diabetic who receives an intermediate-acting insulin each morning.
3. Resident has lost 5 pounds in the past 2 weeks.
4. Resident has an order for a catheterized urine for residual.

Remember. When delegating, clarify that the nursing assistant has accepted the delegation. The nursing assistant's responsibility in delegation includes accepting the delegated duty, as well as safe performance in carrying out the duty.

Tricia Makes Assignments for the Nursing Assistants

See the resident goals on p. 283.

- **Harold:** Tricia has worked with Margarita, CNA, for several years and assigns Margarita to Harold for personal care and assistance with ambulation because Margarita has had training as a restorative aid. Margarita verbally explains that she will make sure Harold gets up from the right side of the bed, does not cross his legs, and does not lean forward while getting up or sitting in the chair. Tricia assigns Margarita to care for Harold and set up for his dressing change. Although Margarita is allowed to change clean dressings, she is to notify Tricia before she starts so Tricia can observe the surgical site because of Harold's temperature and lack of respiratory symptoms.
- **Adelia:** Lenore, CNA, has had training for capillary blood testing. Tricia has worked with Lenore for several months and thinks she has demonstrated proficiency in safely and accurately obtaining samples for glucose testing. Tricia assigns Lenore to Adelia and delegates capillary blood testing. When given information of the need for two fingersticks on the evening shift, Lenore explains she will identify the finger to be used for the fingerstick, warm Adelia's finger under warm water at the sink in the bathroom, and keep that hand down after Adelia sits

before attempting to get the sample. Tricia reminds Lenore that she needs the sample at 6:30 AM before breakfast and 11:30 AM before lunch trays so she can determine if she needs to administer Adelia's sliding scale insulin coverage ½ hour before meals.
- **Blake:** Sergio is a nursing assistant with 7 years' experience, but he is new to Quality Care Home. Sergio has had restorative nursing training and does well with ROM, positioning, and transfers. Sergio has generally been doing well feeding residents. However, last week Tricia saw a resident almost choke on a grapefruit segment while being fed by Sergio. Tricia assigns Sergio for the following care of Blake: Assist with AM care in bed, ROM, positioning, and assist with transfer from bed to chair. Tricia decides to be with Sergio and "care pair" for meals. Tricia will feed Blake and use this as an opportunity to review with Sergio hints and safety techniques for feeding residents with dysphagia.

IMPLEMENTATION

Right Supervision, Feedback, and Evaluation

The National Council (1995) defines *supervision* as "the provision of guidance or direction, evaluation, and follow-up by the licensed nurse for accomplishment of a nursing task delegated to unlicensed assistive personnel." This definition is interpreted to include appropriate monitoring, intervention, and evaluation of the nursing assistant, as needed, while providing the delegated duty and feedback after the delegated duty is completed. The following suggestions also apply to assigning tasks. To comply with the National Council's guidelines, the LPN/LVN charge nurse needs to carry out the suggestions found in the Coordinated Care, Management Hint: Supervision and Feedback box for nursing assistants regarding assigned tasks/delegated duties.

Coordinated Care
Management Hint

Supervision and Feedback

- How often or closely the charge nurse monitors the nursing assistant carrying out the assigned task or delegated duty depends on the resident condition and status and the nursing assistant.
- The LPN/LVN needs to make himself or herself available for questions or concerns as they arise and to provide guidance and assistance when needed. Ask the nursing assistant if assistance is needed.
- Determine if the assigned tasks or delegated duties are being completed. If not, determine the reason for this (e.g., change of condition).
- If necessary, intervene in the situation to ensure carrying out the assigned task or delegated duty safely.

If you fail to supervise adequately and the resident is harmed, the situation could result in a civil suit in a court of law or disciplinary action against your license. See Chapter 12 for information about nursing and the law.

Assessment of residents and functioning of the team by the LPN/LVN charge nurse occurs periodically during the shift. Although clear communication with nursing assistants during assignment helps ensure that helpful information about residents will be collected during the shift, nothing can replace the charge nurse's contact with residents and judgment based on knowledge and experience.

Coordinated Care
Management Hint

Tricia Supervises the Nursing Assistants

At 7:30 AM and 11:30 AM, Lenore reports, without reminder, Adelia's blood glucose levels. Lenore states she had no trouble getting the samples with one fingerstick. Tricia interprets that no sliding scale insulin is required.

Tricia sees Margarita and Harold as they walk to the dining room for breakfast, and Margarita reports that Harold is very careful about getting up. Harold informed Margarita that "I need to keep that new hip in its socket" so he always gets up on the right side of the bed and never crosses his legs. Margarita notified Tricia after she set up for the clean dressing change, and Tricia assessed the incisional line. There was no redness or edema at the area. Harold's lung sounds are clear, and he denies coughing or congestion. Tricia asks Margarita to check Harold's temperature again at noon.

Sergio sets up Blake for breakfast and notifies Tricia when his tray arrives. When Tricia enters Blake's room, she notes that Blake is sitting up in bed. Tricia suggests that they have Blake sit in the chair for meals. When seated, Tricia reminds Blake to keep his head straight and not tilt it back while swallowing. Tricia turns Blake's head to the left (the unaffected side) and starts with a couple of spoonfuls of thickened liquids and explains this will moisten the membranes of Blake's mouth and throat to make swallowing easier. Tricia feeds one-third of a teaspoon at a time of Cream of Wheat and scrambled eggs. Sergio is attentive as Tricia continues with thickened liquids periodically. When done, Tricia arranges with Sergio to be present while he sets Blake up and feeds him his lunch.

EVALUATION

You discovered in Chapters 1 and 20 that clinical evaluation is a two-way process. The information in those chapters applies to this part of the assignment/delegation process. See the Coordinated Care, Management Hint: Evaluation and Feedback box.

Coordinated Care
Management Hint

Evaluation and Feedback

EVALUATION
• Check the completed duty that was assigned/delegated. Was the task/duty completed? Was the task/duty performed safely and correctly?

• Legally, the LPN/LVN charge nurse may not delegate a duty without checking the outcome of that delegation. Have resident goals (outcomes) been met?
• Has something unusual, undesirable, or unexpected occurred? Does the nursing assistant have suggestions to improve carrying out the delegated duty? What went well and what was challenging?
• Did the nursing assistant report as requested?
• Has the nursing assistant documented the activity?

FEEDBACK
• Encourage the nursing assistant to offer input about the assignment/delegation. For example, you might say, "Harper, what problems did you have while assisting Mr. Paul with his shower?" or "Carlos, What suggestions do you have that would make things flow more smoothly during the shift?"
• The LPN/LVN's leadership skills again come into importance during evaluation and feedback. Provide feedback as needed by the nursing assistant.
• Review and use guidelines for performance evaluation from Chapter 20.
• Did the LPN/LVN thank the nursing assistants for their cooperation during the shift?

Tricia's Evaluation of and Feedback from Nursing Assistants

Tricia thanks Margarita, Lenore, and Sergio for their help and for getting back to her with information and notifying her as quickly as they did. She asks each aide how he or she thought the day went. Margarita and Lenore say the day went fine and that Tricia was available when they needed to report. Sergio says the hints for feeding Blake, especially getting him up to eat and giving thickened liquids first to moisten membranes, were very helpful. All three say they hope to get the same assignment tomorrow, and Lenore asks to watch Sergio feed Blake so she can pick up some hints to use with patients with dysphagia.

PUTTING IT ALL TOGETHER

See the exercise in the Critical Thinking: Assigning Residents in Long-Term Care box.

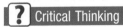

Critical Thinking

Assigning Residents in Long-Term Care

Resource needed:
• As LPN/LVN charge nurse and with available staff, make assignments for the day shift for wing 1 of the nursing home. Include the rationale (reason) for your assignment decisions. Assign and delegate as you feel is appropriate.

STAFF AVAILABLE FOR THE TEAM
• Two student practical/vocational nurses who have completed half of their nursing program. Instructor makes assignments and is present on the clinical area.
• One nursing assistant who has worked at the facility for 10 years (on state registry).

- One nursing assistant who has 7 years' experience and has worked at your facility for 6 months (on state registry).
- One nursing assistant who was sent from a temporary agency to fill the position of a nursing assistant who has the flu. She completed a nursing assistant advanced course 2 months ago (on state registry).

TASKS FOR DAY SHIFT OF WING 1

- *Four showers.* Each of these residents transfers with the help of two nursing assistants. Each of these residents needs to be weighed, have blood pressure checked, and have a complete linen change on shower day. One resident scheduled for a shower says she feels dizzy and has a congested-sounding cough.
- *Sixteen AM cares.* Ten residents are able to wash their own face and hands when set up. Of the remaining six, one has developed a rash over his entire body, one needs electronic glucose monitoring one-half hour before breakfast and lunch on day shift, and four are confused and incontinent of urine and feces. Each of these residents needs one assistant to transfer and ambulate.
- *One complex dressing change for a resident on a Clinitron bed.* (This resident is transferred by a patient-lifting device and requires total care.)
- *One PEG tube intermittent feeding with commercial tube feeding formula and drug administration at 8 AM and 12 noon on day shift.* (This resident is confused and requires two persons to ambulate.)

You have just completed assigning team members, when one of the nursing assistants states that she feels warm and then faints. As it turns out, she has a temperature of 102.2 °F and will not be able to engage in resident care. Reassign the residents on wing 1.

Critical Thinking

Delegating to Nursing Assistants

Resources needed:

- Descriptions of recent clinical assignments for students in your clinical group
- Critical thinking

If your state allows LPNs/LVNs to delegate, use Table 21-2 and the nursing process format in this chapter to practice assigning/delegating recent clinical duties for your clinical group to nursing assistants.

REPORTING AT THE END OF YOUR SHIFT

Giving report at the end of your shift requires planning. As the LPN/LVN charge nurse, you need reports from the nursing assistants before you can tape or give report. This is where the concise, clear directions that you gave to these team members during assignment/delegation will pay off. You will need to set priorities in deciding pertinent information to give to the next shift. Be sure to personally assess residents who have the following:

- Changes in condition
- Current ongoing problems

- New orders (and resident response to new orders)
- Suspected side effects to medications

Use the same sequence of data for each resident. This will make it easier for the oncoming charge nurse to take notes from your report. An example of a suggested sequence of data for reporting to oncoming shift for residents in a long-term care unit can be found in the Coordinated Care, Management Hint: Reporting to Oncoming Shift box.

Coordinated Care
Management Hint

Reporting to Oncoming Shift

THINGS TO REPORT

1. Resident name, room number, and physician
2. New problems/concerns
3. Contact with physician and new orders
4. Progress of current, established problems
5. PRN medication—name of drug, time given, and reason for PRN medication; time follow-up is required
6. *Briefly* describe resident's behavior during shift; include any changes in resident's physical and mental status
7. Resident's voiding, bowel movement (continent versus incontinent)

THINGS TO AVOID DURING REPORT

1. Meaningless chatter that has nothing to do with residents' nursing care and goals/outcomes
2. Routine nursing care, unless it has a bearing on current nursing problems
3. Personal opinions about residents' conditions
4. Value judgments, gossip about residents' lifestyles, behavior, or families

Tricia was very tired and began to put away her textbooks and scrapbook. The review of delegation in her old PVI text proved demanding for Tricia, but it also had been very pleasant reminiscing about her school days and early years as an LVN. She felt good with how far she had come since feeling insecure in those beginning days. At least, she now knew what to question and where to find the answers. It felt good to have a grasp of her LPN/LVN charge nurse position, especially the fine points of delegation of duties. Later, as Tricia was relaxing, a big smile came over her face. Tomorrow would be a big day in her life. Mrs. Kelly had strongly recommended membership in professional organizations. Tricia had been a member of the National Federation of Licensed Practical Nurses at the national, state, and local levels since graduation. Over the years, she had assumed various committee assignments and officer positions at the local level of the organization. Tomorrow she would be installed as the first president of the organization at the state level from her local district! Ticia was proud to be of service to her career and looked forward to promoting and having a say in the direction practical/vocational nursing would take in the twenty-first century.

Get Ready for the NCLEX-PN® Examination!

Key Points

- State Nurse Practice Acts specify requirements needed by LPNs/LVNs to assume first-line manager positions.
- A common first-line manager position is charge nurse in long-term care units and nursing homes.
- Common charge nurse problems include nursing assistants who bring personal problems to work, the need for nursing assistants to be accountable for learning new job skills, and dealing with the residents' demanding/complaining family members.
- Oncoming shift report gives the charge nurse the opportunity to collect data about resident needs, identify resident goals (outcomes) for the shift, and assign nursing tasks to nursing assistants for resident care from *their* job description.
- Assessment of each resident after assignment/delegation identifies changes in condition/circumstances that may require a change in assignment/delegation.
- The charge nurse shares responsibility with nursing assistants for the quality of care that is given.
- Practical/vocational charge nurses routinely assign care to nursing assistants.
- Charge nurses, as part of their jobs, evaluate the thoroughness and safety of all tasks they assign.
- *If allowed in your state's Nurse Practice Act,* and included in facility policies, the LPN/LVN charge nurse may elect to delegate duties from the LPN/LVN job description to nursing assistants.
- Delegation gives the charge nurse time to focus on duties that cannot be delegated.
- Duties can be delegated, but the accountability that goes with those duties remains with the registered nurse, with whom the charge nurse functions under general supervision. The LPN/LVN shares accountability in these situations.
- The charge nurse position is a complex role for LPNs/LVNs. With additional education and experience, many practical/vocational nurses are doing an excellent job in this expanded role position.
- Your license is at stake in the matter of assuming the charge nurse position. Know your state laws regulating nursing.

Additional Learning Resources

evolve Go to your Evolve website (http://evolve.elsevier.com/Hill/Success) for the following FREE learning resources:
- Answers to Critical Thinking and Scenario
- Additional learning activities
- Additional Review Questions for the NCLEX-PN® exam
- Helpful phrases for communicating in Spanish and more!

Review Questions for the NCLEX-PN® Examination

1. Select the defense mechanism that may be present in a family member who continually finds fault and criticizes the care given to a relative by nursing assistants.
   1. Projection
   2. Validation
   3. Introversion
   4. Conversion

2. Select the statement that indicates understanding of delegation.
   1. Nursing assistants cannot refuse a duty delegated to them by the practical/vocational nurse for any reason.
   2. Delegating duties depends on state law, facility policies, resident condition, and the LPN/LVN's desire to delegate.
   3. Any licensed practical/vocational nurse may delegate his or her role to a qualified, dependable nursing assistant.
   4. LPNs/LVNs delegate duties to nursing assistants that are in the facility job description of the nursing assistant.

3. Alfredo, an LPN, has 6 months' experience in a nursing home. He is approached by his employer to perform nursing duties within the expanded role of the practical/vocational nurse as charge nurse. Alfredo knows the expanded role is allowed in his state, but he has not had a leadership component in the basic educational program. Select the best response in this situation.
   1. "I am unable by law to do this, and I could lose my license for functioning in an LPN expanded role."
   2. "I will not function in the expanded role because I did not study this in my student practical nursing program."
   3. "I need some time to contact my board of nursing to clarify state statutes for the LPN expanded role."
   4. "I will assume this role if you will train me for the duties I was not taught and document them in my file."

4. Cindy, LPN, is charge nurse on the evening shift at a nursing home. Select the priority action she will use in making assignments to nursing assistants.
   1. Cindy obtains feedback from the nursing assistants as to the type of procedures for which they feel competent.
   2. Cindy distributes the nursing tasks to be completed on the evening shift equally among the nursing assistants on the team.
   3. Cindy checks job descriptions and skills for nursing assistants to clarify who is competent to perform selected duties.
   4. After report when coming on duty, Cindy establishes patient outcomes for residents for the shift and sets priorities for care.

Alternate Format Item

1. Select from the following sources where permission for the LPN/LVN to delegate in long-term care can be found. *(Select all that apply.)*

   1. BON
   2. NCSBN
   3. NFLPN
   4. FACILITY
   5. NAPNES

2. Which of the following LPN/LVN charge nurses in long-term care facilities are assigning/delegating in a legally sound manner? *(Select all that apply.)*

   1. Lilly did not have classes on delegation in her nursing program but delegates out of fear that if she doesn't, she will lose her job.
   2. Ada clarifies skill levels of nursing assistants by asking the RN to whom she reports to show her where to locate CNA skill lists.
   3. Aiden makes rounds after report to gather data on actual resident condition so he can develop shift outcomes for residents before making assignments.
   4. When making assignments, Alexander provides specific, concrete information for what nursing assistants should do while engaging in resident care.
   5. Whenever a nursing assistant refuses a delegated duty, Brad handles the situation by explaining the effects of insubordination to the CNA.

Critical Thinking Scenario

Sasha, a nursing assistant, has accepted a delegated duty to complete for several evenings. On today's day shift, the LPN/LVN charge nurse says she will do the duty that has been delegated on prior shifts. Sasha complains to the other nursing assistants that the charge nurse doesn't trust her. Comment about this situation.

Objectives

On completing this chapter, you will be able to do the following:

1. List employment opportunities available to licensed practical/vocational nurses (LPNs/LVNs).
2. Determine interpersonal styles and how to use them to achieve interpersonal rapport.
3. Describe and utilize individuals within your job search network.
4. Effectively participate in an informational interview.
5. Discuss how and where to best target job leads.
6. Role-play employer telephone contacts and respond positively to hard interview questions.
7. Practice filling out a job application, including a cover letter.
8. Develop a resume, including a cover letter, that will get an employer's attention.
9. Convey nonverbal messages at the interview.
10. Have insight into the cultural and age differences of the interviewer.
11. Discuss the importance of employer follow-up both at the time of application and after the interview.
12. Anticipate a successful pre-employment physical examination and drug screening.
13. Write an effective resignation letter with style.

Key Terms

conditional job offer (kŏn-dĭ-shŭn-ăl, p. 312)
follow-up illusion (ĭl-oo-shŭn, p. 314)
hidden job market (p. 300)
illegal questions (ĭl-ē-gŭl, p. 305)
informational interviews (ĭn-fŏr-mā-shŭn-ŭl ĭn-tĕr-vūz, p. 298)
interpersonal styles (ĭn-tĕr-pĕr-sŭn-ăl, p. 295)

networking (net-wŭrk-ĭng, p. 296)
reference hierarchy (hī-ĕr-ăr-kē, p. 302)
resignation courtesy (rĕz-ĭg-nā-shŭn, p. 315)
resume (rĕz-ŭh-mā, p. 301)
silence (sī-lĭns, p. 308)
voice control (vŏys kŏn-trōl, p. 299)
work the room (p. 298)

 Keep in Mind

You've decided what you want to be when you grow up; now get out there and do it!

GRADUATION: CLOSER THAN YOU THINK

Twenty to forty million Americans change jobs each year, and due to a struggling economy and increased competition for jobs, the process has not gotten easier (Levinson and Perry, 2009). That said, you are to be congratulated for having chosen to become a licensed practical nurse! In general, health care is expected to be a hot growth area for years to come as baby boomers age. This was recognized as early as 2006 when *Business Week* magazine concluded, "Since 2001, the health care industry has added 1.7 million jobs, while the private sector has added none" (Levinson and Perry, 2009).

According to the *Occupational Outlook Handbook 2010–11 Edition*, "Employment is projected to grow much faster than average, with the best job opportunities in nursing care facilities and home health care services. Employment of LPNs is expected to grow by 21 percent between 2008 and 2018 (Bureau of Labor Statistics, 2011). With respect to where newly licensed LPNs are being hired, the *2009 LPN/VN Practice Analysis: Linking the NCLEX® Practice Examination to Practice* provided the following: 52.1% nursing home, skilled or intermediate care; 14.4% rehabilitation; 11.6% residential care or developmental disability; 10.2% medical-surgical units; 8.6% assisted living; 6.9% home health, including visiting nurses associations; 5.2% hospice care; and 3.2% critical care and emergency departments (NCSBN Research Brief, 2010). Nurses who have had active military combat training may have an edge over other candidates applying for emergency room jobs at hospitals due to already having been acclimatized to the environment (Levinson and Perry, 2009).

WHAT DO I WANT TO DO?

You have a distinct advantage if your educational program included clinical (hands-on) nursing experience in the areas in which you are most interested. These nursing experiences include clinical rotations, special projects, computer work, or work with a temporary permit before taking the NCLEX-PN® examination. If the program did not, it is never too late to contact employers to see about job shadowing their staff members and the work they do, or asking about volunteer opportunities or part-time work in areas you are interested in learning about.

Also, seriously consider taking additional coursework or obtaining certifications to enhance your employability in the areas of basic life support, intravenous therapy, phlebotomy, advanced cardiac life support, behavioral management, and rehabilitation (NCSBN Research Brief, 2009).

◎ Try This

Consider the following questions:
1. What type of environment do I want to work in—direct health care, state/federal government, private duty, insurance-related, sales, industry, or other?

_____

2. What population (i.e., type of client) do I find most rewarding to work with?

_____

3. What kinds of nursing skills do I find most challenging and rewarding? What new areas would I like to be involved in?

_____

_____

USING INTERPERSONAL STYLES TO YOUR BENEFIT

Tony Beshara (2008) suggested that by recognizing your personality type and that of your interviewer, it may be easier to answer questions as well as pose your own. With that, it was noted that in 370 BC, Hippocrates defined four basic personality types:
1. The *analytical* type is highly detail-oriented, can make difficult decisions without all the facts, is perceptive, and may tend to be pessimistic.
2. The *driver* type tends to be blunt, is objective focused, is a hard worker, makes quick decisions, is independent, and is considered a can-do person.

There is a tendency to be assertive, distrusting, impatient, high energy, and motivated by external recognition.
3. The *amiable* type likes to be liked, is easygoing, and is not a big risk taker. He or she likes to blend in, is highly sensitive, has difficulty making firm decisions, and can be quiet and soft-spoken.
4. The *expressive* type is a natural salesperson and storyteller. He or she is gregarious, a good motivator, tends to exaggerate, leaves out facts and details, and is relationship-oriented.

An easier way to remember the four types is to associate them with characters from Charles Schultz's *Peanuts* comic strip: Linus, who is the analytical type; Lucy, who is the driver type; Charlie Brown, who is the amiable type; and Snoopy, who is the expressive type (Personality Types, 2011).

Being able to recognize different personality types around you is a plus. It is recommended that you practice this identification skill with other students and friends so recognizing personality type comes quickly to you. Some examples of conversation responses to individuals with these types of interpersonal styles can be found in Box 22-1.

POTENTIAL REFERENCES

Take a moment to consider who has seen you work and might be willing to confirm in writing and verbally that you are someone employers should hire. Instructors, unit managers, supervisors, team leaders, staff registered nurses (RNs), and LPNs/LVNs are potential sources of references and job openings. With respect to references, ask them in person for permission to use their name as a reference. Do not assume an instructor or anyone will give you a positive reference. Specifically ask, "May I list your name for a positive reference?" If yes, write down the nurse's name (spelled correctly), job title, work address, and work

---

Box 22-1 | **Responding to Individuals through the Four Major Interpersonal Styles**

Analytical type: Tell me how the patient is. (Speak rapidly and to the point about the patient's status.)

Driver type: How is your day going? (Speak slowly and deliberately, hitting the highlights of the shift.)

Amiable type: How are we doing today? (Start off with small talk, such as "The day has been going good," and then go on to highlights of the shift. If there is a problem, present it to them with a solution and ask if they are in agreement.)

Expressive type: Did Mr. Jones get his dinner yet? (Start off with small talk, and leave an opening in the conversation for her to fill, such as "Yeah, but I don't think he was too happy about the peas on his plate.")

Box 22-2	Sample Letter to Reference Writer

May 12, 2014

Ms. Valerie George
Surgical Care Charge Nurse
Veterans Hospital
1000 Veterans Lane
Minneapolis, MN 55402

Dear Ms. George,

Thank you again for agreeing to be a work reference. My experiences on the medical-surgical unit were both challenging and rewarding. I am pleased to have the opportunity to use the skills you taught me.

I am actively seeking employment in medical-surgical units at hospitals within the metro area. A letter of recommendation from you is definitely an asset to my job search.

Knowing your busy schedule, I have enclosed a possible letter of recommendation for your review and signature. However, if you prefer to write your own letter, you may wish to mention my ability to work under pressure, ability to administer medication on time, communication skills with staff and patients, computer proficiency, and willingness to take on new assignments.

Your assistance in helping me secure employment is greatly appreciated. I plan to give you a call next week to let you know how my job search is going and answer any questions you may have regarding the letter. I look forward to talking with you soon.

Cordially,
Katelyn Bieser

2001 Putt Drive
Cottage Grove, MN 55016
612-555-2728 or ktbieser@star.com

ENC: Reference letter

Box 22-3	Sample Letter for Reference Writer to Complete and Place on Facility Letterhead

Dear Employer:

Please accept this as a letter of recommendation for Ms. Katelyn Bieser, whom I supervised during her medical-surgical rotation. Katelyn was enjoyable to work with and displayed a high degree of skill as a student practical nurse.

Specifically, she learned new tasks quickly, measured patient vital signs, was proficient in computer charting, provided nutritional care, and administered medication promptly. Ms. Bieser was able to follow both physician orders and RN instructions and had a keen sense of knowing when to ask for help.

I believe that Katelyn will make a positive contribution to any hospital/company she chooses to work for. Should you have further questions about Katelyn's skills and abilities as a nursing professional, please feel free to contact me.

Cordially,
Valerie George, RN
Surgical Care Charge Nurse

telephone number. Also, take the initiative and ask for a letter of recommendation. Be sure to acknowledge their busy schedule and ask if they'd prefer you to draft a possible letter for their use (see Boxes 22-2 and 22-3). Also consider using managers and employees with whom you have worked as a volunteer or health care worker.

NETWORKING YOUR WAY TO SUCCESS

Smart **networking** of influential people can lead to finding new jobs, better pay, faster promotions, and greater job satisfaction.

- **Placement personnel** are good sources of job opportunities. Register with the school's career service center and local state Job Service/Workforce Centers. Go to the school's placement office frequently, with a smile on your face. This will make them smile as well and store you in their memory job bank. Also, plan to attend job fairs, trade shows, or professional association conferences. Talk to the recruiters, learn about job opportunities, provide your resume, and obtain their business cards.
- **Family and friends with nursing contacts.** Ask them for job leads and names of contacts, and follow up with them every 2 weeks until you get the job. And remember to thank these people for all their help once you get it! You never know if you might need their help again in the future.
- **Media sites.** LinkedIn (www.linkedin.com) is a professional site that can help you find mentors, stay in touch with favorite teachers, and find hiring managers and recruiters in your chosen career. The advantage of LinkedIn is that it allows you to look at others' networks and reach out to them for suggestions and recommendations. LinkedIn has more than 35 million members from 200 countries, has a makeup of 64% male and 36% female, and is considered the must-have tool for ambitious professionals, whether looking for a job now or possibly in the future. Typing in "licensed nurse" or "case manager" will yield some jobs through the associate job search engine Simply Hired (www.simplyhired.com). Today, hospitals, facilities, and government agencies are advertising more through this site, and this is expected to increase in the future. One trick to use is the Advance People Search screen. Type in "nurse," and you will get three links: Companies, Groups, and Skills. As you search through the links, you will find recruiters, companies, and other health

care professionals you can contact about employment. You will also find recent graduates who are looking for jobs and may be picked up by recruiters who use LinkedIn as part of their regular scouting for candidates.

That said, LPNs/LVNs should consider LinkedIn as an investment site like a 401(k) retirement plan. What you do to invest in the plan now (i.e., making sure your profile is 100% complete; adding LPNs/LVNs, nurse managers, recruiters, short- and long-term disability case managers, and any contacts made through active networking with health care and insurance company staff) will help you later in your career when you are looking for new, higher-paying opportunities.

Social media sites like Twitter (twitter.com) and Facebook (www.facebook.com) can be used to expand your job search network. For a Twitter profile, you should list only the basics about who you are because your online "biography" is limited to 160 characters. Twitter will load your address book and show you which of your contacts are already using the site. And, with that, Twitter will give you the option of inviting people in your address book who are not yet registered to join Twitter. Facebook can be used to access the job sites Simply Hired (www.simplyhired.com) and Careerbuilder (www.careerbuilder.com) to search for job openings. Additionally, it can be used for those who want to post their own ads on a daily basis or on specified dates at a nominal rate.

However, because these sites are primarily for social networking, it is first important to find common experiences to talk about with the contact. From there, when talking about yourself, ease into letting them know what job you are seeking and that any assistance they or others can provide would be appreciated. Just a warning: Using LinkedIn's "InMail" system to contact people who are not part of your network can cost you money. Try contacting these individuals via Facebook because you can do that free of charge.

Here are some tips whether you are using professional or social media sites:

1. Do not add your current employer/supervisor to your network of contacts.
2. Be selective about adding coworkers.
3. Do not add someone to your "friends list" unless you know who they are.
4. Never post opinions about any of your employers.
5. Do not post any nonmainstream beliefs, hobbies, or recreational activities.
6. Never let anyone post items on your "wall."
7. Never announce your intention to leave your current employer because this may lead to a rapid termination. *It is not unusual for potential or current employers to browse social medical sites for individuals under age 30 to see if there is a hit and learn what that person's site reveals about them.*

Box 22-4	Internet Sites for Careers

Career site suggestions include typing "practical nurse jobs" into your Internet search engine or visiting the following websites: ajb.dni.us; careerbuilder.com; careers.org; coolworks.com; careerz.com; nurseuniverse.com; hotnursejobs.com; healthsource.com; nursefinders.com; monster.com; nursingjobs.org; webcrawler.com; healthcareers.com; adevia.com; snagajob.com; 50statejobs.com; indeed.com; healthjob.com; afreserve.com; info.com/lpn; workforce50.com; healthcare.Monster.com; nurse-recruiter.com; usa.gov; topusajob.gov; jobvertise.com; aarp.org/work/job-hunting; lpnjobs.com; usajobs.gov; healthcareerweb.com; job-search-engine.com; employmentguide.com; linkup.com; job-hunt.org/state_unemployment_offices; vacareers.gov; health.usnews.com/best-hospitals; abyznewslink.com; twitjobsearch.com; Facebook.com/get.nursing.jobs; latpro.com; travelnursingjobsabroad.com.

Also, for a quick reference on the median wage in the state you are looking at, go to www.bls.gov/oes/current/oessrcst.htm. Find the blue map of the United Stated entitled "Annual Median Wage," and then highlight the state you are interested in. If looking at opportunities in Canada check out careerowl.com or globecareers.com.

General Internet career search sites should be explored to seek job opportunities. Box 22-4 lists several Internet sites for careers that will prove useful.

Locally, check company websites to find current job openings, the facility's mission statement, any specialties, and locations. You can also Google the name of a nursing home, clinic, assisted-living facility, and so on to get their URL. When using the Internet, it often takes a while to locate job and career opportunity links. After entering the career/job area, try using the "search box" and type in "licensed nurse" or "vocational nurse" as a possible shortcut. The beauty of the Internet is that you can search your local area by individual state and in different countries.

Skype Webcam (www.skype.com) consists of free computer software used in conjunction with a webcam (cameras are relatively cheap) in which families and businesses may communicate with one another via voice or video anywhere in the world. It is also a useful tool for interviewing when travel or associated costs are not practical to meet with the employer. For example, the author once met a woman who had been living in Norway and had now found a job in the United States. She explained that when she decided to move to the United States, she contacted several prospective employers. One was willing to download the software, purchase a $50 web camera, and conduct the interview via Skype. Because the Internet is essentially free, she found a job with minimal out-of-pocket expense. In addition to the computer, Skype can be used on an iPhone, an iPod Touch, or an iPad.

Another good way to find employment is to attend professional conferences or training sessions and "**work the room.**" To do this, introduce yourself to someone you don't know or a group of people, learn something about them in 5-10 minutes of time, and then move on to the next new person or group. With this in mind, understand that although these are not formal interview situations, the people you are meeting for the first time are "sizing you up," just as you are doing to them. As such, it is recommended that you wear the same type of clothes that you would to an interview.

Professional Pointer

First impressions count, and you may be talking with the person who does the hiring, has the boss's ear, or knows of job openings.

Here are some more tips for job hunting:
- Don't bring your "significant other" to the conference. Conscientiously or not, he or she will impose on your time during and after the session. You want to be able to focus on the people you are talking to.
- Plan to arrive early, obtain your name badge, and ask the registration people to point out the key representatives who are conducting the conference. It is likely these individuals know who the "movers and shakers" are and who may be hiring.
- Strike up conversations with the key representatives. If they are not available, look for individuals who are professionally dressed. A good way to start a conversation is saying, "Hi, I am ___ (your first name). Are you part of the conference?" and/or "What part of the session did you come for?" Then, as people sit down for the conference, ask if you might join them.
- Don't sit at a table with other students. They can't offer you a job and don't have the networking connections you're seeking.
- After sitting down with the professional, you might ask, "What are your thoughts about _____ (speaker's topic) and best practices?" Whenever possible, use open-ended questions because they will lead to additional conversation and relationship building. Questions that only require yes or no answers can quickly shut down a discussion.
- At the conclusion of the session, tell the professional that it was a pleasure to have met him or her. Request his/her business card, and if none is available, ask where he/she works. If you are feeling brave, ask, "Is it a good place to work, and why or why not?" Then be prepared to listen. Finally, ask, "Would it be okay to call you at work to check on openings?" If yes, ask for the phone number and the best time to call.

Try This
Networking Your Way to Success

Who are potential individuals I haven't yet contacted? List them in the spaces provided.

Name	Telephone
_____	_____
_____	_____
_____	_____

Networking should be a never-ending process whether you are happily employed or looking for another job. The successful person makes a point of meeting someone new each day, knowing there will be openings if they lose their job to downsizing or are looking for an opportunity to increase earnings or advance their position. When doing so, focus on the following:
- Display a positive affect with everyone you meet (i.e., facility staff, patients and their families, technical vendors, professionals at conferences, etc.).
- Seek your supervisor's input on how to build your career.
- Try to build relationships with key facility people where you work.
- Be willing to lend a hand **without** being asked.
- Ask about facility committees you might be able to participate in.
- Join professional organizations; members often know about job openings before they are posted.

INFORMATIONAL INTERVIEWS TO CREATE FUTURE EXPECTATIONS

Chances are, sometime during your educational program you will be asked to visit community health facilities. Your instructor will provide objectives to help make the experience worthwhile. Focus your objectives or questions on the following areas:
- Purpose
- Hours or shifts
- Staffing patterns
- Facility specialty
- The identities of the training staff and their expertise
- Newest technologies being used

Viewing this assignment as an informational interview allows you to find out how the facility works firsthand, assists you in determining whether you would want to work there, and allows you to meet the employer before you actually seek a job.

To obtain an informational interview with an employer, it is important to practice with another individual prior to making that telephone call. It may be tempting to use the example script without practicing in advance, but if you do, remember that this is exactly how you will sound: as though you are reading a script! The following is an example of a telephone request:

1. "Hello, my name is _____ (first and last name)."
2. "Who is the manager for the _____ (specialty floor or area you are interested in)?" (Emphasis is on first learning the name of the right person. Do *not* begin by asking, "May I speak to the manager for _____?") You can also try to bypass human resources and talk directly to the decision maker (i.e., cardiac floor nurse manager).
3. "Please connect me with Mr./Ms. _____."
4. "Hello, Mr./Ms. _____. My name is _____ (first and last name)."
5. "I am a student practical/vocational nurse at (school's name)."
6. "As a part of my learning experience, I would like to visit your facility and meet with you."
7. "Would it be possible to set up an informational interview tomorrow at 9:00 AM or perhaps the following day at 2:00 PM?"
   - *If the answer is yes:* "Great! I'll see you on _____ (day). Thank you!"
   - *If the answer is no:* "Is there someone else you recommend that I contact there?"

Voice control is important as you will be judged on how you sound to others on the telephone and at the interview. It is important to understand that spoken English is broken down into five areas:

- *Low-pitched:* Sounds more mature and truthful
- *Nasal:* Signals a low status and grates on the listener's ears
- *Monotone:* Sounds boring and puts people to sleep
- *Loud:* Viewed as dynamic but shifty
- *Whiny:* Implies a lack of self-confidence—a turnoff

Your friends can help you gain control over your voice by modulating with you, or you can find voice self-help books and/or companies that can help you to speak more clearly and pleasantly.

◎ Try This

Practicing and Getting a Critique of Mock Interviews

With a peer, make a digital recording of you making informational interview requests, using the telephone script in this chapter. Ask them to play the part of the employer on the other end of the telephone line. Evaluate the ease with which you present yourself, how your voice sounds, and the pitch and fluency of your speech. Listen to the recording while they give you feedback. Then practice with them until your voice sounds right with minimal effort on your part.

You should not encounter any difficulties when you speak directly to top nursing management to request an informational interview. Management wants to "get the word out" about their facility and will often give tours and let you meet the training staff. However, do not make the mistake of turning this into a job interview. No one likes to be tricked and management tends to have a long memory about such things.

Arrive looking sharp! This is not a T-shirt, shorts, jeans, and sandals casual meeting. Consider the interview as an opportunity to get insider information about what employers are looking for in potential employees. Keep a copy of the information you obtained with the name, address, and phone number in a safe place (ask for their business card) for the time when your job search begins. Follow up the informational interview with a thank you letter, and mention the staff you met by name. Employers will sometimes share letters like this with their staff, which will bring a smile to their face. Who knows—this may gain you allies should you apply for a job there (Box 22-5).

Box 22-5 | **Follow-Up Letter After Informational Interview**

January 22, 2014

Ms. Elizabeth Ekholm
Director of Nursing
Lyngblomsten Health Care Facilities
1415 Almond Avenue
St. Paul, MN 55118

Re: Informational Interview

Dear Ms. Ekholm:

Thank you so much for meeting with me yesterday. The information you provided was both valuable and interesting. Your suggestions about what employers are looking for and which areas to focus my schooling on were very much appreciated.

I found that the variety of programs offered was progressive and individualized to meet the needs of the resident and their families. The tour that followed supported your comments about the positive interactions between staff and patients. I was pleased to have the opportunity to meet staff trainers Ms. Abbinante and Ms. Wexler, who certainly inspire confidence.

I can only hope to be fortunate enough to work at such a center after my graduation this June. Thank you again!

Sincerely yours,
Katelyn Bieser

2001 Putt Drive
Cottage Grove, MN 55016
612-555-2728 or ktbieser@star.com

SEARCHING FOR EMPLOYMENT OPENINGS

If you expect to work shortly after graduation, it is important to apply for employment approximately 2 months before that date. Obtain a telephone answering machine, use a telephone "voice mailbox" service, or use your cell phone so you do not miss any calls from potential employers. Record a professional-sounding message, such as the following:

> "Hi, this is _____ (first name), and I am not available right now. Please leave your name, telephone number TWICE, and the reason for your call. I will return your call as soon as possible."

If you are not going to graduate until December, do not fret. It is a myth that the November–December holiday season is the worst time to look for a job. Actually, it can be one of the best times. Employers are usually looking at staffing patterns for the new year.

You need to do some homework in preparation for seeking employment. Find out all you can about the facility where you would like to work. Facilities often provide websites or give out free pamphlets as part of their advertising. An easy way to locate company websites is to use search engines like Google, Yahoo!, or MSN and type in the company name. Look for the facility's "mission statement"; determine the number of people they employ and annual profits earned.

Use the Internet to search for news stories/releases so you can work current events into your interview and talk about how your skills relate. A good site is www.healthcarefinancenews.com, which addresses health care business issues that are of interest to employers. Or if considering a move to another community, check into www.abyznewslinks.com, which enables you to visit hometown newspapers for local stories throughout the world.

It is generally accepted that 75% to 85% of all available jobs are not advertised. Do not wait for an ad to appear before seeking employment. Here are some ways to tap the "hidden job market":

- Get assistance from family and friends.
- Get employee/staff recommendations from your school clinical site(s).
- Submit direct applications to employers.
- Do internal job searches. For example, depending on your skills, you could obtain less skilled employment with a health care provider in a different job that would allow you to post for jobs internally before they are released to the public. Jobs might include sterile service technician (process/package surgical instruments), certified nursing assistant, health care coder (ICD-10), or physician's e-scribe (person who follows the doctor to patients' rooms and charts the doctor's notes so the physician is free to serve more patients and make money for the hospital).
- Search company websites, using terms such as "careers," "employment," "jobs," and so on.
- Use State Job Service/Workforce Centers.
- Use Internet job sites (i.e., Careerbuilder.com, Indeed.com).
- Find out about your school's social alumni network sites, or if they don't have one, try Twitter.com to see who may be alumni and then throw out an ice-breaker to get the conversation rolling (i.e., "What dorm did you live in the first year?" or "Was instructor _____ there when you were there, and what did you think about her class?").
- Use private employment or recruiter companies (i.e., type "practical nurse recruiters" into your search engine).
- Search state or federal government websites.
- Read school placement office postings/e-newsletters.
- Do volunteer work, and read professional association newsletters.
- Contact the state's nurses' union and ask about employers who are hiring.
- Use recruiting services. The three types of staffing services are temporary or contract, in which employees work for a specified period of time; temp-to-hire, which allows employees to work with an employer on a trial basis, and if it is a "good fit," they may be offered a permanent job; and direct hire, where the employee is recruited by a staffing service and then hired by the client. Determine which service will best meet your needs.
- Job fairs are typically advertised 2 to 3 weeks before the event, so visit the companies' websites and find out all you can about the companies. You can forward your resume to the fair producers both before and after the event. The producers frequently forward resumes to participating employers at no cost to you. If you attend a job fair, go prepared with a high-energy, *30-second pitch or elevator speech* that covers your key skills, your passion for that type of work, and how it's related to the needs and goals of the recruiter's company. Since most applicants don't have a prepared speech, your presentation will make you stand out.
- Participate in virtual job fairs, such as through www.employmentguide.com/browse-jobfairs.html.
- Beware of scam job ads. Since 2006, phony job ads have increased by 345%. With such a tough job market, people's eagerness to find any job until the right one comes along sometimes overrules their common sense. If you see jobs that include home money transfers (convinces the person to open a bank account as a payment representative and then promises a percentage of the money that comes in), an unidentified employer (only willing to discuss the job in an individual or group presentation), requests for personal information via telephone or website,

such as a Social Security number, address, and driver's license, to "run a background check" before the interview, or promises of high salaries for "simple" work, it is best to avoid them. At worst, you may become a victim of identity theft (Pyrtle, 2009).

It is standard practice to apply directly to employers using website job applications, emails, or cover letters and resumes. Often, a traditional brief, to-the-point cover letter, accompanied by a resume addressed to the director of nursing or nursing recruiter at the facility is best. Box 22-6 provides an example cover letter. Do not include a personal reference list or a photograph of yourself with it. Retain the reference list for your interview and provide it only on request. *Follow through on the cover letter by calling the employer for an interview on the day stated in your letter.*

Box 22-6   Sample Cover Letter for Employment

April 14, 2014

Ms. Cheryl Krutchen
Human Resources Director
Columbus Hospital & Clinics
2031 Lakeside Drive
Columbus, MN 55025

Re: LPN Staff Nurse Position

Dear Ms. Krutchen:

I will graduate from the Rainy Lakes Technical College practical nursing program this June. While doing a medical nursing rotation at your hospital, I was impressed by the quality of client care, staff professionalism, and learning opportunities.

In addition to this rotation, my work experiences have included a focus on electronic patient documentation, care coordination under a multidisciplinary approach, follow-through on individualized patient/family plans, working with a diverse population, patient advocacy, and participation in the evaluation process toward achievement of outcomes.

I am interested in obtaining employment at your hospital and being able to work with your staff again. I will contact you on Tuesday, April 21, to see whether you have received my resume and to determine when we might arrange an interview. Should you wish to contact me before then, I can be reached weekdays after 3:30 PM. I look forward to speaking with you.

Cordially,
Katelyn Bieser

2001 Putt Drive
Cottage Grove, MN 55016
612-555-2728 or ktbieser@star.com

It is best to use Sundays and Mondays to research job opportunities and then contact employers from Tuesday forward. The best time to call employers to schedule interviews or make follow-up contacts is after 9 AM. As a rule, most employers don't have the luxury of contacting every prospective job candidate, owing to time constraints and demands of their own jobs. Candidates who are waiting to hear from employers should not hold their breath or be disappointed when employers do not call.

If your resource for a job opening is the newspaper, call for an interview (unless the ad specifically states emails only). Don't forget that a lot of other people are reading the ad, too, and *the candidate who hesitates is lost.* Ask to speak to the person in charge of hiring. Your conversation needs to reflect the following example:

1. "Hello, my name is _____ (first and last name)."
2. "Who is in charge of hiring?"
3. "May I please speak with Ms. _____?"
4. "Hello, Ms. _____. My name is _____ (first and last name)."
5. "Do you have any practical/vocational nursing positions open now or projected in the near future?"
   a. *If hiring:* "Would it be possible to set up an interview on (date) at 9 AM [pause for a moment]." *If no:* "Would 2 PM tomorrow work?" *If no:* "What would be a better time and date? [Offered time and date.] Great! I will see you then."
   b. If they are not hiring or are under a hiring freeze, catch your breath and don't be put off. An acceptable reply then would be:
      • "Oh, I hadn't heard that. Your facility sounds like a great place to work. Would it be possible to meet with you anyway? I would like to be the first person you consider when an opening occurs or the freeze ends." *If yes,* see 5a. *If no:* "Do you know of anyone who might be hiring?"
      • *If yes:* "Would you also know the contact person and/or have a telephone number?"
      • *If no:* "I appreciate your time. Thank you." Or *if no:* "Thank you for trying. Would it be possible for me to come in for an informational interview?" *If yes,* see 5a. *If no:* "Well, thank you again. Good-bye."

Deflect the employer's interview type of questions until the actual interview. Often when employers do not have an opening, they feel it is kinder to applicants to ask some questions and then tell the applicant that he/she is not what they are looking for. Also, you do not want to be "washed out" by a telephone conversation if the employer does have a job.

If the employer begins to ask you questions about your background, education, or work experience, you might respond, "I have completed an accredited practical/vocational nursing program, passed the NCLEX-PN® examination, obtained my license, and have the necessary work experience. I would like the opportunity to discuss my qualifications during our interview." As in point 5a, say, "Would it be possible to set up an interview on Wednesday at 10:00 AM?"

The tone of your voice can makes a significant difference on the telephone. If you smile while you are talking, you will project a positive tone. Practice the preceding format several times in advance with a friend so there are no hesitations in your presentation and you're prepared for what's thrown at you.

Leaving a Voice Mail Message

At some point you may have to leave a phone message for the employer. Here is a script you can practice beforehand:

> "Ms./Mr. ____, my name is ____, and I am calling about a licensed nurse position. I have clinical skills and am willing to work shifts to get my foot in the door. I would like to meet with you and can be reached at _____ (phone number). Again, this is ____ (name) at _____ (phone number). I look forward to talking with you."

REFERENCES: A TIMELESS TREASURE

Prospective employers will be more interested in certain types of work references than others. There is a reference hierarchy of individuals who act as references. Ranging from most to least important are current or former nursing instructors, clinical staff from your clinical rotations, and supervisors from past nursing-related work or volunteer experiences; past employers or supervisors from non–nursing-related jobs; and personal references or friends. (Employers rarely contact personal references because their opinions are likely to be biased.)

 Try This

Pick Your References

List the people in your reference hierarchy, including the person's name, job title, work address, and telephone number. Most employers request three references. Pick and choose from your list of resources for maximum impression.

The statement "References available on request" can be placed at the end of your resume. It is a matter of personal choice because the employer knows he/she will get them if interested. Letters of recommendation (preferred) or a reference list should be given to the interviewer if requested, so bring them to the interview. References, however, are a "treasure." Avoid giving them out if you are not interested in the job. There is no value in wasting your references' time and in the process upsetting them.

RESUMES: THE CONTRIBUTIONS YOU WILL MAKE

Developing two versions of your resume is a must! First is the traditional *design-focused* document you mail and bring with you to the interview. The second is a scannable or *text-focused* resume, which is good for Internet applications and pasting onto email.

Resumes are not a confession or "tell-all" script, nor should they include reasons for leaving past jobs, salary requirements, or personal photographs. Additionally, listing personal data, such as marital status, race, religion, height, weight, number or age of children, social clubs, and so on, is discouraged.

A list of objectives at the top of a resume went out of fashion more than 20 years ago. Resumes should now include a "Summary" or "Profile" (keyword heavy) section. Also, statements on "personal goals" or "health" are a waste of both time and valuable space on your resume.

Many traditional resumes are never read because they are too cluttered, too wordy, or contain the aforementioned problems. Use short, bulleted sentences of no more than two to four words, which allow employers to compare resume key words to their job description. Plan to modify your resume to contain the keywords from the ads you apply to. This will enhance your chances of being contacted for an interview.

Essentially, all resumes have a format of heading, profile/summary, work and military experience, education, and licenses/professional memberships. With respect to the heading, list your email address so employers can reach you any time of the day or night. Some job searchers, as a time saver or depending on the amount of email traffic they receive, will set up a separate free email account. This can usually be done if your server has a free second email line available or by using free email services such as Gmail or Windows Live Hotmail.

It is recommended that you stop and think about what specific classes or jobs you have performed and record them in your resume. Spell out the job tasks, and do not assume an employer will understand a statement like "Performed nursing duties." It is recommended that military/work experience be listed in years rather than specific dates (i.e., 4 years). Do not list more than 10 years of work history, outdated training (i.e., 2007 CPR certification), or old versions of computer programs (i.e., Windows 2003).

Remember that it is important that your resume be truthful. Human resource departments will look for inconsistencies such as work experiences that are too good to be true or resumes that appears purposely vague. Keep your resume consistent and well balanced.

Box 22-7   Basic Resume Factors

SCANNABLE/ELECTRONIC/EMAIL RESUME FACTORS

For a scannable resume, you want no visual distractions to confuse the OCR (optical character recognition) scanner that reads the resume. As noted previously, a text-focused format is required when completing/submitting online applications or faxing your resume:

- **Length:** Two pages maximum; one page is preferred.
- **Paper:** *Quality bond*. Use colors such as white or off-white only (no designs, textures, or recycled paper). Use matching paper for the cover letter and envelope.
- **Type:** Arial typeface (10- to 14-point type) is preferred; underlining, italics, or graphics should be omitted. Bolding is permitted. Avoid multiple columns, newspaper-style layouts, landscape printing, and designer fonts. Always place your name at the top of the page because scanners assume that whatever is at the top of the top of the page is your name. As such, if your resume has a second page, place your name and a "page 2" designation at the top.
- Use the computer's spell check feature, and then proofread the resume from the bottom up so there are no extra marks or spelling or grammatical errors.
- If you don't have a computer, borrow a friend's or go to the library. Type the resume and save it onto a thumb drive, which is cheap and fits in your pocket. For printing, use a laser printer, which is less likely to smudge, or take your thumb drive to a quick print shop. Avoid standard copy machines because they often provide poor-quality copies.
- **Faxes:** Avoid faxing your resume unless it's specifically requested because faxing degrades the text.
- **Emails:** If asked to email your resume as a nonattachment, use the scannable resume. Simply copy and paste it into an email to the employer. However, before sending it to the employer, send a copy to yourself first to see what the recipient will see and then decide if you can use it or need to go with another option of getting the resume to the employer.

- **Balanced space:** An uncluttered, balanced design is desirable so the resume is easy to read. Also, because most managers don't have time to read, a "bulleted" style is recommended when listing your job skills and past duties.
- **Emphasis:** Whether you have a strong or limited work history, keep in mind that your use of keywords will help answer the employer's question "What can you do for me?"

TRADITIONAL RESUME FACTORS

- **Length:** Two pages maximum; one page is preferred.
- **Paper:** *Quality bond*. Use colors such as white or off-white only (no designs, textures, or recycled paper). Use matching paper for the cover letter and envelope.
- **Type:** Arial typeface (10- to 14-point type) is preferred. Underlining, italics, graphics, and bolding can be used to draw the reader's eyes to points being made. Different resume formats may be used, with conservative design recommended. Multiple columns and newspaper-style layouts are permitted. Make a practice of using your computer's spell check feature, and then proofread the resume from the bottom up so there are no extra marks or spelling or grammatical errors. For printing, use a laser printer, or take your thumb drive to a quick print shop. Avoid standard copy machines because they provide poor-quality copies.
- **Faxes:** If specifically requested to fax your resume, use the scannable one.
- **Emails:** Use a scannable resume instead, or send your traditional resume via U.S. mail (snail mail).
- **Balanced space:** Use an uncluttered, balanced design with a "bulleted" list of job skills.
- **Emphasis:** Whether you have a strong or limited work history, keywords are important.

The initial impression made by the resume is very important. Box 22-7 lists some basic factors to consider for scannable/personal and traditional resumes. Figures 22-1A and 22-1B show sample resumes.

COVER LETTERS: TAILORED TO FIT THE JOB YOU WANT

 Try This

Cover Letters

Why do cover letters need to be sent in with resumes?

It is essential to include a cover letter with each resume, whether submitted by email, fax, snail mail, or dropped off with an employer's application. Cover letters directly respond to the job's requirements and refer to any prior telephone conversation with the employer, including "dropping the name" of the person who referred you. If the employer is located out of town or out of the country, it is also a means to discuss your plans to move there with a request to interview for the job via Skype due to the distance involved. Also, for cover letters, neatness, correct spelling, and proper grammar are mandatory. Each letter should be one page, should be an original (never photocopied), should contain no errors or white correction ink, and should be typed in block letter format. If an employer asks for specific experience, be sure to list this in the cover letter, even if the experiences are not listed on the resume.

You may use the same cover letter you send out by post for your electronic mail. It is recommended that you "paste" your scannable resume to the end of the electronic cover letter and send this out as a whole unit rather than as an attachment. This will help you to avoid running into an employer's computer that can't open your attachment and subsequently lose the opportunity. Boxes 22-8A and 22-8B show sample cover letters to employers through an unsolicited telephone call and Internet advertisement.

Katelyn Bieser
2012 Putt Drive
Cottage Grove, MN 55301
Phone: (651) 555-2728
Email: ktbieser@star.com

SUMMARY OF QUALIFICATIONS

Cardiac-oriented Licensed Practical Nurse with rudimentary Spanish who is patient oriented, has working knowledge of sterile techniques, possesses strong clinical judgment, available night shift, and hardworking.

EXPERIENCE

St. Michael Hospital – Minneapolis, MN
Cardiac Unit – Practical Nurse School Rotation   (Spring 2014)
  • Worked with interdisciplinary health care team including patients, physicians, nursing staff, patient families, and social workers.
  • Performed basic data collection, utilized time management, and infection control.
  • Medication administration, measured vital signs, quality assurance, and charting.
  • Patient/family education, positive attitude, and positive learning attitude.

Forest View Nursing Home – Hastings, MN
Certified Nursing Assistant   (Two Years)
  • Served on memory unit, healthcare intervention, and provided direct patient care.
  • Promoted daily living skills, resident feeding/hygiene, and room sanitizing.
  • Measured/charted vital signs, worked with staff of 10, monitored patients with confusion.
  • Positive family interactions, assisted with patient turning/lifting, and duties as assigned.

The Small Town Café – Bloomington, MN
Waitress   (1 ½ Years)
  • Strong focus on customer service, promotion of specials, and cashiering.
  • Grew café customer base by 20%, participated in marketing strategies, and assisted with food preparation so food served hot.
  • Worked full time, including holidays, and welcomed customers by name.

LICENSE/CERTIFICATION

State of Minnesota Board of Nursing – LPN License   (2014 to present)
American Red Cross - CPR Certification   (2011 to present)
Hmong Cultural Awareness Class – School District 916   (Spring 2014)

EDUCATION

Rainy Lakes Technical College – Practical Nursing Diploma

A

FIGURE 22-1A Sample typed resume scannable/electronic plain text/fax.

Try This

Résumé

Develop a resume, and include a cover letter.

ANSWERS TO APPLICATION QUESTIONS

You will be asked to fill out an application either before or after an interview (see the Evolve site for a sample application). It is important that you answer the questions truthfully. If you have had three or more jobs in the past 3 years, the employer will be concerned about this and expect you to supply good reasons for leaving the jobs. Reasons for leaving might include work interfered with school, a layoff, a relocation, career exploration, job stagnation, and so on. Employment gaps might be explained by responses such as laid off, job hunting, returned to school, travel, or family responsibilities.

If there are questions you wish to defer until the face-to-face interview, write "N/A" (for not applicable) or "Will discuss," or leave the space blank. One such area might include expected wage and wages from former jobs. For current wage expected, write "Open" or "Prevailing wage"; do not specify a dollar amount. With wages in former employment, leave the spaces blank if you know you were underpaid, or tell the truth if the wage was fair.

Note that if applying via the Internet, several companies use software job application programs that are set to reject applicants if all the requested data are not provided. Some job experts recommend listing a midrange salary in the box to position you to get the interview. We recommend entering $00.00 per hour

Katelyn Bieser
2012 Putt Drive, Cottage Grove, MN 55301   (651) 555-2728 • ktbieser@star.com

PROFESSIONAL SUMMARY

Key Strengths

- Cardiac-oriented LPN
- Sterile Tech knowledge
- Willing to move

- Rudimentary Spanish
- Strong clinical judgment
- Quality assurance

- Patient oriented
- Available night shift
- Hardworking

PROFESSIONAL EXPERIENCE

St. Michael Hospital, Minneapolis, MN
Spring 2014
PN School Rotation; Cardiac Unit

- Interdisciplinary H.C. Team
- Time management
- Medication administration
- Quality assurance
- Charted data
- Solicited Sup. feedback

- Basic data collection
- Facilitated Sterile Tech's
- Vital sign measurement
- Patient/family education
- Positive attitude
- Assisted staff as needed

Forest View Nursing Home, Hastings, MN   Two Years
Certified Nursing Assistant; Memory Unit

- Healthcare intervention
- Resident feeding/hygiene
- Charted vital signs
- Coordinated with 10 staff
- Positive communications
- Duties as assigned

- Direct patient care
- Promoted ADLs
- Room sanitization
- Monitored patient activity
- Patient turning/lifting, etc.

The Small Town Café, Bloomington, MN   1 ½ Years
Waitress; Full Time

- Active customer service
- 20% Sales increase
- Time mgmt./memory dev.
- Worked holidays, etc.
- Duties as assigned

- Promotion of specials
- Cashiering/Inventory
- Assisted food preparation
- Cleaned restaurant

LICENSE/CERTIFICATION

State of Minnesota Board of Nursing, St. Paul, MN   2014 to present
Practical Nursing
License (LPN)

American Red Cross, St. Paul, MN   2011 to present
Cardiopulmonary Resuscitation
Certification

School District 916, White Bear Lake, MN   Spring 2014
Hmong Cultural Awareness Class

EDUCATION

Rainy Lakes Technical College, International Falls, MN   Diploma
Practical Nursing   2014

B

FIGURE 22-1B Sample typed traditional resume.

and/or going to the employer's place and obtaining a paper application. Remember, lying on any application is typically grounds for termination.

Be aware that you do not have to answer questions about age, religion, marital status, children, physical data (unless they are specific requirements for the job), workers' compensation injuries, or criminal records (unless related to theft, assault, or use of drugs).

An employer's eyes will naturally gravitate toward any blank spaces. Therefore, answer every question, even if it does not apply to you (i.e., for military experience, write "N/A" in the space if you did not serve). Some employers view blanks or "Will explain" as an automatic screen for someone they do not want to employ. Should you choose to answer illegal questions, the examples in Box 22-9 will be helpful. Do not

Box 22-8A   Sample Cover Letter: Unsolicited Telephone Call

August 12, 2014

Ms. Jana Williams, RN
Director of Nursing
St. Helen General Hospital
8354 177th Lane
St. Paul, MN 55084

Re: LPN Staff Nurse Position

Dear Ms. Williams:

Thank you for taking the time to speak with me about the Practical Nurse position. As we discussed, I believe that my clinical work experiences and skills area a good match for the job.

In addition to two-plus years of Nursing Assistant experience, my education, job skills, and abilities also include direct patient care, electronic charting of observations, verbal/written communications, strong interpersonal skills, being safety oriented, advocating patient/family rights, and the ability to perform efficiently and effectively during emergencies.

I will contact you on Tuesday, August 18, to see if you have had an opportunity to review my resume and to determine when an interview may be arranged. I look forward to speaking with you soon.

Cordially,

Katelyn Bieser
2001 Putt Drive
Cottage Grove, MN 55016
612-555-2728 or ktbieser@star.com

ENC: Resume

Box 22-8B   Cover Letter: Internet Ad Response with No Contact Person Listed

Please accept my resume as application for the Licensed Practical Nurse position advertised in Careerbuilder.com. I believe that my work experiences through the Rainy River Technical College nursing program and clinical rotation at St. Michael Hospital are a good match for the position.

As a recent graduate, I will be taking my NCLEX-PN® examination on September 27. My clinical work experiences include a focus on electronic patient documentation, care coordination under a multidisciplinary approach, follow-through on individualized patient/family care plans, working with a diverse population, patient advocacy, and participation in the evaluation process toward achievement of outcomes. Additionally, I have worked as a Certified Nursing Assistant, which honed a positive attitude when working with seniors.

I will contact your company on Tuesday, August 18, to confirm receipt of my resume and to determine when an interview may be arranged. I look forward to speaking with you soon.

Katelyn Bieser
612-555-2728 or ktbieser@star.com

---

attempt to falsify information, because this will provide grounds for dismissal after hiring. Remember, the personnel department may contact your references, schools, former employers, licensing board, and so on to verify the information on your job application and resume.

 Try This

Job Application

Using the suggestions in the text, fill out a practice job application for a nursing position.

Box 22-9   Sample Answers to Illegal Questions

HAVE YOU BEEN HOSPITALIZED WITHIN THE PAST 5 YEARS?
Answer: I do not have any health problems that would interfere with fulfilling the described position.

HAVE YOU EVER BEEN ON WORKERS' COMPENSATION?
Answer: N/A (not applicable) [Or] I am able to perform all of the described job duties.

DO YOU HAVE A CRIMINAL RECORD?
Answer: I have gotten a speeding ticket, but I have never been convicted of crimes involving drugs, theft, or assault. [Or] I have paid for that error in judgment, taken special classes, and am now wise enough not to repeat it.

PREPARING FOR THE INTERVIEW

During an interview, you should also be interviewing the potential employer to some degree (Box 22-10). If you have prepared adequately, you will be able to evaluate whether your job skills, physical abilities, and interests match the objectives of the facility. Remember to bring a copy of your traditional resume, LPN/LVN license (if you have passed the NCLEX-PN® examination), current CPR card, and medical records documenting tuberculosis skin tests, hepatitis B, and tetanus vaccinations, in case they should be requested.

Box 22-10   Sample Questions to Ask the Interviewer

Use four or five of the following questions:
- Can you explain the scheduling process?
- What types of patients will I work with?
- Do you have 8-, 10-, or 12-hour shifts?
- Will I be floated to other units?
- What type of electronic charting system is used?
- How big is the facility, and how many beds are in the unit?
- How long does orientation last, and what can I expect?
- What is the nurse-to-patient ratio?
- What type of uniform is worn? Who purchases them?
- What can you tell me about the culture and environment here?
- Will there be overtime if I want it?
- Will I be working every other weekend?
- Is testing required before going to the floors?
- Is this a new position, or am I replacing someone?
- Will I be required to do any on-call duty? If so, how often?
- Given my interests the ___ unit, is it possible to move there if an opening occurs?
- Are there annual or review-based bonuses available?
- What opportunities does the facility offer for career development?
- Do you provide support or mentoring for new hires?
- Tell me about your background and why you joined this organization.
- What were the results from the last survey? When is the next one scheduled?

If using the Internet via Skype, remember that it is important to look into the camera to simulate looking into the interviewer's eyes. For those who have difficulty looking into a camera, it is recommended you tape a picture of someone onto the computer monitor, at the same level as the camera, to look at. Then it will be as though you are speaking directly to the person and focused on what he or she is saying.

Interviews are stressful not only for you but also for employers. They have to fit interviews into their regular work duties, justify why one job candidate should be hired rather than another, and be on constant guard not to discriminate in matters of age, sex, race, and so on. Knowing that there are concerns on both sides—yours and the interviewer's—will help you be less defensive and answer in an honest and reassuring way.

Part of your responsibility is to help the interviewer become comfortable with who you are and why you should be selected for the job. There are ways to deal with cultural differences and age when encountered in an interview (Box 22-11).

INTERVIEW QUESTIONS AND ANSWERS: A CHALLENGING OPPORTUNITY

Often the first interview question, "Tell me a little bit about yourself," is an icebreaker designed to make you comfortable and determine what is important to you. Take advantage of the question. Put both you and the interviewer on even ground. Do not use the first question as an opportunity to talk about their

Box 22-11   Tips for Handling Differences between the Interviewer and You

Job seekers near or over the age of 50 may be vulnerable in interviews unless they adopt a vital, energetic, and positive approach. If the interviewer is younger than you and slights your age through a question, then a response like "I'm in excellent health, and as you can see by my resume, I have a solid work history and am not afraid to learn new things" would be appropriate. If the employer representative is older than you, an appropriate response is "I have always been surrounded by workers older than myself, which taught me to work hard and listen to what they had to say."

With respect to cultural background, when there are differences between you and the interviewer, you need to remember that different groups have different norms concerning eye contact, the loudness of your voice, personal distance, body language, joking/teasing, divulging too much information, and other subtle aspects of communication such as the use of metaphors, proverbs, and colloquialisms.

It is recommended you follow the interviewer's lead in the course of communication. Additionally, you can never go wrong by being polite, and if you are unclear about what was said, say, "Excuse me, I'm not quite following what you're asking. Could you ask it in another way?"

illegal job application questions, your dysfunctional family, the bad day you have had because of a fight with your significant other, and so on.

Prepare for your interview by practicing sample responses to typical interview questions (Box 22-12). Do this as role-playing with another person in the role of the interviewer. For better preparation, ask the person to mix up the order of the questions. Have them include so-called illegal questions. This will prepare you to handle these questions effectively and make

you appear confident when the actual interview occurs.

By being prepared, you will not fall victim to the interviewer's most powerful tool: silence. Candidates will usually try to fill the void of silence by providing more information (often revealing details beyond their prepared answers) than they should. If this should happen to you, smile at the interviewer and wait for the next question. An example of "too much information" is:

Box 22-12   Sample Interview Questions and Answers

Tell me about yourself.
Answer: Would you like to know about my work history or personal life? *If work history*, discuss your passion to help care for and treat people. Then provide a brief description of your schooling, past jobs, and goals to work as a staff/long-term care (or whatever) LPN. *For personal*, you might say, I have lived in this area all my life, (or) my plans are to make this area my home. I recently graduated from Rainey River Technical College and am looking for a career I can grow in.

Have you ever done this type of work before?
Answer: Yes, in fact some of my experiences include direct patient care during clinical rotations, volunteer work as a hospital volunteer, experiences as a mother, and. . . .

Why do you want to work here?
Answer: Your company has an excellent reputation in the community and has job opportunities that I am trained in. Additionally, this company's mission statement of _____ reflects my views on _____.

What motivates you?
As a nurse I am motivated by work and its challenge of my skills on a daily basis. I know with the right employer, I will continue to learn new skills as nursing changes.

Why did you leave your last job?
Answer: As you know, I am a recent graduate and am looking for employment in my field of study. *Note:* If you have worked as an LPN/LVN: I am looking for a new position to expand my work skills, keep the job interesting, and provide better advancement opportunities.

Tell me about your last employer.
Answer: I really enjoyed my work at _____, which has an excellent reputation for _____. But now it is time to move on to new opportunities.

What have you done to keep your clinical skills current?
Answer: Well, in addition to participating in several clinical rotations during school, I recently joined the _____ (LPN professional organization) to keep abreast of new developments in nursing.

How do you compare your verbal skills with your writing skills?
Answer: Organizations are more dependent than ever on their employees' communicating well both verbally and in writing. I am constantly taking advantage of opportunities to develop in both areas by asking for feedback and then putting the suggestions into practice.

Why should I hire you instead of someone else?
Answer: I think my references can best answer that question. I am sure when you contact them, they will agree I am hardworking and dependable and get the job done correctly.

When are you available for work?
Answer: Right away. [Or] I would need to give my employer 2 weeks' notice. It will provide me time to tie up loose ends and give my employer time to find a replacement. *Note:* If the interviewer insists you terminate your job immediately, you are witnessing a power play. You need to ask yourself if you really want to work for this individual. This could be the tip of the iceberg for future power plays.

How is your health? Are there any parts of the job you can't perform?
Answer: I have always been in good health. I see myself being able to perform all parts. I think the best approach to any job is to use common sense. If I need help, I am not afraid to ask for it.

What are your greatest strengths?
Answer: I would have to say that my strengths include (1) _____, (2) _____, (3) _____, (4) _____, and (5) _____.
Note: Your responses should be consistent with what your references say about you.

What is your greatest weakness?
Answer: As you know, everyone has weaknesses. My greatest weakness right now is the various computer programs out there for charting on patients. Due to this, I prefer to be shown how to use the facility's program rather than be told to read the manual. I like getting things done right the first time

What are your long-term goals?
Answer: Eventually, I would like to work as a Charge Nurse at this facility. Although my aim is not to replace the current Charge Nurse, it is my goal to learn all I can. This will help me better contribute to the team, and you will feel confident that the work is being taken care of.

Continued

| Box 22-12 | Sample Interview Questions and Answers—cont'd |

Has an employer ever fired you?

Answer: Before going to nursing school and getting my priorities straight, an employer fired me for attendance problems. It was a valuable lesson that I learned from and will never repeat. *Note:* Do not start your response with "Yes"; address the issue.

How do you approach doing things that you don't like to do?

Answer: I tell myself, "Let's get it done, and done right." There is nothing worse than having to go back and redo work that was done incorrectly the first time.

Can you work under pressure?

Answer: Yes, I have experienced working under pressure for many years. This has meant meeting deadlines, dealing with difficult people, and developing employer confidence that the job will be done right.

Will child care be an issue?

Answer: No, I have found a good day care setting for my children. If they cannot go to day care, I have worked out a system of alternating days with another provider or relative to take care of them so that work is minimally affected. *Note:* Although some individuals believe this is an illegal question, I contend the employer has a right to know. A stable staffing pattern is needed to maintain quality patient care.

Would you be willing to work overtime?

Answer: Yes, if it will help the unit.

May we contact your current employer?

Answer: Yes, but only after a firm job offer has been made. I would appreciate it if before you contact my employer, you will allow me to talk with my supervisor first as a courtesy.

Aren't you overqualified for this job?

Answer: I may be more qualified than other individuals you are considering, but this simply means that I will be able to make an immediate contribution. After learning your system, I hope to be eligible for advancement opportunities within the organization.

Is your spouse employed? Will there be a conflict?

Answer: Yes, my spouse has a job. No, I do not see that there would be a conflict. We are both looking forward to my working for you.

What kind of salary or wage do you expect?

Answer: What would a person with my background and qualifications typically earn in this position with your company? [Or] I am ready to consider your best offer. *Note:* If an employer insists you give a wage quote, give a wage using your bottom dollar and a realistic top wage.

Answer: I would think we could agree on a salary between $00.00 per hour and $00.00 per hour. (Note that an hourly wage, not an annual salary, is stated.)

Salary resources include the Internet and labor market sites through your local Job Service/Workforce Centers. Right now, you can use the average median wage because you are new to the profession. Internet sources include www.salary.com; www1.salary.com/Licensed-Practical-Nurse-salary.html; and www1.salary.com/Licensed-Practical-Nurse-Home-Care-salary. html. Also check www.payscale.com/research/US/Job=Licensed_Practical_Nurse_(LPN)/Salary and www.glassdoor.com/Sala ries/licensed-practical-nurse-salary-SRCH_KO0,24.htm. For an idea about the national average median wage, check www.bls.gov. Additionally, if you are considering relocation to another city/state, you are encouraged to use www.salary.com/costoflivingwizard to determine how much salary you will need to maintain your current standard of living. For instance, during the year 2010, an entry-level LPN earning $34,944 in Minneapolis, Minnesota, needed to earn $41,076 in Chicago, Illinois, to break even. The cost of living was 17.5% higher in Chicago. To determine the hourly wage, take the annual wage and divide it by 2080 (hours) for someone working 40 hours per week.

Do you have any questions?

Answer: (See Box 22-10 for questions to ask the interviewer.) After your questions, ask if it would be possible to take a tour of the facility and ask about the date you might start.

How do you deal with criticism, and describe a time you were criticized for poor performance.

Answer: A person who does not make mistakes will never grow. Most recently, in school, I had problems with time management. Due to this, I did not do very well on a couple of tests, and my teachers let me know they were disappointed because I had not done my best work. I agreed they were right and asked for assistance. One of my teachers then showed me how to improve my time management so the problem would not happen again. And it didn't.

How do you vent anger or frustration if your day has been challenging or stressful?

Answer: I am a walker and a talker. My first choice is to burn off the stress by walking/biking/going to the gym/whatever. I always feel better after exercising. If that is not available, I will go outside on my break alone and talk out the problem and associated emotion. It is amazing what talking for 10 minutes will do for getting perspective back.

Do you have a valid driver's license?

Answer: I will use the city bus system to get to work. If the buses aren't running, there is always a taxicab available, plus I have a network of friends who can help me in a pinch. I have never been late to work.

Is there any time when it is okay to break company rules?

Answer: Yes, if someone's life is in danger.

How do you handle change?

Answer: It is all about attitude! If you go in with the thought that the proposed change will help you do your job better and improve patient care, it is easy to embrace it.

Continued

Box 22-12	Sample Interview Questions and Answers—cont'd

ILLEGAL QUESTIONS/RESPONSES

You do not have to answer these questions.

What religious faith are you?

Answer: Religion certainly is a part of this great country of ours, but I prefer to separate religion from work.

That's a nice name. Is it Jewish/Muslim/Irish/other nationality?

Answer: America is a melting pot. That is why it is the greatest country on earth. I feel we are all Americans first and foremost, and that's the most important issue here. Don't you agree?

Have you ever been tested for HIV?

Answer: No, I have never had a reason to test for HIV, nor do I anticipate a reason to do so. [Or] No, has this facility had HIV problems?

You look gay to me. Are you gay?

Answer: I've heard that employers will sometimes ask questions to see if they can make the applicant upset and observe their reaction. Personally I do not care if someone is gay as long as they are professional and do their job. I have always assumed this is important to employers, too. Now, isn't that what this interview is about?

[Male nurse] The supervisor is Janet Smith, who, while being very good, is also very tough and can't seem to keep male staff on her unit. Why do you think you would be different?

Answer: First off, I work well with both male and female bosses. They, like me, have a job to do, want it done right, and want to go home at the end of the day feeling like something was accomplished. So if there is a better or faster way to accomplish job tasks and to communicate with everyone, it is her job to see that it is done that way.

You have applied for a part-time job and appear to be in your forties. Why do you want this job? (Oliver, 2005)

Answer: Sometimes you have to take a step backward to move your career forward. Starting part-time will allow you to see what kind of employee I am and then think of me first when a full-time opportunity becomes available.

I see from your resume that you changed jobs a lot. Do you get bored in a job quickly and find yourself wanting to move? (Oliver, 2005)

Answer: I've enjoyed all my jobs and the challenges they presented. The reason I changed jobs was to bring my salary up to a living wage and to pay for school. My parents were not in a position to help me out financially, so each successive job helped to better pay expenses.

Patients and their families can be pretty mean. Are you sensitive about your weight?

Answer: In my younger days, it was a problem, but now I like who I am and the profession I have chosen. Insults are like emptying bedpans. You flush them away and move on.

Tell me a personal or work story about something that went wrong and what you did about it.

Answer: A friend of mine was celebrating her birthday on a weeknight at one of the local bars. There were folks there I had not seen in a long time, which meant staying longer to get caught up with them. The next thing I knew, it was 3:00 AM, and I had to be at work by 8:00 AM. Needless to say, I was pretty tired and useless that day at work. Never again did I stay out later than 10:00 PM on a work night. It just was not worth it.

It's your lunch break, and you see a resident fall. What would you do?

Answer: I would stop eating, notify another staff member to let the charge nurse know, and then assist the resident as needed. Like CPR, we want help on the way in case the fall is more serious.

Please discuss how you handled a situation when an irate physician, coworker, patient, or patient's family member was involved.

Answer: There was a day at the nursing home when we were short-staffed, had a new resident moving in, and had to remove the belongings of one who had recently passed away. An out-of-town daughter of one resident turned on the call light and began yelling in the hallway that her father needed a drink of water. Upon entering the room, the daughter continued to yell about how her father was being neglected and that she would be making a complaint to the state.

The first thing I did was smile and thank her, in a quiet voice, for letting us know that her father needed assistance. I then went to her father, poured him a glass of water, and asked him how he was doing. When she began to yell again I asked her to lower her voice so I could hear what her father had to say. This was repeated twice more until her voice level dropped. After it was determined that her father was fine and in no distress, I smiled and asked the daughter her name and then introduced myself. Calling the daughter by name, I let her know that her father's care was very important to us, as were all the residents at the facility whose families expected the same. Also, at this point, I reminded her that in the future, if she needed assistance in a similar situation to come to the nurses station and to ask for me rather than to yell down the hallway, which upsets the other residents. She agreed to this, and I then left, letting her know that I needed to care for some other residents and would be back later to check on her father. Following this, I updated my supervisor about the incident.

If you could be doing anything you wanted to right now, what would it be? (Oliver, 2005)

Answer and smile: Celebrating with my friends at a restaurant after getting this job offer. The question now is "When can I make those reservations?"

Question: Why did you leave your last job?

Answer: As you know, I am a recent graduate and am looking for employment in my field of study, *and I have never done anything before but work as a babysitter.* (The italicized portion constitutes "too much information.")

MAKING A LASTING IMPRESSION

 Try This

Impression Counts

The kind of person you are is an additional concern to the interviewer. The impression you make includes everything that has been previously discussed plus your appearance and habits during the interview.

PERSONAL HYGIENE

- Bathe the day of the interview, and wash your hair.
- Make sure your hair is arranged in a moderate style.
- Color your hair. You can let it go back to gray after you get the job.
- Men's hair, mustaches, and beards should be neatly trimmed.
- Keep nails short, clean, and nicely manicured, with clear nail polish (Research has identified long fingernails, fake nails, and nail polish as sites for infection, which subjected some health facilities to litigation.)
- If you are a smoker, remove yellow finger stains with bleach and water.
- Use an unscented or very lightly scented deodorant.
- Floss and brush your teeth, tongue, and palate. Do not consume any food, candy, or drink with a heavy, unpleasant odor or that will stain your teeth or tongue near the time of the interview. Also, carry and use two breath fresheners before you walk into the building.
- Go easy on the aftershave or perfume, and don't sprinkle any on your clothing. Limit yourself to light perfume (a "clean" look and smell go a long way).
- To subtract seven pounds off a middle-age bulge, consider wearing control-top pantyhose.
- To reduce the appearance of skin age, consider using a firming cream for your face and body.
- Smell your clothes; don't go into an interview smelling like you have come from a smoke-filled bar.

CLOTHING

You can contact the human resources department of the prospective employer to ask about interview wear, or you can just take the safe route of interviewing in conservative dress. When choosing clothing, both men and women should try on different suits or blazers to determine which fits best and hangs properly. There should be no overhang or tightness in the shoulder area. Poorly fitting suits look bad and wear out quickly. You will always look your best in conservative clothes that are clean and ironed, with polished shoes. Go to thrift stores and consignment shops; they are resources waiting to be discovered. Additionally, check out www.dressforsuccess.org or Google "clothes closet" for possible sources. When looking for clothing, consider the following points:

Men: Wear a long-sleeved white dress shirt, a solid or pinstripe navy blue or gray suit, and a medallion-patterned red or navy tie that is 3 inches wide and length down to your belt. Wear dark-colored shoes, "long" dark socks, and a belt that matches the color of your shoes.

Women: Choose solid or pinstripe navy, gray, or blue dresses, jacket dresses, or suits. Look for simple, straight or pleated skirts that reach at least knee level and are comfortable to sit in. (Save the sexy, short skirts and/or lack of underwear for other occasions.) If wearing a skirt or suit, consider wearing a white, off-white, or light blue cotton or silk blouse with a conservative neckline and buttons. For women with prominent cleavage, a camisole under the blouse is recommended to keep the focus on your face. Wear dark, polished, low-heeled shoes with closed toes. Women with larger hips will want to avoid wearing short jackets. Short jackets only flatter petite women. Additionally, if wearing a gray jacket, wear a crisp white blouse or a soft beige sweater because gray clothes worn too close to the face will make the complexion look washed out.

MAKEUP

Conservative makeup is always appropriate. Wearing too much makeup is a common mistake; try to keep it at a minimum. Remember: It is the confidence you display in the interview that makes you attractive to the interviewer.

ACCESSORIES

Wear simple jewelry or none at all. Simple necklaces such as a single strand of pearls, colored beads, or a silver or gold chain work well. Avoid drop, dangle, or chandelier-type earrings and noisy charm bracelets that clank or have fake gems. Remove any piercings in the nose, tongue, or lips, and cover tattoos. Also, limit yourself to a small portfolio that is large enough to hold any papers, resumes, and so on. If you have a coat or umbrella, leave it in the car or politely ask where you can hang or lay it. The main point is to avoid holding items or balancing them on your lap. The fewer distractions, the more calm and focused you will be on the interview.

EYEWEAR

Do not wear the latest craze in eyeglasses because they will only serve to distract the interviewer. Wear contact lenses or glasses that contrast the shape of your face.

For a heart-shaped face, consider glasses with a geometric frame that gives some width to the lower half of your face. A square-shaped face benefits from a round or oval frame with some width. A round face should avoid dark frames and use angular and narrow frames—never a square or circle. If the face is oval shaped, use a rectangular frame.

POSTURE

Walk tall and sit erect in the middle of the chair. Both feet should rest on the floor, and your head should be upright. Arms and hands should be in an open position and not crossed. (Remember, you have nothing to hide.) Keep your hands inactive, or if you habitually fidget, consider bringing a paper clip to hold in your hands during the interview.

MANNER

Your manner should be assured. Do not interrupt the interviewer or rush the interview. Pause to think as needed, and then answer without hesitating. Ask for an explanation or repetition of any questions you do not understand. Eye contact is essential, especially when answering questions. If you are uncomfortable with making eye contact, two techniques can be used to correct this: look at the person's nose or look at the space between the interviewer's eyebrows. Both techniques give the illusion of eye contact. Remember to look away periodically so you do not appear to be staring. Avoid making negative statements about your school, former bosses, jobs, current finances, personal problems, and so on. No one likes a whiner!

COURTESY

Arrive for the interview 5 minutes early, and remember to **shut off your cell phone**; don't switch it to mute because the interviewer will still be able to hear it. It is safe to say you can live for 30 or 45 minutes without being able to chat with friends or family. When the employer enters the room, stand, smile, and extend your hand for a firm handshake. Do not use a limp, "dead fish" handshake or "bone-crusher" grip. To get the handshake right, find someone to practice with before the interview. Additionally, if your palms tend to sweat, slide your hands along the top of your thighs, towards your knees, when standing up. It will remove the moisture while appearing very natural.

With a handshake, say, "Hi, Mr. (Ms.) Smith, _____ (your name). I'm pleased to meet you." Similarly, when the interview is over, stand up, look the person in the eyes, and offer your hand for a firm handshake. Address the employer by surname: "Mr. (Ms.) Smith, thank you for the opportunity to interview with you. I am very interested in the job. Would it be all right if I call you next week to see if you have made a decision?" If you want the job, give the employer your work references or letters of recommendation. Last, ask the interviewer for his or her business card. The card will help you when sending your thank you letter (e.g., correct title, name, etc.).

HABITS

Make it a habit to go to bed early the night before so there are no dark circles under your eyes and you appear more energetic. Upon arriving at the employer's, do not chew gum or smoke while in the waiting room or during the interview. Also, do not smoke outside the building and then come in for the interview. Although the nicotine may make you feel calmer, you will be bringing in the fresh smell of smoke, which is often offensive to nonsmokers. Politely refuse an offer of a beverage. In addition, do not attempt to read any materials on the employer's desk or computer screen.

DISCUSSING PREGNANCY ISSUES

 Critical Thinking

Pregnancy

If you are pregnant, what do you need to consider before discussing it with an employer? When should you tell a new employer that you are pregnant? When should you discuss the pregnancy so it doesn't interfere with career advancement?

Even if the Pregnancy Discrimination Act and/or Family and Medical Leave Act will protect your job (FMLA applies if the company has 50 or more employees), pregnancy can lead to some tough questions. It has been this author's observation that women generally wait a couple of months before disclosing the pregnancy. In part, this is to make sure it is a healthy pregnancy, that any financial concerns are addressed, and that the woman is emotionally ready for all the attention.

When you are ready to talk about your pregnancy, be prepared to discuss how long you plan to work, how long you intend to be gone, and possibly how your work will be covered while you are away. Then talk with your coworkers about the pregnancy and enlist their moral support. Expectant mothers will have both good and bad days during the pregnancy, and friends can be a great help.

 Try This

Mock Interview

Enlist a peer to practice traditional and Skype webcam interviews (if planning to move). Take turns in the role of a nurse seeking a job and the employer. Practice asking and answering anticipated questions for an interview. Use the suggestions in this chapter, including appropriate dress and behavior, and stage a mock interview. If possible, arrange with the school's media department or a friend to film the interview. Review the interview and ask your peers to evaluate your performance. Keep an open mind to any criticism given because the goal is to refine your techniques and get you a job.

PREEMPLOYMENT PHYSICAL EXAMINATION, DRUG SCREENING, AND BACKGROUND CHECKS

More and more employers are requiring pre-employment physical examinations as part of conditional job offers. A conditional job offer states that you have been offered the job contingent on your passing a physical examination, drug screening/urine analysis, and/or background check. If you fail, the job offer is withdrawn.

PHYSICAL EXAMINATION

Do not be surprised if you are required to meet with an employer-specified doctor who will perform an examination and can legally ask you about your past medical history. Think about any past surgeries, workers' compensation injuries, allergies, and family history, including cancer and heart trouble. Be prepared to provide the dates of these occurrences and the names of the physicians who provided treatment. If you have any personal concerns about the answers your physician might provide, call the doctor before the pre-employment physical examination to discuss the prospective job and obtain their opinion.

DRUG SCREENING

If you are taking medications, be sure to notify the prospective employer before the screening. You will want to reaffirm in the employer's mind that your treating physician prescribed the medication and its effects will not interfere with your work. Be aware that you may need to provide a copy of your prescription to the employer as verification.

Also, while drug screening accuracy is improving, it is not 100% accurate. False positive drug results may occur if medical conditions such as kidney infection/disease, liver disease, or diabetes exist. Common foods such as anything with poppy seeds, riboflavin in food (vitamin B_2 and hemp seed oil), or vitamin B_2 tablets may trigger false positive results. Additionally, false positive reactions can occur with some prescription medications and over-the-counter medications such as Vicks NyQuil; Contac; Sudafed; Dimetapp; Excedrin IB; Allerest; Robitussin Cold & Flu; Dexatrim; Acutrim; Vicks inhaler; Afrin; cough suppressants with dextromethorphan; asthma medications, including Marax; Bronkaid tablets; and Primatene tablets. If you are taking a prescribed medication, **call your pharmacist** and ask if the medication could trigger a positive drug result.

At this time, it is estimated that there is a 5% to 14% error rate. Due to this, any positive (failed) drug screening test should be followed by a second and more rigorous test. Discuss with the employer that you are aware of reliability problems with initial drug screening tests. State that you would like to take another test but with a different testing service. The employer can name the other service, date, and time for the screening. The key is sincerity; if you want the job, let the employer know you are willing to go the extra mile. If you fail a test and really want the job, you might consider discussing splitting or paying for the cost of the second test.

BACKGROUND CHECKS

Stories abound about individuals who have had successful job interviews, only to lose their opportunity when the employer saw what was on their personal web page or social network site. As such, discussions about partying, recreational drug use, religion, and views about certain classes of people or past employers should be avoided. Additionally, once you have a job, this is not the time to relax and feel you can post anything you'd like. Not long ago, a teacher was fired for trashing her students and community members on Facebook. One of her Facebook friends passed the rant onto the school district, and that was the end of her $92,000/year job! Never forget that others, besides true friends, are reading and developing opinions about what you've written for the world to see.

In 2009, the Society for Human Resource Management (SHRM) (2010) surveyed its employers to see what was being done in the area of employment background checks. The survey showed that 40% did not conduct any checks, 47% checked on select candidates, and 13% conducted checks on all candidates. With respect to employers requesting credit checks, 54% indicated it was to reduce/prevent theft or other criminal activity, 27% to reduce legal liability, 12% to assess the trustworthiness of the candidate, and 7% to comply with applicable state laws.

Oliver (2005) reported that background checks include "employment verification, education verification, criminal records, Social Security trace, basic references, comprehensive references, credit history, and motor vehicle records." Employers may ask you to sign a release of information, or it may be inserted into the job application portion you sign attesting the information you've given is correct. The SHRM found that employers did not extend job offers to prospective employees for the following reasons:

- 64% current outstanding judgments (e.g., lawsuit filed in court)
- 49% accounts in debt collection
- 26% bankruptcy
- 18% high debt-to-income ratio
- 11% foreclosure
- 10% tax lien
- 2% education-related debt
- 1% medical debt
- 3% other

AFTER THE INTERVIEW

Follow-up after a job interview is essential. It is a constant source of amazement to employers that 90% of the people who interview never follow up to see if they got the job. Recent graduates and even nurses who have been working in the field for some time are under the follow-up illusion that it is the employer's responsibility to contact *them*. If you are not interested enough to follow up after the interview, why did you bother to interview in the first place?

Write a handwritten thank you letter (or email, although a letter is preferred) to the interviewer *the same day* you were interviewed. Write it while the information is fresh in your mind and before you become distracted by other projects. Remember, the more often the employer sees or hears your name, the better your chances are of being hired. Do not be the person left waiting for a telephone call. A thank you letter may be as simple as the one provided in Box 22-13.

Remember to follow up with the employer! Call the employer on the date stated in your letter. Make it a practice not to make follow-up contacts on Mondays, which are traditionally full because of staff meetings, weekend concerns, staff discipline, paperwork catch-up, and other duties. The best time to make follow-up calls is after 9:00 AM. The key to a successful

follow-up call is to be courteous but firm with the assistant. Ask to speak with the person who interviewed you.

The following is a sample follow-up contact to an employer:

Assistant: Good morning, Human Resources (do not be surprised if no name is given).

You: Hi, I'm _____ (your name). Is Ms. George available? I am following up on our meeting.

Assistant: One minute, please. (Although the employer might be away from the office or on another line, the assistant will probably check whether he or she wants to take your call.)

Assistant: I am sorry. Ms. George is away from her desk/on another line/in a meeting. May I take a message, or would you like to leave a message on her voice mail?

You: Yes, thank you. Also, when is the best time to typically reach her?

You: (message if transferred to voice mail) Hi, Ms. George, this is _____ (your name), and I am following up on our interview for the LPN staff position to see if you have made a decision. I remain very interested in the job and can be reached at _____ (telephone number). Again, that number is _____ (Say each number of the phone number slowly and clearly.)

You: (If the employer takes your call) Hi, Ms. George, this is _____ (your name), and I am following up on our interview for the LPN staff position. I was wondering if you have made a decision yet? Oh, you have not. Would it be okay to call you next Tuesday to see if you have made a decision? Great! I will call you then. [Or] Oh, you've decided on someone else? Would you please keep me in mind if that person does not work out or if another position becomes available?

 Try This

Thank You Letter

Compose a thank you letter after an employment interview for a nursing position.

RESIGNATION WITH STYLE

 Try This

Keep the Connections

Is there a difference between "burning bridges" and "untying the connection"? What is the value of recapping your accomplishments with a resignation letter?

In today's job market, employers continue to try to hold down their costs by limiting annual raises to 3%

Box 22-13   Letter—Thank You for the Interview

August 12, 2014

Ms. Irene Fedun, RN
Director of Nursing
St. Helen General Hospital
8354 177th Lane
St. Paul, MN 55084

Re: LPN Staff Nurse Position

Dear Ms. Fedun:

Thank you for meeting with me today to discuss the LPN staff position. After our conversation about the job duties and the tour of the hospital floor, I feel that my work experiences and education are a good match for the job. I am especially interested in working on the Memory Unit because this is a special interest of mine. Through our work together, the patients will receive timely, quality care.

I remain very interested in the position. I will contact you on Tuesday, August 18, to see whether you have made a decision or whether a second interview will be arranged. I look forward to speaking with you soon.

Katelyn Bieser
2001 Putt Drive
Cottage Grove, MN 55016

612-555-2728 or ktbieser@star.com

or less. However, in their desire to staff positions, some employers will offer job-hoppers (i.e., frequent job changers) 10% to 20% over their current wages, offer sign-on bonuses, and/or provide higher shift differentials.

If you are contemplating a change, it is recommended that you look at how long you have been with the employer. If you have worked with the company less than 3 months, you can hop right away, remembering not to list the employer on your resume. In the event that you have worked longer than 3 months with the employer, it is recommended that you work a minimum of 1 year to obtain experience and demonstrate stability. (Contact your state board for length of time because it varies from state to state.)

If you have made the decision to leave your employer, it is important to leave the job with class. Perhaps the best expression is "Untie, don't sever, the connection." You never know who may call your former employer as a part of their follow-up.

It is strongly recommended that you have a position secured before leaving. Many employers today have what is called **"at will" employment**. Simply put, you or the employer can terminate your employment at any time for any reason without advance notice. As such, an employer may terminate your job the day you give notice.

That being said, we have found that several "at will" employers have personnel policies requiring that a 2-week notice be given when resigning. The policies typically indicate that if a 2-week notice is given, the employee will be eligible for future rehire.

It is **resignation courtesy** to give 2 weeks' notice whether or not a policy is in place. This is a courtesy to your coworkers and to the employer so a new person might be hired and orientated before you leave.

Use a business format and plain paper, and type the letter of resignation. Even if you are leaving because of unhappy circumstances on the job, do not vent these feelings in the letter. As mentioned before, you may need this employer as a work reference in the future. Additionally, your current supervisor may also leave

in the future, and all there is to remind the employer about you is your personnel file.

Because resignation is part of your permanent record, it provides you with an opportunity to recap your accomplishments or special recognition. The employer may refer to the letter when employers with whom you are seeking employment contact him or her. See the sample resignation letter in Box 22-14.

Box 22-14 Sample Resignation Letter

September 24, 2016

Ms. Sivia Hinkkanen
Director of Nursing
George County Hospital
1515 Rodeo Lane
Minneapolis, MN 55401

Dear Ms. Hinkkanen:

Please accept my resignation as Charge Nurse on Unit 3, to be effective on October 1, 2016. My association with the George County Hospital has been rewarding professionally and personally. It is satisfying to have been able to contribute to the positive reputation of client care.

I am especially pleased to have been a member of the Quality Assurance Committee, which furthered my professional growth. In addition, I remain appreciative of having been honored as "Employee of the Month."

Please accept my thanks for the support you have provided me during the past one and a half years of employment. I wish the members of this hospital the very best.

Cordially,
Katelyn Bieser, LPN,
Alzheimer's Unit

Try This

Letter of Resignation

Compose a letter of resignation from a nursing position.

Box 22-15 Possible Response to Critical Thinking Scenarios [see end of chapter]

From the day we are born until the day we die, we judge people and they judge us on how we look, act, talk, and respond to the environment. Based on this, decisions are made to like, dislike, or not care one way or the other about a person. For the Western culture there is a drive towards being youthful and fit, being a "man's man" or a "woman's woman," and having energy to burn. It is neither good nor bad—it just is! So play the game, get the job, and—afterwards, when you get the job—decide what to let go. Below are checklists for Jeanne and Jack's consideration:

Jeanne:
1. There are always kids' activities. Are you getting a good night's rest before the interview?
2. Did you use some makeup for under the eyes and light blush for the checks?
3. Are there some extra face wrinkles that a little face cream would hide?
4. If there is gray in your hair, wash it away with your favorite natural color.

Continued

| Box 22-15 | Possible Response to Critical Thinking Scenarios [see end of chapter]—cont'd |

5. Will you look a few pounds slimmer with control-top panty hose?
6. Confirm you have a firm handshake and pleasant-sounding voice.
7. Practice quick responses to interview questions and in turn project confidence.
8. Go back through the chapter and review all the job sources other than the newspaper.
9. Check the health care business news, using the suggested website, and incorporate the information into a question for the employer to stand above the other candidates.

Jack:
1. Consider a haircut and check your eyewear (if you wear glasses) for a narrower and stronger masculine look.
2. Consider a man's girdle or control-top panty hose for a firmer look.
3. Confirm you are using a firm handshake and lower tone of voice.
4. Are you looking into the interviewer in the eyes?
5. Practice quick responses to interview questions and in turn project confidence.

6. Research the prospective employer and tie in the company's goals into your interview answers or questions about the company. Doing your homework impresses people.
7. Check the health care business news, using the suggested website, and incorporate the information into a question for the employer to stand above the other candidates.
8. Contact the school/rotation staff that offered to be job references and ask them for letters of recommendation.
9. If you interview for a job you like, offer the letters to the prospective employer and suggest they contact the references if there is any question about what you can do for that employer. Remember, do this only if you really want that specific job.

Last, it would benefit both Jeanne and Jack to contact their references through LinkedIn, which will provide additional personal contacts within different companies. Those contacts will know if there are employment opportunities at their companies and may be used as a "name drop" to get an interview. The old adage is, "It is not what you know, but who you know," so use it.

Get Ready for the NCLEX-PN® Examination

Key Points

- To be successful in your job search, it is important to begin your search with the first day of classes and continue from that day on.
- Opportunities present themselves to those who are willing to put forth a little effort and realize that the world does not owe them a living.
- The methods presented in this chapter have proved successful for graduates, people wishing to make career changes, or those wanting to institute a change in their work. Remember to treat your job search like a job.
- Make contacts by telephone or computer, forwarding resumes or cover letters, or by physically going to the employer to apply and schedule an interview.
- Explore the hidden job market via networking, the Internet, or using the telephone book and then calling employers, whether or not an ad has been placed.
- Dress for the job you want, not the job you have.
- Actively follow up on all interviews! Let the employer know you are interested. Remember, the more often the employer hears or sees your name, the better your chances of getting hired.
- If you are hired, send thank you notes to those who helped you. You may need them again someday. Remember, you are responsible for making your own luck.

Additional Learning Resources

evolve Go to your Evolve website (http://evolve.elsevier.com/Hill/Success) for the following FREE learning resources:
- Answers to Critical Thinking Scenarios
- Additional learning activities
- Additional Review Questions for the NCLEX-PN® exam
- Helpful phrases for communicating in Spanish and more!

Chapter Review Questions

1. What interpersonal style is representative of being easygoing, likes to blend in, has difficulty making decisions, and tends to be quiet and soft-spoken?
   1. Analytical type
   2. Driver type
   3. Amiable type
   4. Expressive type

2. Your employer has an employment policy of at-will employment. Which of the following reflects the meaning of this?
   1. The employer expects a 2-week notice before you leave their employment.
   2. The employer will determine the length or extension of probationary periods.

3. The employer may terminate your job immediately without notice or reason.
4. The employer will continue your job indefinitely, provided job requirements are met.

3. An interviewer asks you a question for which you do not have an answer. Which of the following would be an appropriate response?
   1. Ask the interviewer to please rephrase the question.
   2. Begin to answer and switch to a topic you know about.
   3. Smile pleasantly and say you don't know the answer.
   4. Take a key word from the question, and make up a response.

4. What criminal records would automatically preclude you from employment?
   1. Shoplifting offense
   2. Second-degree assault
   3. Possession of a crack pipe
   4. Graffiti/tagging property

Alternate Format Item

1. Which of the following uses of the Internet are helpful in job hunting? (Select all that apply.)
   1. Perform online interview
   2. Identify salary range
   3. Complete job application
   4. Locate job opportunities
   5. Research facility information
   6. Professional and social networks

2. Which of the following should occur after an interview? (Select all that apply.)
   1. Write down, on paper, information learned and points stressed by the interviewer.
   2. If possible, send out a thank you letter to the interviewer noting some of the points discussed during the interview.
   3. Contact your references immediately after the interview and let them know that they may be contacted. Then discuss points about the job the employer stressed as being important.
   4. Follow up 1 week after the interview with the employer to see if there were additional questions to assist in making their hiring decision.
   5. Continue an active job search until a job offer is made.

Critical Thinking Scenarios

Scenario 1

Jeanne is in her late forties, with gray in her hair and recently divorced. She has three children at home, including a senior in high school who plans to go to college, a sophomore in high school, and a child in the eighth grade. Jeanne's ex-spouse was paying alimony until his manufacturing job went overseas. Wanting the best for her family, Jeanne returned to school and became a licensed practical nurse. Unfortunately, the interviews she has found through the newspaper have gone nowhere. Jeanne has the sense there is something more she can do to put her best foot forward. What would you recommend for a woman in her situation? See box 22-15 for possible responses.

Scenario 2

Jack had been pudgy for as long as he could remember, was a little nerdy, and had a slightly effeminate voice. During his clinical rotations, he was a star, and the staff said to let them know if he needed work references. Because Jack's true passion was helping people, his dream was within reach, but now he had to find a job. Unfortunately, when he went to interviews, he would catch strange looks from the interviewers, who did not seem to care about the lack of references. Jack saw his dream slowly slipping away, until a friend offered some ideas. What suggestions would you make to Jack after reading this chapter? See Box 22-15 for possible responses.

The NCLEX-PN® Examination

Objectives

On completing this chapter, you will be able to do the following:

1. Explain the purpose of the National Council Licensing Examination for Practical Nurses (NCLEX-PN®) examination.
2. Research the requirements of your state board of nursing for eligibility to take the NCLEX-PN® examination.
3. Explain the significance of the Authorization to Test (ATT).
4. Describe how Computerized Adaptive Testing (CAT) determines whether you pass or fail the NCLEX-PN® examination.
5. Explain the process of endorsement.
6. Differentiate between a temporary work permit and licensure.
7. Discuss the proven way of preparing for the NCLEX-PN® examination.
8. Explain the legal implications of ignoring the NCLEX-PN® confidentiality agreement and sharing information about the NCLEX-PN® content with others.

Key Terms

Authorization to Test (ATT) (ĂW-thŏr-ĭ-ZĀ-shŭn, p. 321)
candidate (KĂN-dĭ-dāt, p. 318)
computerized adaptive testing (CAT) (p. 318)
confidentiality agreement (kŏn-fĭ-dĕn-shē-ĂL-ĭ-tē ă-GRĒ-mĕnt, p. 323)

endorsement (ĭn-DŎRS-mĕnt, p. 322)
items (questions) (Ī-tĕms, p. 318)
mock examinations (mŏk ĕg-zăm-ĭ-NĀ-shŭns, p. 324)
NCLEX-PN® examination (p. 318)
state board of nursing (stāt bŏrd, p. 318)

 Keep in Mind

Almost without exception, when student nurses are asked about their goal for the year, they respond by saying they want to pass the "boards," meaning pass the National Council of State Boards of Nursing (NCSBN) practical/vocational licensure examination (NCLEX-PN®) to become a licensed practical or vocational nurse (LPN/LVN).

WHAT IS THE NCLEX-PN® EXAMINATION?

The NCLEX-PN® examination is the National Council Licensing Examination for Practical/Vocational Nursing graduates. It is designed to test minimum knowledge, skills, and abilities needed to safely and effectively practice nursing as a new entry-level LPN/LVN. The NCLEX-PN® examination results provide the basis for licenses granted to practical/vocational nurses by state boards of nursing.

The NCSBN developed a secure method of examination. Since April 1994, practical/vocational nursing graduates (candidates) have taken the NCLEX - PN® examination by computer. This method is called computerized adaptive testing (CAT). All candidates have different questions based on how they answer the previous question. Computer technology makes it possible to choose items from a large pool of questions classified by test category and difficulty to match the candidate's ability and fulfill NCLEX-PN® requirements.

All candidates answer a minimum of 85 items and up to a maximum of 205 items in the 5- hour period of time allotted for the examination. Twenty-five of the items are pretest items (possible future test questions) and are not scored. The time allotted includes the confidentiality agreement, tutorial instruction, and scheduled and unscheduled breaks. All breaks are optional. All answers are scored as right or wrong; no partial credit is given. The computer continues with questions until it determines that the candidate passes or fails the examination. If the candidate runs out of time, and the candidate has not answered the minimum number of questions, the candidate fails. If the candidate has answered the minimum number of questions, the computer evaluates the last 60 items, and if the answers were consistently above the passing standard, the candidate passes.

Computerized adaptive testing administers items with difficulty levels so that each candidate will answer about half correctly. These items provide the most information. All candidates answer about 50% correctly because the computer presents them with questions to match their ability. The next item should not be too easy or too difficult. The computer goes down a "pathway" or "branch," and no candidate has exactly the same test. Items that follow are based on the candidate's previous answer. This is why you *must* answer every item on the computer screen as they show up. You will not be able to go back and answer a previous question. The computer calculates each answer before it can choose the next item.

HOW THE NCLEX-PN® EXAMINATION IS KEPT UP TO DATE

The April 2011 NCLEX-PN® examination reflects the outcome of the *2009 LPN/LVN Practice Analysis: Linking the NCLEX-PN® Examination to Practice* (NCSBN, 2009). Currently this survey is conducted every three years. Of the 12,000 surveys sent out, analyzable response rates were 17.7% for paper surveys and 7.0% for the web. The NCSBN (2011) explains the survey as follows:

Newly licensed practical/vocational nurses are asked the frequency and priority of performing 150 nursing activities. Nursing care activities were then analyzed in relation to the frequency of performance, impact on maintaining safety, and client care settings where the activities are performed.

The 2009 analysis indicated the following:
- 87.9% of participants were female.
- 59.7 were white non-Hispanic.
- 20% were African American.
- 7.7% were Latino or Hispanic.
- 4.3% were Asian.
- The average time of employment since licensure was 4.3 months.
- 56% reported working an average of 4.9% years as a nurse aide.
- Nurse participants worked in long-term care facilities (56.9%), community-based or ambulatory facilities (19.8%), and hospitals (16.8%).
- Almost half worked the day shift. An equal percentage worked evening and night shifts.
- Work of the newly graduated 2009 LPNs/LVNs consisted primarily of pharmacologic therapies:
- Safety and infection control
- Activities related to basic care and comfort
- Physiologic adaptation
- The least amount of time was spent on activities related to coordinated care.
- Nursing care was provided primarily to elderly and adult patients.
- Over half of these patients had a chronic stabilized illness.
- Almost half had behavioral/emotional problems.
- Approximately one third of the LPNs/LVNs worked with patients needing end-of-life care.
- Approximately 45.2% of the LPNs/LVNs had one or more administrative duties.
- The most frequent administrative activity was as charge nurse, primarily in the long-term care facilities. The next most frequent was as team leader.
- 61% had earned one or more certifications or completed additional course work.
- The most common certifications included basic life support, IV therapy, and phlebotomy.
- 39% had no additional course work or certification.
- 25.6% had enrolled in the RN program.
- Only minor changes were made in the 2011 Test Plan for currency and clarification.

The entire study, is available online at www.ncsbn.org or you can Google it by typing in "Report on Findings from the 2009 LPN/LVN Practice Analysis: Linking the NCLEX-PN® Examination to Practice." Use the exact title. The practice analysis can be downloaded from the site.

CORE CONTENT

Four phases (steps) of the nursing process (see Chapter 9) are integrated into all areas of the NCLEX-PN® examination. The four phases are the basis for nursing care plans you developed for each patient assigned to you, prior to beginning nursing care on the clinical unit. The four steps (phases) are:
1. Data collection (assessment)
2. Planning
3. Implementation
4. Evaluation

TYPES OF TEST QUESTIONS

The NCLEX-PN® examination contains items (questions) in the cognitive level of knowledge, comprehension, application, and analysis. Most of the questions are at the application and analysis levels. These questions require prioritizing and decision making. The two main types of test questions are multiple choice and alternate item format.

Multiple Choice

The majority of test questions are multiple choice. Each question describes a client or clinical situation. Four options are given from which to choose the correct response.

Alternate Item Format

The NCLEX-PN® examination also includes alternate item questions, including the following:
- *Fill-in-the-blank*. Medicine and IV rate calculations, intake and output totals.
- *Multiple responses*. Select **all** responses that pertain to the question, with no partial credit given. For

example: Which of the following drugs are antihypertensives?

- *Prioritizing* (ordered response). Options (nursing actions) are numbered as first, second, third, and so on, in order of priority, or the mouse is used to drag and drop options in the ordered priority. For example: When doing the Heimlich maneuver, which of the following actions would you do first, second, third, and so on?
- *Figure or illustration* (hot spot). Questions are asked about a chart or figure. Either an answer is chosen from a list or the mouse is used to point and click a "hot spot" as the answer. For example: Click on the hypochondriac area.
- *Chart/exhibit questions*. A question is included with a chart or exhibit requiring use of the chart/exhibit to answer the question. For example: Which lab result is normal?

An on-screen optional calculator is available for your use during the examination. Any format item, including standard multiple-choice items, might include charts, tables, or graphic images. A tutorial is provided on the computer screen regarding the operation of the computer and how to record answers. For general information about the NCLEX-PN® examination, email nclexinfo@ncsbn.org.

Try This

What Is an Alternate Item Question?

Write an example of an alternate item format using problem solving.

TEST FRAMEWORK: CLIENT NEEDS

The content of the NCLEX-PN® examination is divided into four Client Needs categories. Client Needs provide an overall structure for defining nursing actions and competencies for a variety of patients in many settings and are in agreement with state laws and statutes. Two of the four categories are further subdivided. The percentage of test items assigned to each category and limited examples of content are included. Additional examples of content are found in the *NCLEX-PN® Examination Test Bulletin* and the *2012 NCLEX-PN® Examination Candidate Bulletin*, available at ncsbn.org; type "NCLEX-PN" in the search box. The categories and subcategories are as follows (examples, but not a complete listing):

1. Safe, Effective Care Environment
   a. Coordinated Care: 16% to 22%
   Examples: Advance directives, client rights, concepts of management and supervision, confidentiality/information security, establishing priorities, ethical practice, legal responsibilities
   b. Safety and Infection Control: 8% to 14%
   Examples: Accident/error/injury prevention, handling hazardous and infectious materials, standard precautions/transmission-based precautions/surgical asepsis, restraints and safety devices
2. Health Promotion and Maintenance: 6% to 12%
Examples: Aging process, ante/intra/postpartum and newborn care, data collection techniques, developmental stages and transitions, high-risk behaviors, lifestyle choices, self-care
3. Psychosocial Integrity: 6% to 12%
Examples: Abuse or neglect, behavioral management, crisis intervention, chemical and other dependencies, end-of-life concepts, mental health concepts, stress management, therapeutic communication
4. Physiologic Integrity
   a. Basic Care and Comfort: 6% to 12%
   Examples: Assistive devices, elimination, nutrition and oral hydration, personal hygiene, rest and sleep
   b. Pharmacologic and Parenteral Therapies: 13% to 19%
   Examples: Adverse effects/contraindications/side effects/interactions, medication administration, pharmacologic pain management
   c. Reduction of Risk Potential: 10% to 16%
   Examples: Changes/abnormalities in vital signs, diagnostic tests, laboratory values, potential for complications from surgical procedures and health alterations
   d. Physiologic Adaptation: 11% to 17%
   Examples: Basic pathophysiology, fluid and electrolyte imbalances, medical emergencies, radiation therapy, unexpected response to therapies

? Critical Thinking

Client Need Categories

Provide a "real" example of a patient need for each of the categories and subcategories. Where in the scheduled studies of your program do you expect to learn what is needed for each subcategory? Relate information you give in preconference to the categories and subcategories.

INTEGRATION OF NURSING CONCEPTS AND PROCESSES

Concepts and processes basic to the practice of practical/vocational nursing are integrated into the four categories of patient needs.

- *Clinical problem-solving process* (nursing process): A scientific approach to patient care. It includes data collection, planning, implementation, and evaluation (four phases of nursing process that apply to the practical/vocational nurse).
- *Caring:* Interaction of the practical/vocational nurse and patient, in an atmosphere of mutual trust and respect.
- *Communication and documentation:* Verbal and nonverbal interaction between the practical/vocational

nurse, patient, and others involved with care. Documentation (written or electronic) of all events and activities associated with patient care reflect the standards of practice.

- *Teaching/learning:* Assist the patient to gain information, skills, and attitudes that lead to change in behavior.

 Try This

Categories of Patient Care

Write a one-sentence example of how you might apply each of the four integrated processes in planning patient care.

OVERVIEW OF APPLICATION PROCESS

It is customary for an instructor to introduce you to the application process when it is time to apply to the state board of nursing (the Board) for a license as an LPN or LVN. The process is as follows:

- Complete all eligibility requirements for licensure, as required by the Board (starting with successful completion of the practical/vocational nursing program).
- Send an application for licensure to the state board of nursing or territory in which you plan to be licensed for nursing. Follow the directions of the Board. Rules and fees will vary according to the state or territory.
- NCLEX-PN® examination registration is sent to Pearson VUE (if the Board declares you eligible).
- Pearson VUE acknowledges your registration with a confirmation of registration by postal mail or email.
- Make an appointment to test at any approved Pearson Professional Center (PPC). Pearson Professional Center locations and addresses are found on the NCLEX® Candidate website at www.pearsonvue.com/nclex.

AUTHORIZATION TO TEST

You will receive an Authorization to Test (ATT) from Pearson VUE. The ATT letter has your authorization number, candidate identification number, and an expiration date. The ATT letter is valid for the time specified in the letter (determined by the board of nursing). The time period varies from 60 to 365 days. Once your Board declares you eligible to test, you must test within that period of time. If you do not test within that period, you must reregister and repay to take the examination. If the ATT does not arrive within 4 weeks, call Pearson VUE at the appropriate number listed in the front section of the candidate bulletin. If you are not declared eligible within that time for taking the NCLEX-PN® examination, you forfeit the registration and the fee. To reapply, you must submit a new application and fee. Do not send another registration form before calling about your status. Duplicate registration fees are not refunded.

- Schedule taking the NCLEX-PN® examination at a Pearson Center as soon as possible after receiving the ATT. Test centers may fill up quickly, and attempting to make a last-minute testing appointment may result in missing the ATT validity deadline. Most Pearson Centers are open Monday through Friday, except on holidays, and you may test at any Pearson Center.
- Take the NCLEX-PN® examination on the scheduled day. You must have the ATT and valid identification with you to be admitted to the Pearson Center.
- Validity dates for the ATT will not be extended for any reason. Once approved for testing, the candidate must take the NCLEX-PN® examination within the approved time frame.

 Critical Thinking

Authorization to Test

Explain the significance of attaining the ATT before scheduling your appointment to take the NCLEX-PN® examination.

FEES AND OTHER IMPORTANT INFORMATION

The fee for the NCLEX-PN® is $200. There will be other fees required by the nursing board where you are applying. Fees vary. There is no refund of a registration fee for any reason.

 Try This

List fees required by your state's board of nursing (or by the jurisdiction where you are applying).

HOW TO REGISTER

Internet, mail, or telephone can be used to register. Pearson VUE will confirm receipt of registration and send an ATT to the candidate.

Internet Registration

Visit the NCLEX® candidate website at www.pearsonvue.com/nclex. Select the registration option.

- On the registration form, print your name exactly as it appears on the valid picture identification you will present at the Pearson Center. The name on the ATT that you receive must match the name on the picture identification you present at the testing center.
- Pay for the registration ($200, plus fees if required) with a credit or debit card using VISA, MasterCard, or American Express.
- You may also pay by certified check, cashier's check, or money order.
- Mail the confirmation document and payment made payable to the National Council State Boards of Nursing to NCLEX Operations, PO Box 64950, St. Paul, MN 55164-0950.

U.S. Mail Registration

Obtain a registration scan form by contacting your board of nursing.

- A certified check, cashier's check, or money order payable to the National Council State Boards of Nursing must accompany the registration. Prior to sending in your application, check with your board of nursing in the state or territory if additional fees are required. An incomplete registration form and/or incorrect fee will be returned. Use the envelope included with your registration form.
- Mail to NCLEX Operations, PO Box 64950, St. Paul, MN 55164-0950.

Telephone Registration

Call Pearson VUE NCLEX® Candidate Services at one of the numbers listed on the inside front cover of the candidate bulletin. For those candidates not registering in the United States, telephone numbers for other countries are found at the front of the candidate bulletin.

- Fill out the registration form prior to making the call. The customer representative will ask the same questions that are on the registration form.
- Paying for registration when using the telephone is by VISA, MasterCard, or American Express credit or debit card. Standard questions such as the name shown on the card, the number, and the expiration date are asked, and the credit card is verified before the registration is processed.
- If you provide an email address, correspondence will arrive by email only. This applies to all methods of registering.

NCLEX-PN® ADMINISTRATION IN THE UNITED STATES AND ITS TERRITORIES

The NCLEX-PN® examination is given in the United States, American Samoa, the District of Columbia, Guam, the Northern Mariana Islands, Puerto Rico, and the Virgin Islands. This makes it possible to provide licensure by endorsement from one board of nursing to another within the United States and its territories.

Endorsement means that an LPN/LVN may apply for licensure in a different state or territory without retesting. Taking the same examination in the United States and its territories facilitates endorsement from one nursing board to another.

EXAMINATION SECURITY

The NCLEX-PN® examination ensures *minimal competency* to protect the public, and because of this, strict rules have been established for testing:

- Arrive at the testing center 30 minutes before the scheduled time. If you arrive 30 minutes later than the appointed time, you may be required to forfeit your appointment.
- Avoid bringing children, family, or friends to the Pearson Center. They will not be permitted to wait at the testing center.
- *Name:* Use your name in *exactly* the same form you used when applying for the NCLEX-PN® examination. If your legal name has changed since you applied, the only legal documentation acceptable the day of the test is a marriage license, divorce decree, and/or court action legal name change documents.
- *Proper identification:* Your ATT and a valid form of picture identification in English and signed in English are required. The only proper identification is a valid (not expired) U.S. driver's license; U.S. state identification (issued by the Department of Motor Vehicles); a valid passport; or U.S. Military Identification.
- You will be asked to provide your signature. A digital fingerprint, palm vein scan, and photograph will be taken. No hats, scarves, or coats may be worn while the picture is taken. Hats, coats, or scarves may not be worn in the testing room. Your fingerprint, photograph, and signature accompany the examination results that are sent to the board and can be used to confirm your identity.
- Direct observation by staff and video- and audiorecording of the session occur at all times during the examination.
- Personal belongings are kept in secure storage outside of the classroom during the test. The storage space is small, so plan accordingly. A Pearson staff person escorts you to a secure area. A similar process is followed when you prepare to leave the Pearson Center. At no time does any candidate walk into the secure area without an escort. (Visualize a system similar to accessing a safe deposit box at the bank.)
- All books, papers, unauthorized scratch paper, note boards, food, pens, purses, wallets, watches, beepers, cell phones, handheld computers, and personal digital devices are banned from the test room. The CAT includes both a calculator and a time device that tells you how much time remains to complete the NCLEX-PN® examination. (Refer to your candidate bulletin for a list of other items that are not permitted in the testing room.)
- Erasable note boards are provided for use during the test and collected before you leave the room during a break or at the end of testing. Note boards cannot be taken outside the room.
- Leaving the room is permitted with permission only. A palm vein scan is required each time you leave and return to the testing area after a break. A test administrator (TA) escorts the candidate to and from the room.
- Only medication, food, or beverages may be accessed during a break. Do not attempt to access study materials.

- A classmate or friend will not be seated next to you. Students from other programs will also be taking an examination during the day you are scheduled. This provides additional security for testing.

Violation of center regulations such as attempting to take a test for someone else or inappropriate behavior such as attempting to tamper with the computer will result in dismissal from the testing center. It may also include test results being held or canceled, denial of a license, or denying the candidate future registration for licensure.

 Try This

Security Rules

Explain the significance of each of the security rules. Where will you put your car keys before testing?

Confidentiality Agreement

A confidentiality agreement will appear on the computer, which you must read and sign before beginning the examination. The confidentiality agreement includes not disclosing the contents of the examination items before, during, or after the examination. Disclosure includes, but is not limited to, discussing examination items with faculty, friends, family, and others. Any irregular behavior can result in criminal prosecution, civil liability, and or disciplinary action by the nursing licensing board.

DURING THE TEST

You may ask for assistance with the computer at any time if needed or if the computer does not seem to be functioning properly. Raise your hand for assistance, if you want to change note boards, or if you need a break. Remain in your seat, except when given permission to leave the room. Creating any disturbance can cause you to be dismissed from the room.

After you complete the exam, raise your hand. There will be a brief questionnaire on the computer for you to complete regarding the testing experience. You may also ask for a confidential comment sheet in order to write personal comments to the NCSBN. When all exam requirements are met, the TA will collect and inventory the note boards and dismiss you from the testing room.

REPORTING THE RESULTS OF THE EXAMINATION

The NCSBN Board of Directors voted to raise the passing standard for the NCLEX-PN® Examination. It took effect April 1, 2011 (www.ncsbn.org/Setting_the_NCLEX_Passing_Standard.pdf). The NCLEX-PN® pass rate for first-time U.S.-educated candidates was 87% during July-September 2011.

Although the computer continuously computes the result of your answers, the Pearson Center does not release final results to you directly. The result is available only from the board approximately 1 month after testing. *Do not call the board, the NCLEX® Candidate Services, the Pearson Centers, or the NCSBN for results.* The results will be sent to you by postal mail from the state board of nursing.

Your state's board of nursing (not Pearson Center) notifies you of the test results. Boards are the only agencies that can license a graduate of a practical/vocational program and release the test results to them. Do not contact Pearson VUE for test results; they will not release the results directly to you.

 Critical Thinking

Exam Results

Explain why the state board of nursing (rather than the Pearson Center) provides you with the results of the NCLEX-PN® examination.

 Critical Thinking

Computerized Adaptive Testing

Explain why the CAT method of testing provides a clearer picture of the candidate's competency than does the usual paper/pencil test.

 Try This

Practicing in Other States

Research how to apply for licensure by endorsement in another state. Start by contacting the **state board of nursing** of a state in which you may be interested in applying for a job.

APPLYING FOR A TEMPORARY PERMIT

Your instructor will assist you with an application for a temporary permit so you will be able to work as a graduate practical or vocational nurse (GPN or GVN). Once the result of the NCLEX-PN® examination is in, the temporary permit is automatically revoked. Passing the NCLEX-PN® examination means that you will work as a fully licensed practical or vocational nurse (LPN or LVN). If you fail the NCLEX-PN® examination, you will be required to surrender your temporary permit and work as a nursing assistant.

A WORD ABOUT REVIEW BOOKS AND MOCK EXAMINATIONS

The major nursing publishing companies have developed review books based on the NCLEX-PN® examination format. Each review book basically includes an outline of practical/vocational nursing content, questions with explanations and rationale, and references for the answers. Questions are intended to simulate the NCLEX-PN® examination format. Realize that the test questions of the NCLEX-PN® examination itself are highly guarded and confidential. Actual NCLEX-PN® examination questions are not included in any review book. Some review books contain computer disks with test questions. These disks do not simulate CAT testing, but they do provide computer experience. Silvestri's (2010) book *Q and A Review for the NCLEX-PN® Examination* and its companion CD-ROM contain 3200 NCLEX-PN®-type questions and a comprehensive exam with multiple-choice, alternative item format, and audio questions. Hesi's (2012) book *Comprehensive Review for the NCLEX-PN® Examination* and companion CD-ROM include a study exam CD.

The best preparation is to study faithfully from the beginning of the program to its conclusion, on a regular basis until you take the examination. Merely reading a review book at the end of the program without studying the nursing content throughout the program will rarely help you pass boards. The identified outcome of a nursing program is to learn, understand, and be able to apply basic nursing information in the care of patients on clinical during your student year and when you graduate.

The NLN announced on July 25, 2011, the release of a new and innovative practice test that utilizes the technology used in the NCLEX® examination. It is called ACTION, which stands for Advanced College Testing & Integrated Online Network. The CAT adapts the examiner's ability level just like the NCLEX-PN® and the NCLEX-RN®. This mock examination is available online and provides a student with a way to track areas of needed growth (www. nlnonlinetesting.org/cal.login.pl). The test provides the following benefits:

- Reports generate instantly and include a statement of a candidate's probability of passing the NCLEX-PN®.
- The tests are based on the NCLEX-PN® blueprint.
- Individual performance and class summary reports offer a comprehensive diagnostic profile, detailing areas of strength and weakness on multiple subscales related to the blueprint.
- Correct answer rationales for every question and a reference list are provided after the test is scored.
- Report summaries help educators formulate effective study plans for their classes and individuals and focus their review efforts.
- Provides individuals with valuable test-taking practice.
- Both individual and class reports are available for download and can be retrieved for up to two weeks after the test is scored. Call 800-732-8656, or email CustomerHelp@nln.org.

If you have an idea of your strong and weak areas, you can better focus your study efforts. Be sure to check publishers' offerings of mock examinations. Choose the one that most closely resembles the actual format of the NCLEX-PN® examination. As an SPN/SVN, you can benefit from tests during the year that encourage problem solving, application, and analysis of knowledge. Some publishers provide adaptive testing as used by the NCLEX-PN® examination. Use these experiences as additional means of preparing for your nursing licensure examination. Good luck, and keep a positive mental attitude!

Get Ready for the NCLEX-PN® Examination

Key Points

- Lack of preparation of subject matter (poor studying skills and habits) and poor test-taking skills are the most common reasons for low test scores.
- Occasionally fear and high anxiety are involved in low test scores. If this is an issue, do something about learning habits to reduce test-taking anxiety now. See Chapter 4.
- Graduate practical/vocational nurses (candidates) take the NCLEX-PN® examination to become licensed as an LPN/LVN.
- Before scheduling the NCLEX-PN® examination, all practical or vocational nursing course work must be completed.
- The candidate applies to the board of nursing in the state or territory where he or she wishes to be licensed.
- If the board approves the application, it is sent to Pearson VUE, which sends the candidate a letter acknowledging receipt of the application.
- Pearson VUE also sends an ATT with the authorization number, candidate identification number, and expiration date.

- Candidates may schedule by telephone, U.S. mail, or Internet. Check your candidate bulletin for details.
- Candidates must arrive at the testing center with the ATT and a valid identification.
- A computer administers the NCLEX-PN® examination, using the computerized adaptive testing (CAT) method of testing.
- Each candidate takes a different track (path) during the CAT method of testing. The zigzag track is based on the answer to the content area and difficulty level, not the item type.
- The NCLEX-PN® examination provides all candidates ample opportunity to demonstrate competency in practical/vocational nursing.
- Neither pass nor fail is related to the number of items answered by the candidate.
- The board of nursing to which you applied will provide results in approximately 1 month

Additional Learning Resources

evolve Go to your Evolve website (http://evolve.elsevier.com/Hill/Success) for the following FREE learning resources:

- Answers to Critical Thinking Review Scenarios
- Additional learning activities
- Additional Review Questions for the NCLEX-PN® exam
- Helpful phrases for communicating in Spanish and more!

Review Questions for the NCLEX-PN® Examination

1. Explain how CAT determines that a candidate has passed the NCLEX-PN® examination.
   1. The computer calculates accuracy or inaccuracy of a distracter chosen by a candidate.
   2. The computer subtracts the number of wrong from the number of right questions to determine the score.
   3. The computer zigzags to find questions that will indicate comprehension by the candidate.
   4. The computer determines that the candidate has 50% of the difficult questions correct.

2. How is the NCLEX-PN® examination kept up to date with what LPNs/LVNs are really doing in nursing?
   1. Each nursing school surveys its students during the first year after graduation.
   2. The state board of nursing requires a work survey as a part of license renewal.
   3. The NCSBN sponsors a job analysis of newly licensed nurses throughout the United States.
   4. Each state board of nursing is required to do a work survey and submit questions.

3. A member of the class did not pass the NCLEX-PN® examination and is angry because the temporary work permit was revoked. The member asks, "Why do I have to work as an aide after completing school?" What is the correct response?
   1. "Any graduate who fails embarrasses the nursing school and is punished for it."
   2. "The permit gives you one chance to function as a practical nurse without a license."
   3. "Go work in another state, where licensing laws are not as punitive as they are here."
   4. "If you can provide a 'hardship' excuse, the board will extend the work permit."

4. A candidate attempts to use study aids during the NCLEX-PN® examination. Which of the following is not a consequence of this action?
   1. The Pearson Center notifies the NCSBN of the candidate's action.
   2. The candidate is barred from taking the NCLEX-PN® examination in the future.
   3. Some state boards decide their response on a case-by-case basis.
   4. The Pearson Center may dismiss or cancel the testing result of the candidate.

Alternate Format Item

1. Which of the following are required as security during the NCLEX-PN® examination? (Select all that apply.)
   1. Fingerprint
   2. Observation
   3. No. 2 pencils
   4. Identification
   5. Signature

2. Which of the following are examples of ignoring the confidentiality you signed prior to taking the examination? (Select all that apply.)
   1. Express relief to your family at passing the examination successfully.
   2. Make notes of questions you recall before leaving once out of the testing center.
   3. Contact your nursing program director to give her a list of questions you recall.
   4. Discuss the examination with a friend who has recently entered the PN program.

Critical Thinking Scenarios

Scenario 1
Kara, a friend of yours in another state, is also taking a practical nursing course. She started approximately 3 months after you did. Kara has expressed concern about being prepared for the NCLEX-PN® examination. Kara is a good student, but she is especially concerned about what she should do the night before the examination and wonders what you are planning to do. What are you going to say to your friend?

Scenario 2
Your assignment is to explain the CAT. What are some points you will include?

Future Career Decisions: Choosing What Is Right for You

Objectives

On completing this chapter, you will be able to do the following:

1. Identify areas of licensed practical/vocational nurse (LPN/LVN) employment currently available in your community.
2. Contact the state board of nursing in the state you plan to seek employment to find out which certifications are accepted in the state in which you plan to seek employment.
3. Discuss three advantages of belonging to professional organizations.
4. Describe your postgraduate career goals. (Review your answer periodically.)
5. Investigate opportunities available to you for continuing education.
6. Investigate if Transition to Practice is available for you at the site of employment when you graduate.

Key Terms

career ladder programs (p. 337)
Certification in Managed Care Nursing (CMCN) (p. 336)
Long-Term Care Certification (CLTC) (p. 335)
mobility program (mō-BĬL-ĭ-tē, p. 336)
National Association for Practical Nurse Education and Service, Inc. (NAPNES) (p. 333)
National Certification in Gerontology (jĕ-rŏn-TŎL-ō-jē, p. 335)
National Certification in IV Therapy (p. 335)

National Federation of Licensed Practical Nurses (NFLPN) (p. 334)
National League for Nursing (NLN) (p. 333)
Pharmacology Certification (NCP) (făr-mă-KŎL-ō-jē, p. 335)
podcast (POD-kast, p. 335)
preceptor (p. 327)
residency (p. 326)
Transition to Practice Model (trăn-zĭ-shŭn, p. 327)

 Keep in Mind

Have you developed an appreciation of nursing and the patients you work with? Does the role of LPN/LVN fit for you and your dreams? Are you looking to continue your education in nursing? What is your personal goal?

NURSING OPENS THE DOOR TO A VARIED CAREER

Nursing opens the door to an entirely different world. You enter and touch the lives of many individuals and families. Patients trust you without having to prove yourself. They feel safe in the knowledge that you have pledged to do your best in providing care without passing judgment. Some patients and families will let you know their appreciation for your skill in providing nursing care, but some will never tell you how deeply you touched their life and the lives of their loved ones.

Nursing challenges you throughout your career. As a student, you are expected to learn and use an entirely new language and yet always explain to a patient what you are doing in terms he or she can understand. The

challenge continues when you graduate because you have only scratched the surface of knowledge in nursing. There are many more skills to perfect and a great deal more to learn from courses, in-services, workshops, and skilled nursing practitioners. Every day will provide at least one answer to your question "What did I learn today?"

Approximately one third of those who enter a nursing program do not complete the program for any number of reasons. A major reason is that the course of study demands a great deal of personal discipline, time management, and prioritization of needs (knowing the difference between "I want to" and "I need to"). Nursing changes you: You see and hear more in a short period than you ever imagined. Most of what you see and hear cannot be shared with anyone out of the immediate setting. Nursing is a maturing experience, often beyond your years. Both self-confidence and the ability to say, "I don't know, but I will find out" grow as your professional honesty is tested. Nursing opens doors for you in traditional and atypical careers. Be proud of choosing nursing as a career, and do not keep that information confidential!

Try This

Areas of Interest

Is there a specific area you are interested in at this time? Know that you may change your mind based on classroom and clinical experience in a particular area.

NCSBN TRANSITION TO PRACTICE MODEL

In 2007, in an effort to help new RN and LPN/LVN graduates transition to the work environment from their nursing educational programs, increase retention in their employment, and improve patient outcomes, the NCSBN started to develop the Transition to Practice model. This model, similar to a residency, is a program in addition to orientation to a clinical area. The main parts of the model include:

- A trained nurse (preceptor) to assist the new graduate apply theory to practice, develop clinical reasoning, improve safety, and decrease practice errors in the care of patients.
- Five online modules of study: communication and teamwork, patient-centered care, evidence-based practice, quality improvement, and informatics.

In 2010, the Institute of Medicine called for the implementation and evaluation of nursing residency programs. In 2010, the first of a two-phase, randomized study was conducted in three states (Illinois, Ohio, and North Carolina) involving new RN graduates in hospitals. In 2012 the second phase of the study involving RNs and LPNs/LVNs in non-hospital settings (long-term care, community-based or ambulatory care facilities) in the above states began. The results of these two studies, including the model's effect on patient safety and outcomes, will provide evidence on whether or not to implement the NCSBN model for transition to practice. A full description of the model and study can be found at ncsbn.org or transitiontopractice.org.

 Try This

Transitional Practice

Investigate if your state participates in the Transition to Practice study. Depending on the results of the 2012 study, investigate if health care facilities in your area have a Transition to Practice model for new employees.

WORK SITES AND NURSING CHARACTERISTICS

HELPFUL PERSONAL ATTRIBUTES

LPNs/LVNs must be caring, have an empathic (not sympathetic) nature, and have a genuine concern for the welfare of their patients. Emotional stability is essential because work with sick and injured patients can be stressful. LPNs/LVNs need keen observational, critical-thinking, and decision-making skills and be able to communicate at a patient's level in order to be understood. A comfort level in doing basic nursing skills is absolute. If the LPN has been taught advanced skills that are within the state board's scope of practice for LPNs, then these skills need to be perfected. The condition of a patient may quickly change from stable to acute, and the nurse will have to respond to the situation without panic.

- LPNs/LVNs work as part of a team and will be expected to follow orders and work under close supervision of an RN or physician.
- Assertiveness and patient advocacy are other important attributes.
- Since the LPN/LVN will often hear or see things that cannot be discussed with someone outside of the immediate area, confidentiality is a must.
- The LPN/LVN must also find healthy ways to relieve stress at the end of the shift that will not contribute to his or her personal health problems.

 Try This

Personal Skills and Characteristics

Name some additional nursing skills and personal characteristics you have that enhance your ability to work in an area that currently appeals to you.

 Try This

Availability of Leadership Course

Almost half of the newly licensed practical/vocational nurses who participated in the 2009 Job Analysis regularly assumed administrative responsibility, primarily in long-term care. Inquire whether a postgraduate LPN/LVN leadership/management course is available. Ask for details about the course.

EXTENDED CARE FACILITIES

The growing number of people age 65 and older has a positive impact on the availability of jobs for practical nurses. The extended care population is made up of residents who are:

1. Completing recovery from surgery or trauma and are too well for the hospital but not well enough to go home.
2. Elderly people who are unable to care for themselves because of medical or psychological impairment.
3. Mentally handicapped persons who are unable to live independently or in group homes.
4. Young to middle-aged people with chronic debilitating disease or injuries from accidents.
5. Young, chronically mentally ill persons who need continual supervision and are not candidates for independent living or halfway houses.

LPNs/LVNs who are hired for direct care measure vital signs, collect data, provide physical care and comfort measures, and give oral medications. Many state boards have flexible codes that permit more extensive use of LPN/LVN skills in nursing homes. Other state codes are more restrictive.

There are still several points of contention in the scopes of practice for LPNs and RNs. Some points center around course names (e.g., "mental health nursing" instead of "psychiatric nursing") on terms like *assessment*, *delegation*, and *decision making*. The difference in the terms *assessment* and *data collection* (the preferred term for LPNs/LVNS) is difficult to define. Since critical thinking has been incorporated into the NCLEX-PN®, critical thinking is taught as a part of practical nursing programs and is no longer a point of contention. As noted in the 2009 Practice Analysis, about half of the LPNs/LVNs work as charge nurses, primarily in long-term care facilities; some work as team leaders.

Many states and organizations offer postgraduate courses and certifications. NAPNES offers certification programs in pharmacology, IV therapy, and long-term care (www.napnes.org). NFLPN offers national certifications in IV therapy and gerontology (www.nflpn. org). NFLPN has also partnered with Professional Education, to offer a new Foot Care Certification (www.nflpn.org/cerification.html). The American Board of Managed Care Nursing (www.abmcn.org) offers certification in managed care nursing. Some vocational and technical colleges offer postgraduate courses on being a charge nurse. Some states recognize postgraduate courses and certifications with an increase in salary and permit the LPN/LVN to use the skills they have learned in providing care. A major benefit of postgraduate information is knowledge gained for more effective patient care.

Extended care as an employment option may be available to you if you possess the following characteristics:

- Use solid nursing process skills in gathering data and use the care plan as a guide.
- Use critical thinking throughout the shift.
- Use therapeutic communication skills; differentiate between therapeutic and personal.
- Enjoy longer-term contact with people. (High turnover rates of staff have been associated with lower quality of care in some extended care facilities.)
- Provide excellent nursing care without immediate supervision of an RN or physician.
- Seek assistance or additional instruction as needed.
- Apply information about growth and development changes during illness.
- Willingly seek to learn new skills through continuing education and certification courses needed to take care of a varied population and age group.
- Listen to patients regarding what they see as their needs for care.
- Treat patients of all ages and levels of growth and development with respect.
- Recognize when there is a significant personality clash with a patient to whom you are assigned and ask for a change in assignment. (This statement assumes that you have already tried to talk over differences with the patient and other staffs are available to take over.)

Other special qualities needed include the following:

- Patience
- Ability to see below the surface
- Willingness to listen
- Maturity
- Understand the significance of the work you are doing
- Ability to determine priorities
- Ability to set limits
- Interest in working with people with disabilities
- Willingness to work with other health care givers, significant others, and family members.
- A sense of security in regard to your personal value system

Prior experience on a medical/surgical unit is helpful before working in an extended care facility.

LPNs/LVNs who work in extended care are challenged to assist in providing a homelike atmosphere while dealing with immediate, long-term, and terminal health problems of the residents. The level of responsibility in extended care is great. The LPN/LVN often works in a charge nurse role, and although supervision is available from an RN, during some periods of the day, supervision may be general (i.e., at the other end of a cell phone). Consequently, solid knowledge and skills are essential to understanding when to seek help and from whom. The nursing process and critical thinking provide the basis for skilled, compassionate care.

The charge nurse role also means that the practical/vocational nurse is responsible for managing care given by other LPNs/LVNs, certified nursing assistants, and trained feeding assistants. (Refer to Chapters 20 and 21 for more specific details on leadership and charge nurse skills.)

As the LPN/LVN in an extended care facility, much of your work ultimately relates to assisting the residents to attain or maintain whatever capabilities they have in all areas of health. Through your efforts, residents who are recuperating from surgery or trauma will realize their goal for recovery and discharge. For other residents, your role includes supporting them through the final step of the growth process: a dignified death.

HOME HEALTH NURSING

According to the U.S. Bureau of Labor Statistics, faster-than-average growth is expected in home health services. This is in response to the number of older persons with functional disabilities, preference for home care, and technological advances that make it possible to do more complicated treatments in the home.

Because of shorter hospital stays, patients are receiving an increased amount of care in the home.

The actual care given is under the supervision of an RN, who uses nursing process steps as a guideline to finalize a plan of care approved by the patient. Data from the LPN/LVN involved with care are essential to complete the care plan. Postdischarge (subacute) care fits in well with LPN/LVN basic education, thereby making LPNs/LVNs invaluable in implementing the plan of care. LPN/LVNs' observations of physical and mental changes allow additions to the continuing data collection and evaluation of the plan of care. Because of difficulty in receiving payment from nonprivate sources, some home health agencies use LPNs/LVNs for private-pay patients only. Others employ LPNs/LVNs as home health aides to avoid

restrictions. This is an unfortunate practice because the pay is lower and the LPN/LVN is always held to the standard of his or her highest license in legal situations. Because of the need for the level of LPN/LVN skill, there is some hope the payment plan will be revised.

MENTAL HEALTH NURSING

Mental health nursing facilities include psychiatric hospitals, community mental health centers, day treatment centers, and group homes for the recovering mentally ill. Many community mental health centers and group homes are staffed primarily with LPNs/LVNs and nursing assistants, with RNs in a supervisory role. Many practical/vocational nursing programs have dropped the mental health nursing theory and related clinical experience. Up to 13% of questions in the 2011 NCLEX-PN® examination are in the psychosocial integrity category.

In mental health nursing, LPNs/LVNs are involved in the following:

- Performing treatments
- Administering medications
- Tending to activities of daily living

Furthermore, LPNs/LVNs perform a significant role in developing a therapeutic relationship with the patient and following through with the appropriate interventions, according to the patient's care plan. Mental health facilities practice a team concept in which everyone is expected to contribute to the patient's care plan, know the therapeutic guidelines in a patient care plan, and carry out the plan. A solid knowledge of mental health concepts and nursing process is essential.

Helpful qualities for working in a mental health unit include the following:

Helpful Qualities for Home Health Nurses

- **Flexibility:** You will have to improvise in the home, yet practice sound nursing principles. For example, this may include using makeshift equipment, determining how to clean the equipment, and using it to attain desired results.
- **Communication skills:** You are working in the patient's domain. You have to understand the patient's expression of needs and also make sure that you express yourself clearly and tactfully. For example, you may find yourself having to use words in the patient's vocabulary to be understood.
- **Self-confidence:** An air of insecurity or uncertainty will be picked up by the patient, resulting in lack of confidence in the LPN/LVN. This does not imply that you should fake confidence. Have the knowledge and nursing skills that enable you to perform tasks efficiently. Do not ask for unnecessary reassurance from the patient when performing basic skills. Ask questions away from the patient, unless an emergency exists. For example, you may be tempted to tell the patient, "This is only the second time I have changed a dressing on a foot without contaminating the dressing, and I'm kind of nervous about it." Do not make a comment like this. It will worry the patient.
- **Sensitivity to physical and emotional changes:** Once the initial assessment is completed by the RN, it will be up to you to be alert to any changes of which the RN must be made aware. The RN must be able to depend on your observational skills, for safety's sake. For example, be tuned in to the person's affective communication as well as the verbal and nonverbal. Perhaps the individual is beginning to show signs of agitation that will need to be diffused before continuing the other work you have been assigned.
- **Ability to deal with emergencies:** Staying calm and following agency protocol are essential. For example, the patient may start to bleed from the wound you are dressing. Remembering what you learned to do in basic nursing and during first aid class is more effective than screaming that you can't stand the sight of blood! In an emergency, your motto is "Function now, and shake later."
- **Nonjudgmental attitude:** This is a must because you work in the patient's home. You are providing a service. If you are comfortable with your own values, different values are not personally threatening. For example, the home may not be up to your standards in cleanliness.

 Professional Pointer

Desirable Qualities in a Mental Health Setting

- Basic knowledge of dealing with psychiatric behaviors
- Keen observational skills regarding behavioral change
- Knowledge of basic self-defense
- Experience with medical/surgical patients prior to working in a mental health unit
- Calm and able to make quick decisions
- Empathic rather than sympathetic
- Therapeutic communication skills
- Separates personal and professional life
- Nonjudgmental and respectful
- Sound mental health
- Excellent nursing process and critical-thinking skills
- Contributes to patient care plan
- Follows established patient goals
- Sets patient-centered limits assertively
- Functions as a team member
- Observes and reports patient changes
- Does not take unnecessary risks with a patient who is acting out and knows when to seek assistance

MILITARY SERVICES

As a practical/vocational nurse, you will take basic training if you volunteer for military service in the reserves or for active duty. Contact recruiters for all branches of the military services, including the National Guard. Compare the differences in available nursing careers to determine which branch best fits your needs. The U.S. Army, for example, cross-trains LPNs/LVNs to be able to work in any area of the hospital. The benefits of military service also provide the financial means to continue education, and some LPNs/LVNs have taken advantage of this benefit to become an RN and an officer. Others have gone on to get advanced degrees in nursing.

 Professional Pointer

Desirable Qualities in Military Service Nursing

- Interest in teamwork
- Strong ego
- Ability to cope with changing situations
- Emotional stability
- Good communication skills
- Self-directed
- Desire for adventure
- Flexible
- Adaptable
- Empathetic (rather than sympathetic) with patients
- Self-directed, but knows when to seek help
- Healthy personal stress-relieving habits

A desire for a challenging career and an ability to adjust quickly to new situations are handy prerequisites for this kind of nursing.

HOSPITAL NURSING

The acute care experience in most practical/vocational nursing programs is found in the medical and surgical units of hospitals. In some areas of the country, hospital-based jobs have decreased and are available primarily to replace nurses who leave. Some of the ads for nurses are written for RN or LPN/LVN positions, so be sure to check that the job description is within the LPN/LVN scope of practice. Often the LPN/LVN is underutilized in the hospital setting because the RN is not familiar with what the LPN/LVN is permitted to do legally. LPNs/LVNs are often overheard complaining to one another that they do the same work as nursing aides. Your responsibility is to know what your scope of practice is in your state. Make this information, plus information on continuing education (including certifications you have earned), known to your RN supervisor. Some RNs do not trust LPNs/LVNs primarily because they have never worked with them. Do your nursing care with skillful professionalism and help pave the way for other LPNs/LVNs to be fully accepted in this important hospital nursing role.

If you consider working in a specialty area, it is helpful to have both theory class and clinical experience, or additional education. Areas with complex nursing duties mean that additional postgraduate education such as in-service, workshops, or courses related specifically to the area are required. Previous nursing experience may also be listed as a requirement. Refer to your state's Nurse Practice Act to see how performance of nursing acts beyond basic nursing care is handled. These acts are referred to as the expanded role of the practical/vocational nurse or performance of acts in complex patient situations (see Chapters 20 and 21). The anticipated pay scale is approximately two-thirds that of the RN pay scale. Other benefits vary according to agency policy.

 Professional Pointer

Desirable Qualities in Hospital Nursing

- Strong technical skills
- Organizational skills
- Nursing process and critical-thinking skills
- Strong ego
- Copes well during emergencies
- Teamwork: knows own and others' scope of practice
- Knows own limits and asks for help as needed

OUTPATIENT CLINICS, DOCTORS' OFFICES, AND CHIROPRACTIC OFFICES

Outpatient clinics and doctors' offices continue to provide jobs for many LPNs/LVNs. Most clinics and offices are open Monday to Friday. The day begins later and, consequently, runs a little later. Assigned work varies, but it generally includes the following:
- Checking supplies
- Greeting patients
- Measuring vital signs
- Weighing patients
- Limited data collection about the purpose of the appointment
- Preparing the patient for an examination
- Assisting the doctor with the examination
- Performing additional duties delegated by the physician

Cross-training (learning to do jobs other than nursing) is expected in some of these facilities. For example, you might be expected to do basic lab tests, x-rays, and clerical work, including answering telephones and making appointments.

If you are working as a private nurse for a physician, you can also expect to accompany the physician on hospital rounds and assist with examinations and treatments as needed. When patients remain with the same physician, these nurses develop rapport with the patients, which is an asset to both the patient and the physician.

Professional Pointer

Desirable Qualities in Outpatient Nursing and Doctors' Offices

- Has good communication skills
- Pays attention to details
- Enjoys routine
- Has excellent organizational skills
- Applies nursing process and critical-thinking skills
- Adapts and is self-directed when patient load is small
- Treats all patients and their families with respect and empathy
- Practices confidentiality and is respectful of patient's right to privacy
- Maintains a sense of humor and uses it appropriately
- Uses a well-modulated voice throughout the work period
- Is flexible and willing to learn

Previous work experience in a medical-surgical unit is advised to prepare you for data collection, administering medications, doing select treatments as assigned by the physician, and keeping records, as required.

OPERATING ROOM NURSING

Operating room (OR) technicians who have been hired as OR nurses for cost-cutting reasons are not nurses. Technicians are not licensed and lack the extensive training that is required of LPNs/LVNs. For example, technicians do not possess knowledge of the steps of the nursing process and critical thinking. Gathering data and skill in observation are not part of technician training. Technician training is limited to learning particular OR functions. LPNs/LVNs who have worked in the OR for years describe their work as assisting the surgeon with instruments and equipment, collecting data, doing preoperative and postoperative patient care, and supporting postoperative education. They strongly urge that if you are interested in this line of work, stress your education and clinical skills as an LPN/LVN to your future employer.

In some states, LPNs/LVNs can become trained to become an operating room technician. There is the combined value of being an LPN/LVN and operating room technician. If the operating room is your passion, it may be worth researching the possibility.

Professional Pointer

Desirable Qualities for Operating Room Nurses

- Has good manual dexterity
- Applies personal stress management skills
- Separates personal and professional feedback from physicians and supervisors
- Possesses a sense of self-worth
- Accepts and follows directions
- Uses nursing process
- Maintains composure in a crisis

- Differentiates between empathy and sympathy
- Practices standard precautions; maintains sterile technique where needed
- Maintains good personal health practices
- Treats patients and their families with respect
- Maintains a willingness to learn

VETERANS ADMINISTRATION CAREERS

Working with the nation's veterans in VA hospitals or veterans retirement homes are additional options for LPNs/LVNs. You do not have to be a veteran to apply for employment. More LPNs/LVNs are hired in veterans nursing homes than in acute care veterans facilities.

Facilities generally provide new nurses an extensive orientation during duty hours regardless of the shift you are assigned. Veterans care includes medicine, surgery, spinal cord injury, alcohol/drug treatment, psychiatry, intensive care, hemodialysis, ambulatory care, and long-term care. Minimum qualifications include U.S. citizenship, graduation or pending graduation from an accredited nursing school, and English language proficiency. Benefits are normally generous and are based on civil service grades. LPNs/LVNs with no experience start at GS-3 level. Salary rates are based on the grade, performance, and promotion to higher grades, overtime, and shift differential. If interested, go to the "Job Search" section of the VA Careers website at www.vacareers.va.gov/lpn.cfm.

HOSPICE

Hospice care is for terminally ill patients of any age, whether in institutional settings or their homes. The same qualities that are important in an extended-care facility are important in a hospice setting. The nurse's role is to keep the patient comfortable and administer pain medication as ordered. In the past, nurses sometimes withheld pain medication from the patient, even when ordered, in the mistaken belief that they might cause the patient to become addicted.

Critical Thinking

Pain Medication for the Terminally Ill Patient

Think about the statement "You should withhold pain medication from a terminally ill patient so he or she does not become addicted." Does that statement make sense to you? Explain your response.

OTHER JOB OPPORTUNITIES

Health Insurance Companies

Health insurance companies provide in-depth orientation for the work required. Some companies prefer to hire practical/vocational nurses immediately on graduation so the LPN/LVN is taught the company routine and does not have to unlearn previous practices.

Travel Nursing

There are a variety of ways to inquire about travel nursing as a career. Many health care–related websites include information on their site. Another option is to make your search selective. Use any search engine available to you on the computer and type in "travel nurse," "travel nursing," "travel health care," "travel nursing career," or "travel nurse information." Placing the words in quotes makes the search more selective.

Veterinary Clinics and Hospitals

For some LPNs/LVNs, this is an opportunity to combine a love of nursing with a love of animals. In some states you may work as an assistant to the veterinarian in the care and treatment of animals. Other states, such as California, require a special training program and a passing grade in a state test to assist veterinarians.

Pharmaceutical/Medical Equipment Sales

Some pharmacies select LPNs/LVNs to staff this particular area. For example, a former student practical nurse became the colostomy care expert in her city and gives seminars on the topic to agencies, patients, and health professionals. She enjoys the backing of the drugstore management and a pharmaceutical company.

Coroner's office

A former student practical nurse working with a coroner commented, "I never saw myself as doing this, but it is so interesting. I've learned a lot about people, pain, compassion, and myself. The doctor I work with is a born teacher and is always respectful of the person on whom he is doing the autopsy. He has helped me accept the life cycle."

Private Duty Nursing

LPNs/LVNs have been employed for years as private duty nurses. This is frequently a long-term commitment on the part of an LPN/LVN. The most common responsibility is for ill, elderly individuals who wish to be cared for in their home rather than in an institution. Some private duty nurses accompany the person on extended trips. Private duty nursing can also involve a child or adult with a long-term chronic illness. The LPN/LVN may be part of an around-the-clock care system with nurses on opposing shifts. Responsibilities vary according to the shift involved and include basic nursing skills. The LPN/LVN works under the general supervision of the patient's physician.

Parish Nursing

Some church parishes employ their own nurse to take care of the basic health needs of the congregation. The work includes basic nursing skills such as measuring blood pressure, temperature, pulse, and respirations and contacting a physician as needed. Foot care under the supervision of a podiatrist is sometimes included. Some parish nurses provide presentations on basic health care issues to the parishioners.

Temporary Help Agency

Temporary help agencies are listed under a variety of names. They supply nurses when requested by a health facility. Some provide temporary help exclusively for certain kinds of health facilities (e.g., long-term care). The need for help may be related to a shortage of nurses, lack of availability in the area, need for temporary coverage, and so on. Assignments are intended to be short term. Sometimes the facility decides to hire the temporary nurse. Nurses who work for temporary agencies must be ready to "hit the floor running." Consequently, the temporary agency rarely hires a newly licensed nurse. They prefer a nurse with at least 1 year of experience in a clinical hospital setting. The nurse must be competent in doing the required procedures. The temporary agency handles the contract for the health facility and for the nurse. Because of the immediate need for a nurse, the temporary agency usually pays the nurse a higher salary than usual. A former student used this method of nursing employment to pay for continuing education to become an RN. The ability to grasp information quickly, good nursing process skills, and good critical-thinking skills are essential. Some temporary help agencies hire nurses for other countries and states.

Assisted Living Facility

Although adults who live in assisted living facilities do not need 24-hour skilled nursing care, they benefit from an LPN/LVN with good nursing process and critical-thinking skills. The LPN/LVN is constantly gathering data on the medical and psychological condition of the client. A skilled LPN/LVN, for example, will be able to pick up soft signs such as an early cough before it goes on to become pneumonia. Assisted living facilities are often a part of a nursing complex. The RN in charge evaluates the needs of the resident at the time of admission and assigns specific duties to the LPN/LVN. The RN also identifies the chain of command for the LPN/LVN should there be an emergency. If you like the human connection and you function well with less supervision, this may be an area to consider.

Additional possibilities for employment to consider include the following:

- Residential treatment centers
- Medical management companies
- State, federal, or private prison systems
- Corporate short- or long-term disability benefit administration case manager
- Day care centers for adults and children
- Weight loss clinics
- Social service agencies
- Ambulance and emergency medicine staff

- Dentist office
- Blood bank
- Substance abuse clinics
- Schools
- Adult day care
- Welfare and religious organization
- Specialized mobile units (e.g., bloodmobile)
- Fitness centers
- VISTA or the Peace Corps
- Certified Hearing Instrument Dispenser (additional education needed to attain certification)
- School nurse
- Industrial/occupational health
- Your own other areas of interest. Dare to apply!

 Try This

Area Job Opportunities

Investigate nursing job opportunities in your area. Add ideas to the list in the "Assisted Living Facility" section.

PROFESSIONAL ORGANIZATIONS

Becoming a part of and participating in at least one professional nursing organization is essential for career development. Becoming an active member permits you to have a voice in the future of nursing. It is an opportunity to meet nursing leaders, learn about current issues that affect your career, and take part in education opportunities, as well as serve on committees that influence nursing policy.

NATIONAL LEAGUE FOR NURSING

The National League for Nursing (NLN) membership is open to all levels of nurses and anyone interested in nursing issues. One of the goals of the NLN is to lead in setting standards that advance excellence and innovation in nursing education. The NLN's "Excellence in Education Model" has relevance for all levels of nursing education programs, from practical/vocational nursing to doctoral level nursing. The position statement urges nursing faculty to base their curriculum designs, teaching/learning strategies, and evaluation methods on research rather than on politically driven pronouncements (www.nurseuniverse.com/Nursing-Job/2454.html). The NLN is available to help with changes with both workshops and individual programs.

Due to changes in health care, the NLN (2010) has developed a national model for nursing education that includes competencies that graduates of all levels of nursing programs should be able to do to meet workforce needs and the needs of an increasingly diverse population. The following are NLN competencies for graduates of practical/vocational nursing programs:

- Promote the human dignity, integrity, self-determination, and personal growth of patients, oneself, and other members of the health care team.
- Provide a rationale for judgments used in the provision of safe, quality care and for decisions that promote the health of patients within a family context.
- Assess how one's personal strengths and values affect one's identity as a nurse and one's contributions as a member of the health care team.
- Question the basis for nursing actions, considering research, evidence, tradition, and patient preferences (National League for Nursing, 2010).

The NLN Centers of Excellence in Nursing Education (www.nln.org) is designed to recognize schools of nursing that have achieved a level of excellence in specific areas. The application for accreditation is voluntary, has specific criteria, and requires fees.

THE AMERICAN NURSES ASSOCIATION

The American Nurses Association (ANA) only represents registered nurses (RNs). State affiliates of the ANA are altering bylaws to allow LPNs/LVNs to join the association at the state level and pay dues but not have a voice or vote in the organization. The ANA does not represent licensed practical/vocational nurses and has attempted to limit their scope of practice. In 1965, the ANA set policy to eliminate LPNs/LVNs (Mahan, 2007) and attempted to do so again in the 1980s.

NATIONAL ASSOCIATION FOR PRACTICAL NURSE EDUCATION AND SERVICE, INC

The National Association for Practical Nurse Education and Service, Inc. (NAPNES) was founded in 1941. The multidisciplinary composition of its membership includes LPNs/LVNs, RNs, students, and schools of practical nursing, organizations, and public members promoting the ideals of NAPNES. It was the first organization dedicated to protecting practice and education and regulation of LPNs/LVNs, nursing educators, practical nursing schools, and practical nursing students. Membership in NAPNES provides the following benefits:

- A year's subscription to the *Journal of Practical Nursing* (*JPN*), the oldest journal devoted entirely to practical/vocational nursing. This quarterly, peer-reviewed journal keeps you up to date with nursing articles, news about NAPNES, infection control, nursing law, and legislation and regulations affecting LPNs/LVNs. The journal also includes feature articles about practical/vocational nursing, information about certification in pharmacology and long-term care, and other educational opportunities.
- The *eJournal of Practical Nursing* is also a publication of NAPNES. e-Members have all the rights and privileges of regular members, except they do not receive a printed copy of the *JPN*. Instead, they access *eJPN* as a PDF download. Regular membership that includes the printed *JPN* is $75 and $25

for students. e-Membership is $35 per year and $10 for students. Because of savings to NAPNES through e-Membership, the savings is passed on to members. A vast majority of income for NAPNES is provided by membership dues.

- NAPNES has launched an online continuing education program called Continuing Education Record Keeping System (CERKS). This program is available to LPN/LVN and PN educators. Registration is free and includes an online record-keeping system and instant certificate printing.
- The NAPNES website (www.napnes.org) includes information about certifications, regulation news and updates, clinical articles, CEUs, podcasts, webinars, blogs, and jobs.
- The online bookstore offers members a 10% discount and free handling and shipping.
- Networking with other LPNs/LVNs through the constituent state members throughout the United States.
- The NAPNES technology department has developed a tool for making nursing updates and education on line faster and easier.
- National representation and a say for the future of nursing.
- NAPNES Standards of Practice for LPNs/LVNs (see Appendix A).

NATIONAL FEDERATION OF LICENSED PRACTICAL NURSES

The **National Federation of Licensed Practical Nurses (NFLPN)** was organized in 1949 (www.nflpn.org). It is the policy-making body for LPNs/LVNs. NFLPN is made up of LPNs/LVNs, SPNs/SVNs, and affiliate members. Affiliate members receive all communications and may attend all meetings but do not have the right to vote or hold office. NFLPN was formed by LPNs/LVNs who wanted an organization to work for and speak on their behalf. It is the only nursing organization governed entirely by LPNs/LVNs. It is recognized by other national nursing organizations as the official voice of LPNs/LVNs. The NFLPN motto is "The Spirit of Care—The Heart of Nursing."

NFLPN membership includes the following benefits:

- Student membership fee: $25; LPN/LVN membership: $100
- National certification in IV therapy, gerontology, and foot care (new: partnered with Professional Education LLC).
- Authorized free continuing education unit (CEU) classes online through NFLPN
- CEU databank to track your CE credits
- NFLPN scholarships
- MBNA credit card
- NSO insurance

- Other merchant discounts, including Global Fitness, Tire Kingdom, Merchant's Auto Center, NTB, Hertz, Coast to Coast, and Healthcare Workwear
- Annual convention and trade show offering CE courses
- Legislative watchdog on issues affecting LPNs/LVNs
- Networking opportunities through your chapter meetings
- Student Honor Society for achieving PN students
- Monthly scholarship toward tuition for upward mobility through RUE Education
- Bachelor of science program for LPNs/LVNs through Medical University of the Americas
- Annual LPN/LVN Recognition & Awareness Week (first week in October each year)
- Discounted convention registration for members

RUE Education in partnership with NFLPN is sponsoring websites for participating LPN/LVN associations. The websites make it possible to follow the work being done on your behalf. The quarterly *Visions* newsletter informs what is happening in regard to NFLPN and Rue Education opportunities. See Appendix B for NFLPN Practice Standards for Licensed Practical/Vocational Nurses.

CONTINUING EDUCATION

Historically, LPNs/LVNs have a reputation for being apathetic in pursuing continuing education classes. This is difficult to believe because many LPNs/LVNs have gone on to learn complex nursing skills after graduation. Continuing education classes are available through many agencies. If the education benefits the agency, they may be willing to pick up part or the entire fee. Some agency courses are free and are part of continuing service within the agency. Initial licensure is being questioned as providing competency for life. Your continued study helps keep you up to date and ensure competency as an LPN/LVN. Continuing education includes the following.

IN-SERVICE TRAINING

In-service training is information chosen to meet specific needs in a facility. Attendance at some in-service programs, such as a yearly update on bloodborne pathogens, is required. Offer suggestions for content to your employer. Usually a specified amount of time is required for in-service programs, such as 1 hour per month or three times per year, according to the agency policy. Depending on the credentials of the instructor, continuing education credits may be available.

WORKSHOPS

Workshops present information and an opportunity to practice what is being taught. Workshops provide opportunities to learn new skills. Workshop length varies according to content. Some agencies pay the workshop fee or expenses if the topic is specific to, and enhances, your nursing skills. Workshops are also a major source of continuing education credits that are required by many states as a part of continued licensure in nursing.

CONTINUING EDUCATION UNITS

Classes are often taught involving complex nursing skills such as intravenous therapy, physical assessment, LPN or LVN charge nurse (leadership/management), mental health concepts, nursing process for LPNs/LVNs, and so on. Many vocational schools and community colleges will provide any course you are interested in if you request it and if enough people are available to make up the required minimum enrollment. Many of these classes provide continuing education units (CEUs) as opposed to course credit. You receive a certificate if you complete course work satisfactorily.

One of the most valuable benefits of continuing education classes is the opportunity to get together with other working LPNs/LVNs. You discover similarities in challenges and satisfactions. Ideas are shared on how to deal with difficult situations in the work setting. It is a good idea to keep a running record of all in-service programs, seminars, and workshops taken—including dates, CEUs, and topics—for future reference. Ask for these records to be included in your file at your place of employment, and keep a copy for your own file. Some states require that you list the CEUs when you apply for license renewal. Other state boards of nursing want you to have the file available in case the board decides to check the accuracy of what you stated in your renewal application.

Continuing education contact hours are also available through your professional organizations. For example, RueCEU in association with NFLPN offers unlimited contact hours for 1 year for a one-time fee of $29.99 or $8.00 per contact hour (www.RueCEU.com). The member is allowed to read any course and take the test at no cost. Tests are only paid for if they are passed. Tests are graded immediately, and incorrect answers are shown. A test can be retaken at no cost if not passed (www.nflpn.org/education.htm).

INTERNET RESOURCES

Numerous sources are available online depending on what fits your needs:
- **Advance for Nurses** (including Advance for LPNs) is available online with a free subscription (www.advanceweb.com). Current updates and nursing articles are available at the tip of your finger.
- Podcasts A podcast is a digital recording of audio and visual information on the Internet that can be downloaded to a personal media player (for example, an iPod) or a computer. The term "pod" is derived from iPod of Apple Computer, Inc, but an iPod is not necessary to listen to a podcast. The term "cast" is derived from "broadcast," as many podcasts are radio-style shows. However, they are commercial-free, of interest to the listener, and can be listened to when convenient. Google "Nursing Podcasts" for a wide selection of podcasts; Google "iTunes Nursing Podcasts" for examples of free podcasts. Medscape also provides these programs by medical experts. Remember, anyone can upload anything to the Internet. Check podcasts for relevancy and accuracy (see Chapter 5) and check with your instructors for further suggestions and the accuracy of podcasts you discover. A good primer to understand podcasting is "How to Podcast" at www.how-to-podcast-tutorial.com/what-is-apodcast.htm.
- **Medscape** offers information on health care changes, new guidelines for care, emerging infectious diseases, sudden disasters, and more through daily summaries. Medscape offers partial CE hours through their Medscape Medical News service. Although the focus is primarily RNs, there is useful information for all nurses on a daily basis. The subscription is free through www.Medscape.com.

CERTIFICATION OPPORTUNITIES

Take advantage of knowledge available during certification seminars and self-study courses. Knowledge is the basis for improved nursing skills and safety in patient care. In many states/agencies, certification is also the basis for salary increases and advancement. Some states do not recognize the significance of the certifications. Avoid using this as an excuse to avoid certification. Enhancing your competence as a nurse increases both personal and professional satisfaction. Use the extended title you have earned and wear your pin(s) proudly.

NAPNES CERTIFICATION PROGRAMS

NAPNES offers Long-Term Care Certification (LPN CLTC or LVN CLTC), Pharmacology Certification (LPN NPC or LVN NPC) and IV Therapy (LPN IVT or LVN IVT), all of which are available online (www.napnes.org/certifications/index.htm). The website offers specific directions for each certification. After NAPNES notifies you of successful completion of the examinations, you may use the preceding title that applies in your signature/title.

NFLPN CERTIFICATION PROGRAMS

NFLPN offers National Certification in Gerontology (LPN GC or LVN GC) and National Certification in IV Therapy (LPN IVC or LVN IVC). A new Foot Care Certificate is available to become a Foot Care Specialist. It includes online training, internship, and an application for certification and testing. Check out the website at www.nflpn.org/certification.html. Program details to complete the certification you desire are explained. NFLPN notifies you after successful completion of the examination. You will be able to use the appropriate initials as part of your signature/title.

Recertification is required every 2 years to maintain a valid certificate. Do not assume that requirements are the same for all certifications. Check the website for full details.

ABMCN CERTIFICATION IN MANAGED CARE

American Board of Managed Care Nursing (ABMCN) **Certification in Managed Care Nursing (CMCN)** is available to LPNs/LVNs through a home study course. Order the course materials through ABMCN (www.abmcn.org). An option is to provide an affidavit of equivalency of a course taken elsewhere. The examination is provided through a proctor. Application is done online and requires the following:

- Completed official registration form
- Proctor agreement form
- Copy of your current nursing license
- Registration fee: $250

The examination includes basic knowledge of managed care, health care economics, health care management, and patient issues. Upon successful completion of the examination, the nurse is certified and may use the title Certification in Managed Care in Nursing (CMCN).

Certification is valid for 3 years beginning January 1, following the completion of the certification exam. Proof of 25 CEUs, verification of current nursing licensure, and a $55 licensing fee are required for renewal.

MOVING UP

If you are an LPN/LVN who says, "I want to be an LPN/LVN, but I have no desire to be an RN," you have obviously given careful consideration to your personal goals. Satisfaction in nursing, both for you and patients you care for, is closely related to clear-cut goals. If you decided you want to be an LPN/LVN, chances are you will be satisfied with your choice and will provide satisfactory care to your patients. If, however, someone else decided you should be a nurse, chances are you will never be entirely satisfied with the choice. This lack of satisfaction will be mirrored in the care you give to patients. The same process is true in regard to making a decision to become an RN. If you do not want to become an RN, avoid letting anyone push you into it. Only when a goal is truly your own will you be motivated to do your best both in the educational process and in the care of patients.

If you want to enter an RN program, learn what programs of study are available. There are numerous reasons (beyond personal choice) for considering additional nursing education:

- You have investigated job opportunities in the area in which you plan to live and find that jobs for LPNs/LVNs are limited.
- The salary available is inadequate to support you and your family.
- Your current place of employment will assist you in paying for additional schooling.

[?] Critical Thinking Exercise

What are some other reasons you can think of to pursue additional education and become an RN?

MOBILITY

A major problem in developing upward **mobility programs** for LPNs/LVNs is the belief held by some educators that a practical nursing course is terminal in nature—that some state boards of nursing will not permit upward mobility programs, nor will credit be given by some professional nursing programs. Although the same reasoning continues to be held in some parts of the country, other directors of nursing have successfully negotiated with state boards of nursing to develop progressive LPN/LVN-to-RN programs. Contact your state's board of nursing for a list of available accredited nursing programs in your state. Also, talk to your current school counselor about accredited nursing programs available to you. Find out how to apply and if additional courses are needed for admission; the costs; the availability of grants, if local; and if transfer of credits is possible.

Educational Mobility for Nurses

In her book *Career Ladder*, Ahl (1975) states the following:

> I believe that historically the Helene Fuld School of Nursing at the Hospital of Joint Diseases and Medical Center [New York City] is the first program to demonstrate the belief that practical/vocational nursing is indeed a part of the nursing profession and that a curriculum can be constructed that effectively articulates with one that prepares for registered nurse licensure with minimal repetition.

The program, initially a 15-month course trimmed down to 47 weeks, was initiated in 1964. Justine Hannan, hospital director of nursing, worked with the board of nursing in New York State's Education Department. By 1968 the department granted full registration to the program, and by 1970 it was accredited by the NLN. Ahl goes on to say:

> The school has had an impact on the quality of nursing in its home hospital and has sent graduates into dozens of

other health care facilities throughout New York and 15 other states. It has willingly shared its experience with educators who have made inquiries about its work and has demonstrated that career ladder education is both valid and appropriate for a large number of persons who have the aptitude and commitment to such a goal.

Career ladder programs (seamless programs) are carefully planned to avoid duplication of content. In her book *Career Mobility*, Story (1974) describes her nursing program.

> The curriculum is a practical nursing curriculum for the first year and an associate degree nursing curriculum for the second. It is a totally new curriculum designed in terms of essential learning for beginning nursing competencies. It allows the student to be a competent practical nurse at the end of the program and a competent registered nurse at the end of an additional year.

Career ladder programs (seamless programs) exist in many areas of the country. The costs of programs vary considerably. Your state board of nursing is an excellent resource for information about programs in your area.

Minneapolis Community and Technical College Mobility Program.
Minneapolis Community and Technical College (MCTC) has one of the oldest nursing programs in the country, and it has continued to evolve with the times. Its major nursing program is a seamless program for nursing assistant/home health aide to practical nurse to associate in science degree in Nursing (A.S.D.N.). MCTC has an articulation agreement with the Metropolitan State University and Minnesota State College and Universities (MNSCU) consortium and many private institutions. This gives you an opportunity to transfer upon completion of the ASDN to complete a bachelor of science in nursing degree (BSN). The program is accredited by the NLN and is approved by the Minnesota State Board of Nursing.

Distance Learning Nursing Program at Excelsior College.
Excelsior College (previously known as Regents College), of Albany, New York, is the first in the United States to have a distance learning nursing program (online). The associate degree in nursing program began in 1972 and has been continuously accredited by the National League for Nursing Accrediting Council (NLNAC). There are no classes to attend; the student can study when convenient and take examinations when ready. Interest-free financing is available.

LPNs/LVNs must apply for admission and be accepted to the School of Nursing before enrolling. Requirements are found on their website at www. excelsior.edu. Licensed LPNs/LVNs are eligible to apply (except for California residents). The college is founded on the premise that what you know is more important than where you learned it. College faculty evaluate all previous credits you have earned. Possible credits include courses you have taken from other regionally accredited colleges and universities, military training, continuing education programs, and Internet-based programs. Generous learner support is made available to students from full-time advisors and nursing faculty. Students are able to study and prepare at their own pace while maintaining their jobs. Because there is no residency requirement, you will not have to repeat courses you have already taken.

iStudySmart.com.
iStudySmart.com is an educational partners to help LPNs/LVNs continue their nursing education to become an associate of science RN or a bachelor of science nurse. iStudySmart helps you test out of college classes and receive college credit.. You determine the testing time when you are ready. Some local universities accept 30 to 45 semester hours of credit by exam. Fully accredited schools may accept more. Course work is available for purchase at www.iStudySmart.com. Course work is done online, in workbook format, or with a CD-ROM. After purchasing the textbook, complete all the assignments. Work through the practice exams, and when ready, go to the local test site to have your examination for the course. Send the passing score to the university or college.

NONCREDIT REGISTERED NURSE PROGRAMS

Turf issues continue to exist in all levels of nursing—CNA to LPN/LVN to ADN to BSN to MSN to a Doctorate in Nursing (see Chapter 15). Plan to be a part of the solution, not the problem, when you are in a position to make a difference. This is an area where you, as a member of your professional nursing organization, can make your voice heard.

Some RN programs continue to ignore the value of practical/vocational education. These programs insist that LPNs/LVNs start from the beginning and repeat all previously covered theory and skills courses, including basic nursing skills. The bottom line is that a number of programs are available throughout the country that the LPN/LVN can use to become an RN—with credit given for being an LPN/LVN.

The state boards of nursing are an excellent source for locating approved nursing programs. Many of the programs have websites that make it possible to get information about a program before inquiring directly. Ask your board for a list of board-approved professional nursing programs preparing for registered nurse licensure that are open to the LPN/LVN.

Get Ready for the NCLEX-PN® Examination

Key Points

- A majority of 2009 newly licensed LPNs/LVNs work in long-term care facilities and a smaller number in rehabilitation units and other settings. Care was primarily for adults and elderly patients. Over half of the patients had chronic, stable illnesses, and almost half had behavioral/emotional problems.
- NCSBN's Transition to Practice Models Phase I and II studied the use of standardized evidence-based models on patient safety and quality outcomes.
- Desirable nursing characteristics for work areas vary according to the work involved. Overall, nurses must know how to think critically and problem solve and to be emotionally stable, physically healthy, caring, and empathetic.
- Postgraduate certification courses are available for LPNs/LVNs through NAPNES, NFLPN, American Board of Managed Care, and other organizations. Certifications increase knowledge and skill and, in many states, salary and position.
- LPN/LVN to associate degree programs in nursing are available throughout the United States. Contact your state board of nursing for a current listing of approved programs.
- Belonging to at least one professional nursing organization (e.g., NAPNES, NFLPN, NLN) provides benefits and, most important, a voice in the future of nursing.
- Turf issues continue in all levels of nursing: CNA to LPN/LVN to ADN to BSN to MSN to a nursing doctorate. When you are in a position to make a difference, plan to be part of the solution, not the problem.

Additional Learning Resources

evolve Go to your Evolve website (http://evolve.elsevier.com/Hill/Success) for the following FREE learning resources:
- Answers to Critical Thinking Review Scenarios
- Additional learning activities
- Additional Review Questions for the NCLEX-PN® exam
- Helpful phrases for communicating in Spanish and more!

Review Questions for the NCLEX-PN® Examination

1. What is the current major area of employment for LPNs/LVNs?
   1. Military
   2. Nursing homes
   3. Hospitals
   4. Clinics

2. Why should you become certified in nursing-related areas after becoming an LPN/LVN?
   1. The certifications are designed to increase your nursing knowledge and skill.
   2. You will gradually be able to assume the work of an RN without an RN license.
   3. Use of the extended title(s) will greatly improve your status among other employees.
   4. Unless your state board acknowledges the certification, it serves no purpose.

3. After a visit to an NFLPN meeting, you evaluate critically the major benefit to you as an LPN/LVN. Which benefit has long-term value to you and to nursing?
   1. Obtaining IV Therapy and Gerontology certifications through the organization.
   2. Working toward reform in nursing curricula and methods of teaching in nursing.
   3. Receiving reduced rates on insurance, continuing education, and credit cards.
   4. Being part of the policy-making body for LPNs/LVNs, governed by LPNs/LVNs.

4. When seeking employment, you want to find out whether the health facility has a Transition to Practice model. What is a Transition to Practice model?
   1. A series of courses that are a shortcut to becoming an RN.
   2. Assistance in learning for "how things are really done" here.
   3. Trained staff assigned to assist in applying theory into practice.
   4. A system of perks for model employees during the first 6 months.

Alternate Format Item

1. Using critical thinking, which of the following will enhance your career when choosing your first job as an LPN/LVN? (Select all that apply.)
   1. Learn if the work you are expected to do is within your scope of practice.
   2. Take the least challenging job because you are just beginning your career.
   3. Check the availability of orientation, RN supervision, and instruction as needed.
   4. Know the hours of work, salary, benefits, types of patients, in-service, and staffing.

2. What are some benefits of joining an LPN/LVN-affiliated nursing organization? (Select all that apply.)
   1. It will give you a vote on nursing issues.
   2. There are discounts on certification programs.
   3. It helps keep you up to date on nursing issues.
   4. It provides an opportunity to network with peers.

Critical Thinking Scenarios

Scenario 1
Susan has been receiving a lot of pressure from her parents to become an RN. How should she decide?

Scenario 2

Richard has been employed at the local nursing home as a staff LPN. He finds the job stressful because he has to make so many decisions. His dad keeps telling him, "Richard, if you can't make it in civilian life, join the army. You'll have food, shelter, and clothing, and they will tell you what to do and when to do it."

Today was Richard's day off. He walked into the army recruiting office and signed up! What is your impression of Richard's decision?

NAPNES Standards of Practice and Educational Competencies of Graduates of Practical/Vocational Nursing Programs

These standards and competencies are intended to better define the range of capabilities, responsibilities, rights, and relationship to other health care providers for scope and content of practical/vocational nursing education programs. The guidelines will assist:

- Educators in development, implementation, and evaluation of practical/vocational nursing curricula.
- Students in understanding expectations of their competencies upon completion of the educational program.
- Prospective employers in appropriate utilization of the practical/vocational nurse.
- Consumers in understanding the scope of practice and level of responsibility of the practical/vocational nurse.

A. PROFESSIONAL BEHAVIORS

Professional behaviors, within the scope of nursing practice for a practical/vocational nurse, are characterized by adherence to standards of care, accountability for one's own actions and behaviors, and use of legal and ethical principles in nursing practice. Professionalism includes a commitment to nursing and a concern for others demonstrated by an attitude of caring. Professionalism also involves participation in life long self-development activities to enhance and maintain current knowledge and skills for continuing competency in the practice of nursing for the LP/VN, as well as individual, group, community, and societal endeavors to improve health care.

Upon completion of the practical/vocational nursing program, the graduate will display the following program outcome:

Demonstrate professional behaviors of accountability and professionalism according to the legal and ethical standards for a competent licensed practical/vocational nurse.

Competencies which demonstrate this outcome has been attained:

1. Comply with the ethical, legal, and regulatory frameworks of nursing and the scope of practice as outlined in the LP/VN nurse practice act of the specific state in which licensed.
2. Utilize educational opportunities for life-long learning and maintenance of competence.
3. Identify personal capabilities and consider career mobility options.
4. Identify own LP/VN strengths and limitations for the purpose of improving nursing performance.
5. Demonstrate accountability for nursing care provided by self and/or directed to others.
6. Function as an advocate for the health care consumer, maintaining confidentiality as required.
7. Identify the impact of economic, political, social, cultural, spiritual, and demographic forces on the role of the licensed practical/vocational nurse in the delivery of health care.
8. Serve as a positive role model within healthcare settings and the community.
9. Participate as a member of a practical/vocational nursing organization.

B. COMMUNICATION

Communication is defined as the process by which information is exchanged between individuals verbally, non-verbally, and/or in writing or through information technology. Communication abilities are integral and essential to the nursing process. Those who are included in the nursing process are the licensed practical/vocational nurse and other members of the nursing and healthcare team, client, and significant support person(s). Effective communication demonstrates caring, compassion, and cultural awareness and is directed toward promoting positive outcomes and establishing a trusting relationship.

Upon completion of the practical/vocational nursing program, the graduate will display the following program outcome:

Effectively communicate with patients, significant support person(s), and members of the interdisciplinary health care team, incorporating interpersonal and therapeutic communication skills.

Competencies which demonstrate this outcome has been attained:

1. Utilize effective communication skills when interacting with clients, significant others, and members of the interdisciplinary healthcare team.
2. Communicate relevant, accurate, and complete information.
3. Report to appropriate health care personnel and document assessments, interventions, and progress or impediments toward achieving client outcomes.
4. Maintain organizational and client confidentiality.
5. Utilize information technology to support and communicate the planning and provision of client care.
6. Utilize appropriate channels of communication.

C. ASSESSMENT

Assessment is the collection and processing of relevant data for the purposes of appraising the client's health status. Assessment provides a holistic view of the client which includes physical, developmental, emotional, psychosocial, cultural, spiritual, and functional status. Assessment involves the collection of information from multiple sources to provide the foundation for nursing care. Initial assessment provides the baseline for future comparisons in order to individualize client care. Ongoing assessment is required to meet the client's changing needs.

Upon completion of the practical/vocational nursing program, the graduate will display the following program outcome:

Collect holistic assessment data from multiple sources, communicate the data to appropriate health care providers, and evaluate client responses to interventions.

Competencies which demonstrate this outcome has been attained:

1. Assess data related to basic physical, developmental, spiritual, cultural, functional, and psychosocial needs of the client.
2. Collect data within established protocols and guidelines from various sources, including client interviews, observations/measurements, health care team members, family, significant other(s), and review of health records.
3. Assess data related to the client's health status, identify impediments to client progress, and evaluate response to interventions.
4. Document data collection, assessment, and communicate findings to appropriate member(s) of the healthcare team.

D. PLANNING

Planning encompasses the collection of health status information, the use of multiple methods to access information, and the analysis and integration of knowledge and information to formulate nursing care plans and care actions. The nursing care plan provides direction for individualized care and assures the delivery of accurate, safe care through a definitive pathway that promotes the clients and support persons's(s') progress toward positive outcomes.

Upon completion of the practical/vocational nursing program, the graduate will display the following program outcome:

Collaborate with the registered nurse or other members' of the health care team to organize and incorporate assessment data to plan/revise patient care and actions based on established nursing diagnoses, nursing protocols, and assessment and evaluation data.

Competencies which demonstrate this outcome has been attained:

1. Utilize knowledge of normal values to identify deviation in health status to plan care.
2. Contribute to formulation of a nursing care plan for clients with non-complex conditions and in a stable state, in consultation with the registered nurse and as appropriate in collaboration with the client or support person(s), as well as members of the interdisciplinary health care team, using established nursing diagnoses and nursing protocols.
3. Prioritize nursing care needs of clients.
4. Assist in the review and revision of nursing care plans with the registered nurse to meet the changing needs of clients.
5. Modify client care as indicated by the evaluation of stated outcomes.
6. Provide information to client about aspects of the care plan within the LP/VN scope of practice.
7. Refer client as appropriate to other members of the health care team about care outside the scope of practice of the LP/VN.

E. CARING INTERVENTIONS

Caring interventions are those nursing behaviors and actions that assist clients and significant others in meeting their needs and the identified outcomes of the plan of care. These interventions are based on knowledge of the natural sciences, behavioral sciences, and past nursing experiences. Caring is the "being with" and "doing for" that assists clients to achieve the desired outcomes. Caring behaviors are nurturing, protective, compassionate, and person-centered. Caring creates an environment of hope and trust, where client choices related to cultural, religious, and spiritual values, beliefs, and lifestyles are respected.

Upon completion of the practical/vocational nursing program, the graduate will display the following program outcome:

Demonstrate a caring and empathic approach to the safe, therapeutic, and individualized care of each client.

Competencies which demonstrate this outcome has been attained:

1. Provide and promote the client's dignity.
2. Identify and honor the emotional, cultural, religious, and spiritual influences on the client's health.
3. Demonstrate caring behaviors toward the client and significant support person(s).
4. Provide competent, safe, therapeutic, and individualized nursing care in a variety of settings.
5. Provide a safe physical and psychosocial environment for the client and significant other(s).
6. Implement the prescribed care regimen within the legal, ethical, and regulatory framework of practical/vocational nursing practice.
7. Assist the client and significant support person(s) to cope with and adapt to stressful events and changes in health status.
8. Assist the client and significant other(s) to achieve optimum comfort and functioning.
9. Instruct client regarding individualized health needs in keeping with the licensed practical/vocational nurse's knowledge, competence, and scope of practice.
10. Recognize client's right to access information, and refer requests to appropriate person(s).
11. Act in an advocacy role to protect client rights.

F. MANAGING

Managing care is the effective use of human, physical, financial, and technological resources to achieve the client-identified outcomes, while supporting organizational outcomes. The LP/VN manages care through the processes of planning, organizing, and directing.

Upon completion of the practical/vocational nursing program, the graduate will display the following program outcome:

Implement patient care, at the direction of a registered nurse, licensed physician, or dentist, through performance of nursing interventions or directing aspects of care, as appropriate, to unlicensed assistive personnel (UAP).

Competencies which demonstrate this outcome has been attained:

1. Assist in the coordination and implementation of an individualized plan of care for clients and significant support person(s).
2. Direct aspects of client care to qualified UAPs commensurate with abilities and level of preparation and consistent with the state's legal and regulatory framework for the scope of practice for the LP/VN.
3. Supervise and evaluate the activities of UAPs and other personnel as appropriate within the state's legal and regulatory framework for the scope of practice for the LP/VN, as well as facility policy.
4. Maintain accountability for outcomes of care directed to qualified UAPs.
5. Organize nursing activities in a meaningful and cost-effective manner when providing nursing care for individuals or groups.
6. Assist the client and significant support person(s) to access available resources and services.
7. Demonstrate competence with current technologies.
8. Function within the defined scope of practice for the LP/VN in the health care delivery system at the direction of a registered nurse, licensed physician, or dentist.

NFLPN Nursing Practice Standards for the Licensed Practical/Vocational Nurse

Nursing Practice Standards is one of the ways that the NFLPN meets the objective of its bylaws to address principles and ethics and also to meet another Article II objective: "To interpret the standards of practical (vocational) nursing."

In recent years, LPNs and LVNs have practiced in a changing environment. As LPNs and LVNs practice in expanding roles in the health care system, *Nursing Practice Standards* is essential reading for LPNs, LVNs, PN, and VN students and their educators, and all who practice with LPNs and LVNs.

NURSING PRACTICE STANDARDS FOR THE LICENSED PRACTICAL/VOCATIONAL NURSE

PREFACE

The Standards were developed and adopted by the NFLPN to provide a basic model whereby the quality of health service and nursing service and nursing care given by LPs/VNs may be measured and evaluated.

These nursing practice standards are applicable in any practice setting. The degree to which individual standards are applied will vary according to the individual needs of the patient, the type of health care agency or services, and the community resources. The scope of licensed practical nursing has extended into specialized nursing services. Therefore, specialized fields of nursing are included in this document.

THE CODE FOR LICENSED PRACTICAL/ VOCATIONAL NURSES

The Code, adopted by the NFLPN in 1961 and revised in 1979, provides a motivation for establishing, maintaining, and elevating professional standards. Each LP/VN, upon entering the profession, inherits the responsibility to adhere to the standards of ethical practice and conduct as set forth in this Code:

1. Know the scope of maximum utilization of the LP/VN as specified by the Nurse Practice Act and function within this scope.

2. Safeguard the confidential information acquired from any source about the patient.
3. Provide health care to all patients regardless of race, creed, cultural background, disease, or lifestyle.
4. Uphold the highest standards in personal appearance, language, dress, and demeanor.
5. Stay informed about issues affecting the practice of nursing and delivery of health care and, when appropriate, participate in government and policy decisions.
6. Accept the responsibility for safe nursing by keeping oneself mentally and physically fit and educationally prepared to practice.
7. Accept responsibility for membership in the NFLPN, and participate in its efforts to maintain the established standards of nursing practice and employment policies that lead to quality patient care.

INTRODUCTORY STATEMENT

Definition

Practical/vocational nursing means the performance for compensation of authorized acts of nursing that utilize specialized knowledge and skills and that meet the health needs of people in a variety of settings under the direction of qualified health professionals.

Scope

Licensed practical/vocational nurses represent the established entry into the nursing profession and include specialized fields of nursing practice. Opportunities exist for practicing in a milieu where different professions combine their particular skills in a team effort in order to preserve or improve an individual patient's functioning and to protect health and safety of patients.

Opportunities also exist for career advancement in the profession through academic education and for lateral expansion of knowledge and expertise through both academic/continuing education and certification.

STANDARDS

Education

The licensed practical/vocational nurse:

1. Shall complete a formal education program in practical nursing approved by the appropriate nursing authority in a state.

2. Shall successfully pass the National Council Licensure Examination for Practical Nurses.
3. Shall participate in initial orientation within the employing institution.

Legal/Ethical Status

The licensed practical/vocational nurse:

1. Shall hold a current license to practice nursing as an LP/VN in accordance with the law of the state wherein employed.
2. Shall know the scope of nursing practice authorized by the nurse practice act in the state wherein employed.
3. Shall have a personal commitment to fulfill the legal responsibilities inherent in good nursing practice.
4. Shall take responsible actions in situations wherein there is unprofessional conduct by a peer or other health care provider.
5. Shall recognize and have a commitment to meet the ethical and moral obligations of the practice of nursing.
6. Shall not accept or perform professional responsibilities that the individual knows he or she is not competent to perform.

Practice

The licensed practical/vocational nurse:

1. Shall accept assigned responsibilities as an accountable member of the health care team.
2. Shall function within the limits of educational preparation and experience as related to the assigned duties.
3. Shall function with other members of the health care team in promoting and maintaining health, preventing disease and disability, caring for and rehabilitating individuals who are experiencing an altered health state, and contributing to the ultimate quality of life until death.
4. Shall know and utilize the nursing process in planning, implementing, and evaluating health services and nursing care for the individual patient or group.
   a. Planning: The planning of nursing includes:
      (1) Assessing and collecting data on the health status of the individual patient, the family, and community groups
      (2) Reporting information gained from the assessment/data collection
      (3) Identifying health goals
   b. Implementing: The plan for nursing care is put into practice to achieve the stated goals and includes:
      (1) Observing, recording, and reporting significant changes that require intervention or different goals

      (2) Applying nursing knowledge and skills to promote and maintain health, to prevent disease and disability, and to optimize functional capabilities of an individual patient
      (3) Assisting the patient and family with activities of daily living and encouraging self-care as appropriate
      (4) Carrying out therapeutic regimens and protocols prescribed by personnel pursuant to authorized state law
   c. Evaluating: The plan for nursing care and its implementations are evaluated to measure the progress toward the stated goals and will include appropriate persons and/or groups to determine:
      (1) The relevancy of current goals in relation to the progress of the individual patient
      (2) The involvement of the recipients of care in the evaluation process
      (3) The quality of the nursing action in the implementation of the plan
      (4) A reordering of priorities or new goal setting in the care plan
5. Shall participate in peer review and other evaluation processes.
6. Shall participate in the development of policies concerning the health and nursing needs of society and in the roles and functions of the LP/VN.

Continuing Education

The licensed practical/vocational nurse:

1. Shall be responsible for maintaining the highest possible level of professional competence at all times.
2. Shall periodically reassess career goals and select continuing education activities that will help achieve these goals.
3. Shall take advantage of continuing education and certification opportunities that will lead to personal growth and professional development.
4. Shall seek and participate in continued education activities that are approved for credit by appropriate organizations, such as the NFLPN.

Specialized Nursing Practice

The licensed practical/vocational nurse:

1. Shall have had at least 1 year's experience in nursing at the staff level.
2. Shall present personal qualifications that are indicative of potential abilities for practice in the chosen specialized nursing area.
3. Shall present evidence of completion of a program or course that is approved by an appropriate agency

to provide the knowledge and skills necessary for effective nursing services in the specialized field.

4. Shall meet all of the standards of practice as set forth in this document.

GLOSSARY

Authorized (acts of nursing) Those nursing activities made legal through state Nurse Practice Acts.

Lateral expansion of knowledge An extension of the basic core of information learned in the school of practical nursing.

Peer review A formal evaluation of performance on the job by other LPs/VNs.

Special nursing practice A restricted field of nursing in which a person is particularly skilled and has specific knowledge.

Therapeutic regimens Regulated plans designed to bring about effective treatment of disease.

Career advancement A change of career goal.

LPN/LVN A combined abbreviation for licensed practical nurse and licensed vocational nurse. The LVN is the title used in California and Texas for the nurses who are called LPNs in other states.

Milieu One's environment and surroundings.

Protocols Courses of treatment that include specific steps to be performed in a stated order.

Glossary

A

Abandonment Leave patient unit without a nurse of equal skill and education assigned to provide care for your assigned patient.

ABMCN Certification in managed care (CMCN). Offered by the American Board of Managed Care Nursing. Certification valid for 3 years.

Abstract Summary of a research article.

Accountability Obligation to answer for personal actions.

Acculturation Adopting the culture of a different group.

Active learning Taking charge of own education.

Active listener Listener who is open minded and curious and is always asking questions about content.

Active listening Hearing sounds and searching for information relevant to those sounds so the sounds may be understood.

Acute care Higher level of care required for seriously ill patients.

Adult ADHD Adult form of attention deficit hyperactivity disorder (ADHD). Includes undependable memory and learning system.

Adult care home Assistive and health care services provided in the home.

Adult day care center A service that provides mental stimulation, socialization, assistance with some activities of daily living (ADLs), and basic observation. Services often include transportation, meals, therapeutic activities, nursing interventions, and rehabilitation activities. The service is hospital based or freestanding.

Advance directives Written documents to state personal wishes regarding future health care.

Advanced practice Post registered nurse (RN) degree, resulting in an expanded role (e.g., clinical nurse specialist, nurse practitioner, certified nurse midwife, nurse anesthetist).

Affective communication Sending or receiving information through feeling tone.

Aggressive An attacking type of behavior that occurs in response to frustration and hostile feelings.

Agnostic A person who holds the belief that the existence of God can neither be proved nor disproved.

Allah Muslim name of the one supreme being; God of Islam.

Alliances New partnerships among hospitals, clinics, laboratories, health care systems, and physicians. They coordinate the delivery of care, contain costs, and attempt to provide a seamless system.

Almshouses Homes for the poor and sick in the seventeenth and eighteenth centuries.

Ambulatory care facilities Primary health care services for walk-in patients. Also known as Urgent Care, Express Care, and Quick Care.

Ambulatory surgery centers One-day surgery centers that perform surgery at a scheduled date and time. Patient discharged home when recovered from surgery and is stable.

Analysis Break down complex information into its basic parts and relate it to the whole picture.

Anger management A way to deal with unjustified or inappropriately displayed anger.

Application Use learned information in new situations.

Apps Abbreviation for applications—programs that can be stored on an electronic device.

Artful vagueness Responding without implying either party is wrong, for example, saying, "You've got a point" or "You may be right."

Assault An unjustified attempt or threat to touch someone.

Assertiveness A way of accepting responsibility for oneself by expressing thoughts and feelings directly and honestly, without blaming oneself or others.

Assigning (assignment) Allotting tasks that are in the job description of workers. Assigned tasks are the ones that workers are hired and paid to perform.

Assimilation Giving up parts of your own culture and adopting parts of the culture of the dominant group.

Assisted care Residences that provide "a home with services."

Assisting LPN/LVN role in 4 phases (steps) of nursing process.

Associate degree nursing A 2-year community college or technical school program. The title RN is used after passing the NCLEX-RN®.

Atheist A person who does not believe the supernatural exists and therefore does not believe in God.

Attitude Nonverbal expression of the way a person thinks or feels.

Audiovisual (AV) materials Films, videotapes, or CD-ROMs.

Auditory learner Talks to himself or herself or hears sounds when thinking. Learns best by hearing.

Authorization to test (ATT) Denotes that the graduate practical/vocational nurse has met the requirements for eligibility to take the NCLEX-PN® examination. ATT applied for and obtained from the testing center.

Authorized consent Parents cannot give informed consent for medical care of a child but can give authorized consent instead.

Automatic responses Both passive and aggressive responses result from being caught by an emotional hook. These responses are not based on choice.

Autonomy Control over personal decisions.

Ayatollah A high-ranking religious and political leader in Islam.

B

Baccalaureate nursing program A 4-year college or university nursing education program.

Barton, Clara Founder of the American Red Cross.

Basic nursing skill Nursing procedure learned by the practical/vocational nursing student and suitable for providing nursing care to a patient whose clinical condition is predictable.

Basic patient situation Patient's clinical condition is predictable. Medical and nursing orders are not changing continuously. No complex modifications of nursing care is needed.

Battery Causing acute physical harm to someone.

Belittling Mimicking or making fun of person in some way.

Beneficence Doing good.

Beneficent paternalism Health care provider making decisions for the patient based on "I know what's best for you." Discounts patient autonomy.

Biomedicine Belief that abnormalities in structure and function of body organs are caused by pathogens, biochemical alterations, and/or environmental factors.

Blended course A course that combines face-to-face instruction with online learning.

Board and care homes Offer housing and custodial care. Also known as adult care homes or group homes.

Boards The NCLEX-PN® examination.

Bodily/kinesthetic learner Learns best by touching, moving, and processing knowledge through bodily sensations.

Border recognition agreement Agreement among select states to permit licensed nurses to practice in their states without additional criteria.

Breach of duty One of the elements needed to prove negligence. Means that the nurse did not adhere to standards of care.

Bridge program Associate degree nursing program that admits LPNs/LVNs to their course of study after they fulfill certain requirements.

Bucket theory Suggests that merely by lecturing, the teacher can transfer knowledge from the teacher's mind to the student's mind.

Buddha The enlightened one; Siddhartha Gautama, founder of Buddhism.

Bullying Negative acts perpetrated by one at a higher level.

Burnout Negative attitude and behavioral change about one's career, working with patients, and self-care.

C

Cadet Nurse Corps 1943 Bolton Act was the basis of the government subsidizing schools to teach nursing skills in 2½ years. More than 150,000 nurses graduated from these programs. Discontinued in 1948.

Call number Series of letters and numbers used to identify library materials and assist in locating materials.

Candidate Graduate practical/vocational nurse who will take (or is taking) the NCLEX-PN® examination.

Capability Ability or capacity.

Capitation Set fee for health care, paid annually regardless of the number of health services provided.

Care bundle Set of interventions that when used together significantly improve patient outcomes.

Career ladder programs Nursing programs planned to avoid duplication of content. The student may progress from a position as a nursing assistant to a practical/vocational nurse to an associate degree nurse to a bachelor degree nurse in approximately 4 years.

Case management method Focus is on quality, service, and cost.

Case method A method of patient care in which one nurse is assigned to give total care to one patient.

Case scenarios A printed or computer patient story that brings reality to theory in the form of a clinical situation.

C. difficile (*Clostridium difficile*) Illness caused by fecal matter from one patient entering another patient's mouth. Using an alcohol-based hand cleaner does not destroy this organism.

CD-ROM Computer disk that contains information.

Centers for Medicare and Medicaid Services (CMS) Formerly Health Care Financing Administration (HICFA). Federal agency of Department of Health and Human Services. Certifies nursing homes for Medicare and Medicaid reimbursement.

Certification Certificate awarded to an RN or LPN/LVN after passing a comprehensive examination in a select area of practice.

Certification in Long-Term Care (CLTC) Postgraduate course offered by NAPNES. Replaces previous gerontology certification. Recertification is every 5 years.

Certification in Managed Care Nursing Postgraduate course including basic knowledge of managed care, health care economics, health care management, and patient issues.

Certification in Pharmacology (NCP) Postgraduate course offered by NAPNES. Recertification is every 5 years.

Change-of-shift report Report on patient condition at beginning and end of shift.

Chemical dependency Abuse of alcohol and/or other drugs.

Chiding Scolding.

Choice Act of choosing. For example, to speak assertively is to speak out of choice.

Civil action (related to individual rights) Involves the relationships between individuals and the violation of those rights.

Clark, Mildred L Chief of Army Nurse Corps from 1963-1967.

Clerk receptionist Assumes responsibility for many clerical duties in the patient care area.

Clinical pathway Blueprint for patient care. Includes time frame of significant events that are expected to occur each day a patient with a specific diagnosis is in the hospital.

Closed-ended questions Questions that require specific answers from a patient.

Clustering A form of mapping is a method of note making.

Cochrane Collaboration An international, not-for-profit organization that prepares, maintains, and promotes the accessibility of systematic reviews of the effects of health care.

Cochrane Reviews Systematic reviews of research in health care prepared by the Cochrane Collaboration and that are freely accessible.

Codependency Situation in which a person allows another person's behavior to affect him or her and is obsessed with controlling that person's behavior.

Cognitive level Intellectual level of functioning.

Coinsurance Percentage of total bill paid for by insurance company once deductible is paid.

Commitment Pledge to do one's best.

Common law Judge-made law, which has its origins in the courts.

Communication blocks Stops meaningful conversation. Examples include chiding, belittling, probing, giving advice, and providing pat answers.

Community health nursing Nursing that focuses on improving the health status of communities or groups of people through public education, screening for early detection of disease, and providing services for people who need care outside the acute care setting.

Community health nursing services Nurses work with many people and groups on prevention and modification of health issues. Exist as part of clinic service or HMO, or is freestanding.

Community resources Include city library, museums, and health care facilities that offer programs and exhibits of interest to nurses.

Compensation Coping mechanism used to cover for real or imagined inadequacy by developing or exaggerating a desirable trait.

Complementary and alternative medicine (CAM) Focus is on assisting the body's own healing powers and restoring body balance.

Complex nursing situation Patient's clinical condition is not predictable. Medical and nursing orders are likely to involve continuous changes or complex modifications.

Comprehension Basically understand information, recall it, and identify examples of that information.

Computer-aided instruction An increasingly used teaching strategy in nursing education.

Computerized adaptive testing (CAT) Method by which the NCLEX-PN® examination is administered to the candidate (a nursing graduate who has fulfilled requirements for testing).

Computer simulation Learning activities on a CD-ROM or floppy disc that use an imaginary patient situation. The student uses the nursing process as he or she would in an actual clinical situation.

Conditional job offer Job offer contingent on passing physical, drug screening, and/or background check.

Confidentiality Avoid sharing patient information with anyone not directly involved in care without the patient's permission.

Confidentiality agreement Prior to taking NCLEX-PN examination, read and sign agreement not to disclose contents of examination.

Conflict resolution A method of resolving differences in a peaceful way.

Constructive evaluation Critique directed toward performance and behavior; has no bearing on one's value as a person.

Content management system (CMS) A platform for constructing an online course.

Continuous care retirement community Provides a continuum living option from independent living, assisted living, and skilled nursing home, all on one campus.

Continuous quality improvements (CQIs) Search for new ways to improve patient care, prevent errors, and identify and fix problems.

Continuum A way to look at two extremes (from least complex to most complex.)

Control group Subjects in a quantitative research study who do not receive the treatment. This group is compared to the experimental group.

Cooperative learning Emphasis on individual accountability for learning a specific academic task while working in small groups.

Copayment Percentage of the bill that is paid by a person (subscriber) who is enrolled in a health insurance plan.

Copyright laws These laws permit a single copy of an article for personal use. Instructors may not make copies of articles, chapters, or books for distribution to each student.

Cost containment Holding costs within fixed limits.

Course outlines Up-to-date listings of what is covered in a course. Provided by the instructor.

Criminal action Involves persons and society as a whole, for example, murder.

Critical thinking Used to resolve problems and find ways to make improvements, even when no problem exists.

CRKP Carbapeneme-resistant pneumoniae is a drug-resistant bacteria known to cause pneumonia, bloodstream infections, and meningitis. It is resistant to most antibiotics.

Cross-training Health care workers are trained to provide specific skills outside their area of assignment/education in an attempt to use workers more efficiently and to reduce costs.

Cultural bias Unquestioned, unproved way of thinking.

Cultural competence The continuous attempt of practical/vocational nurses to gain the knowledge and skills that will allow them to effectively provide care for patients of different cultures.

Cultural differences Elements found in one culture that may not be found in another.

Cultural diversity Differences in elements of culture in groups of people.

Cultural sensitivity Learning about other cultures and being respectful of their customs, rites, and beliefs.

Cultural uniqueness Differences such as family structure, food preferences, religious beliefs, concept of time, communication, education, economic status, wellness and illness beliefs, and so on.

Cultural universality Similarities that all people share regardless of culture, for example, basic needs.

Culture The total of all the ideas, beliefs, values, attitudes, communication, customs, traditions, and objects that a group of people possess. Culture includes ways of doing things.

Customs Ways of doing things that are common to a group of people of the same culture.

D

Damages One of four elements needed to prove negligence. Patient must be able to show the nurse's negligent act injured the patient in some way.

Database Data gathered provides basis for developing and evaluating care plan.

Data collection Phase 1 of nursing process for practical/vocational nurses. Involves systematic gathering and reviewing of information about the patient.

Decentralized The idea to locate centralized service departments, such as the x-ray department and the laboratory, on patient units. Health care workers are cross-trained to provide a variety of services for the patient. The goal is patient-focused care.

Deductibles Amount the subscriber must pay before health insurance begins to cover costs.

Defamation Damage to someone's reputation through false communication or communication without permission.

Delano, Jane of the American Red Cross began to recruit and train nurses for overseas duty in WWI.

Delegated medical act Physician's orders given to an RN, LPN, or LVN by a physician, dentist, or podiatrist.

Delegating (delegation) Generally, duties within the LPN/LVN job description that can be given to another worker to perform.

Denial Coping mechanism that includes rejection of events as they really are. Eliminates need for anxiety.

Department of Health and Human Services (DHHS) A federal agency funded by taxes. Advises president on national health matters.

Dependent role The LPN/LVN functions with supervision in a dependent role to the RN, physician, or dentist.

Depositions Gathering information under oath. One of the steps in bringing legal action.

Desired patient outcome Observable result. Focuses directly on what the patient will accomplish (not what the nurse will do).

Diagnosis-related group (DRG) Prospective payment system. Specifies number of days for which Medicare will pay, based on illness category.

Dietary Guidelines for Americans 2010 Based on the most recent scientific evidence for choosing healthy eating patterns.

Differentiated practice System of assigning patients for care according to patient needs, using skill mix of nursing staff.

Diploma nurse RN who has received his or her education in a 3-year hospital-based nursing program.

Diploma program A 3-year nursing educational program conducted by a hospital-based school of nursing.

Direct supervision Supervisor is continuously present to coordinate, direct, or inspect nursing care. Supervisor is in building.

Directed (or focused) thinking Purposeful and outcome-oriented thinking. Focuses on particular problem to find solution.

Discrimination Rights and privileges are withheld from those of another cultural group.

Discussion buddy Another student with whom you discuss a topic to comprehend the information.

Distance learning A course in which the teacher and student are separated by physical distance, using such tools as two-way television, videotapes, audiotapes, and the Internet.

Distracters Incorrect options for multiple-choice items.

Dix, Dorothea Lynde Appointed Superintendent of Nurses during Civil War in order to organize a corps of nurses to tend to wounded soldiers.

Do-not-resuscitate (DNR) Order written by physician. Patient will not recover. Patient may have signed an advance directive regarding end-of-life care that states personal wishes.

Durable medical power of attorney Identifies who will make decisions regarding future care, extent of treatment, and kinds of treatment if the person is unable to make his or her own decisions. Written while the person is mentally competent.

Duty One of four elements needed to prove negligence. Refers to nurse's responsibility to provide care in an acceptable way. As used in the text, responsibilities directly related to nursing licensure and scope of practice. Usually not delegated to someone with less education and nursing skill.

E

eBook Electronic, digital textbook. See *virtual textbook.*

Effectiveness Choosing the most important thing to do, and doing it accurately.

Efficiency Getting tasks done in the shortest time possible.

Electronic Controlled by a computer.

Electronic database a collection of information on a computer, for example, articles on a specific nursing topic from several sources.

Electronic device Smartphone (BlackBerry, Android, iPhone), notebook, tablet, laptop, computer.

Electronic medical record Patient records stored on a computer.

Emotional mind Site of positive feelings, such as love, caring, kindness, and compassion.

Emotional needs How people respond and deal with feelings of joy, anger, sadness, guilt, remorse, sorrow, love, etc.

Empathizer A person who intuitively figures out how people are feeling and how to treat them with sensitivity.

Empathy Respectful, detached concern.

Empower Enable, permit, and give power or authority.

Enculturation Process of learning your culture: the way your group does things, resulting in a worldview.

End-of-life principles Support core principles for end-of-life care.

Endorsement Agreement among states that nurses licensed in one state may become licensed in another if they meet the state nursing board criteria.

Entitlement program Those eligible because of age, disability, or economic status are entitled by law to benefits of certain programs, namely, Social Security, Medicare, and Medicaid.

Ethics Rules or principles that govern correct conduct.

Ethnic groups Cultural groups composed of people who are members of the same race, religion, or nation or who speak the same language.

Ethnocentrism The belief that one's own culture is best; the belief that one's way of doing things is superior/right/best.

Euthanasia Physician or other person administering lethal dose of medication to end life; illegal in the United States and Canada.

Evaluation Phase 4 of nursing process for LPNs/LVNs. Compares actual patient outcomes to expected outcomes.

Evidence-based practice Nursing procedures/interventions that have been proven to be effective.

Experimental group Subjects in a research study who receive the experimental treatment.

External distractions Interruptions in concentration from outside oneself, such as background sounds, lighting, peers, and so forth.

Extrovert A person who prefers action with others, talks more than listens, and learns by teaching others.

F

Face-to-face class A learning situation that takes place in real time.

Facilitator Instructor who creates a learning environment by arranging for a variety of activities and experiences.

False reassurance Promising patient something you cannot deliver, such as saying, "You'll be just fine."

Feedback Response to sender's message as a part of meaningful conversation.

Fee-for-service Patient pays the physician a fee for each service provided.

Felony Serious offense, with a penalty that ranges from 1 year in prison to death.

Fidelity In nursing, to be faithful to the charge of acting in the patient's best interest when the capacity to make free choice is no longer available.

Fight-flight mind When feeling threatened, the mind is activated and person begins to defend self.

First Amendment Guarantees freedom of expression as long as it is not at the expense of harming others.

Focused questions Questions that require definitive, precise information from a patient.

Follow-up illusion Irrational belief that it is the employer's responsibility to contact applicants after an interview.

Formal education Planned, organized learning, such as the nursing course of study.

Free clinic Used by persons who cannot afford traditional health care. May have an age and income range. The clinic charges a minimal fee.

Freestanding Health facility not attached to a hospital.

Functional method A method of patient care that is task-oriented and involves dividing the tasks to be done among staff members according to their abilities.

Fundamentalism A conservative form of a religion.

G

General hospitals Set up to treat a variety of medical/surgical problems.

General (implied) consent By entering a health facility voluntarily, a patient gives permission for treatment with noninvasive procedures. However, a patient may revoke this consent verbally and refuse to be treated.

General supervision Supervisor regularly coordinates, directs, or inspects nursing care and is within reach either in the building or by phone.

Generalization Broad, sweeping statements made about a group.

Generational personality Personality of people born around the same period of time and shaped by a common history of cultural events, images, and experiences.

Gerontology Certification (GC) Postgraduate education in gerontology through NFLPN and ERI. Certification effective for 2 years.

Giving advice Telling someone what to do.

Global thinkers Also known as right-brain dominant.

Goals (outcomes) Realistic, measurable, time-limited statements of resolution of a problem or need.

Good Samaritan Act Stipulates that a person who provides emergency care at the scene of an accident is immune from civil liability for actions done in good faith. There is some variation of the law within states.

Goodacres, Glenna Designed and sculpted Vietnam Women's Memorial. Located on the National Mall in Washington, D.C.

Goodrich, Anna helped form the National Emergency Committee on Nursing during WWI.

Green House Designed to deinstitutionalize longterm care by eliminating large nursing facilities. These are homes with 6–12 elders in a residential setting.

Gretter, Lystra modified the Hippocratic Oath in 1893 and named it The Nightingale Pledge.

Group home Provides personal care services (custodial) for 3 to 16 residents. Provides help with ADLs, self-administration of medication, meal preparation, and transportation.

Guest speakers Nurses or other health professionals invited to present up-to-date information on areas of expertise.

Guidelines Specific practice recommendations derived from the summary of research articles.

H

Habits Established patterns of behavior.

Halal Lawful or legal; anything allowable by Islamic law.

Haram Anything forbidden by Islamic law.

Hard copy Data from a computer that is printed out to be read, rather than reading from the computer screen.

Hard wiring Biologically a part of brain development.

Hayes, Colonel Anna Mae Led Army Nurse Corps during the Vietnam War. First woman to become a brigadier general and first woman in American military to attain general officer rank.

Healthcare Associated Infections (HAIs) Infections patients develop in a hospital or other facility.

Health care provider A licensed health care person, such as a physician, dentist, or nurse practitioner, whose health care services are covered by a health insurance plan.

Health Insurance Portability and Accountability Act (HIPAA) 2003 Federal law commonly called the Privacy Act.

Health maintenance organization (HMO) A comprehensive care system of medical services based on a set, prepaid fee.

Hidden job market Unadvertised jobs.

Higbee, Lenah S. World War I Navy nurse. Received the Navy Cross. Was the first nurse to have a destroyer named in her honor.

Home health nursing Provides health services supervised by a licensed professional in a patient's home. Examples include visiting nurse associations, health departments, home health agencies, etc.

Honesty To not deliberately deceive in order to present oneself in a better light.

Hospice care End-of-life care for the terminally ill. The philosophy is to maintain comfort as death approaches.

Howlett Hierarchy Hierarchy of work motivators. Adapted from Maslow's Hierarchy of Needs.

Humor Communication characteristic to help "lighten up" a situation.

Hybrid course A course that blends face-to-face instruction with online learning.

I

Idea sketches Representing a verbal concept with a picture.

Illegal questions Interview questions that do not have to be answered, such as age, marital status, number of children, and health problems, unless directly related to job.

Illiteracy Inability to comprehend meaning of what is read.

Impaired nurse One who is addicted to alcohol or other drugs.

Implementation Phase 3 of the nursing process for LPNs/LVNs. Provides required nursing care to accomplish established patient goals.

Incident report Federally required brief narrative of incident, written by person who witnessed it. Purpose is in-house improvement of care.

Incremental method Changes that occur here and there without affecting the system as a whole.

Independent Function without supervision, for example, the RN role in the nursing process.

Informal education Obtained through school of life.

Informational interview By appointment, meet with an administrator to learn about a facility. This is not a job interview, although it is treated with the same courtesy.

Informed consent Obtained by physician for invasive procedures after physician has provided patient with facts about effects, side effects, alternative treatments, prognosis, and so on. May be revoked verbally at any time up to time of procedure.

Insidious aggression Involves incivility and hostile acts that are note obvious to others.

Institute of Medicine An independent, nonprofit organization that advises the public and decision makers with ways to improve health.

Institutional liability Form of vicarious liability. Health setting sued for negligence of employee.

Intentional tort Intent to do a wrongful act.

Interdependent Both RNs and LPNs/LVNs collaboratively carry out orders for treatments and medications written by a physician.

Interlibrary loan services Allows libraries to borrow materials from other libraries that are not a part of their holdings.

Intermediate care facility (ICF) Recognized under Medicare program. Provides services for people who have physical or mental conditions but do not require acute or skilled nursing services.

Internal distractions Interruptions in concentration from inside oneself, such as daydreaming and boredom.

Internet Physical infrastructure that allows the electronic circulation of vast amounts of information to computer users. This information is unregulated and cannot always be taken at face value.

Interpersonal learner Learns best by sharing, comparing, cooperating, and interviewing.

Interpersonal styles Four major styles: analytical type, driver type, amicable type, and expressive type.

Interstate endorsement Agreement among states that licensed nurses do not have to repeat the NCLEX-PN® examination if they meet criteria for working in the state.

Intervention Action taken to reach a patient outcome.

Intrapersonal learner Learns best by working alone, self-paced instruction, and having own space.

Introvert A person who listens more than talks, concentrates; a reflective thinker who wants to understand the world.

Irrational thinking Based on Ellis (1994). Self-talk is often irrational thinking: Judgments are subjective and have no bearing on facts. Leads to negative emotions and stress.

IV Therapy Certification (IVC) Postgraduate education on intravenous therapy, offered through NFLPN and ERI.

J

Jesus Christ Founder of Christian religion.

Justice Giving patients their due and treating them fairly.

K

Key Correct option(s) for a multiple choice or alternate item format question.

Kinesthetic/tactual learner Have 2 sub channels: movement and touch.

Kinkela-Keil, Captain Lillian Member of the Air Force Nurse Corps. Flew over 200 air evacuation missions during World War II, as well as 25 transatlantic crossings. Went back to civilian flying until the Korean War. Flew several hundred more missions as a flight nurse in Korea. Numerous decorations. Inspiration for the movie *Flight Nurse*.

Knowledge Repeat information exactly as read or told. Does not imply an understanding of the information.

Kosher Prepared or served according to Jewish ritual dietary laws.

L

Lateral violence Between nursing colleagues. Includes both overt and covert physical, verbal, and emotional abuse by one nurse against another.

Law Nursing law is based on each state's Nurse Practice Act.

Leadership Manner in which the leader gets along with coworkers, with the goal of producing workplace changes to meet the goals of the employing agency.

Learning resource center (LRC) The library.

Lecture-discussion strategy A strategy in which the instructor shares several ideas with the class and then stops to let the class discuss the ideas.

Left-brain dominant A person who is more orderly, is logical, reads and writes well, and excels at analytical thinking.

Leininger's Culture Care Theory Recognition of the link between a person's cultural background and his or her response to nursing care.

Liability Legal responsibility of a person to account for wrongful acts by making financial restitution.

Libel Damage to someone's reputation through written communication or pictures.

Librarian College-educated specialist in what the library has to offer.

Linguistic learner Learns best by saying, hearing, and seeing words.

Living will Written directive stating personal wishes regarding future health care. Not recognized as a legal document in every state or other countries.

Logical learner Learns best by using an organized method of study.

Long-term care Range of medical care to assist persons with disability or chronic care needs.

Long-term goal A general realistic statement of what one hopes to attain ultimately.

LRC holdings Library materials including books, periodicals, catalogued materials, CDs, DVDs, audiotapes, videotapes, etc.

M

Malpractice (professional negligence) A part of negligence that relates to lack of skill or misconduct by professional persons.

Managed care A system of controlling cost of health care by arranging health care at predetermined rates. An HMO is an example of managed care.

Management Organizing all care required for patients in a health care setting for a specific period.

Manipulation An indirect way of dealing with issues that may be positive or negative. Negative (maladaptive) manipulation occurs if the feelings of others are disregarded or other people are treated as objects.

Map Care maps are a combination of care plans and critical pathways.

Mapping A form of note making in which information and its relationships are put in a visual pattern.

Maslow's Hierarchy of Human Needs and Evolving Hierarchy of Needs A way to look at identifying patient care priorities and responding to the patient's needs according to the patient's level of functioning.

Medicaid Financial assistance provided by the federal government for states and counties to pay for medical services for eligible poor.

Medicare Federally sponsored and supervised health insurance plan for persons 65 years of age and older and persons under 65 years who are totally and permanently disabled.

Medicare Advantage Government-approved health plan options to original Medicare offered by private insurance companies.

Medicare Quality Improvement Organizations (QIOs) Formerly known as peer review organizations. Under the direction of Centers for Medicare and Medicaid Services.

Melting pot The United States became known as the "melting pot" in the nineteenth century, when immigrants would assimilate into the dominant culture.

Mental imagery Uses the right side of the brain to generate pictures of an idea; the left side supplies the script.

Message The idea being conveyed or the question being asked.

Minitask Simple to do and takes no more than 5 minutes. An unpleasant, difficult, time-consuming task can be divided into a series of minitasks.

Misdemeanor Least serious infraction of the law. Can result in a fine or up to 1 year in jail.

Mission statement A statement that defines the purpose and goals of a health care organization.

Mississippi, 1914 First state to pass a law licensing practical nurses.

Mnemonic devices Memory aids such as rhymes or acronyms.

Mobile device PDA, smartphone (iPhone, BlackBerry), iPod Touch, ebook reader, and tablet.

Mobility program Seamless program of study from CNA to LPN/LVN to associate degree RN to BSN to MSN to Doctorate Degree in Nursing.

Mock Examination NCLEX-PN type examination but does not include actual NCLEX questions.

Mock examinations Prelicensure and readiness tests in the NCLEX-PN® examination format. Does not contain actual NCLEX-PN® examination questions.

Morals Dealing with right and wrong behavior.

MRSA Methicillin-resistant *Staphylococcus aureus*. Sometimes called the original superbug: dangerous, deadly, and highly transmissible.

Multiculturalism Mix of cultures.

Multistate licensure (Nursing Licensure Compact) Legislation in some states that renders a nursing license obtained in that state valid for practice in other states with multistate legislation. Each state's individual regulations must still be followed.

Musical learner Learns best by humming, singing, or playing an instrument.

MyPlate Replaces the MyPyramid food guideline. Introduced June 2011 by the Department of Agriculture and U.S. Health and Human Services. Provides a reasonable way to make healthy food choices.

N

NANDA-I North American Nursing Diagnosis Association.

NAPNES National Association for Practical Nurse Education and Service, Inc.

National Certification in IV Therapy Postgraduate course through NAPNES.

National Certification in Gerontology Postgraduate NFLN program leading to certification in gerontology.

National Patient Safety Foundation (NPSF) An organization that aims to improve safety in health care.

Naturalistic system Beliefs developed from the traditional medical practices of the ancient civilizations of China, India, and Greece.

NCLEX-PN® examination National Council Licensing Examination for Practical Nursing.

Negligence Conduct that falls below the standard of care established by law for the protection of others.

Networking Building relationships with instructors, employers, and peers for the purposes of finding new jobs, better pay, faster promotions, and greater job satisfaction.

NFLPN National Federation of Licensed Practical Nurses.

NIC Nursing Interventions Classification.

Nightingale, Florence Founder of modern nursing who is known as "The Lady with the Lamp" because of her after-hours rounds with her lamp during the Crimean War.

Nightingale's Environmental Model Often considered the first nursing theory. Nightingale believed strongly that environmental issues such as ventilation, warming, noise, light, cleanliness of rooms and walls, personal cleanliness, food, and so on influenced the outcome of an illness.

NLN National League for Nursing.

NOC Nursing Outcomes Classification.

Nonassertive (passive) Fear-based, emotionally dishonest, self-defeating type of behavior. Gives message of "I don't count, but you count."

Nonjudgmental Taking at face value. Accepting people as they are.

Nonmaleficence First, do no harm.

Nonverbal communication Sending or receiving information by facial expressions or body language.

Notes on Nursing Written by Florence Nightingale.

Nurse Practice Act Governs the practice of nursing.

Nursing assistant Minimum 75-hour course prepares nursing assistant to give bedside care. Successful completion makes Certified Nursing Assistant eligible for state registry.

Nursing research An organized way of finding information that supports existing knowledge and develops new knowledge for clinical practice, nursing education, and nursing services.

Nursing diagnosis Second step of the nursing process for RNs: Actual and high-risk problems that nurses can respond to. Exclusive responsibility of RN in nursing process.

Nursing ethics System of principles governing conduct of nurses.

Nursing home Offers personal and skilled nursing care (if needed) 24 hours a day.

Nursing organizations Groups for nurses focused on nursing issues of importance.

Nursing process An orderly way of developing a plan of care for the individual patient. RN is responsible for developing the nursing diagnosis.

Nursing research Developing new knowledge through observation and experimentation.

Nursing skills lab Resource that allows student nurses to practice and develop nursing skills.

Nursing standard of care Guideline for good nursing care. Standards are based on what an ordinary, prudent nurse with similar education and nursing experience would do in a similar situation.

Nursing theories Often used as a basis for developing nursing curricula.

Nutrient-dense foods Foods high in nutritional value.

Nutting, Adelaide helped form the National Emergency Committee on Nursing during WWI.

O

Objective information Data that can be observed and verified. Data obtained by seeing, hearing, touching, smelling, tasting, measuring, counting, and so on. Does not include subjective judgment.

Official (government) health care agencies Local, state, and federal health agencies supported by tax dollars.

Omnibus Reconciliation Act of 1987 (OBRA) Major federal legislation that addresses the quality of life, health, and safety of residents.

One-way communication When the sender controls a situation and offers no opportunity for feedback from the receiver; used to give a command.

Online catalog Computerized card catalog in the library.

Open-ended questions Questions that permit the patient to respond in a way most meaningful to him or her. These type of questions often begin with what, where, when.

Options Choices—for example, choices for an answer in a multiple-choice item.

Oregon Death with Dignity Act Allows terminally ill Oregonians to end their lives through voluntary self-administration of lethal medication.

Orem's Self-Care Deficit Theory This nursing theory has three subtheories: self-care, self-care deficit, and the nursing system. Nursing data collection can be used to identify the particular deficit in order to choose interventions that will have the desired outcomes for the patient.

Original Medicare Part A (hospital insurance; no premium required), and Part B (medical insurance) and Part D (prescription insurance). Plan B and D are optional and require a monthly fee.

Outcome Identifies the degree of progress made (or not made) by the patient toward reaching a goal.

Outpatient clinic Provides health care outside of the hospital setting. Staffed by physicians and nurses.

Outlining method Especially popular method of note making for left-brain dominant persons.

Out-of-pocket Fee a patient pays directly.

P

Paradigm A way of thinking.

Paradigm shift Change in the way of thinking.

Parish nurse Works in various church settings in a health ministry.

Passive learning Dependent on instructor to provide information, for example, through lecture.

Passive listener A person who receives sounds with little recognition or personal involvement.

Pastoral care team Members of the health team who assist nurses in meeting the spiritual needs of the patients.

Pat answers General responses. Communication block. Discounts patient as a person.

Patience Willingness to put up with waiting and being okay about doing so.

Patient Bill of Rights Mandated by federal and state laws. Spell out patient rights while hospitalized.

Patient-centered care Care that is responsive to patient preferences, needs, and values.

Patient competency Relates to ability to understand and make decisions. Has both legal and clinical meaning.

Patient-focused care Attempt to improve the quality of care by using hospital resources more efficiently to meet the patient's needs (e.g., decentralizing services).

Patient outcomes Focus on whether patient has accomplished what was desired during treatment. Does not focus on what the nurse did.

Patient Self-Determination Act (PSDA) Basis for advanced directives. Federal law mandates that Medicare and Medicaid patients must be told of their right to formulate advance directives.

Peer-reviewed Information reviewed by others in a subject for accuracy, quality, and appropriateness.

Peplau's Interpersonal Relations Theory Basis for developing a therapeutic relationship with a patient (especially useful for working with adult or child psychiatric patients). The relationship has certain parameters that are a major part of the treatment. The overlapping phases are orientation, identification, exploitation, and resolution.

Perceptual learning style Refers to learning by three main sensory receivers: visual, auditory, and kinesthetic.

Performance evaluation Evaluation of clinical performance that involves input from the instructor and the student.

Periodical indexes List of periodicals by author, title, and subject.

Periodicals Magazines published weekly, monthly, and quarterly.

Personal ethics Provide personal guidelines for living.

Personal liability Holds person (nurse) responsible for own actions.

Personalistic system Belief that a deity, ghost, god, evil spirit, witch, or angry ancestor is punishing the sick person.

Physician-assisted suicide Name tagged onto "Oregon Death with Dignity Law." Physician writes prescription for medication to end life but does not administer it. Patient self-administers lethal medication.

Planning Phase 2 of the nursing process for LPNs/LVNs. Involves assisting the RN in development of the nursing diagnosis, goals, and interventions for the patient's plan of care and maintaining patient safety.

Podcast A digital audio/visual recording of information on the Internet that can be downloaded to a personal media player or a computer.

Positive mental attitude Expectation to succeed combined with hard work.

Postacute care (PAC) Also known as subacute care or transitional care. Patient discharged from hospital to lower-level, less expensive care. Will be discharged home when deemed ready.

PQRST method A method of reading to increase understanding by developing comprehension. Stands for preview, question, read, state, and test.

Practical/vocational nurse A person who performs, for compensation, any basic acts in the care of convalescent, subacutely, or chronically ill, injured, or infirm persons, or any act or procedure in the care of the acutely ill, injured, or infirm under the specific direction of a registered nurse, physician, podiatrist, or dentist.

Preceptor An experienced nurse who guides a newly licensed nurse to adjust/learn how to "tie it all together" in the first job.

Preferred provider organizations (PPOs) Similar to HMOs, except that physicians maintain their own practice and continue to be part of their own physician group. Part of the day is spent treating patients enrolled in a PPO.

Prejudice The opinion that a person has about something, even though facts dispute the opinion.

Premium Monthly fee a subscriber must pay for health care insurance coverage.

Preponderance Evidence that is beyond a reasonable doubt.

Primary care The point at which a person enters the health care system.

Primary care method A method of patient care in which one nurse is responsible and accountable for care given to patients on all shifts from admission to discharge.

Priorities What is most important, as in determining priorities when planning patient care.

Privacy Both a legal and ethical issue. Patient's right to choose what is done to his or her body, based on personal beliefs, feelings, and attitude.

Private health care agencies Agencies that are generally proprietary (for profit) and that charge a fee for service. The primary focus is curing illness.

Private pay The patient pays out of pocket for services received.

Probing Pushing for information beyond what is medically necessary to know.

Problem solving A series of steps used to solve problems long before the nursing process was developed.

Problem-oriented thinking Focus on a particular problem to find a solution (e.g., planning your school, work, and home schedule).

Procrastination Putting off tasks that must be done.

Projection A coping or mental mechanism in which an individual attributes his or her own weaknesses to others.

Proprietary hospitals (for profit) For-profit hospitals.

Prospective payment system (PPS) A system in which the federal government announces to a hospital in advance what it will pay for health care costs.

Provider The organization providing health care services.

Proximate cause One of four elements needed to prove negligence. Refers to reasonable cause-and-effect relationship between omission and commission of nursing act and harm to patient.

Public health care agencies Made up of official and voluntary health care agencies.

Purpose Reason.

Q

Qualitative research study Subjective study that gathers data as a narrative description of the "lived experience" of individuals.

Quantitative research study Objective study that collects numerical data that are measured using statistics. Establishes a cause-effect relationship.

R

Randomized controlled trial An experiment in which two or more interventions, possibly including a control intervention or no intervention, are compared by being randomly allocated to participants in the research study.

Rapport A harmonious relationship.

Rationalization A coping or mental mechanism in which the individual offers a logical but untrue reason as an excuse for his or her behavior.

Receiver Person receiving the message, idea, or question.

Recycled adult learner Adult person starting a new career by enrolling in practical/vocational nursing.

Reference hierarchy Ranking of references from best to least by employers: current and former supervisors from work and volunteer experiences, unit managers, and teachers; workers who have seen your work; and personal references or friends.

Reference materials Includes medical and nursing dictionaries, almanacs, yearbooks, atlases, encyclopedias, handbooks, and so on. Generally cannot be checked out, but needed material can be copied.

Referral Send or direct for help.

Reflective thinking Thinking about what you are thinking about.

Registered nurse A member of the nursing team who has gone to nursing school for two, three, or four years and has passed the NCLEX-RN® to be registered. The person on the nursing team who functions independently in decision making regarding the nursing care of patients.

Rehabilitation After acute care is completed, treatment may continue in order to bring person up to maximum functioning.

Reincarnation Belief in rebirth of the soul in many bodies as many times as necessary to achieve enlightenment.

Religion Attempts to give form to spiritual beliefs by adopting specific beliefs and rituals.

Religious denomination An organized group of persons with a philosophy that supports their particular concept of God.

Repatterning Deliberately working to change a pattern that is not working. Pattern can be a way of thinking, feeling, or doing.

Research and teaching hospital Facility that treats patients with unusual or serious conditions. Training site for physicians, nurses, and other health professionals. Does research on illness and treatment. Develops new methods of treatment.

Residency Further "training" in nursing after initial schooling and licensure.

Residential care Broadly defined as 24-hour supervision of persons, for reasons of age or impairments. Falls between skilled care and intermediate care facilities.

Resignation courtesy A two-week notice of ending employment is considered courteous even if not part of the contract.

Respect Consideration, regard.

Responsible Reliable and trustworthy.

Restructuring Changing something that is not working out as planned.

Resume Summary of what you have accomplished—work, skills, education, experience, and sometimes personal achievements. Used to persuade an employer that you are the right person for the job. Limit to one or two pages.

Returning adult learner A learner in the age bracket of the mid-twenties or older who has entered an educational program and has not experienced formal education for a period of time.

Right-brain dominant This person shows more advanced spatial relationships, recognizes negative emotions more quickly, is less verbal, adds tone and inflection to voice, and sees the total picture.

Rituals Religious practices that affirm believers' connection to a higher power.

Rosenstock's Health Belief Model A theory that attempts to explain why a person will or will not take action to prevent or detect illness.

Rosenstock's Health Belief Theory Attempts to explain why a person will or will not seek help to prevent or detect illness.

S

SBAR A method of clear communication between nurses and physicians. S = situation, B = background, A = assessment, and R = recommendation.

Schedule A plan that identifies what needs to be done, who is doing it, and when it must be completed.

Scope of practice What the nurse is able to do legally.

Seacole, Mary Black nurse from Jamaica, West Indies. Helped Florence Nightingale during Crimean War. Used knowledge of tropical medicine, herbs, and natural plant medicines to treat soldiers with cholera, yellow fever, malaria, and diarrhea.

"Seamless" nursing systems Provide progressive nursing programs without the need to repeat courses as the person goes from certified nursing assistant, to LPN/LVN to associate degree RN to BSN to MSN to Doctorate in Nursing degrees; provide ease of movement from one nursing education program to another.

Self-directed learner Takes responsibility for own learning and performance.

Self-esteem Special sense that it is okay to receive credit for something you did well.

Self-evaluation Objective look at personal performance with a plan for improvement.

Self-proclaimed nurse Informally trained person who chooses to or was appointed to care for people who were ill, injured, dying, or pregnant.

Self-worth Sense of self. Crediting self for what you do well.

Semmelweis, Ignaz Philipp Hungarian physician credited with developing the first antiseptic method to combat death from "childbed fever by washing hands."

Sender Person conveying an idea or asking a question.

Sensitivity Awareness of what others are feeling. Tunes in on affective and nonverbal communication.

Service, quality, and cost control Major concerns in the area of providing health care.

Sexual harassment A form of assault. Abuse of power. Not about sex or passion.

Shi'ite An Islamic sect that believes that Muhammad designated a relative to be his successor.

Short-term goal A smaller, more reasonable and manageable unit of a long-term goal that is a small step toward attaining a long-term goal.

Silence Avoid filling the interviewer's void of silence by providing information beyond what is needed.

Simulation A learning activity that uses imaginary patient situations and mimics the reality of the clinical environment.

Single-payer system Comprehensive health care for everyone regardless of past medical history. Payment comes from a single fund, such as the U.S. Medicare system.

Sister Callista Roy's Adaptation Model Describes the patient as a holistic adaptive system influenced by both internal and external stimuli.

Sisters of Charity Organized by St. Vincent DePaul to care for the poor and the sick.

Skill mix Health care staff made up of workers with different levels of education and training.

Skilled care Trained medical professionals provide a higher level of care.

Skilled nursing facility (SNF) Patients with more serious problems need a higher level of care by skilled and well-trained staff.

Slander Damage to someone's reputation by verbalizing untrue or confidential information.

Socialization How a person of one culture learns how to function in another culture.

Social media Ways of using the Internet for interactive dialogue, such as Facebook, Twitter, and LinkedIn.

Social networking Gathering of individuals to share information; specifically used in this book as online communities.

Spatial learner Learns best by studying diagrams, boxes, and special lists.

Specialized hospital Limited to one type of patient, such as women or children.

Spirit Life force that penetrates the person's entire body. Gives meaning to life.

Spirit of inquiry Trait of LPNs/LVNs that challenges traditional and existing practices and seeks creative approaches to problems.

Spiritual caring Recognize and support spiritual need of the patient in the health care setting.

Spiritual dimension That which gives insight into the person's meaning of life, suffering, and death.

Spiritual distress Observed in patients who are unable to practice their rituals or seen in those who experience conflict between their religious or spiritual beliefs and prescribed medical regimen.

Spiritual needs Requirements that arise out of the desire of human beings to find meaning in life, suffering, and death.

Spirituality Pertaining to the soul, one's life force.

Stacks Place in library where material that can be checked out is located.

Standards of care What a prudent nurse is expected to do.

State board of nursing Develops and enforces Nurse Practice Act, which is the basis for nursing law. There is some variation among states.

Static mannequins Full-size body models or models of specific parts of the body made to be realistic.

Statutory law Law developed by the legislative branch of state and federal governments.

Stem First line of a multiple-choice item.

Stereotype Casting all people in a culture as being the same in regard to thinking, feeling, and acting.

Stoic Seemingly unaffected by joy, sorrow, pain, and so on.

Stress management Maintenance of stress at a moderate level. The reaction to both high and low levels of stress may be overwhelming.

Student nurse Person involved in a course of study to become a nurse.

Study group Peers who are actively involved in understanding information by discussing it in a small group.

Study skills lab A place where schools provide services to assist a student with academic problems.

Subacute care Short-term transitional care. Known as postacute care (PAC).

Subjective information Information based on a patient's opinion.

Subjective versus objective Subjective relates to patient's opinion about his or her condition (symptoms). Objective relates to what can be verified (signs).

Subungual zone Area in crook between the fingertip and the nail. Collects largest number of hand pathogens.

Sunni An Islamic sect comprised of the majority of Muslims. Sunnis believe that Muhammad did not designate a successor.

Support system Individuals who are available to assist the patient when ill or dying, usually family and/or friends. Support may range from emotional to physical to spiritual. Also applies to personal support system.

Systematic review A rigorous overview of research on a particular research question that tries to identify, select, synthesize, and appraise all high-quality research evidence relevant to that question in order to answer it.

Syllabus Up-to-date course document distributed at the beginning of a course. This document usually includes a course description, course objectives, course requirements, required text, grading scale, and instructor information.

Sympathy Feel the person's pain.

Systemizer A person who intuitively figures out how things work and what underlying rules control the system.

T

Tactual learner Learns best by doing.

Tasks Activities carried out by nursing assistants. As used in this book, basic skills the certified nursing assistant has learned to do, for example, activities of daily living. Tasks can be assigned.

Taxonomy Standardized, orderly, systematic language (example, NANDA-I).

Teaching Originally thought of as lecturing to students. All responsibility was on the instructor. Current method equalizes responsibility between student and instructor and encourages a wide range of learning/teaching methods.

Teaching and research hospital Private or public hospitals that focus on treating patients; training physicians, nurses, and other health professionals; and research and development.

Team building Working toward cohesion with staff so mission statement of health facility can be carried out in the course of patient care.

Team method A method of patient care in which small teams of nursing personnel are assigned to give total care to groups of patients.

The Joint Commission (TJC) Sets the standards of care for hospitals and long-term care agencies. Agencies receive accreditation if they elect to be reviewed and meet standards.

The Patient Cure Partnership: Understanding Expectations, Right, and Responsibilities Previously called the Patient's Bill of Rights.

Therapeutic Having healing properties, results of treatment.

Therapeutic communication Between the patient and the nurse. The focus is on the patient.

Thinking mind Creativity, reasoning, and analytical thinking occur in this part of the brain, the thinking cap.

Third-party coverage Health insurance.

Time management The effective use of time to meet goals.

TJC National Patient Safety Goals 2003 federally mandated safety rules for health facilities.

Total quality management (TQM) A method by which continuous quality improvement (CQI) is carried out.

Traditional adult learner A learner who comes to an educational program directly from high school or from another program of study, usually in his or her late teens or early twenties.

Transitional care Subacute care at a lower, level facility after acute (hospital) care is completed but patient is not ready to go home.

Transitional practice model Helps new graduate nurses transition from their educational program to the work environment.

Trust Rely on, depend on.

Tutoring Select study group. Student arranges for special help through instructor referral or self-referral.

Two-way communication When there is feedback or discussion between the sender and receiver; the usual form of conversation.

U

Uncompensated care Provider does not receive full payment for services because of free care, bad debt, or difference in what is charged and what insurance reimburses.

Understanding Comprehension. Able to recall and provide examples.

Unintentional torts Nurse did not intend to injure patient. Negligence and malpractice are examples.

Unit manager Has supervisor and management functions for patient units.

United Nations (UN) International organization that deals with world issues. Has representatives of many countries.

Universal coverage Health insurance coverage for all persons; usually paid through taxes.

Unlicensed assistive personnel (UAP) Trained by health care organizations to function in an assistive role to RNs and LPNs/LVNs. Also known as patient care technicians, patient care associates, nurse extenders, and multiskilled workers.

U.S. Public Health Service (USPHS) Division of Department of Health and Human Services. Made up of six agencies.

V

Validate information Verify data.

Values Assigned to an idea or action. Freely chosen and affected by age, experience, and maturity.

Variable Characteristic in a research study that is measured.

Verbal communication Sending or receiving communication through the spoken or written word.

Vertical violence Occurs between persons of unequal power, for example, an instructor and a student.

Vicarious liability Responsible for actions of another because of a special relationship with the other person.

Virtual clinical excursion A real clinical experience simulated on a computer, including changing physician orders.

Virtual Simulated by a computer.

Visual learner Generates visual images, that is, thinks primarily in pictures. Learns best by watching a demonstration first.

Visual/Linguistic Learner Learns best through reading and writing.

Visual/Spatial Learner Learns best through charts, demonstrations, videos, and other visual materials.

Vocalization Verbalization.

Voice control Be aware of how your voice sounds. A well modulated voice makes a better impression.

Voluntary community hospital Nonprofit hospital operated by community association or religious organization.

Voluntary health care agencies Not-for-profit, nonofficial health care agencies that complement official health agencies and meet the needs of persons with a specific disease.

W

Wahhabism An ultraconservative form of Islam.

Wald, Lillian Began Henry Street Settlement visiting nurse service in New York in 1893 to care for indigent persons.

Watson's Theory of Human Care Health is a harmony among body, mind, and spirit. It involves self-perception and how the self is experienced. Illness is a lack of harmony within the self and the soul.

Wellness and illness Relative terms. Have different meanings for different cultures.

Wellness center Promotes wellness. Includes nutritional counseling, exercise programs, stress reduction, and weight control programs.

Working the room Identify and contact people in a position to hire you (e.g., during meetings or workshop breaks).

World Health Organization (WHO) International health agency of the United Nations, located in Geneva.

Worldview Shared by persons with same cultural background.

References and Suggested Readings

Chapter 1

Billings, D., & Halstead, J. (2009). *Teaching in Nursing: A Guide for Faculty.* St. Louis: Elsevier/Saunders.

Borrello, S. (January/February 2011). Nursing as a Second Career. *Nursing made Incredibly Easy, 9*(1), 6–7.

Chenevert, M. (2011). *Mosby's tour guide to nursing school: A Student's Road Survival Kit.* St Louis: Mosby.

deWit, S. (2010). *Saunders student nurse planner: a guide to success in nursing school.* Philadelphia: Elsevier Saunders.

Galbraith, M. (2003). *Adult learning methods: a guide for effective instruction.* Melbourne, FL: Krieger Publishing.

Halfer, D., & Saver, C. (2008). Bridging the Generation Gaps. *Nursing Spectrum/Nurse Week.* Retrieved June 8, 2008 from http://www.nurse.com.

Hartner, K. (February 20, 2007). Generational Diversity. *ADVANCE Newsmagazines for LPNs.* Retrieved September 20, 2007 from http://lpn.advanceweb.com.

Hislop, J. (Oct. 2010). Paper Chart Nurse. *American Journal of Nursing, 110*(10), 72.

Keepnews, K., et al. (May/June, 2010). Generational Differences Among Newly Licensed Registered Nurses. *Nursing Outlook, 58*(3), 155–163.

Knowles, M., Holton, E., & Swanson, R. (2005). *The adult learner: the definitive classic in adult education and human resource development* (6th ed.). New York: Butterworth-Heinemann.

Lieberman, S., & Berardo, K. (March 31, 2008). Closing Age Gaps. *ADVANCE for Nurses.* Retrieved April 1, 2008 from http://lpn.advanceweb.com.

Oblinger, D., & Oblinger, J. (2005). *Educating the next generation.* Page last updated August 20, 2007. Retrieved March 14, 2007 from www.educause.edu/educatingthenet.

Olson, M. (Jan., 2009). The Millennials: First Year in Practice. *Nursing Outlook, 57*(1), 10–17.

Palfrey, J., & Gasser, U. (2008). *Born Digital: Understanding the First Generation of Digital Natives.* NY: Basic Books: A Member of the Perseus Books Group.

Sanoff, A. (2005, May 8). Survey: High school fails to engage students. *USA Today.* Retrieved March 1, 2007 from http://www.usatoday.com/news/education/2005-05-08-high-school-usat_x.htm.

Skiba, D. The Net Generation: Implications for Nursing Education and Practice. Retrieved November 16, 2010 from http://www.electronicvision.com/nln/chapter01/chapter_01.htm.

Chapter 2

Chenevert, M. (2011). *Mosby's tour guide to nursing school.* St Louis: Mosby.

deWit, S. (2010). *Saunders student nurse planner: a guide to success in nursing school.* Philadelphia: Elsevier Saunders.

Lakein, A. (1973). *How to get control of your time and your life.* New York: New American Library-Dutton.

Landsberger, J. (2011). Time Management. *Study Guides Strategies.* Retrieved December 1, 2010 from, http://www.studygs.net/timman.htm.

Chapter 3

Barsch, J. (1999). *Understanding your learning preference.* Ventura, CA: Ventura College Learning Disability Clinic.

Byrne, M. (2001). Uncovering racial bias in nursing fundamentals textbooks. *Nurse Health Care Perspect, 22*(6), 299–303.

Chatterbean. *Are you a right-brain thinker?* Retrieved February 18, 2007 from http://www.chatterbean.com/right_brain_thinker/1/.

Clinton, P. (2000). The crisis you don't know about. In Book 4th anniversary issue. (pp. L4–L11).

Dryden, G., & Vos, J. (2010). *Check Your Personal Thinking Style.* Retrieved July 28, 2010 from http://www.thelearningweb.

Dryden, G., & Vos, J. (2010). *Learning Styles: Learning methods to identify and build on your strengths.* Retrieved July 28, 2010 from http://www.thelearningweb.

Eagleman, D. (2007). 10 unsolved mysteries of the brain. In Discover. (pp 54–75). PARS International.

Felder, R., & Soloman, B. *Learning styles and strategies.* Retrieved April 11, 2007 from http://www.ncsu.edu/felder-public/ILSdir/styles.html.

Felder-Silverman Model. Learning styles. Retrieved April 11, 2007 from http://www.ncsu.edu/felder-public/Learning_Styles.com.

Gardner, H., & Hatch, T. (1990, March). *Multiple intelligences go to school: Educational implications of the theory of multiple intelligences.* (Technical Report No. 4). New York: Center for Technology in Education.

Gardner, H. (1999). *Intelligence reframed: Multiple intelligences for the 21st century.* Basic Books: a member of the Perseus Books Group.

GSU master teacher program: on learning styles. Retrieved February 18, 2007 from http://www2.gsu.edu/~dschjb/wwwmbti.html.

Guardian Unlimited. *They just can't help it.* Retrieved February 18, 2007 from http://www.guardian.co.uk/life/feature/story/0,13026,937913,00.html.

Gurian, M. (1997). *The Wonder of boys.* New York: Jeremy P. Tarcher/Putnam.

Hallowell, E., & Ratey, J. (2010). *Adult ADHD: 50 Tips on Management.* Retrieved November 16, 2010 from http://www.addresources.org/.

Hallowell, E., & Ratey, J. (2010). *50 Tips on the Management of Adult Deficit Disorder.* Retrieved November 16, 2010 from http://www.faslink.org/adhdtips.htm.

Houghton Mifflin College. (2010). *Thinking and Learning Styles.* Retrieved July 28, 2010 from http://college.hmco.com/.

ISD-Development. *Learning styles or, how we go from the unknown to the known.* Retrieved April 8, 2007 from http://www.nwlink.com/~donclark/hrd/learning/styles.html.

Jensen, E. (1998). The learning brain. In *Teaching with the brain in mind.* Alexandria, VA: Association for Supervision and Curriculum Development.

Kelly, K., & Ramundo, P. (1993). *You mean I'm not lazy, stupid or crazy?!* New York: Scribner.

King, V. (2010). *Learning & Thinking Styles.* Retrieved July 28, 2010 from http://www.hoagiesgifted.org/.

Learning Styles and Thinking Styles. (2010). Retrieved July 18, 2010 from http://www.targetlearning.

Lisa-Angelique, L., & Cheong, E. (2004, January). Learning Styles. *CDTL Brief, 7*(1). Retrieved February 18, 2007 from http://www.cdtl.nus.edu.sg/brief/v7n1/default/html.

Paul, R., & Elder, L. (2002). *Critical thinking: tools for taking charge of your personal and professional life.* Upper Saddle River, NJ: Financial Times Prentice Hall.

Reis, R. *Learning styles. Tomorrow's professor listserv.* Retrieved February 18, 2007 from http://sll.stanford.edu/projects/tomprof/newtomprof/postings/216.htm.

Shirley, R. (2010). *Which One Are You?* Retrieved November 16, 2010 from http://www.worldwide.

Springer, S., & Deuttsch, G. (1997). *Attempts at applying asymmetry: Hemisphericity, education, and culture.* In *Left brain right brain: A perspective on cognitive neuroscience* (5th ed.). New York: W.H. Freeman & Co.

Thinking and Learning Styles: What type of Learner are you?. (2010). Retrieved July 28, 2010 from http://www.new-oceans.uk/.

Wade, N. Scans show different growth for intelligent brains. *The New York Times.* Retrieved March 30, 2006 from http://www.nytimes.com/2006/03/30/science/39brain.html.

Chapter 4

2011 NCLEX-PN® Detailed Test Plan (Candidate Version). (2011). National Council of State Boards of Nursing. Retrieved from NCSBN.org.

Carey, B. (Sept. 6, 2010). Forget What You Know About Good Study Habits. *The New York Times.* Retrieved on December 1, 2010 from http://www.nytimes.com/2010/09/07/health/views/07mind.html?pagewanted=all. t.

Pauk, W., & Owens, J. (2010). *How to study in college* (10th ed.). Wadsworth Publishing.

Silvestri, L. (2010). *Comprehensive Review for the NCLEX-PN® Examination.* St Louis: Saunders/Elsevier.

Skiba, D. The Net Generation: Implications for Nursing Education and Practice. Retrieved November 16, 2010 from http://www.electronicvision.com/nln/chapter01/chapter_01.htm.

Staton, T. (1959). *How to Study.* Circle Pines, MN: American Guidance Service, Inc..

Chapter 5

Billings, D., & Halstead, J. (2009). *Teaching in Nursing.* St. Louis: Elsevier/Saunders.

Burke, M., & Harper, J. (May/June, 2010). I've Arrived in Cyberspace: Have You Seen My Lecture? *Nurse Educator, 35*(3), 101–102.

Board of Governors, Position Statement, Preparing the Next Generation of Nurses to Practice in a Technology-Rich Environment: an Informatics Agenda. NLN, May 9, 2008.

Chenevert, M. (2011). *Mosby's tour guide to nursing school: a student's road survival kit.* St Louis: Mosby.

Craig, E. (September 23, 2009). Personal Digital Assistants and Smartphones: Clinical Tools for Nurses. *From Medscape Business of Medicine.* Retrieved January 5, 2010 from http://medscape.com/viewarticle/709144_print.

Cunningham, D. (Spring 2010). Incorporating Medium Fidelity Simulation in a Practical Nurse Education Program. *Journal of Practical Nursing, 60*(1), 2–5.

Delpier, T. (2006, July/Aug). Cases 101: learning to teach with cases. *Nurs Educ Perspect, 27*(4), 204–209.

deWit, S. (2006). Virtual clinical excursions—general hospital. In Fundamental concepts and skills for nursing. St Louis: Elsevier.

Duffy, M. (April 2011). Facebook, Twitter, and LinkedIn, Oh My! *American Journal of Nursing, 111*(4), 56–59.

Filer, D. (July/August 2010). Using Technology to Increase Classroom Participation. *Nursing Education Perspectives, 31*(4), 247–250.

How Private Is Your Facebook? (May/June 2011). *Nurse Educator, 36*(3), 102.

Levine, J., & Young, M. (2010). *The Internet for dummies.* Indianapolis, IN: Wiley.

Lim, F. (Sept. 2010). I Simulate. Therefore I Am Nursed *AJN, 110*(9), 72.

National Council of State Boards of Nursing. (Effective April 2011). *NCLEX-PN examination test plan for the National Council Licensure Examination for licensed practical/vocational nurse.* Chicago: NCSBN.

NCSBN. (2011). *White Paper: A Nurse's Guide to the Use of Social Media.* Retrieved September 6, 2011 from https://www.ncsbn.org/11_NCSBN_Nurses_Guide_Social_Media.pdf.

Silvestri, L. (2010). *Comprehensive Review for the NCLEX-PN® Examination.* St Louis: Saunders/Elsevier.

Social Networking for Student Nurses. *Nursing Times.net.* Retrieved April 15, 2011 from http://www,nursingtimes.net/whats-new-in-nursing/students/social.

Staton, T. (1962). *How to study* (5th ed.). Circle Pines, MN: Publisher's Building, American Guidance Service.

Williams, M., & Dittmer, A. (July/August 2009). Textbooks on Tap: Using Electronic Books Housed in Electronic Devices in Nursing Clinical Courses. *Nursing Education Perspectives,* 220–229.

Wink, D. (May/June 2010). Online Lectures. *Nurse Educator, 35*(3), 95–97.

Wink, D. (March/April 2010). Social Networking Sites. *Nurse Educator, 35*(2), 49–51.

Wink, D. (July/August 2010). Teaching With Technology: Automatically Receiving Information from the Internet and Web. *Nurse Educator, 35*(4), 141–143.

Wink, D., & Killingsworth, E. (March/April 2011). Organizing Use of Library Technology. *Nurse Educator, 36*(2), 48–51.

Chapter 6

ACE. (2007). *Exercise you can't do without.* Retrieved February 20, 2007 from http://www.acefitness.org/fitfacts/fitbits_display.aspx?items=231.

Aleccia, J. (2008). *Hey, doc, wash your hands: Patients shouldn't be shy about asking providers to hit the sink, experts say.* Retrieved January 27, 2008 from http://www.msnbc.com/id/22827499/print1./displaymode/1098/.

Almost 100,000 People Die Every Year From Hospital Infections. (2010). Retrieved December 1, 2010 from http://www.articlebase.com/medicine-articles/almost-000000.

Associated Press. (2007, April 26). *Study: Overweight workers cost employers more.* Retrieved July 14, 2008 from http://www.usatoday.com/news/health/2007-04-23-overweight-worker-study_N.htm.

Barber, P. (2003). Scratch That. *NurseWeek.* Retrieved [May 09, 2003] from http://www.nurseweek.com/news/features/03-06/nails.asp.

Baron, J. (2007). *Stress: A trigger for disease in advance for nurses.* Retrieved February 24, 2007 from http://nursingadvanceweb.com.

Baxley, S., & Ibitayo, K. (2009). *De-stress for success!.* Retrieved April 21, 2009 from http://www.nursingsociety/org.

Beattie, M. (1992). *Codepend no more: How to stop controlling others and start caring for yourself.* Center City, MN: Hazelton.

Burnout: signs, symptoms, and prevention. Retrieved April 8, 2007 from www.Helppguide.org/mental/burnout_signs_symptoms.htm.

Calfee, D. (2009). *Emergence of Carbapenem-Resistant Klebsiella pneumoniae as a Significant Healthcare-Associated Pathogen.* Presented at Jacksonville, FL.

CDC. *General information on hand hygiene.* Retrieved April 8, 2007 from http://www.cdc.gov/nceh/vsp/cruiselines/hand_hygiene_general.htm.

Cohen, M. (2008). The next best thing. *Real Simple,* 173–178.

Converso, A., & Murphy, C. (2004). Winning the battle against back injuries. *RN, 67*(2), 52–57.

Crocker, E. *Learning to save your back.* Advance NewsMagazine for LPNs. King of Prussia, PA: Merion Publications, Retrieved August 1, 2006 from www.advanceweb.com.

Delahanty, K., & Myers, F. (2010). 3 bad bugs. *Nursing 2010*, 24–30.

DeNoon, D. (2010). *Healthy Aging Center Hospital Infections Kill 48,000 Each Year.*

DeNoon, D. (2011). USDA Ditches Food Pyramid for a Healthy Plate. Retrieved June 2, 2011 from http://www.medscape.com/viewarticle/743889?ssdmh=dm1.692731&src=nidn.

Dietary Guidelines for Americans 2010. USDA and HHS.

Dunbar, C. (2006, July 31). Infection squads. *Nurs Spectr.*

Dunbar, S., & Levitt, S. (2006, September 24). Freakonomics: selling soap. *The New York Times.*

Edmunds, M., & Scudder, L. (2009). *Do Nurses Practice What They Preach?* Retrieved December 15, 2009 from http://www.medscape.com/viewarticle/712966_print.

Emery, C. (2006). *Simple measures to reduce infections: Hopkins study finds catheter rules, clean hands aid hospitals.* Retrieved from http://www.baltimoresun.com/news/health/bal-te.infection   28dec28.0.7609251.story?coll=bal-home-headlines.

Felegas, M., et al. *Risk factors of carbapenem-resistant Klebsiella pneumoniae infections: a matched controlled study.* Retrieved March 26, 2011 from http://jac.oxfordjournals.org/content/60/5/1124.full.

Gerber, S. Associate Medical Director (2009). *Public Health and Long-Term Care: A Cautionary Tale.* Chicago: Cook County Department of Public Health.

Girou, E., et al. Efficacy of hand rubbing with alcohol based solution versus standard hand washing with antiseptic soap: randomized clinical trial. *BJM.* Retrieved April 8, 2007 from http://www.bmj.com/content/325/7360/362.full.

Goldman, D. (2006). System failure versus personal accountability: the case for clean hands. *N Engl J Med, 355*(2), 121–123.

Haas, J., & Larson, E. (August 2008). Compliance with Hand Hygiene. *AJN, 108*(8).

Hand hygiene and multidrug-resistant organisms. (2004). *AJN, 104*(8), 51.

How to Deal with Stress. (2010). Retrieved September 6, 2010 from http://www.studygs.net/stress.htm.

Illustrated Health Encyclopedia, (2007). *Physical Activity.* Retrieved February 20, 2007 from http://stateman.com/health/healthfd/shared/health/adam/ency/article/001941.html.

Infections Caught in Hospitals Kill 48,000 in U.S. Every Year. (2010). Retrieved December 1, 2010 from http://www.newsinferno.com/health-concerns/infections-caught-in-hospitals-kill-48000-in-u-s-every-year.

Leung-Chen, P. (August 2008). Everybody's Crying MRSA. *AJN, 108*(8).

Maxworthy, J. (2008). *The dirty hands of health care: What would Florence think?* Retrieved June 3, 2008 from http://www.nursingsociety.org/pub/rnl/pages/vol34_2_maxworthy.asps.

McCaughey, B. (2005). Coming clean. *The New York Times.* Retrieved June 7, 2005 from http://www.nytimes.com/2005/06/opinion/06mccaughey.html?th=andemc=thandpages wanted=print.

McCaughey, B. (November 2008). A Hospital Germ on the Warpath. *AARP Bulletin, 49*(9).

MyPlate from http://opinion.latimes.com/opinionia/2011/06/myplate=the-food-pyramid-for-dummies.html.

Nelson, A., Fragala, G., & Menzel, N. (2003). Myths and facts about back: injuries in nursing. *Am J Nurs, 103*(2), 32–41.

NIAAA. *A snapshot of annual high-risk college drinking consequences.* Retrieved May 2, 2007 from http://www.collegedrinkingprevention.gov/StatsSummaries/snapshot.aspx.

Rettner, R. (March 25, 2011). *Deadly Drug-Resistant Bacteria Found in L.A.* Retrieved March 27, 2011. Retrieved from http://www.myhealthnewsdaily.com/drug-resistant-bacteria-los.

Rothrock, J. (2006). What are the current guidelines about wearing artificial nails and nail polish in the healthcare setting? *Medscape Nurses, 8*(2).

Tierro, P. (2007). *Germ-fighting secrets: a leading microbiologist tells how to stay healthy.* Boulder, CO: Bottom Line.

U.S. Department of Health and Human Services. (2003, May). *FDA Fact sheet on hand hygiene in retail and food service establishments.* Retrieved April 8, 2007 from http://vm.cfsan.fda.gov/~comm/handhyg.html.

University of Maryland Medical Center. (2007). *What are some specific stress reduction methods?* Retrieved March 25, 2007 from http://www.umm.edu/patended/articles/.

USDA Press Release. (June 2, 2011). *USDA and HHS Announces New Dietary Guidelines to Help Americans Make Healthier Food Choices and Confront Obesity Epidemic.* USDA. http://www.choosemyplate.gov.

USDA. (June 2, 2011). *First Lady and Agriculture Secretary Vilsack to Launch New Food Icon as a Reminder to Help Consumers Make Healthier Food Choices.*

USDA. *DietaryGuidelines.gov. Guidelines for Americans.* Retrieved June 2, 2011 from http://www.usda.gov/DietaryGuidelines.htm.

WebMD. Retrieved from http://webmd.com/healthy-aging/news/20100222/hospital.

Weiss, B. (2005). Winning the battle with addiction. *RN, 68*(7), 63–66.

What Are Hospital-Acquired Infections? (2010). Retrieved December 1, 2010 from http://www.wisegeek.com/what-are-hospital-acquired-infections.htm.

Yamamoto, L., & Marten, M. (December, 2007). Listen up, MRSA The bug stops here. *Nursing.*

Chapter 7

Afghanistan: Nursing in a War Zone. Retrieved December 15, 2010 from http://www.medscape.com/viewarticles/433919.

ANA Report. (1944). Trained attendants and practical nurses. *Am J Nurs, 44*, 7–8.

Backer, B. (1993, March). The Nightingale pledge: a commitment that survives the passage of time. *Nurs Health Care, 14*, 3.

Bolvin, J. *War on the Mind, Part 1: Nurses Deployed in Iraq and Afghanistan struggle with PTSD.* Retrieved December 15, 2010 from http://news.nurse.com/article/20101004/NATIONAL.02/109270040.

Brown, E. (1948). *Nursing for the future.* New York: Russell Sage Foundation.

Carlson, M. *Women, the Unknown Soldiers.* Retrieved December 15, 2010 from http://www.deanza.edu/.

Cherry, B., & Jacob, S. (2011). *Contemporary Nursing: Issues, Trends, and Management.* St. Louis: Mosby.

D'Antonio, P. (1997). Nineteenth century nursing: Science, and the values of duty, will and power. *Reflections, 23*(75th Anniversary Commemorative Issue), 16–17.

Delougherty, G. (1998). *Issues and trends in nursing* (3 rd ed.). St Louis: Mosby.

Deming, D. (1944). Practical nurses—a professional responsibility. *Am J Nurs, 44*, 36–43.

Desch, E., & Doherty, M. E. (2010). Experiences of U. S. Military Nurses in Iraq and Afghanistan Wars, 2003-2009. *Nursing Scholarship, 42*(1).

Donahue, M. P. (1985). *Nursing, The Finest Art.* St. Louis: C.V. Mosby.

Donley, R. (2002). Revisiting the American Nurses Association first position on education for nurses. *2002 Online J Issues Nurs.* Retrieved May 31, 2002 from http://nursingworld.org/ojin/topic18/tpc18_1.htm.

Dryden, P. *Nursing in Iraq: Starting from Sratch*. Retrieved December 3, 2010 from http://www.medscape.com/viewarticle/470849.

Fahy, E. (1993, March). Covering the history of nursing. *Nurs Health Care, 14*(3).

Florence Nightingale. (2009). *Notes on Nursing*. Reprinted New York: Fall River Press.

Frantz, A. (1998, Oct). Nursing pride: Clara Barton in the Spanish-American War. *Am J Nurs, 98*(10).

Go, P. (2009). Role of Canadian Nurses in World War One. Retrieved December 30, 2010 from http://ezinearticles.com/?Role-of-Canadian-Nurses-in-World-War-One&id=2631265.

Goldsmith, J. (1942). New York's practical nurse program. *Am J Nurs, 42*, 1026–1031.

Goldstein, J. (excerpts from Chapters 2, 5, and 6), *War and Gender*. Retrieved December 30, 2010 from http://www.warandgender.com/wgwomww1.htm.

Gosnell, D. (2002). Overview and summary: The 1965 Entry into Practice Proposal—Is It Relevant Today? *2002 Online J Issues Nurs*. Retrieved May 31, 2002 from http://nursingworld.org/ojin/topic18/tpc18ntr.htm.

James, E. *Legacy lives on in advance for nurses*. Retrieved February 17, 2005 from http://Nursing.advanceweb.com/common/editorial/PrintFriendly.aspx?CC=49113.

Joel, L. (2002). Education for entry into nursing practice: revisited for the 21st century. *2002 Online J Issues Nurs*. Retrieved from http://nursingworld.org/ojin/topic18/tpc18_4htm.

Kalish, P., & Kalish, B. (1995). *The advance of American nursing* (3 rd ed.). Boston: Little, Brown.

Kinder, J. (1986, Nov). President NLN. *Letter*.

LeVasseur, J. (1998). Plato, Nightingale, and contemporary nursing. *IMAGE: Journal of Nursing Scholarship*, Indianapolis: Sigma Theta Tau, *30*(3).

Longfellow, H. W. (1975). *The political works of Longfellow*. Cambridge ed. Boston: Houghton-Mifflin.

Martinez, O. L. (posted April 24, 2010). *The Honor Society of Vietnam War Nurses*. Retrieved January 31, 2011 from http://www.experienceproject.com/stories/Am-A-Registered-Nu.

McGuane, E., & Bullough, B. (1992, Dec). Proud history, promising future. *Pract Nurs*, 40–42.

Metules, T. (1998, Dec). Pins and pinning-the traditions continue. *RN*, 12.

NLN Research and Policy. (1994). Practical nursing's role in a community-based health care system. *Prism: NLN, 2*, 1–8.

Philips, E. (1944). Practical nurses in a public agency. *Am J Nurs, 44*, 974–975.

Pillitteri, A. (1994, June). One nursing curriculum 100 years ago: a retrospective view as a prospective necessity. *J Nurs Ed, 33*(6), 286–287.

Records of Nurse Casualties in the Korean War. National Archives and Records Administration. Retrieved December 3, 2010 from http://www.archives.gov/research/korean-war/nurses.html.

Romanoff, B. (2006, May). Facts about Flo you may not know. *Nurse Week, 7*(3), 32–33.

Russel, L. (1987). *Women in Vietnam*. Retrieved December 15, 2010 from http://www.tourofdutyinfo.com/Notebook/Essay3-women.htm.

Server, S. (1998). The story of the lamp. *Am J Pract Nurs, 5*(1).

Seymour, M. (2004). 'Nightingale's nurses aides. *The New York Times*. Retrieved October 25, 2004 from, http://www.nytimes.com/2004/10/24/books/review/24SETMOUR.html?8bu=8pageswanted=printandposition=.

Sigma Theta Tau International. (2006, Nov 5). *Helping nurses help others*. Indianapolis: Nursing Knowledge International. Sigma Theta Tau, 3 rd/4th Quarter, 3:3.

The Army Nurse Corps in World War 11. Retrieved December 15, 2010 from http://www.history.army.mil/books/wwii/72–14/72–14HTM.

Thompson, M. (1955). *The cry and the covenant*. New York: Signet Books.

Vansasson, C. (February, 2011). Letters from Afghanistan. *AJN, 111*(2).

West, I. J. *The Women of the Army Nurse Corps During the Vietnam War*. U.S. Army Center of Military History.

Widerquist, J. (1992). The spirituality of Florence Nightingale. *Nurs Res, 41*(1), 49–55.

Wilde, R. *Women in World War 1*. Retrieved December 30, 2010 from http://europeanhistory.about.com/od/worldwar1/a/ww1women.htm.

Wilson, B. (2011). Women in the Korean Conflict. *Women in War*. Retrieved December 30, 2010 from http://userpages.aug.com/captbarb/femvets6.html.

Women's roles in the World Wars. Retrieved December 15, 2010 from http://en.wikipedia.org/wik9/Women's_roles_in_the_World_Wars.

Wilson, B. (2011). WWI Thirty Thousand Women Were There. *Women in War*. Retrieved December 30, 2010 from http://www.userpages.aug.com/captbarb/femvets4.html.

Yourk, D. (2008). *American Nurse Today. Nursing in Afghanistan: A cultural perspective*. Retrieved February 1, 2011 from http://www.americannursetoday.com/article.aspx?id=4256&1256 &fid.

Chapter 8

A key to critical thinking habits of the mind: what are habits of the mind? Retrieved February 18, 2007 from http://hsc.unm.edu/consg/media/pdf/critical/habits.pdf.

Alfaro-LeFevre, R. (2000). *Applying nursing process: promoting collaborative care* (5th ed.). Philadelphia: Lippincott.

Alfaro-LeFevre, R. (2003, July). Improving your ability to think critically. *Healthcare Traveler, 11*(1), 72–76.

Alfaro-LeFevre, R. (2006). *Critical thinking indicators*™. Available at www.AlfaroTeachSmart.com.

Alfaro-LeFevre, R. (2009). *Critical thinking and clinical judgment: a practical approach* (4th ed.). Philadelphia: WB Saunders.

Austhink Software Pty Ltd. Australia. *Augment mapping and critical thinking*. Retrieved February 18, 2007 from http://www.austhink.com/augmentmap/thinking/?gclid=CKnku92auYoCFQbmYAod0Te.

Bauer, B., & Hill, S. (2000). *Mental health nursing: an introductory text* (2nd ed, pp 69–70. Philadelphia: WB Saunders).

Critical Thinking in Nursing. Retrieved July 28, 2010 from http://wps.prenhall.com/chet_kozier_fundamentals_8/61/156881.

Foundation of Critical Thinking. (2009). *Nursing and Health Care*. Retrieved July 28, 2010 from http://www.criticalthinking.org/starting/nurse_health.cfm.

Heaslip, P. (2008). *Critical Thinking: To Think Like a Nurse*. Retrieved July 28, 2010 from http://www.com.criticalthinking.org/resources/HE/ctandnursing.cfm.

Ignatavicius, D., & Workman, M. L. (2011). *Medical surgical nursing* (6th ed.). Philadelphia: WB Saunders.

Khosravani, S., & Memarian, R. (2005). Developing Critical Thinking Skills in Nursing Students by Group Dynamics. *The Internet Journal of Advanced Practice Nursing*™, ISSN: 1523-6064, *7*(2).

Martin, C. (2002). *The Theory of Critical Thinking in Nursing in Nursing Education Perspectives*. Retrieved July 28, 2010 from http://findarticles.com/p/articles/mi_hb3317/is_5_23/ai_n2894.

National Council of State Boards of Nursing. (effective April 2010). *NCLEX-PN test plan*. Chicago: NCSBN, Inc.

National Council of State Boards of Nursing (2007). *NCLEX Examination candidate bulletin*. NCSBN at *www.ncsbn.org*.

National Council of State Boards of Nursing. (2007). *NCLEX-PN test plan for the National Council Licensure Examination for Practical/Vocational Nurses.* Chicago: NCSBN, Inc.

NCLEX-PN Examination effective (2011). Chicago: NCSBN.

Silvestri, L. (2010). *Saunder's Q & A Review for the NCLEX-PN® Examination* (4th ed).

University of New Mexico Health Sciences Center. *What is critical thinking?* Retrieved February 18, 2007 from http://hsc.unm.edu/consg/conct/whatis.shml.

Chapter 9

Wendt, K. (2010). *Report on findings from the 2009 LPN/LVN practice analysis: linking the NCLEX-PN examination to practice.* Chicago: National Council of State Boards of Nursing, Inc.

Alfaro-LeFevre, R. (2002). *Applying nursing process: promoting collaborative care* (5th ed.). Philadelphia: Lippincott.

ANA continuing education: nursing nomenclature and needed taxonomies for health care. (2000). Nursing Classification 1. Retrieved February 3, 2000 from http://nursingworld.org/mod7/cec1full.htm#accumulate.

Christensen, B., & Kockrow, E. (2011). *Foundations and adult health nursing* (6th ed.). St Louis: Mosby.

Critical Thinking Strategies: Concept Mapping. Retrieved July 28, 2010 from http://cord.org/txcollabnursing/onsite_conceptmap.htm.

Frederick, J., et al. (2002). *Speaking a common language. AJN,* 101(3), 2400.

Ham, K. (2002). *From LPN to RN: role transitions* (Ch. 7). Philadelphia: WB Saunders.

International Journal of Nursing Terminologies and Classifications, 19(1), (January-March 2008).

Johnson, M., Bulechek, G., Dochterman, J., et al. (2006). *Nursing diagnoses, outcomes, and interventions: NANDA, NOC and NIC Linkages* (2nd ed.). St Louis: Mosby.

Johnson, M., Bulechek, G., Doterman, J., Maas, M., et al. (2006). *NANDA, NOC, and NIC LINKAGES* (2nd ed.). St. Louis: Mosby-Elsevier.

Maslow, A. (1943). A theory of human motivation. *Psych Rev, 50,* 370.

McCloskey, J. C., & Bulechek, G. M. (2000). *Nursing interventions classification* (3 rd ed.). St Louis: Mosby.

MEDI-SMART. *Study tips from former nursing students.* Retrieved April 13, 2007 from http://medi-smart.com/study-tips.htm.

NAPNES (2007). Standards of practice and educational competencies of graduates of practical/vocational nursing programs. *JPN,* 57(2).

National Council of State Boards of Nursing. (1998). Implementation of the 1999 NCLEX-PN test plan. In *Issues* (pp. 4–5). Chicago: NCSBN.

National Council of State Boards of Nursing. (2007). *NCLEX-PN® test plan for the National Council Licensure Examination for Practical Nurses.* Chicago: NCSBN.

National Council of State Boards of Nursing. (2010). *NCLEX-PN® test plan for the National Council Licensure Examination for Practical/Vocational Nurses.* Chicago: NCSBN.

Peseit, D. J., & Herman, J. (1998). OPT: Transformation of nursing process for contemporary practice. *Nurs Outlook, 46.*

Chapter 10

Ackley, B., et al. (2008). *Evidence-Based Nursing Care Guidelines.* St. Louis: Elsevier/Mosby.

Alligood, M. (2010). *Nursing Theory: Utilization and Application* (4th ed). Mosby, Elsevier.

Burns, N., & Grove, S. (2011). *Understanding Nursing Research: Building an Evidence-Based Practice.* St. Louis: Elsevier/Saunders.

Cherry, B., & Jacob, S. (2011). *Contemporary Nursing: Issues and Trends, and Management.* St. Louis: Elsevier/Mosby.

Chinn, P., & Kramer, M. (2011). *Integrated Theory and Knowledge Development in Nursing* (8th ed.). Philadelphia: Elsevier.

The Cochrane Collaboration. *Working Together to Provide the Best Evidence in Health Care.* Retrieved on June 12, 2011 from http://www.cochrane.org/about-us.

deWit, S. (2009). *Fundamental Concepts and Skills for Nursing* (3 rd ed.) Philadelphia: Saunders/Elsevier.

Massey, V. (1998). Theories and Models in Nursing Practice. In J. Leahy & P. Kizilay (Eds.), *Foundations of Nursing Practice.* Philadelphia: WB Saunders.

Mazurek, B., & Fineout-Overholt, E. (2011). *Evidence-Based Practice in Nursing and Healthcare: A Guide to Best Practice.* Philadelphia: Walters Kluwer Health/Lippincott Williams and Wilkins.

Motacki, K., & Burke, K. (2011). *Nursing Delegation and Management of Patient Care.* St. Louis: Elsevier.

Nightingale, F. (1860). *Notes on Nursing: What It Is, and What It Is Not.* New York: D. Appleton and Company.

Chapter 11

Armstrong, R. M. (2003). *Turning to Islam: African-American conversion stories.* Chicago: Christian Century.

Carpenter, A. (2007). Ethical suspicion and Katrina's nurses. *AJN,* 107(3), 15.

Christensen, B., & Parker-Feliciano, K. (2011). Legal and Ethical Aspects of Nursing. In *Christenson & Kockrow's Foundations and Adult Health Nursing* (6th ed.). St. Louis: Mosby/Elsevier.

deWit, S. (2009). *Fundamental Concepts and Skills for Nursing* (3 rd ed.). Philadelphia: Saunders/Elsevier.

Haddad, A. (2005). Ethics in action. *RN,* 68(5).

Ham, K. (2000). Legal/ethical components of nursing. In *From LPN to RN role transitions.* Philadelphia: WB Saunders.

Health workers can refuse to participate in procedures. (2003). *In Midwest/Heartland NurseWeek,* 4, 3.

Rumbold, G. (2002). *Ethics in nursing practice.* Edinburgh: Elsevier Science Ltd.

Shannon, J. (2003). *Legal and ethical issues in counseling: a primer for mental health and substance abuse professionals.* Duluth, MN: Workshop.

Soglin, B. (2005). *Teaching medical students to examine ethics.* Spectator: University of Iowa.

Tyson, S. (2002). Ethical issues with age. In *Gerontological nursing care.* Philadelphia: WB Saunders.

Venes, D. (Ed.) (2005). *Taber Cyclopedic Medical Dictionary.* (20th ed, pp. 679–680). Philadelphia: FA Davis.

Ulrick, B. *(1992). Florence Nightingale Leadership and Management.* Appleton and Lange, p.22. Norwalk, CT.

Chapter 12

2001 Partnership in Caring, Inc. (2003). *Choice in dying honoring a legacy.* Retrieved August 11, 2003 from www.partnershipforcaring.org/Aboutus/choice_content.html.

A Rules 101. *Frequently asked questions on HIPAA.* Retrieved May 23, 2007 from http://www. hipaarules101.com/hipaa-faq.htm.

Alfaro-LeFevre, R. (2009). *Critical thinking and clinical judgment: a practical approach* (4th ed.). Philadelphia: WB Saunders.

American Hospital Association. (2003). *The patient care partnership: understanding expectations, rights and responsibilities.*

Anderson, F. (2007, February). Finding HIPPA in Your Soup. *AJN,* 107(2), 66–71.

Assisted Suicide. Tread Carefully When You Help to Die: assisted suicide laws around the world. Retrieved February 27, 2011 from http://www.asistedsuicide.org/suicide_laws.html.

Bioethics. *Policy on do not resuscitate.* Retrieved May 25, 2007 from http://www.clevelandclinic.org/bioethics/policies/dnr.html.

Brekken, S. *MN Board of Nursing.* Retrieved 3/4/11 from http://www.nursingboard.state.mn.us/.

Charting Checkup. (2006). Making it clear with an incident report. *LPN2006*, 2(3), 17–19.

Christensen, E., & Kockrow, E. (2011). *Foundations and adult health nursing* (6th ed.). St Louis: Elsevier: Mosby.

Daly, B. J., Berry, D., Fitzpatrick, J. J., et al. (1997). Assisted suicide: implications for nurses and nursing. *Nurs Outlook*, 45, 209–214.

Dempski, K. (2000). If you have to give a deposition. *RN*, 63(1), 59–60.

deWit, S. (2009). *Fundamental concepts and skills for nursing* (2nd ed.). Philadelphia: Elsevier Saunders.

DHS Oregon Department of Human Services. (2003). *Physician-assisted suicide: Oregon's Death with Dignity Act.* Retrieved August 11, 2003 from www.dhs.state.or.us/publichealth/chs/pas/pas.cfm.

Ethics in Medicine. *Physician-assisted suicide.* Retrieved May 25, 2007 from http://depts.washington.edu/bioethx/topics/pas.html.

FamilyDoctor. *Advance directives and do not resuscitate orders.* Retrieved May 25, 2007 from http://familydoctor.org/online/famdocen/home/patadvocacy/endoflife/003.html.

Glazer, G. *Legislative and policy issues related to interstate practice.* Retrieved May 17, 2007 from http://www.nursingworld.org/ojin/tpclg/leg_7.htm.

Glazer, G. *Multistate licensure: overview and summary.* Retrieved May 17, 2007 from http://www.nursingworld.org/ojin/topic9/tpc.htm.

Hanawalt, A. (2001). End of life issues advanced directives-a health professional's guide to their use. *NFLPN*, 1(1), 8–11.

Helm, A., & Kihm, N. (2006). Liability insurance: is it for you? *LPN2006*, 2(3), 14–15.

Main, A., & Todd, F. (2005, Oct 7). *Depositions 101.* Louisville, KY: American Bar Association Young Lawyers Division.

McNeil, D. (2003). *First study on patients who fast to end their lives.* Retrieved August 2, 2003 from www.nytimes.com/2003/0731/sciences/31DIE.html.

MedlinePlus. *Advance directives.* Retrieved May 25, 2007 from http://www.nlm.nih.gov/medlineplus/advancedirectives.html.

NAPNES standards of practice for licensed practical/vocational nurses. Silver Spring, MD: NAPNES.

National Council of State Boards of Nursing. *Complaints.* Retrieved May 18, 2007 from http://www.ncsbn.org/163.htm.

NiCastro, D. HIPAA proposed rule–a breakdown. Retrieved March 4, 2011 from http://blogs.hcpro.com/hipaa/2010/07/hipaa-proposed-rule-a-breakdown/.

O'Keefe, M. (2001). *Nursing practice and the law: avoiding malpractice and other legal risks.* Philadelphia: FA Davis.

Oregon. *Death With Dignity Act.* Retrieved May 25, 2007 from http://www.oregon.gov/DHS/ph/pas/faqs.stml.

Oregon's Death with Dignity Law. Retrieved May 25, 2007 from http://theocracywatch.org/oregon_death_dignity.htm.

Phillipsen, N., & Haynes, D. (2007). *The multi-state licensure compact: making nurses mobile.* Retrieved May 17, 2007 from http://www.medscape.com/viewarticle/551037.

Quickinfo. (2007). *National Practitioner Data Bank.* Retrieved May 18, 2007 from acnm.org.

Ryan, B., Sullivan, G., Mackay, T., et al. (2007 January). *RN*, 70(1), 26–31.

U.S. Department of Health and Human Services. (2003). *OCR privacy brief: summary of the HIPAA privacy rule.* Retrieved June 29, 2008 from www.hhs.gov/ocr/privacysummary.pdf.

U.S. Department of Health and Human Services, Office for Civil Rights-HIPAA. *National standards to protect privacy of personal health information.* Retrieved June 29, 2008 from www.hhs.gov/ocr/hipaa.

Ventura, M. J. (1999). Report tracks impact of Oregon's assisted suicide law. *RN*, 62(5), 16.

Ventura, M. J. (1999). When information must be revealed. *RN*, 62(2), 61–64.

Gelfand, J. (2010). *The Living Will and Durable Power of Attorney for Health Care.* Retrieved February 28, 2011 from http://www.webmd.com/a-to-z-guides/frequently-asked-questions-about-advance-directives.

You're on trial: how to protect yourself. (2007, March/April). *LPN2007*, 3(2), 16–18.

Zittel, B. (2007, May 21). Profession update in teaching techniques. *ADVANCE for LPNs.* New York Tri-State Area, 7(5).

Chapter 13

Alessandra, T. Sixteen common-sense listening tips. *ADVANCE for LPNs.* Retrieved March 3, 2005 from http://LPN.advanceweb.com/common/Editorial/Editorial.aspx?CC=4953.

Arnold, E., & Boggs, K. U. (2003). *Interpersonal relationships: professional communication skills for nurses* (4th ed.). Philadelphia: WB Saunders.

Banotai, A. Simplified strategies. *ADVANCE for LPNs.* Retrieved January 25, 2007 from www.advanceweb.com.

Carey, B. (10/16, 2005). In the hospital, a degrading shift from person to patient. *The New York Times.* Retrieved August 17, 2005 from http://www.nytimes.com/2005/08/16/health/16dignity.html?ex=1124942400anden=dlc1749.

Carson, V. B. (2000). The vehicle for healing: communication as part of a therapeutic relationship. In *Mental health nursing, the nurse-patient journey* (2nd ed., Ch. 10). Philadelphia: WB Saunders.

Christenson, B., & Kockrow, E. (2011). *Foundations and Adult Health Nursing* (6th ed.). St. Louis: Elsevier.

Federwische, A. (2007). *RN and physician communication: from conflict to collaboration.* Spring Med/Surg Specialty Guide.www.nurse.com.

Fuimano, J. (2004, Dec 13). Language matters. *ADVANCE for LPNs.* Retrieved June 11, 2004 from http://www.advanceforlpn.com/common/editorial/PrintFriendly.aspx?CC=35819.

Gurian, M. (1997). *The wonder of boys.* New York: Jeremy P. Tacher/Putnam.

Holman, J. (2001, May). *Providing age appropriate care in healthcare organizations: infancy to adolescence.* NFLPN.

Mascioli, S., et al. (2009). Improving Handoff Communication. February, *Nursing. 2009*, pp. 52–55.

Pagana, K. (2008). *Indianapolis: The Nurse's Etiquette Advantage.* Sigma Theta Tau.

Pope, B. B., et al. (March, 2007). Raising the SBAR. *Nursing 2007*, 41–43.

Tannen, D. (1990). *You just don't understand.* New York: Ballantine Books.

Tokarski, C. (2005). Better communication needed to reduce medical errors. *Medscape Medical News.* Retrieved February 4, 2005 from http://www.medscape.com/viewarticle/498276_print.

Ustun, B. (2006, Oct). Communication skills training as part of a problem-based learning curriculum. *J Nurs Educ*, 45(10), 421–424.

Chapter 14

Bast, M. Collaboration (vs. manipulation, coercion, or throwing your hands up in despair) Self-assessment. Retrieved April 1, 2007 from http://www.breakoutofthebox.com/manipula.htm.

Bast, M. *Communicating Assertively.* Retrieved April 1, 2007 from http://www.breakoutofthebox.com/assert.htm.

Belanger, D. (2000). Nurses and Suicide:The Risk is Real. *RN. 63,* (10) 61–64.

California Department of Industrial Relations. *Guidelines for security and safety of health care and community service workers.* DOSH publications. Retrieved April 3, 2007 from http://www,dir.ca.gov/DOSH/dosh_publications/heworker.html.

Carrol, V. (March 1997). Health and Safety in Workplace Violence. *Sm J Nurs,* 99(3).

McKay, D. (2011). *Job Burnout: Causes, Symptoms and Cures.* About.com. Retrieved April 8, 2007 from http://careerplanning.about.com/od/workrelated/aburnout.htm.

Center for American Nurses: Serving the Needs of Nurses Today & tomorrow. *Lateral Violence and Bullying in Nursing.* Retrieved 7/2011 from www.centerforamericannurses.org.

Frequently Asked Questions/Patient Rights Council. Retrieved July 13, 2011 from www.patientrightscouncil.org/site/frequently-asked-questions/.

HealthDay. (March 8, 2008). *Aggression on Job More Harmful Than Sexual Harassment.* Retrieved from http://health.yahoo.com/news/healthday/aggressiononjobmoreharmfu….

HealthyPlace.com. *Depression community. assertiveness, non-assertiveness, and assertive techniques.* Retrieved April 1, 2007 from http://www.healthyplace.com/Communities/Depression/suicide/assertingourselves.asp.

Improving communications. Assertiveness vs. passive and aggressive behavior. Retrieved April 1, 2007 from http://www.arthritis.ca/tips%20for%20living/communicating%20your%needs/develop%2.

In which states is euthanasia or assisted suicide legal? Retrieved July 13, 2011 from www.sharecare.com/.../in-which-states.euthanasia-assistedsuicide-le.

International Journal for Quality in Health Care, Nurse Staffing and Patient Safety. *Current knowledge and implications for action.* Retrieved February 19, 2007 from http://inqhc.oxfordjounals.org/cgi/contents/full/15/4/275.

Jahner, J. (February 1, 2011). *Building Bridges: An Inquiry into Horizontal Hostility in Nursing Culture and the Use of Contemplative Practices to Facilitate Cultural Change.* Retrieved 7/2011 from www.upuya.org/uploads/pdfs/Jahnersthesis.pdf.

King, S. (1996, August). *Top ten signs you are approaching burnout.* Retrieved February 8, 2007 from http://webpages.charter.net/stormking/topten.html.

Kurz, J. (2002, July). Combating sexual harassment. *RN,* 65(7), 65–68.

Levine, P., Hewitt, J., & Misner, S. (1998). Insights of nurses about assault in hospital-based emergency rooms. *Image J Nurs Schol,* 30(3), 9–10.

Lipson, J., & Dibble, S. (2006). *Culture and clinical care.* San Francisco: UCSS Nursing Press.

Montana/Patients Rights Council. Retrieved July 13, 2011 from http://www.patientrightscouncil.org/site/montana/.

National Council State Boards of Nursing (2012). The Nurse Licensure Compact. Retrieved March 5, 2012 from http://www.ncsbn.org/nlc.htm.

New York State Nurse Association. *NYSNA position statement. workplace violence.* Retrieved April 3, 2007 from http://www.nysna.org/programs/nai/practice/positions/position39.htm.

Pagana, K. (2008). *The Nurse's Etiquette Advantage.* Indianapolis, IN: Sigma.

U.S. Department of Labor. (2004). *OSHA guidelines for preventing workplace violence for health care and social service workers.* Retrieved April 4, 2007 from www.osha.gov.

Chapter 15

About the IOM. (2010). Retrieved on 3/4/11 from http://www.iom.edu/About-IOM.aspx.

AANC Nurse Certification. (2011). Retrieved on April 4, 2011 from http://www.nursecredentialing.org/Certification.aspx#.

Aiken, L. (2011). News for the Future. *New England Journal of Medicine,* 364(3), 280–281.

American Nurses Association, (2011). *Nursing World.* Accessed on 28.01.2011 from http://www.nursingworld.org/EspeciallyForYou/StudentNurses/Wh….

Bureau of Labor Statistics, U.S. Department of Labor. *Occupational outlook handbook* (2010-11 ed.). Licensed Practical and Licensed Vocational Nurses. Retrieved June 26, 2008 from http://www.bls.gov/oco/print/ocos102.htm.

Clark, A. (January 2009). Advanced Practice Nursing. *American Journal of Nursing Career Guide,* 109(1), 17.

Cherry, B., & Jacob, S. (2011). *Contemporary Nursing: Issues, Trends, and Management.* St. Louis: Elsevier.

Dumrose, C. (2010). Where's the Shortage? New RNs Find Difficult Job Hunting. *Nurse.com. Retrieved September 15, 2010 from* http://news.nurse.com/apps/pbcs.dll/article?AID=20100912/N.

Gibson, S. (January/February, 2009). Intergenerational Communication in the Classroom: Recommendations for Successful Teacher-Student Relationships. *Nursing Education Perspectives,* 30(1), 37–39.

Hader, R. (2009). Is Being a Chief Nursing Officer in Your Future? *NSNA imprint,* Retrieved July 24, 2011 from www.nsna.org.

Henderson, V. (1966). *The nature of nursing: a definition and its implications for practice, research and education.* New York: Macmillan.

How Old Is Too Old to Work? Economic woes add a twist to the age-old question. (April 10, 2009). *Nursing Knowledge International,* Retrieved May 22, 2009 from http://www.nursingknowledge.org/Portal/main.aspx?PageId=5….

Kennedy, M. (June 2010). Don't Call Us, We'll Call You: But Will new nurses be available when we need them? *American Journal of Nursing,* 110(6), 7.

Licensed Practical and Licensed Vocational Nurses, Occupational Outlook Handbook (2010-11 ed.). Retrieved March 4, 2011 from http://www.bls.gov/oco/ocos102.htm#outlook.

Mahaffey, E. (May 31, 2002). The Relevance of Associate Degree Nursing Education: Past, Present, Future. *Online Journal of Issues in Nursing,* 7(2), Manuscript 2.

Mitchell, P. H. (2008). Patient-centered Care – a New Focus on a time-honored concept. *Nursing Outlook,* 56(5), 197–198.

National Council of State Boards of Nursing (NCSBN). (2009). *LPN/VN Practice Analysis:Linking the NCLEX-PN® Examination to Practice.* Chicago: NCSBN.

National Council of State Boards of Nursing. (effective April 2011). *NCLEX-PN® Examination Test Plan for the National Council Licensure Examination for Licensed Practical/Vocational Nurses.* Chicago: NCSBN.

National League for Nursing. (2010). *Outcomes and Competencies for Graduates of Practical/Vocational, Diploma, Associate Degree, Baccalaureate, Master's, Practice Doctorate, and Research Doctorate Programs in Nursing.* New York: NLN.

Northam, S. (June 2009). Conflict in the Workplace (Part 1): Sex, age, hierarchy, and culture influence the nursing environment. *American Journal of Nursing,* 109(6), 70–73.

Seago, J., et al. (2004, Nov. 1). *Supply, demand, and use of licensed practical nurses.* Health Resources and Services Administration, Bureau of Health Professions, National Center for Health Workforce Analysis.

Sorrentino, S. (2011). *Mosby's Textbook for Long-term Care Nursing Assistants.* St Louis: Elsevier/Mosby.

Stokowski, L. (2008). Old, But Not Out: The Aging Nurse in Today's Workplace. *Medscape.* Retrieved January 7, 2009 from http://www.medscape.com/viewarticle/585454_print.

The Clinical Nurse Leader. (Jan. 2010). *American Journal of Nursing,* 110(1), 22 and 23.

The Registered Nurse Population: Findings from the 2004 National Sample Survey of Registered Nurses. (2004). U.S. Department of Health and Human Services, Health Resources and Services Administration. Retrieved January 11, 2010 from http://bhpr.hrsa.gov/healthworkforce/rnsurvey04/3.htm.

UWM to Offer Doctorate of Nursing Practice. (January 2009). *Nursingmatters*, 20(1), 1 and 7.

Willard, K., Haley-Moyer, C., & Arbour, R. (2009). *Synergy Model, Role of Clinical Nurse Leader and Optimal Care Delivery*. Retrieved January 13, 2011 from www.aacn.org.

Chapter 16

Carroll, R. The evil eye. *The skeptic's dictionary*. Retrieved March 1, 2011 from http://skepdic.com/evileye.html.

Cook, L. (March 2010). Convicted: The job description doesn't say you get to choose your patients. *American Journal of Nursing*, 110(3), 72.

Culver, V. (1974). *Modern bedside care* (8th ed.). Philadelphia: WB Saunders.

D'Avanzo, C., & Geissler, E. (2008). *Pocket guide to cultural assessment*. St Louis: Mosby.

deWit, S. (2007). *Medical-surgical nursing: concepts and practice*. Philadelphia: WB Saunders.

Darrah, J. (February 2009). Expanding the Diversity Definition: LTC facilities are learning how to better accommodate the LGBT population. *Advance for LPNs*, 9(2), 9.

Dibble, S., & Robertson, P. (2010). *Lesbian Health 101: a Clinician's Guide*. San Francisco: UCSF Nursing Press.

Eliason, M., Dibble, S., DeJoseph, J., & Chinn, P. (2012). "LGBTQ issues in Nursing," *Nursing made Incredibly Easy*. March/April, 10(2), 4.

Explore the Form. U.S. Census 2010. Retrieved March 22, 2011 from http://2010.census.gov/2010census/about/interactive-form.php.

Fadiman, A. (1997). *The spirit catches you and you fall down*. New York: Farrar, Strauss, and Giroux.

Foster, G. (1978). *Medical anthropology*. New York: John Wiley and Sons.

Goulette, C. Cultural Competence and Kids: Sensitivity to patients' needs is a must for pediatric nurses. *Advance for Nurses*. Retrieved June 25, 2010 from http://nursing.advanceweb.com/Editorial/Content/PrintFriendly.as....

Hall, E. (1973 Reissue). *The silent language*. Westport, CT: Greenwood Press.

Hall, E. (1966). *The hidden dimension*. New York: Doubleday.

Honer, D., & Hoppie, P. (2004, Aug). The enigma of the Gypsy patient. *RN*, 67(8), 33–36.

Jackson, L. (1993). Understanding, eliciting and negotiating patients' multicultural health beliefs. *Nurse Pract*, 18(4), 30–32, 37–43.

Joyce, E., deGonzalez, M. (2004). *Say it in Spanish*. Philadelphia: WB Saunders.

Kutner, M., et al. (2006). *The health literacy of America's adults: results from the 2003 National Assessment of Health Literacy*. National Center for Education Statistics. Retrieved March 13, 2011 from http://nces.ed.gov/pubsearch/pubsinfo.asp?pubid= 2006483.

Leininger, M., & McFarland, M. (2002). *Transcultural nursing: concepts, theory, research, and practice*. New York: McGraw-Hill.

Lipson, J., & Dibble, S. (2006). *Culture and clinical care*. San Francisco: UCSF Nursing Press.

Minority Nurse magazine. *The career and educational resource for the minority nurse professional*. Retrieved March 13, 2011 from http://www.minoritynurse.com/.

Murphy, K. (March/April 2011). The importance of cultural competence. *Nursing Made Incredibly Easy*, 9(2), 5.

Narayan, M. (April 2010). Culture's Effects on Pain Assessment and Management: Cultural patterns influence nurses' and their patients' responses to pain. *American Journal of Nursing*, 110(4), 38–45.

Pagana, K. (2008). *The Nurse's Etiquette Advantage*. Indianapolis: Sigma Theta Tau International.

Randall-David, E. (1992). *Strategies for working with culturally diverse patients*. Bethesda, MD: Association for the Care of Children's Health.

Reinhardt, E. (1995). *Through the eyes of others—intercultural resource directory for health care professionals*. Minneapolis: Hennepin County Medical Society, United Way Intercultural Awareness.

Roberts, S. Projections Put Whites in Minority by 2050. NYTimes.com. Retrieved February 27, 2011 from http://www.nytimes.com/2009/12/18/us/18census.html.

Rodriguez, B. (1995, May 18). *Understanding and integrating cultural awareness and related issues into specialized health curricula*. Green Bay, WI: Seminar at Northeast Wisconsin Technical College.

Spector, R. (2003). *Cultural diversity in health and illness*. Englewood Cliffs, NJ: Prentice Hall.

Srivastava, R. (Ed.). (2007). *The healthcare professional's guide to clinical cultural competence*. Canada: Elsevier.

Tang, G. (March 31, 2008). Bridging Languages and Culture: Using a healthcare interpreter linguistic competence optimizes quality and patient safety. *Advance for Nurses*, Retrieved April 1, 2008 from http://nursing.advanceweb.com/Editorial/Content/PrintFriendly.asp....

Task Force, Junior League of Minneapolis, and University of Minnesota School of Public Health. *Transcultural nursing: basic concepts and case studies, 1997-2005*. Retrieved April 25, 2007 from www.culturediversity.org/.

Transcultural nursing: basic concepts and case studies 1997–2005. Retrieved April 25, 2007 from www.culturediversity.org/.

Varcarolis, E., & Shoemaker, N. (2006). *Foundations of psychiatric-mental health nursing* (5th ed.). Philadelphia: Elsevier/Saunders.

Yen, H. (February 3, 2011). Census Estimates Show Big Gains for U.S. Minorities. Associated Press. Retrieved February 3, 2011 from http://www.msnbc.msn.com/id/41402130/ns/politics/.

Yoder-Wise, P. (2011). *Leading and managing in nursing*. St Louis: Mosby.

Chapter 17

Anonymous. (29 January 2007). Om. *ReligionFacts*. Retrieved February 13, 2011 from http://www.religionfacts.com/hinduism/symbols/aum.htm.

Anonymous. (14 April 2010). Christian Crosses. *ReligionFacts*. Retrieved February 13, 2011 from http://www.religionfacts.com/christianity/symbols/cross.htm.

Anonymous. (23 November 2010). Islamic Symbols. *ReligionFacts*. Retrieved February 13, 2011 from http://www.religionfacts.com/islam/symbols.htm.

Atwood, D., Mead, F., & Hill, S. (2010). *Handbook of denominations in the United States*. Nashville, TN: Abingdon Press.

A View on Buddhism. (2011). Retrieved February 28, 2011 from http://viewonbuddhism.org/4_noble_truths.html.

Armstrong, K. (2001). *Buddha*. New York: Penguin Group Penguin Putnam.

Armstrong, K. (2000). *Islam*. New York: Random House.

Baha'ism. (2007). *The Columbia Electronic Encyclopedia* (6th ed.). Columbia University Press.

Bauer, B., & Hill, S. (2000). *Mental health nursing: an introductory text*. Philadelphia: WB Saunders.

Bowker, J. (Ed.). (2007). *The Oxford dictionary of world religions*. Cambridge, MA: Oxford University Press.

Carson, V. (1989). *Spiritual dimensions of nursing practice*. Philadelphia: WB Saunders.

Compendium of the Catechism of the Catholic Church. (2006). Washington, D.C.: USCCB Publishing.

D'Avanzo, C., & Geissler, E. (2003). *Pocket guide to cultural assessment*. St. Louis: Mosby.

Christian Science. (2011). *The Columbia Electronic Encyclopedia* (6th ed.). Columbia University Press. Retrieved February

22, 2011 from http://www.infoplease.com/ce6/society/A0812103.html.

Singer, D., & Grossman, L. (Eds.). (2006). NY: American Jewish Committee.

Pennington, R. (2009). Do Muslims Observe the Sabbath? Retrieved February 13, 2011 from http://muslimvoices.org/do-muslims-observe-the-sabbath/.

Episcopal Church. (2011). *The Columbia Electronic Encyclopedia* (6th ed.). Columbia University Press. Retrieved February 22, 2011 from http://www.infoplease.com/ce6/society/A0817503.html.

Esposito, J. (1998). *Islam: the straight path*. New York: Oxford University Press.

Friends, Religious Society of. (2011). *The Columbia Electronic Encyclopedia* (6th ed.). Columbia University Press. Retrieved February 22, 2011 from http://www.infoplease.com/ce6/society/A0819726.html.

Gellman, M., & Hartman, T. (2002). *Religion for Dummies*. New York: Wiley.

Gerardi, R. (1989). Western spirituality and health care. In V. Carson (Ed.), *Spiritual dimensions of nursing practice*. Philadelphia: WB Saunders.

Gritsch, E. (2002). *A history of Lutheranism*. Minneapolis: Augsburg Fortress.

Grossman, C. (January 27, 2011). Number of U.S. Muslims to Double. *USA Today*. Retrieved February 6, 2011 from www.usatoday.com/news/religion/2011-01-27-1Amuslim27_ST_N.htm.

Hinduism: The world's third largest religion. (2010). Retrieved February 28, 2011 from http://www.religioustolerance.org/hinduism.htm.

LargestReligious Groups in the United States of America. (2005). Retrieved February 28, 2011 from http://www.adherents.com/rel_USA.html.

Leininger, M., & McFarland, M. (2002). *Transcultural Nursing: concepts, theory, research, and practice*. New York: McGraw-Hill.

Lewis, B. (2003). *The crisis of Islam*. New York: The Modern Library.

Lindner, E. W. (2010). *Yearbook of American and Canadian Churches 2010*. Nashville, TN: Abingdon Press.

Lipson, J., & Dibble, S. (2006). *Culture and nursing care: a pocket guide*. San Francisco: The Regents of the University of California.

McCurdy, D. (May 2008). Ethical Spiritual Care at the End of Life. *American Journal of Nursing*, 108(5), 11.

Mennonites. (2011). Retrieved February 22, 2011 from http://mbsoft.com/believe/text/mennonit.htm.

Mormon Underwear. Retrieved February 15, 2011 from http://www.ldschurchtemples.com/mormon/underwear/.

National Council of Churches. (2011). *.Yearbook of American and Canadian Churches, 2011*. Abingdon Press.

Nomani, A. (2005). *Standing alone in Mecca*. New York: HarperCollins Publishers, Inc.

Pentecostalism. (2011). *The Columbia Electronic Encyclopedia* (6th ed.). Columbia University Press. Retrieved February 22, 2011 from http://www.infoplease.com/ce6/society/A0838204.html.

Rocca, F. (2011). Vatican: Number of Catholics Is Up, Still Behind Muslims. *USA Today*. Retrieved on February 24, 2011 from http://www.usatoday.com/news/religion/2011-02-23-catholic_vatican_22_ST_N.htm?csp=34&utm_source=feedburner&utm_medium=email&utm_campaign=Feed%3A+Religion-TopStories+%28News+-+Religion+-+Top+Stories%29.

Schoenbeck, S. (1994). Called to care: addressing the spiritual needs of patients. *J Pract Nurs*, 44, 19–23.

(2005). *Seventh-Day Adventists*. Retrieved February 22, 2011 from http://www.adventist.org/beliefs/index.html.

Sheskin, I., & Dashefsky, A. Jewish Population of the United States, 2006. In *the American Jewish Year Book 2006* (Vol. 106).

Star of David. Retrieved February 14, 2011 from http://www.jewishvirtuallibrary.org/jsource/Judaism/star.html.

Sumner, C. (1998). Recognizing and responding to spiritual distress. *Am J Nurs*, 98(1), 26–30.

United Church of Christ. (2011). Retrieved February 22, 2011 from http://www.ucc.org/beliefs/.

United Methodist Church. (2011). Retrieved on February 22, 2011 from http://www.infoplease.com/ce6/society/A0850064.html.

Wahhabi. (2011). *The Columbia Electronic Encyclopedia* (6th ed.). Columbia University Press. Retrieved February 22, 2011 from www.infoplease.com/ce6/society/A0851259.html.

What Is Halal? Retrieved February 13, 2011 from http://www.ifanca.org/halal/.

What is the Society of St. Pius X? (2011). Retrieved on February 28, 2011 from http://www.sspx.org/SSPX_FAQs/q1_sspx.htm.

Why Do Some Muslim Women Wear Head Scarves? (2011). Retrieved March 23, 2011 from http://www.wisegeek.com/why-do-some-muslim-women-wear-head-scarves.htm.

Yearbook of American and Canadian Churches. (2011). National Council of Churches in the USA: Abingdon Press.

Chapter 18

Bauer, J. (April 14, 2009). *Green House Concept Combines Best New Thinking for Elderly*. The Grand Rapids Press. Retrieved May 17, 2011 from http://ww.globalaging.org/elderrights/us/2009/green.htm.

Callantine, P. (2011). Sheridan, WY: Green House Board, Task Force, and Chair of Operations Committee.

Christensen, E., & Kokrow, B. (2011). *Foundations of Adult Health Nursing* (6th ed.). St. Louis: Mosby.

Day, T. *What Is Long-Term Care?* Retrieved May 7, 2011 from http://www.longtermcarelink.net/eldercare/long_term_care.htm.

Eden Values: The 10 Principles. Retrieved May 15, 2011 from http://www.edenalt.org/our-10-principles.

Gale Encyclopedia of Public Health. http://www.answers.com/topic/united-states-public-health-service.

Chapter 19

Bihari, M. (April 2, 2010). Cost of Health Insurance: What Determines Your Costs and What the Average American Pays. Retrieved June 24, 2011 from http://healthinsurance.about.com/od/healthinsurance   basics/a/cost_of_health_insurance.htm.

Cherry, B., & Jacob, S. (2011). *Contemporary Nursing: Issues, Trends, and Management*. St. Louis: Elsevier.

Chester, H. (March/April 2011). What Does Health Care Reform Mean For You. *Nursing Made Incredibly Easy!* 9(2), 6–9.

DeParie, N. (April 20, 2011). The Facts About the Independent Advisory Board. *The White House Blog*. Retrieved June 20, 2011 from http://whitehouse.gov/blog/2011/04/20/facts-about-independe....

Fact Sheet: The Affordable Care Act's New Patients Bill of Rights. (2010). Retrieved July 3, 2011 from http://www.healthreform.gov/newsroom/new_patients_bill_of_rights.html.

Federal Officials Try Again to Bolster Plans for People with Medical Conditions. (July 6, 2011). Kaiser Health News. Retrieved July 6, 2011 from http://www.kaiserhealthnews.org/Features/Insuring-Your-Health/Michelle-Andrews-on-high-risk-plans.aspx.

Frakt, A. (June 14, 2010). *Medicare Advantage: You Get What You Pay For*. Kaiser Health News. Retrieved June 14, 2010 from http://www.kaiserhealthnews.org/Columbus/2010/June/061410Frakt....

Health Reform Quiz. The Henry J. Kaiser Family Foundation. (2011). Retrieved July 3, 2011 from http://healthreform.kff.org/quizzes/health-reform-quiz.aspx.

Gawande, A. (2009). *The Checklist Manifesto: How to Get Things Right*. NY: Metropolitan Books.

Highlights from the National Healthcare Quality and Disparities Reports. (2010). *Agency for Healthcare Research and Quality* Retrieved July 13, 2011 from http://www.ahrq.gov/qual/nhqr10/Key.htm.

Holly, C. (March/April 2011). What Does Healthcare Reform Mean to You? *Nursing Made Incredibly Easy*, 9(2), 6–9.

How does the new health reform law change the Medicare Part D coverage gap, sometimes called the "doughnut hole"? (2011). The Henry J. Kaiser Family Foundation. Retrieved July 4, 2011 from http://healthreform.kff.org/faq/how-does-law-change-the-medicare-part-d-donut-hole.aspx.

Institute of Medicine. (2001). *Report Brief: Crossing the Quality Chasm: A New Health System for the 21st Century*. Retrieved July 5, 2011 from http://www.iom.edu/Reports/2001/Crossing-the-Quality-Chasm-A-New-Health-System-for-the-21st-Century.aspx.

Institute of Medicine. (1999). *Report Brief: To Err is Human: Building a Safer Health Care System*. Retrieved July 5, 2011 from http://iom.edu/Reports/1999/To-Err-is-Human-Building-A-Safer-Health-System.aspx.

Ip, G. (2010). *The Little Book of Economics*. N.J.: John Wiley and Sons.

Kovner, C., & Spetz, J. (2011). The Future of Nursing: An Interview with Susan B. Hassmiller. *Medscape*. Retrieved April 5, 2011 from http://www.medscape.com?viewarticle/739963_print.

Medicaid and Chip. (2011). The Henry J. Kaiser Family Foundation. Retrieved July 4, 2011 from *http://healthreform.kff.org*.

Medicare and You. (CMS Publication Number 10050). Baltimore, MD: U.S. Department of Health and Human Services, Sept. 2007.

Masson, D. (Jan. 2011). What Future for the Affordable Care Act? *The American Journal of Nursing*, 111(1).

National Health Expenditure (NHE) Fact Sheet. Retrieved June 23, 2011 from https://www.cms.gov/NationalHealthExpendData/25_NHE_Fact_Sheet.asp.

National Patient Safety Foundation. Retrieved July 29, 2011 from http://www.npsf.org/.

Prater, C. (2008). *15 tips for paying high medical bills: Negotiate before using credit cards to finance medical expenses.* credit cards.com. Retrieved July 4, 2011 from http://www.creditcards.com/credit-card-news/medical-bill-payment-tips-1266.php.

Schorn, D. FAQs on Hospital Bills (2009). *Sixty Minutes*. Retrieved July 4, 2011 from http://www.cbsnews.com/stories/2006/03/03/60minutes/main1369185.shtml.

What Will Happen to Medicare Advantage Plans. (2011). Retrieved July 3, 2011 from http://healthreform.kff.org/faq/what-happens-to-medicare-advantage-plans.aspx.

Will everyone have to buy health insurance? What happens if they don't? How will people prove they have health insurance?. (2011). The Henry J. Kaiser Family Foundation. Retrieved on July 4, 2011 from http://healthreform.kff.org/faq/will-everyone-have-to-buy-health-insurance.aspx.

Chapter 20

Akrani, G. (June 26, 2010). Frederic Herzberg's Two Factor Theory–Motivation Hygiene. Retrieved June 26, 2010 from http://kalyan-city.blogspot.com/2010/06/frederick-herzberg-two-factor-theory.html.

Bennis, W. (2003). *On becoming a leader: the leadership classic—updated and expanded*. Boulder, CO: Perseus Publishing.

Blanchard, K., et al. (1994). *Leadership and the one minute manager*. UK: Clays Ltd.

Blanchard, K., et al. (2009). *The one minute manager builds high performance teams*. New York: Morrow.

Blanchard, K., & Johnson, S. (2000). *The one minute manager*. New York: Berkeley Publishing.

Cherry, B., & Jacob, S. (2011). *Contemporary Nursing: Issues, Trends, and Management*. St. Louis: Mosby, Inc.

Ellis, A. (1994). *Reason and emotion in psychotherapy*. New York: Carol Publishing Group.

Fisher, R., Ury, W., & Patton, B. (1991). *Getting to yes: negotiating agreement without giving in*. New York: Random House Business Books.

Frederick Herzberg's Motivation and Hygiene Factors. Retrieved May 10, 2011 from http://www.businessballs.com/herzberg.htm.

Hearthfield, S. (2011). What People Want From Worrk: Motivation. Retrieved May 10, 2011 from http://humanresources.about.com/od/rewardrecognition/a/needs_work.htm.

Herzberg, F. (1993). *The motivation to work*. New Brunswick, NJ: Transaction Pubs.

Huber, D. (2010). *Leadership and nursing care management*. St Louis: Elsevier.

Klaus, P. (March 3, 2010). When You Can't Show Them the Money: How to Motivate and Appreciate Employees in a Recession. Retrieved May 10, 2011 from http://www.85broads.com/experts/peggy-klaus-2/when-you-cant-show-them-the-money-how-to-motivate-and-appreciate-employees-in-a-recession.

Javitch, D. (June 19, 2009). 5 Employee Motivation Myths Debunked. Retrieved on May 12, 2011 from http://www.entrepreneur.com/humanresources/employeemanagementcolumnistdavi djavitch/article202352.html.

Maslow, A. (1998). *Maslow on management*. New York: John Wiley and Sons.

Murray, J. (March 24, 2009). Motivating Employees in a Down Economy. Retrieved May 10, 2011 from http://everyjoe.com/work/motivating-employees-in-a-down-economy/.

NCSBN Research Brief. (March 2010). *2009 LPN/VN Practice Analysis: Linking the NCLEX-PN® Examination to Practice* (Vol. 44).

Pink, D. (2009). *Drive: The Surprising Truth About What Motivates Us*. New York: Riverhead Books.

Quality Improvement Organizations. (April 15, 2011). U.S. Department of Health and Human Services, Centers for Medicare & Medicaid Services. Retrieved May 10, 2011 from https://www.cms.gov/QualityImprovementOrgs/.

Rewarding your Employees with Recognition Beats Rewarding With Money. Retrieved May 12, 2011 from http://www.biztrain.com/motivation/stories/rewarding.htm.

Sorrentino, S. (2011). *Mosby's textbook for long-term care assistants*. St Louis: Mosby.

Yoder-Wise, P. (2011). *Leading and managing in nursing*. St Louis: Mosby.

Chapter 21

Bauer, B., & Hill, S. (2000). *Mental health nursing: an introductory text*. Philadelphia: Elsevier.

Blancharf, K., Oncken, W., & Burrows, H. (1991). *The One Minute Manager Meets the Monkey*. New York: William Morrow and Co.

Blanxhard, K., Fowler, S., & Hawkins, L. (2005). *Self Leadership and the One Minute Manager: Increasing Effectiveness through Situational Self-Leadership*. NY: William Morrow/Harper Collins Publishers, Inc.

Covey, S. (2004). *The 7 Habits of Highly Effective People*. New York: Free Press.

Hansten, R., & Jackson, M. (2008). *Clinical delegation skills: a handbook for professional practice*. Boston: James and Bartlett.

Hansten, R., & Washburn, M. (2001, March 12). Delegating to UAPs—making it work. *NurseWeek*, 2(3), 21–22.

Huston, C. (March, 2009). 10 Tips for Successful Delegation. *Nursing 2009*, 54–56.

LaCharity, L., Kumagai, C., & Bartz, B. (2006). *Prioritization, delegation, assignment*. St Louis: Elsevier.

Linton, A. (2007). *Introduction to medical-surgical nursing*. St Louis: Elsevier.

Motacki, K., & Burke, K. (2011). *Nursing Delegation and Management of Patient Care*. St. Louis: Elsevier/Mosby.

NCSBN Research Brief. (March 2010). *2009 LPN/VN Practice Analysis: Linking the NCLEX-PN® Examination to Practice*. (Vol. 44).

National Council of State Boards of Nursing. (2006). *ANA and NCSBN Joint Statement on Delegation*. Chicago: IL.

Nightingale, F. (1946). *Notes on nursing. What it is, and what it is not*. Philadelphia: Edward Stern and Co.

Rachels, M. (1994, Aug 24). President of the National Council of State Boards of Nursing. *Letter*.

Safer Healthcare Partners (2010). *SBAR: A Communication Technique for Today's Healthcare Professional*. Retrieved September 30, 2010 from http://www.saferhealthcare.com/cat-shc/sbar-a-communication-technique.

The Joint Commission. *2007 National patient safety goals*. Retrieved June 1, 2007 from http://www.jcrinc.com/13474/.

Ulrich, B. (1992). *Leadership and management according to Florence Nightingale*. Norwalk, CT: Appleton and Lange.

Ury, W. (1993). *Getting Past No: Negotiating Your Way from Confrontation to Cooperation*. New York: Bantam Books.

Working with others: a position paper. Attachment A of the NCSBN 2005 Annual Meeting. *Mission impossible: building a safer workforce through regulatory excellence*. Retrieved from ncsbn.org under delegation.

Wywialowski, E. (2004). *Managing patient care*. St Louis: Mosby.

Yoder-Wise, P., Hansten, R., & Jackson, M. (2011). *Leading and managing in nursing*. St Louis: Mosby.

Chapter 22

Background Checking: The Implications of Credit Background Checks on the Decision to Hire Society for Human Resource Management Poll. (Sept. 22, 2010). Retrieved from http://www.shrm.org/research/survey/findings/articles/pages/background.

Beshara, T. (2008). *Acing the Interview: How to Ask and Answer the Questions That Will Get You the Job* (pp. 20–22). New York: AMACON.

Bureau of Labor Statistics, U.S. Department of Labor. (May 15, 2011). *Occupational Outlook Handbook*. (2101- ed.). Licensed Practical and Licensed Vocational Nurses. Retrieved from http://www.bls.gov/oco/ocos102htm.

Elsenpeter, R. (August 30, 2009). *Opportunities in Staffing Service*. Star Tribune Newspaper. Section W, WI.

Levinson, J., & Perry, D. E. (2009). *Guerilla Marketing for Job Hunters 2.0: 1001 Unconventional Tips, Tricks, and Tactics for Landing Your Dream Job* (pp. 1, 7, 118). Hoboken, New Jersey: John Wiley & Son, Inc.

NCSBN Research Brief: 2009 LPN/VN Practice Analysis Linking the NCLEX–PN® Examination to Practice (Vol. 44, pp. 15, 17). (March 2010). Chicago, IL.

Oliver, V. (2005). *Smart Answers to Tough Interview /Questions* (pp. 47, 64, 143, 144). Naperville, IL.: Source Books, Inc.

Payne, N. (July 21, 2011). *Cross Culture Interviews*. Retrieved from http://www.career-bytes.com/Articles/7865.php.

Personality Types. (June 01, 2011). Retrieved from http://www.2h.com/Articles/personality-tests/personality-type.html.

Pyrtle, B. (July 12, 2009). *Tips To Recognize Scam Job Ads*. Star Tribune Newspaper. Section W., WI.

Shepp, B., & Debra, (2010). *How to find a Job on Linkedin, Facebook, Twitter, MySpace and Other Social Networks* (pp. 5-6, 157, 173). New York,N.Y. McGraw-Hill.

Teacher Fired Over Facebook Post (Aug. 20, 2010). Retrieved from http://video.foxnews.com/v/4316834/teacher-fired-over-facebook-post.

Chapter 23

Heisel, J. (2012). *Comprehensive Review for NCLEX-PN Examination*. St. Louiis: Elsevier Saunders.

NCSBN. (2011). *NCSBN Currently Accepting Study Site Applications for Phase 11 of NCSBN Transition to Practice Study*. Retrieved 7/28/11 from http://mail.google.com/mail/?ui=2&ik= 9621232bcde&view=pt.

NCSBN. (2011). *Dispelling NCLEX Myths*. Retrieved December 1, 2011 from http://mail.google.com/mail/?ui=2&ik=9621232bde&view=pt&se.

NCSBN. *NCLEX Pass Rates*. (July-September). Retrieved November 4, 2011 from http://mail.google.com/mail/?ui=2&ik=9621232bde&view=pt.

NCSBN. (2010). *Report of Findings from the 2009 LPN/LVN Practice Analysis: Linking the NCLEX-PN® Examination to Practice*. Chicago: NCSBN.

NCSBN. (2011). *NCLEX-PN® Test Plan*. Chicago: NCSBN. Available online at www.ncsbn.org/testplan.

NCSBN. The NCSBN Board of Directors Voted to Raise the Passing Score for the NCLEX-PN Examination at its December 8 meeting. Retrieved December 13, 2011 from www.ncsbn.org/setting_the_NCLEX_passing_standard.pdf. Accessed March 5, 2012.

NCSBN. (2012). *NCLEX® Examination Candidate Bulletin*. Chicago: NCSBN. Available online at https://www.ncsbn.org/1213.htm.

NLN. *PN-Pre-NCLEX® Readiness Tests*. Retrieved May 4, 2011 from http://wwwdev.nln.org/testproducts/pas_gradnurse. htm.

Chapter 24

ABMCN. *What is the American Board of Managed Care Nursing?* Retrieved August 16, 2007 from http://www.abmcn.org/right_pageframe.htm.

Ahl, M. E. (1975). In C. Lemburg (Ed.), *Open learning and career mobility in nursing*. St Louis: Mosby.

American Board of Managed Care Nursing. (2009). *Candidates Guide for Certification in Managed Care Nursing*. apatrick@abmcn.org.

Department of Veterans Affairs. *Licensed Practical Nursing*. Retrieved May 15, 2011 from http://www.vacareers.va.gov.

Doctorate, and Research Doctorate Programs in Nursing. New York: NLN.

Mahan, P. Is it worth the price? *Jrnl of Pract Nurs*, 57(4), 22 and 25.

NAPNES Certifications for Licensed Practical/Vocational Nurses and Unlicensed Assistive Personal. Retrieved May 20, 2011 from http://www.napnes.org/certifications/index.html.

NAPNES Certifications for LPNs /LVNs in Pharmacology and Long Term Care. Retrieved 5 May 15, 2011 from http://www.napmes.org/certifications.htm.

NAPNES Long-Term Care Certification Testing Content Outline. Retrieved May 20, 2011 from http://www.napnes.org/index.htm.

NAPNES Nursing Certifications. NAPNES Certificate FAQs. Retrieved from http://www.nursingcerts.com/faqs.aspx.

National Council State Boards of Nursing. (2011). Transition to Practice accessed on 12/20/11 @ncsbn.org.

National League for Nursing. (2010). Outcomes and Competencies for Graduates of Educational Programs in Practical Nursing. New York: NLN.

NCSBN. (2009). *Description of NCSBNs Transition to Practice Model.* www.ncsbn.org.

NCSBN. (2011). *Currently Accepting Study Site Applications for Phase ll of NCSBN Transition to Practice Study.* Accessed on 12/19/11 @ http://www.ncsbn.org/2993htm.

NFLPN Certification Programs. *NFLPN Education foundation IV therapy and Gerontology certifications.* Retrieved May 15, 2011 from http://www.nflpn.org/certification.html.

NFLPN. *Education.* Retrieved May 15, 2011 from http://www.nflpn.org/edcation.htm.

NFLPN. *National Federation of Licensed Practical Nurses Membership Information and Benefits.* Retrieved May 20, 2011 from http://www.nflpn.org/membership.htm.

NFLPN. *National Federation of Licensed practical Nurses What Is NFLPN?.* All About the NFLPN. Retrieved from http://www.nflpn.org/about.htm.

Nursing Mobility Program Option A: Practical (P.N.) Nursing Diploma and Associate Science Degree (A.S.D.N.) Nursing Program for MCTC first Year P.N. students.

Nursing Mobility Program Option B: Associate in Science Degree Program for Licensed Practical nurses (LPN).

Spector, N. (Nov/Dec 2009). *Deans Notes,* Anthony J. Jannett.Inc. *31*(2).

Story, D. (1974). *Career mobility.* St Louis: Mosby.

Illustration Credits

CHAPTER 6

Figure 6-1: Copyright United States Department of Agriculture (www.choosemyplate.gov).

CHAPTER 7

Figures 7-1, 7-2, 7-3, 7-5, and 7-6: Courtesy National Library of Medicine.
Figure 7-4: Courtesy U.S. Naval Historical Center.
Figure 7-7: Courtesy U.S. Army Center of Military History.
Figure 7-8: Photo courtesy Barbara Smith, U.S. Army.
Figure 7-9: Photo courtesy Cpl. M. M. Bravo, United States Marine Corps.

CHAPTER 9

Figure 9-1: From Ignatavicius D, Workman L (2006). Medical-Surgical Nursing: Patient-Centered Collaborative Care, 5e. St. Louis: Elsevier.

CHAPTER 10

Figure 10-1A: Redrawn from Maslow, AH; Frager, RD; Fadiman, J (1987). Motivation and personality, 3e. Reprinted and Electronically reproduced by permission of Pearson Education Inc., Upper Saddle River, New Jersey.
Figure 10-1B: From deWit S (2009). Fundamental Concepts and Skills for Nursing, 3e. St. Louis: Elsevier.

CHAPTER 15

Figure 15-1: Courtesy Cleveland Clinic Foundation, Department of Advanced Practice Nursing, Cleveland, Ohio.

Index

Note: Page numbers followed by *b* indicate boxes, *f* indicate figures and *t* indicate tables.

NCLEX-PN® Answer Key

CHAPTER 1

1. 1
2. 3
3. 1
4. 4

ALTERNATE FORMAT ITEM

1. 1, 4
2. 1, 5

CHAPTER 2

1. 1
2. 2
3. 3
4. 2

ALTERNATE FORMAT ITEM

1. 1, 3, 4, 5
2. 4, 1, 2, 3

CHAPTER 3

1. 1
2. 2
3. 3
4. 4

ALTERNATE FORMAT ITEM

1. 1, 3
2. 1. Draw idea sketches.
   2. Use color to direct attention to information.
   3. Make your own diagram as you read.

CHAPTER 4

1. 4
2. 1
3. 3
4. 1

ALTERNATE FORMAT ITEM

1. 1, 2, 3, 4
2. 1, 2, 4

CHAPTER 5

1. 3
2. 4
3. 1
4. 1

ALTERNATE FORMAT ITEM

1. 1, 4
2. 1, 4, 5

CHAPTER 6

1. 3
2. 2
3. 1
4. 4

ALTERNATE FORMAT ITEM

1. 4
2. 2, 3, 5, 6

CHAPTER 7

1. 1
2. 4
3. 3
4. 1

ALTERNATE FORMAT ITEM

1. 1, 3
2. 1, 2, 3, 4

CHAPTER 8

1. 4
2. 2
3. 4
4. 2

ALTERNATE FORMAT ITEM

1. 1, 2
2. 2, 3, 4

CHAPTER 9

1. 3
2. 2
3. 1
4. 1

ALTERNATE FORMAT ITEM

1. 2, 4
2. 3, 4, 2, 1, 5

CHAPTER 10

1. 4
2. 3
3. 4
4. 1

ALTERNATE FORMAT ITEM

1. 2, 1, 3, 4
2. 3, 4, 5

CHAPTER 11

1. 3
2. 1
3. 4
4. 2

ALTERNATE FORMAT ITEM

1. 1, 4
2. 3, 4

CHAPTER 12

1. 2
2. 4
3. 1
4. 4

ALTERNATE FORMAT ITEM

1. 1, 3, 5
2. 2, 4
3. 1, 2, 3, 4

CHAPTER 13

1. 4
2. 1
3. 3
4. 2

ALTERNATE FORMAT ITEM

1. 3, 4
2. 1, 3, 4

CHAPTER 14

1. 4
2. 4
3. 3
4. 1

ALTERNATE FORMAT ITEM

1. 1, 2
2. 1, 2, 3

CHAPTER 15

1. 4
2. 2
3. 1
4. 4

ALTERNATE FORMAT ITEM

1. 2, 4
2. 1, 2, 3, 4, 5, 6

CHAPTER 16

1. 1
2. 1
3. 4
4. 3

ALTERNATE FORMAT ITEM

1. 1, 4

CHAPTER 17

1. 3
2. 2
3. 4
4. 1

ALTERNATE FORMAT ITEM

1. 5
2. 1, 2, 4, 5

CHAPTER 18

1. 1
2. 4
3. 2
4. 3

ALTERNATE FORMAT ITEM

1. 1, 4
2. 3

CHAPTER 19

1. 1
2. 3
3. 2
4. 2

ALTERNATE FORMAT ITEM

1. 2, 4, 5
2. 2, 4

CHAPTER 20

1. 1
2. 4
3. 3
4. 1

ALTERNATE FORMAT ITEM

1. 1, 3, 4, 5
2. 1, 3

CHAPTER 21

1. 1
2. 2
3. 4
4. 4

ALTERNATE FORMAT ITEM

1. 1
2. 2, 3, 4

CHAPTER 22

1. 3
2. 3
3. 1
4. 2

ALTERNATE FORMAT ITEM

1. 1, 2, 3, 4, 5, 6
2. 1, 2, 3, 4, 5

CHAPTER 23

1. 4
2. 3
3. 2
4. 2

ALTERNATE FORMAT ITEM

1. 1, 2, 4, 5
2. 2, 3, 4

CHAPTER 24

1. 2
2. 1
3. 4
4. 3

ALTERNATE FORMAT ITEM

1. 1, 3, 4
2. 1, 2, 3, 4